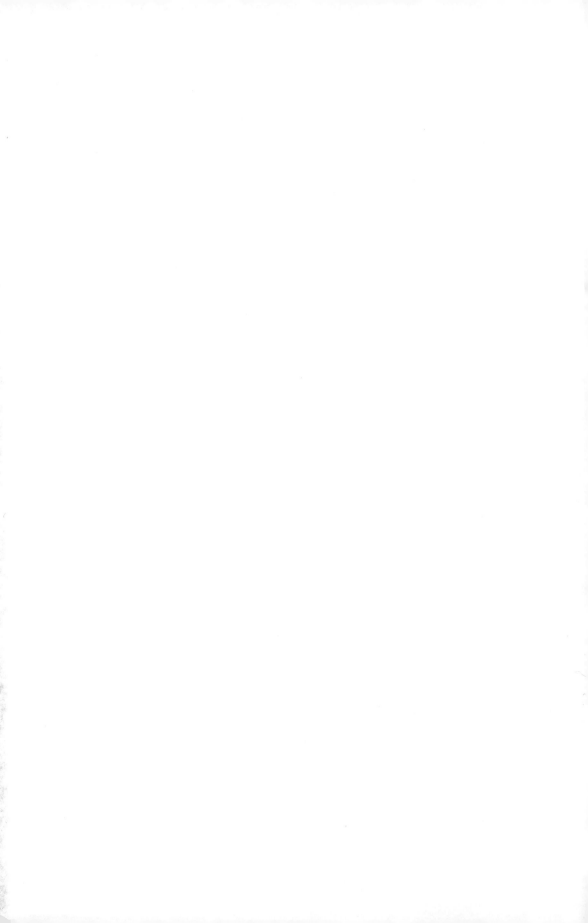

Encyclopedia of Arthropod-transmitted Infections of Man and Domesticated Animals

Encyclopedia of Arthropod-transmitted Infections of Man and Domesticated Animals

Edited by

M.W. Service

Liverpool School of Tropical Medicine, Pembroke Place, Liverpool L3 5QA, UK

Advisers

R.W. Ashford (parasitology)
Liverpool School of Tropical Medicine, Pembroke Place, Liverpool L3 5QA, UK

C.H. Calisher (arboviruses)
Arthropod-Borne and Infectious Diseases Laboratory, Department of Microbiology, Colorado State University, Fort Collins, Colorado 80523, USA

B.F. Eldridge (entomology)
University of California Department of Entomology, Davis, California 95616, USA

T.W. Jones (veterinary parasitology)
University of Edinburgh, Centre for Tropical Veterinary Medicine, Easter Bush, Roslin, Midlothian EH25 9RG, UK

G. Wyatt (medicine)
Liverpool School of Tropical Medicine, Pembroke Place, Liverpool L3 5QA, UK

CABI *Publishing*

CABI is a trading name of CAB International

CABI Head Office
Nosworthy Way
Wallingford
Oxfordshire OX10 8DE
UK

CABI North American Office
875 Massachusetts Avenue
7th Floor
Cambridge, MA 02139
USA

Tel: +44 (0)1491 832111
Fax: +44 (0)1491 833508
Email: cabi@cabi.org
Web site: www.cabi.org

Tel: +1 617 395 4056
Fax: +1 617 354 6875
Email: cabi-nao@cabi.org

A catalogue record for this book is available from the British Library, London, UK

Library of Congress Cataloging-in-Publication Data
The encyclopedia of arthropod transmitted infections / edited by M.W. Service; advisors, R.W. Ashford ... [et al.].
  p. cm.
 Includes bibliographical references.
 ISBN 0-85199-473-3 (alk. paper)
 1. Arthropod vectors—Encyclopedias. I. Service, M. W. II. Ashford, R.W.
RA641.A7 E53 2001
614.4'3—dc21

2001025065

ISBN-13: 978-0-85199-473-4
ISBN-10: 0-85199-473-3

First published 2001
Transferred to print on demand 2006

Printed and bound in the UK by CPI Antony Rowe, Eastbourne.

Contributors

B.E. Anderson, College of Medicine, MDC10, Department of Medical Microbiology and Immunology, University of South Florida, Tampa, FL 33612-4799, USA. E-mail banderso@coml.med.usf. edu

R.C. Anderson (deceased), Department of Zoology, University of Guelph, Guelph, Ontario, Canada N1G 2W1. E-mail randerso@uoguelph.ca

R.W. Ashford, Liverpool School of Tropical Medicine, Pembroke Place, Liverpool L3 5QA, UK. E-mail ashford@ liverpool.ac.uk

C.T. Atkinson, USGS–Biological Resources Division, Pacific Island Ecosystems Research Center, PO Box 218, Hawaii National Park, HI 96718, USA. E-mail Carter_Atkinson@usgs.gov

A.F. Azad, University of Maryland, School of Medicine, Department of Microbiology and Immunology, 655 West Baltimore Street, Baltimore, MD 21201, USA. E-mail aazad@maryland.edu

G. Baneth, Hebrew University of Jerusalem, School of Veterinary Medicine, PO Box 12, Rehovot, 76100, Israel. E-mail baneth@agri.huji.ac.il

A.D.T. Barrett, Department of Pathology and Center for Tropical Diseases, University of Texas Medical Branch, Galveston, TX 77555-0605, USA. E-mail abarrett@utmb.edu

B.J. Beaty, Arthropod-Borne and Infectious Diseases Laboratory, Foothills Campus, Department of Microbiology, Colorado State University, Fort Collins, CO 80523, USA. E-mail bbeaty@colostate. edu

R.J. Birtles, Department of Pathology and Microbiology, School of Medical Sciences, University of Bristol, University Walk, Bristol BS8 1TD, UK. E-mail richard.birtles@bristol.ac.uk

M. Bouloy, Groupe des Bunyaviridés, Institut Pasteur, 25 rue du Dr Roux, 75724 Paris Cedex 15, France. E-mail mbouloy@pasteur.fr

A.S. Boyd, Vanderbilt University, Departments of Medicine and Pathology, 1301 22nd Avenue South, 3900 The Vanderbilt Clinic, Nashville, TN 37232-5227, USA. E-mail EyeBacon@aol.com

T. Butler, Department of Internal Medicine, Texas Tech University Health Sciences Center, 3601 4th Street, Lubbock, TX 79430, USA. E-mail medtcb@ttuhsc. edu

C.H. Calisher, Arthropod-Borne and Infectious Diseases Laboratory, Department of Microbiology, Colorado State University, Fort Collins, CO 80523, USA. E-mail calisher@cybercell.net

P. Cattand, World Health Organization (CDS), 20 Avenue Appia, CH-1211 Geneva 27, Switzerland. E-mail cattandp@wanadoo.fr

Chao-chin Chang, School of Veterinary Medicine, Department of Population Health and Reproduction, 1021 Haring Hall, University of California, Davis, CA 95616, USA. E-mail joechang@ucdavis.edu

B.B. Chomel, School of Veterinary Medicine, Department of Population Health and Reproduction, 1021 Haring Hall, University of California, Davis, CA 95616, USA. E-mail bbchomel@ucdavis.edu

J.A. Comer, Viral and Rickettsial Zoonoses Branch, National Center for Infectious Diseases, Centers for Disease Control and Prevention, Atlanta, GA 30333, USA. E-mail jnc0@cdc.gov

B.D. Cooke, CSIRO Sustainable Ecosystems, GPO Box 284, Canberra ACT 2601, Australia. E-mail brian.cooke@cse.csiro.au

W. Crewe, 24 Ranelagh Drive North, Liverpool L19 9DS, UK.

J.B. Davies, Liverpool School of Tropical Medicine, Division of Parasite and Vector Biology, Pembroke Place, Liverpool L3 5QA, UK. E-mail daviesjb@liverpool.ac.uk

A.J. Della-Porta, CSIRO, Livestock Industries, Australian Animal Health Laboratory, Private Bag 24, Geelong, Victoria 3220, Australia. E-mail Antony.Della-porta@li.csiro.au

V. Deubel, Centre de Recherche Mérieux Pasteur à Lyon, 21 avenue Tony Garnier, 69365 Lyon Cedex 7, France. E-mail vdeubel@cervi-lyon.inserm.fr

D.C. Dragon, 5602 51A Avenue, Yellowknife, Northwest Territories X1A 1G4, Canada. E-mail dcdragon@internorth.com

B.F. Eldridge, University of California, Department of Entomology, Davis, CA 95616, USA. E-mail bfeldridge@ucdavis.edu

S.A. Ewing, College of Veterinary Medicine, Department of Veterinary Pathobiology, 250 McElroy Hall, Oklahoma State University, Stillwater, OK 74078, USA. E-mail saewing@okstate.edu

F. Fenner, The John Curtin School of Medical Research, The Australian National University, PO Box 334, Canberra, ACT 2601, Australia. E-mail fenner@jcsmr.anu.edu.au

I.N. Gavrilovskaya, Department of Medicine/GI, SUNY at Stony Brook, NY 11794/8173, USA. E-mail IRINA@mail.som.sunysb.edu

E.P.J. Gibbs, Department of Pathobiology, Box 110880, College of Veterinary Medicine, University of Florida, Gainesville, FL 32610, USA. E-mail pgibbs@ufl.edu

E.A. Gould, Centre for Ecology and Hydrology, Institute of Virology and Environmental Microbiology, Mansfield Road, Oxford OX1 3SR, UK. E-mail eag@ceh.ac.uk

E.C. Greiner, Department of Pathobiology, College of Veterinary Medicine, Box 110880, University of Florida, Gainesville, FL 32611-0880, USA. E-mail Greinere@mail.vetmed.ufl.edu

D.E. Griffin, Department of Molecular Microbiology and Immunology, Johns Hopkins University Bloomberg School of Public Health, 615 N. Wolfe Street, Room E5132, Baltimore, MD 21205, USA. E-mail dgriffin@jhsph.edu

P.R. Grimstad, Department of Biological Sciences, University of Notre Dame, Notre Dame, IN 46556-0369, USA. E-mail Paul.R.Grimstad.1@nd.edu

C.A. Hart, The University of Liverpool, Department of Medical Microbiology and Genitourinary Medicine, Duncan Building, Daulby Street, Liverpool L69 3GA, UK. E-mail C.A.Hart@liverpool.ac.uk

T. Hatchette, Department of Medicine, Queen Elizabeth Second Health Sciences Center – VG site, 1278 Tower Road, Halifax, Nova Scotia, Canada B3H 2YG. E-mail t_hatchette@hotmail.com

K.E. Hechemy, Office of Epidemiology, Wadsworth Center, PO Box 509, Albany, NY 12201-0509, USA. E-mail hechemy@wadsworth.org

F.X. Heinz, Institute of Virology, University of Vienna, Kinderspitalgasse 15, A-1095 Vienna, Austria. E-mail franz.x.heinz@univie.ac.at

J.E. Hillerton, Institute for Animal Health, Compton Laboratory, Compton,

Newbury, Berkshire RG20 7NN, UK. E-mail eric.hillerton@bbsrc.ac.uk

H. Holzmann, Institute of Virology, University of Vienna, Kinderspitalgasse 15, A-1095 Vienna, Austria. E-mail heidemarie.holzmann@univie.ac.at

F.W. Huchzermeyer, Veterinary Consultant: Crocodiles and Ostriches, PO Box 12499, 0110 Onderstepoort, South Africa. E-mail crocvet@mweb.co.za

C.J. Issel, University of Kentucky, Gluck Equine Research Center, Lexington, KY 40546-0099, USA. E-mail cissel@pop.uky.edu

T.W. Jones, University of Edinburgh, Centre for Tropical Veterinary Medicine, Easter Bush, Roslin, Midlothian EH25 9RG, UK. E-mail T.W.Jones@ed.ac.uk

R.M. Kinney, Division of Vector-Borne Infectious Diseases, National Center for Infectious Diseases, Centers for Disease Control and Prevention, PO Box 2087, Fort Collins, CO 80522, USA. E-mail rmk1@cdc.gov

K.M. Kocan, Department of Veterinary Pathobiology, College of Veterinary Medicine, Oklahoma State University, Stillwater, OK 74078-2007, USA. E-mail kmk285@okstate.edu

L.D. Kramer, The Arbovirus Laboratories, Wadsworth Center, New York State Department of Health, 5668 State Farm Road, Slingerlands, New York 12159, USA. E-mail ldk02@health.state.ny.us

T. Kumanomido, Equine Research Institute, JRA, 321-4 Tokami-cho, Utsunomiya, Tochigi 320-0856, Japan. E-mail takeshi@center.equinst.go.jp

K. Kurtenbach, The Wellcome Trust Centre for Epidemiology of Infectious Diseases, Department of Zoology, University of Oxford, South Parks Road, Oxford OX1 3PS, UK. E-mail klaus.kurtenbach@ceid.ox.ac.uk

M. Labuda, Institute of Zoology, Slovak Academy of Sciences, Dubravska cesta 9, 84206 Bratislava, Slovakia. E-mail uzaelabu@nic.savba.sk

E.T. Lyons, Department of Veterinary Science, Gluck Equine Research Center, University of Kentucky,

Lexington, KY 40546-0099, USA. E-mail elyons1@pop.uky.edu

J.S. Mackenzie, Department of Microbiology and Parasitology, The University of Queensland, Brisbane, Queensland 4072, Australia. E-mail jmac@biosci.uq.edu.au

P.J. McCall, Liverpool School of Tropical Medicine, Pembroke Place, Liverpool L3 5QA, UK. E-mail mccall@liverpool.ac.uk

D.M. McLean, Department of Pathology and Laboratory Medicine, University of British Columbia, Rm GF 227-2211 Wesbrook Mall, Vancouver, British Columbia, Canada V6T 2B5. (Fax 001 604 263 0220)

T.J. Marrie, Department of Medicine, University of Alberta, 2F1.30 Walter C. Mackenzie Health Sciences Center, 8440–112 Street, Edmonton, Alberta, Canada T6G 2B7. E-mail tom.marrie@ualberta.ca

I.D. Marshall, Department of Microbiology, John Curtin School of Medical Research, Australian National University, Canberra, Australia. E-mail iankathleen@ozemail.com.au

P.S. Mellor, Department of Arbovirology, Institute for Animal Health, Ash Road, Pirbright, Woking, Surrey GU24 0NF, UK. E-mail philip.mellor@bbsrc.ac.uk

C.J. Mitchell, Division of Vector-Borne Infectious Diseases, National Center for Infectious Diseases, Centers for Disease Control and Prevention, PO Box 2087, Fort Collins, CO 80522, USA. E-mail cjm2@lamar.colstate.edu

T.P. Monath, Acambis Inc., 38 Sidney Street, Cambridge, MS 02139, USA. E-mail thomas.monath@acambis.com

B. Murgue, Unité des Arbovirus et Virus des Fièvres Hèmorragiques, Institut Pasteur, 25–28 rue du Docteur Roux, 75724 Paris Cedex 15, France. E-mail bmurgue@pasteur.fr

M.B. Nathan, World Health Organization (CDS/CPE), 20 Avenue Appia, CH-1211 Geneva 27, Switzerland. E-mail nathanm@who.int

H. Neimark, Department of Microbiology and Immunology, Morse Institute of Molecular Genetics, State University of New York, 450 Clarkson Avenue, Brooklyn, NY 11203, USA. E-mail neimah25@hscbklyn.edu

P.A Nuttall, Natural Environmental Research Council, Institute of Virology and Environmental Microbiology, Mansfield Road, Oxford OX1 3SR, UK, E-mail pan@wpo.nerc.ac.uk or pan@ceh.ac.uk

S. Pampiglione, Dipartimento di Sanità Pubblica Veterinaria e Patologia Animale, Università degli Studi di Bologna, Laboratorio di Parassitologia, Via Tolara di Sopra, 50–40064 Ozzano Emilia (Bologna), Italy. E-mail jacq. pampi@libero.it

P. Parola, Unité des Rickettsies, CNRS UMR A6020, Université de la Méditerranée, Faculté de Médecine, 27 boulevard Jean Moulin, 13385 Marseilles Cedex 5, France. E-mail phparola@yahoo.fr

J.S. Malik Peiris, The University of Hong Kong, Department of Microbiology, University Pathology Building, Queen Mary Hospital Compound, Hong Kong. E-mail malik@hkucc.hku.hk

D.B. Pence, Department of Pathology, Texas Tech University, Health Sciences Center, 3601 4th Street, Lubbock, TX 79430, USA. E-mail pthdbp@ttuhsc. edu

M. Pfeffer, Institute for Medical Microbiology, Epidemic and Infectious Diseases, Veterinaerstr. 13, D-80539 Munich, Germany. E-mail Martin. Pfeffer@micro.vetmed.uni-muenchen. de

P.M. Preston, The University of Edinburgh, Institute for Cell, Animal and Population Biology, The King's Buildings, West Mains Road, Edinburgh EH9 3JT, UK. E-mail ppreston@srv0.bio.ed.ac.uk

D. Raoult, Unité des Rickettsies, CNRS UMR A6020, Université de la Méditerranée, Faculté de Médecine, 27 Boulevard Jean Moulin, 13385 Marseilles Cedex 05, France. E-mail Didier.Raoult@medecine.univ-mrs.fr

W.K. Reisen, Arbovirus Field Station, Center for Vector-borne Disease Research, School of Veterinary Medicine, University of California, Davis, CA 95616, USA. E-mail arbo123@pacbell.net

M. Renshaw, UNICEF, Avenida do Zimbabwe 1440, PO Box 4713, Maputo, Mozambique. E-mail melanierenshaw@ hotmail.com

A. Renz, Universität Tübingen, Friedhofstrasse 73, 72074 Tübingen, Germany. E-mail AlfonsRenz@uni-tuebingen-de

F. Rivasi, Dipartimento di Scienze Morfologiche e Medico Legali, Università di Modena e Reggio Emilia, via del Pozzo 71, 41100 Modena, Italy. E-mail rivasi@ unimo.it

S.M. Schäfer, The Wellcome Trust Centre for Epidemiology of Infectious Diseases, Department of Zoology, University of Oxford, South Parks Road, Oxford OX1 3PS, UK. E-mail Stefanie. Schafer@ceid.ox.ac.uk

C.J. Schofield, ECLAT Coordinator, Department of Infectious and Tropical Diseases, London School of Hygiene & Tropical Medicine, London WC1 7HT, UK. E-mail C.J.Schofield@lshtm.ac.uk

M.W. Service, Liverpool School of Tropical Medicine, Pembroke Place, Liverpool L3 5QA, UK. E-mail mservice@ liverpool.ac.uk

D.J. Sexton, Department of Medicine, Division of Infectious Diseases, Duke University School of Medicine, Durham, NC 27710, USA. E-mail sexto002@mc.duke.edu

J.B. Silver, UNICEF, Avenida do Zimbabwe 1440, PO Box 4713, Maputo, Mozambique. E-mail melanierenshaw@ hotmail.com

R.D. Smith, College of Veterinary Medicine, University of Illinois, 2001 South Lincoln Avenue, Urbana, IL 61802, USA. E-mail rd-smith@uiuc.edu

D. Strickman, Walter Reed Army Institute of Research, Building 503, Robert Grant Avenue, Silver Spring, MD 20910, USA. E-mail daniel.strickman@na. amedd.army.mil

K. Sumption, Centre for Tropical Veterinary Medicine, University of Edinburgh,

Easter Bush, Roslin, Midlothian EH25 9RG, UK. E-mail keiths@vet.ed.ac.uk

O. Tomori, World Health Organization, Regional Office for Africa (WHO-AFRO), PO Box BE 773, Belvedere, Harare, Zimbabwe. E-mail tomorio@whoafr.org

G. Uilenberg, 'A Surgente', route du Port, 20130 Cargèse, France. E-mail uilenber@club-internet.fr

M.G.R. Varma, Department of Farm Animal and Equine Medicine and Surgery, The Royal Veterinary College, Boltons Park, Hawkshead Road, Potters Bar, Hertfordshire EN6 1NB, UK. E-mail rvarma@rvc.ac.uk

D.A. Warrell, Centre for Tropical Medicine, University of Oxford, John Radcliffe Hospital, Headington, Oxford OX3 9DU, UK. E-mail david.warrell@ndm.ox.ac.uk

S.C. Weaver, Center for Tropical Diseases and Department of Pathology, University of Texas Medical Branch, 301 University Boulevard, Galveston, TX 77555-0609, USA. E-mail sweaver@utmb.edu

W.S.S. Wijesundera, University of Colombo, Department of Biochemistry and Molecular Biology, Faculty of Medicine, PO Box 271, Colombo 8, Sri Lanka. E-mail wssw@eureka.lk

J. Woodall, Universidade Federal do Rio de Janeiro, Instituto de Ciencias Biomedicas, Departamento de Bioquimica Medica, Bloco D Subsolo, Sala 16, Cidade Universitaria, 21941-590 Rio de Janeiro – R.J, Brazil. E-mail woodall@bioqmed.ufrj.br

Rongman Xu, Institute of Microbiology and Epidemiology, AMMS, 20 Dongdajie, Fengtai, Beijing 100071, China. E-mail xurm@nic.bmi.ac.cn

H. Zeller, Unité des Arbovirus et Virus des Fièvres Hèmorragiques, Institut Pasteur, 25–28 rue du Docteur Roux, 75724 Paris Cedex 15, France. E-mail hzeller@pasteur.fr

Preface

This ambitious project has involved the cooperation of 88 authors from 19 countries. I have been ably advised by the five international advisers. However, the final choice of infections included, and those omitted, was my decision. It was, for example, considered impractical to describe the transmission of some 300 arboviruses, so I have had to be selective. Similarly, a few rare and/or obscure non-arboviral infections of humans and domesticated animals have also been excluded. There can be several criteria for inclusion, such as the impact of a veterinary or medical infection on the health of the hosts, its economic importance, or because of interesting ecological or immunological considerations. Parasites such as *Dipylidium caninum* have not been included because I regard fleas as intermediate hosts, not vectors involved in transmission.

This is an encyclopedia, not a specialized medical or veterinary textbook, and so the aim has been to present up-to-date basic information on the transmission of a broad range of infections. It is hoped that the encyclopedia will prove useful for a wide readership, including not only those in the medical field but those interested in finding out, for example, what transmits an infectious agent, where it is found and whether it can be cured or prevented. Those wishing for more detailed or specialized information should be guided by the list of publications under 'Selected bibliography' found at the end of most entries.

Efforts have been made to obtain balanced entries but, as these were written by physicians, veterinarians, parasitologists, immunologists and entomologists, not unexpectedly, different entries emphasize different aspects of infections. Some contributors have chosen to give detailed drug regimens, others have not; I have left this to their personal choice. Moreover, some infections required additional headings and a different format. There has, therefore, been some flexibility in the approach.

Although the encyclopedia is concerned with infections, and the role of arthropods in their transmission, I have nevertheless included separate brief accounts of various categories of arthropods, such as biting midges, lice and ticks. This is so that the relevant points of their classification, biology and control need not be repeated in the entries on named infections. Likewise, short accounts of some of the more important categories of infective organisms, such as arboviruses, rickettsiae and filarial worms, are included.

A few words on nomenclature. I give the scientific names of mammals found in *Mammal Species of the World* (1993), edited by D.E. Wilson and D.M. Reeder, National Museum of Natural History, Smithsonian

Institution, Washington, DC (scientific names can also be found using www.nmnh.si.edu/msw). I have used vernacular names given by the authors in their contributions, or where appropriate those listed in *A World List of Mammalian Species* (1980), written by G.B. Corbet and J.E. Hill, British Museum (Natural History), London. Mule deer and Black-tailed deer are usually regarded as the same species, *Odocoileus hemionus*. I have used the vernacular names chosen by the authors, except that when an author refers to both Mule deer (*Odocoileus hemionus hemionus*) and Black-tailed deer (*O. h. columbianus*) I treat them as subspecies.

I have used various recent ornithological books for scientific and vernacular names of birds, sometimes giving more than one vernacular name when I considered this appropriate.

J.E. Reinert (*Journal of the American Mosquito Control Association* (2000) 16, 175–188) raised the subgenus *Ochlerotatus* of *Aedes* to generic rank. Although inevitably this will cause some confusion, I have adopted this change in anticipation that it will become generally accepted. I have placed a numerical indicator against the first mention of the genus *Ochlerotatus* in all relevant contributions and inserted a brief note just before the Selected bibliographies explaining its elevation to generic status.

There are differences of opinion concerning several issues of viral nomenclature.

After consultations with arbovirologists and medical entomologists I have decided not to italicize family names or so-called species names, such as yellow fever. I have used the capital letter abbreviations given in the third edition of the *International Catalogue of Arboviruses Including Certain Other Viruses of Vertebrates* (1985), edited by N. Karabatsos, The American Society of Tropical Medicine and Hygiene, Texas, USA, for arboviruses. The two exceptions are that I have used BT instead of BLU for bluetongue virus and OHF instead of OMSK for Omsk haemorrhagic fever virus; this is because these abbreviations are more widely used. The letter V is not appended after arbovirus abbreviations to denote virus, so, for example, West Nile virus is abbreviated to WN virus, not WNV. Furthermore, abbreviations of virus names are not used for the diseases they cause. I recognize that not all these actions will be universally acceptable; the main motivation has been to reach an acceptable compromise between different procedures.

Dosages are given using superscripts: thus 25 mg chloroquine/kg/day is given as 25 mg chloroquine kg^{-1} day^{-1}, and 200 mg permethrin/m^2 is written as 200 mg permethrin m^{-2}.

Some of the more specialized textbooks relevant to many of the entries in this encyclopedia are given below.

Selected bibliography

Bowman, D.W. and Lynn, R.C. (1999) *Georgis' Parasitology for Veterinarians*, 7th edn. W.B. Saunders, Philadelphia, 414 pp.

Cook, G.C. (ed.) (1996) *Manson's Tropical Diseases*, 20th edn. W.B. Saunders, London, 1779 pp. (21st edn in preparation).

Eldridge, B.F. and Edman, J.D. (eds) (2000) *Medical Entomology. A Textbook on Public Health and Veterinary Problems Caused by Arthropods*. Kluwer Academic Publishers, Dordrecht, 659 pp.

Guerrant, R.L., Walker, D.H. and Weller, P.F. (eds) (1999) *Tropical Infectious Diseases: Principles, Pathogens and Practice*, 2 vols. Churchill Livingstone, Edinburgh, 1644 pp.

Kettle, D.S. (1995) *Medical and Veterinary Entomology*, 2nd edn. CAB International, Wallingford, UK, 725 pp.

Lane, R.P. and Crosskey, R.W. (eds) (1993) *Medical Insects and Arachnids*. Chapman & Hall, London, 723 pp.

Marcondes, C.B. (2001) *Entomologia Média e Veterinária*. Atheneu, São Paulo, 432 pp.

Murphy, F.A., Gibbs, E.P.J., Horzinek, M.C. and Studdert, M.J. (1999) *Veterinary Virology*, 3rd edn. Academic Press, San Diego, California, 629 pp.

Palmer, S.R., Soulsby, L. and Simpson, D.I.H. (1998) *Zoonoses*. Oxford University Press, Oxford, 948 pp.

Pstoret, P.-P. (coordinator) (2000) An update on zoonoses. *OIE Scientific and Technical Review* 19(1), 1–336.

Schoonbaer, D. (2000) Tropical medicine, the internet and current trends in biomedical communication. *Annals of Tropical Medicine and Parasitology* 94, 661–674.

Service, M.W. (2000) *Medical Entomology for Students*. Cambridge University Press, Cambridge, 283 pp.

Sewell, M.M.H. and Brocklesby, D.W. (eds) (1990) *Handbook on Animal Diseases in the Tropics*, 4th edn. Baillière-Tindall, London, 385 pp.

Soulsby, E.J.L. (1982) *Helminths, Arthropods and Protozoa of Domesticated Animals*, 7th edn. Baillière-Tindall, London, 809 pp.

Strickland, G.T. (ed.) (2000) *Hunter's Tropical Medicine and Emerging Infectious Diseases*, 8th edn. W.B. Saunders, Philadelphia, Pennsylvania, 1192 pp.

Urquhart, G.M., Armour, J., Duncan, D.L. and Jennings, F.W. (1987) *Veterinary Parasitology*. Longman Scientific & Technical, Harlow, 268 pp.

Wall, R. and Shearer, D. (1997) *Veterinary Entomology*. Chapman & Hall, London, 439 pp.

White, D.O. and Fenner, F.J. (1994) *Medical Virology*, 4th edn. Academic Press, San Diego, California, 603 pp.

Williams, R.W., Hall, R.D., Broce, A.B. and Scholl, P.J. (eds) (1985) *Livestock Entomology*. John Wiley & Sons, New York, 335 pp.

M.W. Service
January 2001

Acknowledgements

Professor Barry J. Beaty, author of the La Crosse virus contribution, wishes to acknowledge that his research has been supported by NIH grant AI 32543 and the John D. and Catherine T. MacArthur Foundation. He also gratefully acknowledges the many colleagues who have contributed to the studies on La Crosse over the years, especially Dr Laura Chandler, Dr Len Wasieloski, Dr Jennifer Woodring, Ms Dawn Dobie, Mr Mike McGaw, Ms Cindy Oray and Mr Ryan Mackie.

Dr P.R. Grimstad, author of the Cache Valley virus contribution, acknowledges that research in Indiana and Michigan on Cache Valley virus, especially the work of Dr Robert Boromisa, Dr Philip Heard and Dr Mingbao Zhang, was supported in part by NIH grants AI-02793, AI-19679, AI-07030, a contribution of Federal Aid in Wildlife Restoration, Michigan Project W-127-R and the University of Notre Dame.

Dr P.M. Preston wishes to thank Professor C.G.D. Brown for helpful discussions concerning her entry on Theilerioses.

Dr W.S.S. Wijesundera, author of the contribution on setariosis, wishes to express his gratitude to Dr C. Shoho for his expert advice on *Setaria* infections.

Abbreviations

ABR	annual biting rate	CT	computerized tomography
AG	arthrogryposis	CTC	capillary tube centrifugation
AGH	arthrogryposis with hydranencephaly	DALY	disability-adjusted life years
		DDT	dichlorodiphenyl-trichloroethane
AGID	agar gel immunodiffusion	DEC	diethylcarbamazine
APOC	African Programme for Onchocerciasis Control	DEET	diethyl-methylbenzamide, formerly *N, N*-diethyl-m-toluamide
ASM	American Society for Microbiology		
		DHFR	dihydrofolate reductase
ATP	adenosine triphosphate	DIMP	dimethylphthalate
ATP	annual transmission potential	DNA	deoxyribonucleic acid
AUG	translation initiation codon, e.g. methionine	DRC	Democratic Republic of Congo
		dsRNA	double-stranded RNA
BHK-21	baby hamster kidney cell line	EDTA	ethylenediamine tetra-acetic acid
BKA	baby hamster kidney cell line	EEG	electroencephalogram
BS-C-1	African green monkey cell line	EIA	enzyme immunoassay
BSK	Barbour–Stoenner–Kelly medium	ELISA	enzyme-linked immunosorbent assay (same as EIA)
Bti	*Bacillus thuringiensis* subsp. *israelensis*		
		ESS	erythrocyte-sensitizing antigen
CAM	chorioallantoic membrane	Fab	fragment of immunoglobulin
CATT	card agglutination trypanosomiasis test	FAT	fluorescent antibody test
		Fc	crystallization fragment
CDC	Centers for Disease Control and Prevention	FDA	Food and Drug Administration (USA)
cDNA	complementary DNA	FEMS	Federation of European Microbiological Societies
cELISA	competitive enzyme-linked immunosorbent assay		
		G6PD	glucose-6-phosphate dehydrogenase
CF	complement fixation		
CIS	Commonwealth of Independent States (former Soviet Union)	HCH	benzene hexachloride (= BHC)
		HE	hydranencephaly
CNS	central nervous system	HEL	human embryonic lung cell line
CPE	cytopathic effects	HeLa	human cervix epithelioid carcinoma cell line
CSF	cerebrospinal fluid		

HGE	human granulocytic ehrlichiosis	nsPs	non-structural proteins
HI	haemagglutination inhibition	NSs	small-sized segment of DNA encoding a non-structural gene
hnRNA	heterogeneous nuclear RNA		
IATA	International Airline Transport Association	NT	neutralization test
		OCP	Onchocerciasis Control Programme
i.c.	intercranial or intracerebral		
IFA	indirect immunofluorescent antibody	OIE	Office International des Epizooties
IFN	interferon	Omp	outer membrane protein, such as rOmpA and rOmpB
IgG	immunoglobulin isotype G; others are IgM, immunoglobulin isotype M, etc.	ORF	open-reading frame, on chromosomes
IGR	insect growth regulator	OspA, OspB, OspC, etc.	outer surface proteins
IHA	indirect haemagglutination assay		
IHR	International Health Regulations	OX2, OX19, OXK	names of strains of *Proteus* antigens
IIP	indirect immunoperoxidase assay		
IL	interleukin	$PaCO_2$	arterial partial pressure of CO_2
i.p.	intraperitoneal	PARP	procyclic acidic repetitive protein
ITN	insecticide-treated net		
i.v.	intravenous	PBL	peripheral blood leucocytes
J-HR	Jarisch–Herxheimer reaction	PCR	polymerase chain reaction
kb	kilobase	PK15	pig kidney cell line
kbp	kilobase pair	PNG	Papua New Guinea
kDa	kilodalton	PrM	pre- (or precursor) membrane protein
L929 cells	mouse fibroblasts, clone 929		
LD_{50}	lethal dose for 50% of population	PRN	plaque reduction neutralization
LLC-MK2	Rhesus monkey (*Macaca mulatta*) kidney cell line	PS	pig kidney cell line
		PS-C1	porcine kidney stable cell line
MA-104	human heteroploid cell line	QBC	quantitative buffy coat
MA-111	human diploid cell line	R_0	basic reproduction rate
Mab	monoclonal antibody	rDNA	ribosomal DNA
MAC-ELISA	IgM antibody-capture enzyme-linked immunosorbent assay	RFLP	restriction fragment length polymorphism
		RIA	radioimmunoassay
m-AECT	miniature anion exchange centrifugation technique	RNA	ribonucleic acid
		rRNA	ribosomal RNA
MCA	monoclonal antibody (more usually abbreviated as Mab)	RT-PCR	reverse transcription–polymerase chain reaction
MDa	megadalton	s.c.	subcutaneous
MHC	major histocompatibility complex	SDS-PAGE	sodium dodecyl sulphate polyacrylamide gel electrophoresis
MID	mosquito infectious dose		
MIR	minimum infective rate (number of arthropods tested/number isolations obtained)	SIT	sterile insect technique
		s.l.	sensu lato
		ssRNA	single-stranded RNA
MRC5	human diploid lung cell line	s.str.	sensu stricto
MRI	magnetic resonance imaging	TCID	tissue culture infective dose
mRNA	messenger RNA	TGF	tumour growth factor
MSP	major surface protein	TNF	tumour necrosis factor
NSm	medium-sized segment of DNA encoding a non-structural gene	TOT	transovarial transmission
		ULV	ultra-low-volume

VERO	African green monkey (= Vervet monkey) (*Chlorocebus aethiops**) kidney cell line	Vmps	variable membrane proteins
		VN	virus neutralization
		VSG	variable surface glycoprotein

---

*   This monkey was formerly placed in the genus *Cercopithecus*.

Aegyptianella pullorum *see* **Aegyptianellosis**

Aegyptianellosis

F.W. Huchzermeyer

Infection of birds and poikilotherms with *Rickettsiae* of the genus *Aegyptianella*.

Aegyptianellosis, avian

While aegyptianellae have been found in a number of avian species, clinical disease has only been observed in domestic poultry, notably chickens, ducks and geese.

Distribution

Found in all of Africa, southern Europe, the Middle East and the Indian subcontinent. An *Aegyptianella* found in Wild turkeys (*Meleagris gallopavo*) in the USA and described as *A. pullorum* appears, however, to be a different species, specific to turkeys. Another species, *A. botuliformis*, has been isolated from Helmeted Guinea fowl (*Numida meleagris*) in South Africa.

Parasite

Aegyptianella pullorum (*Rickettsiales*: *Anaplasmataceae*) is found in the erythrocyte cytoplasm, where it is seen as small round bodies, larger solid round bodies and ring shapes (Fig. 1).

Clinical symptoms

The main clinical symptom is paleness of wattles and mucosae, caused by a severe anaemia. This may be accompanied by

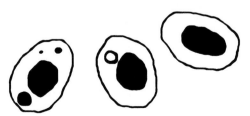

Fig. 1. Small and large round bodies and ring shape of *Aegyptianella pullorum* in the cytoplasm of chicken erythrocytes.

weakness, somnolence and diarrhoea. This picture may be complicated by the neurotoxic effects of the tick vectors, which can cause a severe paralysis, particularly when large numbers of argasid (soft tick) larvae have attached, as well as by a concomitant infection with *Borrelia anserina* (see Avian borreliosis). The latter frequently occurs in the northern range of its distribution but rarely in southern Africa. There is a marked age resistance, which causes the symptoms to be more severe and the pre-patent period (8–14 days) to be shorter in younger birds. In uncomplicated cases, mortality is seen only in chicks under 4 weeks of age. Recovery from anaemia is also quicker in older birds. Ducks and geese are equally susceptible to the infection with *A. pullorum*, while Guinea fowl (*N. meleagris*) and turkeys are generally regarded as resistant.

Diagnosis

The disease is diagnosed by demonstrating the presence of the intraerythrocytic round and ring shapes of the agent on a stained blood smear. However, one has to bear in mind that the anaemia persists longer than the parasitaemia. Consequently even a few parasites found in a highly anaemic blood smear are sufficient to confirm the diagnosis. Finding attached argasid larvae on the bird, as well as the presence of argasid ticks in the fowl run, further helps to confirm the diagnosis. If the disease is suspected or found in an uncommon host, the transmission by the injection of infected blood into one or several suitable clean birds should be attempted and the recipient(s) be monitored by taking blood smears for 3–4 weeks.

Post-mortem lesions

Anaemia, in late cases also icterus, splenomegaly and a certain degree of right ventricular hypertrophy of the heart, are the main post-mortem findings. Hydropericardium may also be seen in cases of advanced anaemia.

Transmission

Argasid ticks are the vectors, *Argas persicus* in the northern range of distribution and *A. walkerae* in southern Africa, while *A. reflexus* has also been incriminated. Three reproductive cycles take place in the argasid host, in the gut epithelial cells, in the haemocytes and in the salivary glands, and all developmental stages of the ticks can become infected and transmit the infection in the following stage or at the next feeding. That is there is trans-stadial transmission. The developmental cycle in the tick vector takes about 30 days, and transmission is by the tick's bite.

While argasid nymphs and adults only feed at night and leave the host immediately after the small blood meal, the larvae remain attached for up to 10 days and thereby can play a major epidemiological role, being able to be transported with their host over long distances. This can then start new foci of infection at their new destination. However, the mode of transmission limits outbreaks of aegyptianellosis to backyard flocks. The disease does not occur in intensive poultry production.

Treatment

The agent is susceptible to tetracycline and other broad-spectrum antibiotics administered orally or by injection.

Control

Control is achieved by ridding the fowl house and run of nymphs and adult ticks and the birds themselves of attached larvae. The house and run can be sprayed with carbamates or similar acaricides while the birds can be dusted or bathed with appropriate acaricides. The choice of acaricide depends on what is registered for the specific use in the country as well as on availability and size of packaged products. Because the adults and nymphs hide under stones and in cracks and crevices, it is important to apply the acaricides very thoroughly. The treatment must be repeated 2–3 weeks later to reach the newly hatched larvae. Newly acquired fowl should be quarantined, thoroughly examined and if necessary treated before introduction to the flock. Depopulation of the fowl run is not an option, because the ticks can survive fasting for more than a year.

Selected bibliography

Castle, M.D. and Christensen, B.M. (1985) Isolation and identification of *Aegyptianella pullorum* (Rickettsiales, Anaplasmataceae) in wild turkeys from North America. *Avian Diseases* 29, 437–445.

Gothe, R. (1967) Ein Beitrag zur systematischen Stellung von *Aegyptianella pullorum* Carpano, 1828. *Zeitschrift für Parasitenkunde* 29, 119–129.

Huchzermeyer, F.W. (1967) Die durch künstliche *Aegyptianella pullorum*-Infektion beim Haushuhn hervorgerufene Anämie. *Deutsche Tierärztliche Wochenschrift* 74, 437–439.

Huchzermeyer, F.W., Cilliers, J.A., Diaz Lavigne, C. and Bartkowiak, R.A. (1987) Broiler pulmonary hypertension syndrome. I. Increased right ventricular mass in broilers experimentally infected with *Aegyptianella pullorum*. *Onderstepoort Journal of Veterinary Research* 54, 113–114.

Huchzermeyer, F.W., Horak, I.G., Putterill, J.F. and Earlé, R.A. (1992) Description of *Aegyptianella botuliformis* n. sp. (Rickettsiales: Anaplasmataceae) from the helmeted guineafowl, *Numida meleagris*. *Onderstepoort Journal of Veterinary Research* 59, 97–101.

Ristic, M. and Kreier, J.P. (1974) Family III. Anaplasmataceae Philip, 1957. In: Buchanan, R.E. and Gibbons, N.E. (eds) *Bergey's Manual of Determinative Bacteriology*, 8th edn. Williams & Wilkins, Baltimore, Maryland, pp. 906–914.

African horse sickness

P.S. Mellor

African horse sickness is a non-contagious, infectious, insect-borne disease of equids that was first recognized in Africa in the 16th century. The effects of the disease, particularly in susceptible populations of horses, can be devastating, with mortality rates often in excess of 90%. Although African horse sickness is normally restricted to Africa the disease has a much wider significance as a result of its ability to spread, without warning, beyond the borders of that continent. For these reasons it has been allocated Office International des Epizooties (OIE) list A status (i.e. communicable diseases which have the potential for very rapid spread, irrespective of national borders, which are of serious socio-economic or public health consequence and which are of major importance in the international trade of livestock or livestock products).

Distribution

African horse sickness is widely distributed across sub-Saharan Africa and is enzootic in a band stretching from Senegal and The Gambia in the west to Ethiopia and Somalia in the east, and reaching as far south as northern parts of South Africa. It is probably also enzootic in northern Yemen, the only such area outside the African continent. From these zones the disease makes seasonal extensions both northwards and southwards to a degree dependent mainly upon the climatic conditions and how these affect the abundance and prevalence of the vector insects. More rarely, the disease has spread much more widely and has extended as far as Pakistan and India in the east and Spain and Portugal in the west. However, prior to the 1987–1991 Spanish, Portuguese and Moroccan outbreaks, African horse sickness had been unable to persist in any area outside sub-Saharan Africa or Yemen, for more than 2–3 consecutive years, at most.

Aetiological agent

African horse sickness (AHS) virus is a member of the genus *Orbivirus* in the family Reoviridae. It is an unenveloped virus 65–80 nm in diameter with a core containing ten segments of double-stranded RNA (dsRNA) surrounded by a double-layered capsid. Nine distinct serotypes of the virus have been identified. The core particle contains five proteins that make up the group-specific epitopes, while the outer capsid contains two further proteins that comprise the type-specific determinants. Three non-structural proteins have also been identified in infected cells. African horse sickness virus serotypes 1–8 are typically found only in restricted areas of sub-Saharan Africa, while serotype 9 is more widespread and has been responsible for virtually all epizootics of African horse sickness outside Africa. The only exception is the 1987–1990 Spanish–Portuguese outbreak, which was due to AHS virus serotype 4.

African horse sickness virus is relatively heat-resistant and is stable at 4°C and −70°C; however, it is labile between −20°C and −30°C. It is partially resistant to lipid solvents but is rapidly inactivated at pH levels below 6.0.

Clinical signs

The virus can cause four forms of disease in equids and in ascending order of severity these are: horse sickness fever, cardiac, mixed and pulmonary forms. Horse sickness fever is the mildest form of disease, involving only a rise in temperature and possibly oedema of the supraorbital fossae; there is no mortality. It occurs following the infection of horses with less virulent strains of virus or when some degree of immunity exists. It is usually the only form of disease exhibited by the African donkey and zebra (*Equus* species).

The cardiac or subacute form has an incubation period of about 7–14 days and then the first clinical sign is fever. This is followed by oedema, first of the supraorbital fossae and eyelids, and then extending to other areas of the head, neck and chest. Petechial haemorrhages may appear in the conjunctivae and ecchymotic haemorrhages on the ventral surface of the tongue. Colic is also a feature of the disease. The mortality rate in horses from this form of disease may be as high as 50% and death usually occurs within 4–8 days of the onset of fever.

The mixed form of African horse sickness is a combination of the cardiac and pulmonary forms of the disease, with mortality rates, in horses, as high as 80%.

The pulmonary form is peracute and may develop so rapidly that an animal can die without previous indication of disease. Usually there will be marked depression and fever (39–41°C), followed by onset of respiratory distress. Coughing spasms may also occur, the head and neck are extended and severe sweating develops. There may be periods of recumbence and, terminally, quantities of frothy fluid may be discharged from the nares and mouth. Death is from congestive heart failure or asphyxia and the mortality rate in horses is frequently over 90%. During epizootics in naïve populations of horses all forms of disease can occur but the mixed and pulmonary forms usually predominate so mortality rates well in excess of 80% are likely, making African horse sickness one of the most lethal of all horse diseases.

Pathology and post-mortem findings
The lesions caused by AHS virus differ in accordance with the form of disease. With the pulmonary form the most conspicuous lesions are likely to be oedema of the lungs (which remain fully distended after death) and hydrothorax. The subpleural and interlobular tissues are infiltrated with yellowish gelatinous exudate and the entire bronchial tree may be filled with a surfactant, stabilized froth (i.e. froth that does not deliquesce). Ascites can occur in the abdominal and thoracic cavities and the

mucosa of the fundic part of the stomach may be reddened and oedematous.

In the cardiac form the most obvious lesions are gelatinous exudates in the subcutaneous, subfascial and intramuscular tissues and lymph nodes. Hydropericardium is seen and haemorrhages are found on the epicardial and/or endocardial surfaces. Petechial haemorrhages and/or cyanosis may also occur on the serosal surfaces of the caecum and colon. As in the pulmonary form, ascites may be found but oedema of the lungs is either slight or absent.

In the mixed form of African horse sickness, lesions common to both pulmonary and cardiac forms are found.

The histopathological changes that are seen in cases of African horse sickness are a result of increased permeability of the capillary walls and consequent impairment in circulation. The lungs exhibit serous infiltration of the intralobular tissue with distension of the alveoli and capillary congestion. The central veins of the liver are distended and interstitial tissues contain erythrocytes and blood pigments, while the parenchymal cells show fatty degeneration. Cellular infiltration can be seen in the cortex of the kidneys, while the spleen is heavily congested. Congestion may also be seen in the intestinal and gastric mucosae and cloudy swelling in the myocardial and skeletal muscles.

Diagnosis
In enzootic areas the typical clinical features of African horse sickness, as described earlier, can be used to form a presumptive diagnosis. Laboratory confirmation should then be sought. In regions where African horse sickness is usually absent, all suspicious cases should be referred to an appropriately qualified laboratory. The specimens likely to be required are as follows:

1. Blood for virus isolation: collected during the early febrile stage into an anticoagulant such as heparin or ethylenediamine tetra-acetic acid (EDTA) and kept cool (4°C) but not frozen.[1]
2. Tissues for virus isolation (or for antigen detection by enzyme-linked immunosorbent assay (ELISA) or for RNA detection by

polymerase chain reaction (PCR)-based assays). Spleen is best followed by lung, liver, heart and lymph nodes. Tissues should be collected at autopsy and kept and transported to the laboratory at 4°C.

3. Serum for serological tests. Preferably, paired samples should be taken 14–28 days apart and should be kept frozen at –20°C.

Confirmation of African horse sickness is by one or more of the following:

1. Identification of the virus directly from submitted samples by a group-specific antigen detection ELISA or by PCR-based assays.

2. Isolation of infectious virus in suckling mice or embryonating hens' eggs, followed by adaptation to cell culture and identification first by the group-specific agar gel immunodiffusion (AGID) test or antigen detection ELISA, and then by the serotype-specific virus neutralization or reverse-transcription PCR (RT-PCR) tests.

3. Identification of AHS virus-specific antibodies by the group-specific antibody detection ELISA, complement fixation (CF) or serotype-specific virus neutralization test.

Transmission

African horse sickness virus is transmitted between its vertebrate hosts almost exclusively via the bites of haematophagous arthropods. Various different types of arthropods, ranging from mosquitoes to ticks, have been implicated over the years, but certain species of *Culicoides* midges are considered to be by far the most significant. These biting midges act as true biological vectors and support virus replication by up to 10,000-fold of the infectious units ingested. Subsequent to feeding upon a viraemic equid, susceptible species of *Culicoides* become capable of transmission after an incubation period of 8–10 days at 25°C, though this period lengthens as the temperature falls, and becomes infinite below 15–18°C. The incubation or pre-patent period in the vector is the time interval necessary for ingested virus to escape from the gut lumen by entering and replicating in the midgut cells, and then for progeny virus particles released

into the haemocoel to reach and replicate in the salivary glands. Transovarial or vertical transmission of AHS virus by vector midges does not occur.

Culicoides imicola, a widely distributed species found across Africa, southern Europe and much of Asia, is the major vector of AHS virus and has long been considered to be the only important field vector. However, a closely related species, *C. bolitinos*, has recently been identified as a second vector in Africa, and the North American *C. variipennis* is a highly efficient vector in the laboratory. Further additions to this list are likely.

In general, *Culicoides* species have a flight range of a few kilometres or less. However, in common with many other groups of flying insects, they have the capacity to be transported as aerial plankton over much greater distances. In this context, a considerable body of evidence exists to suggest that the emergence of AHS virus from its enzootic zones may sometimes be due to long-range dispersal flights by infected vector *Culicoides* carried on the prevailing winds.

Vertebrate hosts

Equids are by far the most important vertebrate hosts of AHS virus and the horse is the species most susceptible to disease, with mules and European donkeys somewhat less so. African donkeys are fairly resistant to clinical African horse sickness, while Zebra (e.g. *Equus burchellii*) are usually only affected subclinically.

Dogs may occasionally be infected with AHS virus by ingesting virus-contaminated equid meat and can die from the disease. Some reports also suggest that they can be infected by insect bite but most authorities believe that dogs play little or no part in the epidemiology of African horse sickness and are merely dead-end hosts.

African horse sickness is not a zoonosis, though at least four human cases of severe disease have been documented. These were all infections acquired in an AHS virus vaccine plant under conditions unlikely to be duplicated elsewhere.

Incubation period and viraemia

Under natural conditions the incubation period of African horse sickness is less than 9 days, although experimentally it has been shown to range from 2 to 21 days. Viraemia in horses usually lasts from 4 to 8 days, with a maximum duration of 18 days, and can reach a peak titre of around 10^5 tissue culture infective dose for 50% ($TCID_{50}$) of virus per ml. In zebra, viraemia occasionally extends for as long as 40 days but peaks at only $10^{2.5}$ $TCID_{50}$ of virus per ml. Viraemia in donkeys is intermediate in titre and duration between that in horses and zebra, while in dogs it is considered to be very low-level and transitory.

Treatment

Apart from supportive treatment, there is no specific therapy for African horse sickness. Affected animals should be nursed carefully, fed well and given rest as even the slightest exertion may result in death. During convalescence, animals should be rested for at least 4 weeks before being returned to light work.

Prevention and control

Importation of equids from known infected areas to virus-free zones should be restricted. If importation is permitted, the animals should be quarantined for 60 days in insect-proof accommodation, prior to movement.

Following an outbreak of African horse sickness in a country or zone that has previously been free of the disease, attempts should be made to limit further transmission of the virus and to achieve eradication as quickly as possible. It is important that control measures are implemented as soon as a suspected diagnosis of African horse sickness has been made and without waiting for the diagnosis to be confirmed. In epizootic situations the following measures should be taken:

- Delineate the area of infection, taking into consideration topographical features such as mountain ranges and rivers.
- Prevent the movement of all equids within, into and out of the infected area.
- All equids should be stabled in insect-proof buildings if possible, at least from dusk to dawn, which is the period of major activity for the *Culicoides* vectors. The use of insect repellents inside the stables may enhance protection.
- Vector abatement measures should be implemented, e.g. insecticide treatment in and around animal holdings and of suspect *Culicoides* breeding sites, elimination of breeding sites through improved water management and waste disposal (see Biting midges).
- The rectal temperatures of all equids should be taken twice a day to detect infected animals as early as possible because overt disease is generally preceded by viraemia for about 3 days. Animals with a fever should be slaughtered or housed in insect-proof stables to prevent access by vectors and further spread of disease.
- All susceptible animals should be immediately vaccinated with polyvalent vaccines until the causative virus has been serotyped and the relevant monovalent vaccine has become available. Depending upon the severity of challenge, up to 20% of horses may still contract African horse sickness subsequent to vaccination with a polyvalent vaccine. All vaccinated animals should be identified.
- The virus serotype responsible for the outbreak should be determined as soon as possible and a suitable monovalent vaccine produced and administered. The use of a monovalent vaccine is the most successful control measure available, as it induces effective and enduring immunity in most animals within 3 weeks of vaccination.
- The OIE should be notified immediately of all cases of the disease because

African horse sickness is on their A list of notifiable diseases.

In enzootic situations and in regions where African horse sickness occurs almost every year, regular annual vaccination with live, attenuated polyvalent vaccines, effective against all known local serotypes of AHS virus, is strongly recommended. Such vaccines are only available from the Onderstepoort Veterinary Institute, South Africa. Two polyvalent vaccines are produced, one containing serotypes 1, 3, 4 and 5, and the other containing serotypes 2, 6, 7 and 8. These serotype formulations may vary from time to time. No serotype 9 is included since immunization with serotype 6 is cross-protective.

Note

[1] While in the circulation, most AHS virus is sequestered in immunologically privileged sites in the erythrocyte membranes and is protected from the effects of humoral antibody. Virus and antibody, therefore, may coexist in the circulatory system. Consequently, blood and tissue samples collected for virus isolation should be kept cool but must not be frozen; otherwise, upon defrosting, the erythrocytes will lyse and the released virus will be neutralized by serum antibody. Washing protocols have been devised to remove antibody from non-lysed blood prior to virus isolation procedures.

Selected bibliography

Coetzer, J.A.W. and Erasmus, B.J. (1994) African horsesickness. In: Coetzer, J.A.W., Thomson, G.R. and Tustin, R.C. (eds) *Infectious Diseases of Livestock with Special Reference to Southern Africa*, Vol. 1. Oxford University Press, Cape Town, pp. 460–475.

Hess, W.R. (1988) African horse sickness. In: Monath, T.P. (ed.) *The Arboviruses: Epidemiology and Ecology*, Vol. II. CRC Press, Boca Raton, Florida, pp. 1–18.

Howell, P.G. (1963) African horsesickness. In: *Emerging Diseases of Animals*. Agricultural studies, Food and Agriculture Organization, Rome, pp. 71–108.

Lagreid, W.W. (1996) African horsesickness. In: Studdert, M.J. (ed.) *Virus Infections of Equines*. Vol. 6 in the series Virus Infections of Vertebrates, Horzinek, M.C. (series ed.), Elsevier, Amsterdam, pp. 101–123.

Meiswinkel, R., Nevill, E.M. and Venter, G.J. (1994) Vectors: *Culicoides* spp. In: Coetzer, J.A.W., Thomson, G.R. and Tustin, R.C. (eds) *Infectious Diseases of Livestock with Special Reference to Southern Africa*, Vol. 1. Oxford University Press, Cape Town, pp. 68–89.

Mellor, P.S. (1993) African horse sickness: transmission and epidemiology. *Veterinary Research* 24, 199–212.

Mellor, P.S. (1994) Epizootiology and vectors of African horse sickness virus. *Comparative Immunology Microbiology and Infectious Diseases* 17, 287–296.

Mellor, P.S., Baylis, M., Hamblin, C., Calisher, C.H. and Mertens, P.P.C. (1998) *African Horse Sickness*. Springer, Vienna, 342 pp.

Sellers, R.F. (1980) Weather, host and vectors: their interplay in the spread of insect-borne animal virus diseases. *Journal of Hygiene* 85, 65–102.

Walton, T.E. and Osburn, B.I. (1992) *Bluetongue, African Horse Sickness and Related Orbiviruses*. CRC Press, Boca Raton, Florida, 1042 pp.

African swine fever

E. Paul J. Gibbs

African swine fever is a frequently fatal and epidemic disease of domesticated swine and European wild boar (*Sus scrofa*), characterized by haemorrhage and caused by a DNA virus that can be transmitted to susceptible pigs through close contact with other infected pigs, the ingestion of contaminated food or the bite of infected soft (argasid) ticks. The natural life cycle of African swine fever (ASF) virus, in its ancestral home in southern and East Africa, involves the soft tick, *Ornithodoros moubata porcinus* and the African Warthog (*Phacochoerus aethiopicus*). Other species of wild pig, such as the Bushpig (*Potamochoerus porcus*), are also involved. The infections in the Warthog and Bushpig are subclinical.

The introduction of the virus from infected Warthogs to domesticated pigs in Africa provided the springboard for the dissemination of the virus first to Europe and subsequently to the western hemisphere. Infection of domesticated pigs has apparently allowed the virus to 'escape' from the dependency of the arthropod vector for perpetuation. African swine fever is an example of an emerging disease resulting from the interspecies transfer of a virus. It is important to recognize this feature to fully understand the current geographical distribution and epidemiology of the disease. Whether the virus can perpetuate itself indefinitely in domesticated pigs without arthropod involvement is open to question.

Distribution

African swine fever was first reported as a disease of domesticated pigs in Kenya in East Africa in 1921. Subsequently, other countries in East and southern Africa reported similar outbreaks of the disease. The start of an outbreak was commonly traced to pigs being fed with tissue scraps from hunted Warthogs or from close contact with Warthogs or their burrows. Sporadic outbreaks of African swine fever continue to this day in this region.

The disease remained confined to Africa until 1957 when African swine fever was diagnosed for the first time in Europe, in Portugal. The virus was believed to have been introduced from Angola, possibly by Portuguese settlers returning to Portugal with infected pork products. The disease was apparently eradicated, but in 1960 it was believed to have been reintroduced to Portugal, from where it subsequently spread to Spain. The virus became endemic in Spain and Portugal because it was able to establish infection in *Ornithodoros erraticus*, a species of soft tick that inhabits the pigpens of peasant farms in the south-west of the Iberian Peninsula. An aggressive campaign to eradicate African swine fever has, in recent years, dramatically reduced the numbers of disease outbreaks in both Spain and Portugal. No outbreaks have occurred in Spain since 1994. Until a single herd outbreak was reported in late 1999, Portugal had

been free of African swine fever since 1993. (In contrast, in 1977 in Spain alone there had been 1780 outbreaks affecting 309,110 pigs.)

The large number of outbreaks of African swine fever in the 1960s, 1970s and 1980s in the Iberian Peninsula is believed to have led to 'spillover' into France in 1964, 1967 and 1974, Belgium in 1985 and The Netherlands in 1986. An outbreak in Malta in 1978 might also have been caused by the virus being introduced from Spain or Portugal. In each country, the disease was eradicated relatively quickly by slaughtering clinically diseased pigs and also pigs believed to have been exposed to infection.

African swine fever was first seen in mainland Italy in 1967 and in Sardinia in 1978. The virus was successfully eradicated from mainland Italy, but African swine fever persists in Sardinia, partly because the disease has become established in the free-ranging pigs and wild boar in the mountains.

In 1971, African swine fever was diagnosed in Cuba. This represented the first incursion of the disease into the Americas. The source of infection has never been determined. Although there has been a fanciful suggestion that the virus was introduced intentionally to aid in the downfall of President F. Castro through economic pressure, it is most likely that the virus was introduced in infected pork products from Spain or Portugal. The disease was efficiently eradicated by slaughtering over 450,000 pigs in the province of Havana. Seven years later in 1978, African swine fever devastated the pig population of the neighbouring island of Hispaniola. The source of this infection was also believed to have been pork products from Spain or Portugal. The disease was first recognized in the Dominican Republic, but it soon spread across the border to Haiti. By 1984, the disease had been eradicated, but, because it had spread so widely across the island, it had been necessary to slaughter the entire domesticated pig population (estimated at 2 million) and then repopulate with pigs from overseas. During the time when African swine fever was present in Haiti, it was once again diagnosed in Cuba, the result, it is believed, of refugees from

Haiti trading pig meat for petrol as they sailed for the USA.

The first diagnosis of African swine fever in South America occurred in the same year (1978) as the disease was seen in the Dominican Republic, a year that followed a high incidence in Spain (see above). The disease was seen in Brazil and the first outbreaks were in herds fed food waste from the international airport at Rio de Janeiro. Once again, it is highly likely that the origin of the virus lay in the Iberian Peninsula. The presence of disease in Brazil was alarming, as it was feared that it could rapidly extend to infect other parts of the continent. Although it was initially thought that the virus had spread widely in Brazil, eradication was successful.

The pig populations of several countries of West Africa, from Senegal to Gabon, have been affected by epidemics of African swine fever. Cameroon, for example, has seen its pig industry all but destroyed by the disease. The origins of the various epidemics have not been clearly traced, but in some cases the virus is considered to have been introduced in infected pig products imported from Europe. It is not known whether ASF virus is present in ticks in West Africa.

Aetiological agent

African swine fever virus is classified as the only member in its own family, the Asfaviridae. It is a large enveloped virus that has a genome of a single molecule of double-stranded linear DNA. The complete genome has been sequenced; it is 170–190 kbp in size and encodes for approximately 200 proteins. Replication occurs mainly in the cytoplasm, but the nucleus is required for DNA synthesis. Virions are released by budding or cell lysis.

Restriction endonuclease analysis of the DNA of isolates of ASF virus from Africa, Europe and the Americas permits classification into five groups. All European and American isolates fall within one group, whereas the African isolates show greater variation. This is probably because only one or two genotypes were introduced to Europe from Africa, where the virus has been circulating for a long time and has diverged

extensively. The analyses support the epidemiological conclusion that the strains of ASF virus that have occurred in the Americas originated in Europe.

Clinical signs

African swine fever virus infects domesticated pigs, European wild boar (*S. scrofa*) and other members of the family Suidae, such as the Warthog and Bushpig. Clinical disease, however, is only seen in domesticated pigs and wild boar. After an incubation period of 5–15 days, pigs develop high fever (40.5–42°C), which persists for about 4 days. Starting 1–2 days after the onset of fever, pigs lose their appetite, show signs of incoordination and may have diarrhoea. They often huddle as a group to keep warm. Some may die at this stage without further clinical signs. As the disease progresses, many pigs develop dyspnoea; they may vomit and exhibit reddening of the skin and cyanosis of the ears. Haemorrhage from the nose and anus is frequently seen before death. Pregnant sows may abort. Mortality is often 100%, with most affected animals dying a few days after the onset of fever.

The above description is typical of African swine fever in domesticated pigs in Africa that have been exposed to infected Warthogs or their tissues. However, in those geographical areas of Europe and the Americas where soft (argasid) ticks do not appear to be involved in virus transmission, the course of disease has usually been rapid and fatal at first, but rapidly diminishing in severity, until finally it becomes predominantly chronic and even subclinical.

Pathogenesis, pathology and immunity

At autopsy, haemorrhage characterizes the gross pathology seen in pigs dying in the acute stage of the disease. Haemorrhages are seen most prominently in the lymphatic and vascular systems. The spleen is often grossly enlarged, the kidneys and heart show petechial haemorrhage, and the visceral lymph nodes may resemble blood clots. Domesticated pigs with chronic disease exhibit pneumonia, pleuritis, pericarditis and arthritis.

Studies of the pathogenesis of ASF virus in domesticated and feral pigs have shown that the virus replicates in several cell types of the reticuloendothelial system causing a severe leucopenia. Infected swine are believed to die through the indirect effects of viral replication on platelets and complement functions rather than by direct cytolytic effect. Genomics has established that there are a number of genes associated with virulence and host range. Some have never been seen in viruses before and several are completely novel. For example, one gene, *A238L*, codes for a protein that acts as an analogue of the immunosuppressant drug cyclosporin A. These studies are providing the tools to a better understanding as to why domesticated pigs and Warthogs differ in their clinical susceptibility.

Domesticated pigs infected with ASF virus may become persistently infected. While diseased pigs are more easily recognized as possibly being persistently infected, development of clinical disease is not a prerequisite for persistent infection. The duration of persistence is unknown, but low levels of virus have been detected in tissues for more than a year after infection. This feature of the disease is one reason why eradication of African swine fever has often involved removal of large numbers of pigs from the national herd (even the entire population in some countries, such as Malta, the Dominican Republic and Haiti).

One of the most striking aspects of ASF virus infection in pigs is the absence of a neutralizing antibody response. Infected pigs develop antibodies in their sera that bind to the virus, but the humoral immune response confers no protection. This has bedevilled the development of effective vaccines.

Diagnosis

Any febrile disease in swine associated with haemorrhage and death should raise suspicion of African swine fever. The clinical signs of African swine fever are similar to those of several diseases, such as poisoning with anticoagulants (for example, rat poisons), erysipelas and acute salmonellosis, but the major diagnostic problem lies in the differentiation of African swine fever from a similar virus disease, namely, hog cholera or European/classical swine fever. African swine fever and hog cholera are both notifiable diseases in most countries and veterinary regulatory authorities should be contacted upon any suspicion of either disease. Laboratory confirmation is essential and samples of blood, spleen and visceral lymph nodes should be collected for virus isolation and for detection of antigen. Virus isolation is done in swine bone marrow or peripheral blood leucocyte (PBL) cultures, in which haemadsorption can be demonstrated and a cytopathic effect seen within a few days after inoculation. From this point, the virus can be adapted to grow in various cell lines such as pig kidney (PK15) and VERO cells. Antigen detection is done by immunofluorescence staining of tissue smears or frozen sections, by immunodiffusion, using tissue suspensions as the source of antigen, and by enzyme immunoassay.

Transmission

African swine fever virus can be transmitted between susceptible pigs by several routes. Once the virus is introduced to domesticated pigs, it can be transmitted by close contact, fomites, food containing scraps of meat from infected pigs and the bite of infected soft ticks of the genus *Ornithodoros* (Fig. 1B). The introduction of the virus to a previously unaffected country is usually by the feeding of infected scraps of pork products to pigs, as outlined earlier in the section on geographical distribution. The focus of this section will therefore be on the arthropod transmission of the virus. Only soft ticks of the genus *Ornithodoros* are considered to be vectors.

Africa

In its natural ecosystem in southern Africa, the virus is biologically transmitted between Warthogs by the soft tick *O. moubata porcinus* within the ecological niche of the Warthog burrow. The infection of the Warthog is a consequence of being bitten by an infected tick and there is no evidence for horizontal or vertical transmission between

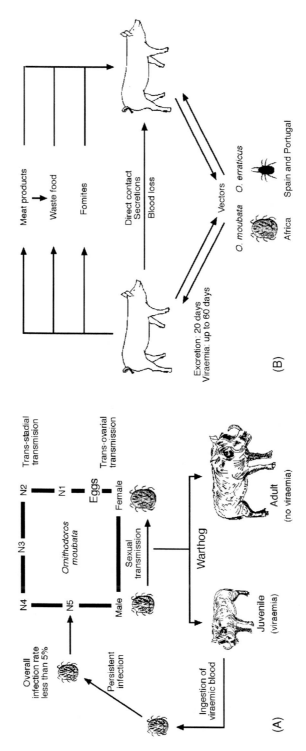

Fig. 1. Transmission of African swine fever. (A) Sylvatic cycle of virus between Warthogs and *Ornithodoros moubata* ticks. In ticks there is transovarial, venereal and trans-stadial transmission of the virus. (B) Cycle in domestic pigs by direct contact, meat products and scraps, fomites, and through *Ornithodoros* species of ticks. (Courtesy of P.J. Wilkinson, Pirbright Laboratory, Institute for Animal Health, UK.)

Warthogs (Fig. 1A). Surveys have shown that adult Warthogs are commonly persistently infected with ASF virus, with the virus being mainly limited to the lymph nodes. Persistently infected adult Warthogs are not usually viraemic; however, young Warthogs develop a viraemia when first infected. While the level of this viraemia is not high (up to 4.0 $\log_{10}$ haemadsorbing units per ml), it has been shown to be above the threshold of infection for uninfected ticks. After a tick has fed on an infected host, ASF virus first replicates in the gut and then spreads to the haemocoel, from which the virus infects the salivary glands and reproductive system (Fig. 1). The virus is transmitted to susceptible pigs by the bite of the infected tick. The infection of the reproductive organs allows sexual transmission of virus between male and female ticks. Trans-stadial and transovarial transmission also occur. *Ornithodoros moubata porcinus*, in common with most soft ticks, usually feeds on its hosts at night. During the day it remains hidden in crevices of the walls of the burrow. It is an opportunistic and multiple feeder; individual soft ticks have been shown to be capable of transmitting the virus several years after their initial infection with it. Through these mechanisms the virus is perpetuated within the soft tick populations resident within a Warthog burrow; however, not all Warthog populations or tick populations are infected with the virus. The role of Bushpigs in the epidemiology of the virus is unknown.

Europe

The rural economy of the south-western area of the Iberian Peninsula relies heavily upon the cork forests; here domesticated pigs are allowed to range in search of fallen acorns of oak trees (*Quercus* species). *Ornithodoros erraticus* is found in this region in the rock walls of traditional pigpens and under the bark of trees. When, in the 1960s, ASF virus was introduced to swine in the region, *O. erraticus* became infected and maintained the virus in a cycle paralleling that of *O. moubata porcinus* and the Warthog in Africa. This has made the eradication of ASF virus from the pig population of Spain and Portugal far more difficult.

The Americas

When African swine fever was confirmed in the Americas, the possibility that ASF virus could establish itself in indigenous species of *Ornithodoros* was considered. Although species such as *Ornithodoros turicata* and *O. puertoricensis* were experimentally shown to be potential biological vectors and could play a role smilar to that of *O. moubata porcinus* and *O. erraticus* in the Old World, no soft ticks were ever found to have become naturally infected, despite the extensive outbreaks of disease that occurred in the late 1970s and early 1980s.

Treatment

There is no treatment for swine with ASF virus.

All attempts to develop a commercial vaccine have been unsuccessful. However, recent genomic studies have indicated that, after inoculation into pigs, some gene-deleted strains of ASF virus can protect them from subsequent infection with lethal strains of ASF virus.

Control

Within a global context, African swine fever is considered to be the most important epidemic disease that affects the pig industry. When the pigs of a country becomes infected, the economic loss is substantial, due to the costs of disease control, lost production and ban on exports. The control and prevention of African swine fever are difficult because of the biology of the disease and the virus. Summarized these are as follows:

- Biological transmission by soft ticks occurs; infection in soft ticks can remain undetected for many years and can re-emerge.
- There are no vaccines available.
- Some pigs can become persistently infected.
- The virus is present in fresh meat from infected pigs.

- The virus is robust and resistant to the curing process used to prepare several pork products.
- The clinical disease can be confused with hog cholera.

Accordingly, countries free of disease have restrictions on the importation of live pigs and pork products from countries where African swine fever exists. All food waste from seaports and airports is destroyed.

When African swine fever is confirmed in a country, most veterinary authorities elect to eradicate the virus by depopulating the affected herd(s). When disease is extensive within a country, it may be necessary to depopulate a region of domesticated swine. On those occasions when disease is extensive on an island (for example, Malta), the cost-effective approach has been to kill all the pigs and restock with disease-free pigs from overseas.

When ASF virus is present in the tick population of a country, it is extremely difficult to eradicate the virus. In Spain and Portugal, it has been found that constructing pens of concrete is far more effective than attempting to control ticks with acaricides. In Africa, where the virus exists in a sylvatic cycle, the problem is even more difficult. Disease control relies upon not feeding food waste to pigs and by separating ticks and Warthogs from domesticated swine by double fences extending beneath the ground.

Selected bibliography

Butler, J.F. and Gibbs, E.P.J. (1984) Distribution of potential soft tick vectors of African swine fever in the Caribbean Region. *Preventive Veterinary Medicine* 2, 63–70.

Gibbs, E.P.J. (1984) African swine fever: an assessment of risk for Florida. *Journal of the American Veterinary Medical Association* 184, 644–647.

Hess, W.R. (1988) African swine fever. In: Monath, T.P. (ed.) *The Arboviruses: Epidemiology and Ecology*, Vol. II. CRC Press, Boca Raton, Florida, pp. 19–37.

Martinez, P.F. and Espinosa, J. (1997) Role of *Ornithodoros erraticus* in the epidemiology of African swine fever. *Medicina Veterinaria* 14, 197–200.

Murphy, F.A., Gibbs, E.P.J., Horzinek, M.C. and Studdert, M.J. (eds) (1999) African swine fever. In: *Veterinary Virology*, 3rd edn. Academic Press, San Diego, California, pp. 293–300.

Plowright, W., Thomson, G.R. and Neser, J.A. (1994) African swine fever. In: Coetzer, J.A.W., Thomson, G.R. and Tustin, R.C. (eds), *Infectious Diseases of Livestock with Special Reference to Southern Africa*, Vol. 1. Oxford University Press, Cape Town, pp. 568–599.

Wilkinson, P.J. (1981) African swine fever. In: Gibbs, E.P.J. (ed.) *Virus Diseases of Food Animals: a World Geography of Epidemiology and Control*, Vol. 2. Academic Press, London, pp. 767–786.

Wilkinson, P.J. (1984) The persistence of African swine fever in Africa and the Mediterranean. *Preventive Veterinary Medicine* 2, 71–82.

Wilkinson, P.J. (1989) African swine fever virus. In: Pensaert, M.B. (ed.) *Virus Infections of Vertebrates*, Vol. 2. Elsevier, Amsterdam, pp. 15–36.

African tick-bite fever see **Tick-borne typhuses**

African trypanosomiasis, human

Pierre Cattand

Although long known by the indigenous population and reported in ancient writings by Arab merchants, as well as slave traders in the 18th and 19th centuries, sleeping sickness aetiology was only elucidated in the early part of the 20th century. Shortly after this discovery, the transmission cycle was described, along with the role of the tsetse-fly (*Glossina*) as the vector. The occupation of Africa by European settlers is claimed to have been the cause of the spread of the disease through the opening of trade paths and population movements. It is not unlikely that behavioural changes of local populations under the colonial times enhanced disease transmission. Very rapidly thereafter, in less than 10 years, the essential factors were known about the epidemiology of African trypanosomiasis. Following the dramatic epidemics in East and West Africa (Uganda and Cameroon) in the early 1900s, fearing the loss of human resources necessary to develop their colonies, the local administrations established extensive control programmes. The unfailing effort, organization, dedication and motivation of the staff of these programmes achieved the elimination of the disease in some 35 years (1930–1965). By the mid-1960s only sporadic cases occurred throughout the continent. Since then, political instability, wars and diminishing financial means have brought health services virtually to a halt and the disease has reappeared in almost all ancient foci. In the subsequent 35 years the disease returned to levels comparable to those of the beginning of the 20th century and, by 1999, the number of new cases soared to some 45,000 (Fig. 1). Today, major outbreaks are reported from the Democratic Republic of Congo (DRC), Angola, Sudan and Uganda.

Impact

The importance of human sleeping sickness in terms of public health lies not in the annual incidence, but in its potential for development of explosive epidemics, causing thousands of deaths. If incidence alone is considered, the disease appears as a minor health problem compared with other parasitic diseases, such as malaria (see Malaria, human) and helminthic infections. However, because of its severity, the occurrence of a case in a family will affect all members. Moreover, outbreaks place a major burden on whole communites, reducing the labour force, interrupting agricultural activities, disrupting the local economy and jeopardizing food security. In the past, thousands of people died during large-scale epidemics. If the disability-adjusted life year (DALY) figures (i.e loss of healthy life years by premature mortality and disability) are considered, the social and economic impact of trypanosomiasis ranks third of all parasitic diseases behind malaria and schistosomiasis in sub-Saharan Africa. The number of deaths each year is estimated at 100,000. Populations fleeing sleeping sickness leave behind them vast deserted regions. A comparable exodus due to a disease can only be found in regions where river blindness (see Onchocerciasis, human) has occurred.

Distribution

Sleeping sickness is focal and concerns only part of the population in 36 African countries south of the Sahara desert. Only some 60 million people are at constant risk of infection. Today, active transmission

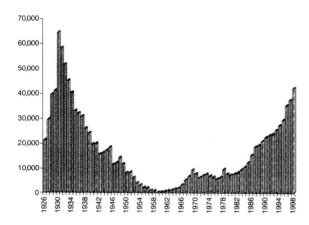

Fig. 1. The evolution of the number of new cases per year identified in the central African region between 1926 and 1999.

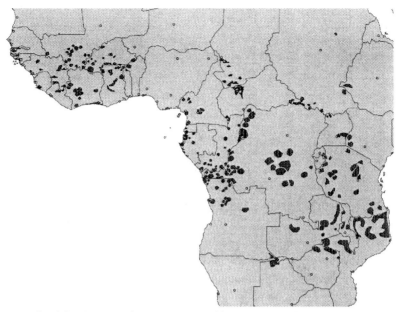

Fig. 2. Geographical distribution of the 259 present and former human African trypanosomiasis foci (1930–1999). Present epidemiological status of each focus ranges from inactive to epidemic. Inactive foci, however, remain risk areas where the disease can reappear at any time.

takes place in at least 20 countries. Various levels of endemicity are found in the 259 discrete known foci, but not more than 3–4 million people are under adequate surveillance (Fig. 2).

The World Health Organization (WHO) estimates that at least 300,000 individuals are now infected, but only 10–15% are diagnosed and treated. In the DRC, where some 10,000 cases were diagnosed annually in the late 1980s, control activities ceased following the withdrawal of external technical and financial aid due to political problems. After only 4 years with little or no control the number of reported cases rose to 30,000, but it is estimated that at least 150,000 individuals have the disease. In Uganda an outbreak in 1986 produced more than 4000 cases. In Angola, cases rose sixfold following interruption of control operations due to war and social upheavals. In 1999, for the first time in the history of the disease, urban and peri-urban transmission was reported (Kinshasa, DRC; Luanda, Angola). Throughout Africa some 40,000 new cases were reported in both 1998 and 1999.

Parasite

The protozoans that cause sleeping sickness belong to the genus *Trypanosoma*, subgenus *Trypanozoon*. They are classified in the phylum Euglenozoa (formerly classified in the Sarcomastigophora), the order Trypanosomatida (formerly placed in Kinetoplastida) and the family Trypanosomatidae. Although morphologically indistinguishable, only two subspecies of *Trypanosoma brucei*, namely. *T. b. gambiense* and *T. b. rhodesiense,* are infective for humans. The former causes an acute form of the disease found in East Africa, while *T. b. gambiense*, a chronic form, is widespread in West and Central Africa. These parasites are transmitted to humans by bites of tsetse-flies (*Glossina* species). Following the bite of the fly the parasites invade the blood and lymph and, as the disease progresses, they cross the blood–brain barrier to enter the central nervous system.

Biochemical and molecular characterization

Biological, biochemical and molecular criteria can be used to distinguish the various subspecies. The subgenus *Trypanozoon* can be identified on the basis of isoenzyme and DNA characteristics. *Trypanosoma b. gambiense* isolates fall into two groups, known as Types I and II. Type I is characterized by low virulence in humans, while Type II produces an acute rhodesiense-like disease syndrome. A clear separation between sympatric populations of *T. b. rhodesiense* and *T. b. brucei* is now possible.

Antigenic variation
The surface of trypanosomes consists of a layer of variable surface glycoprotein (VSG), which is sequentially replaced by another, composed of an antigenically distinct VSG that is not recognized by existing antibodies. The host responds against the new VSG, and the cycle of antigen switching and antibody response is repeated. The repertoire of VSGs is very large. The steady accumulation of antibodies in the host is manifested as hypergamma-globulinaemia. When trypanosomes enter the tsetse-fly, the VSG coat is replaced with a coat of invariable glycoprotein, procyclic acidic repetitive protein (PARP) or procyclin, which is thought to be present only in the procyclic and epimastigote parasite stages in the tsetse-fly. Variable surface glycoprotein expression reoccurs at the infective metacyclic stage in the fly's salivary glands. The metacyclic bloodstream population is composed of a mixture of VSGs and, because its repertoire changes, it precludes the development of a classical vaccine against African trypanosomiasis.

Clinical symptoms
Despite the close biological relationship of the two parasite species infecting humans and the fact that both forms of the disease are lethal if untreated, there are important differences in their epidemiology and clinical features. Sleeping sickness due to *T. b. gambiense* is characterized by a slow progressive course, which may last from a few months to several years before death occurs. In the form due to *T. b. rhodesiense* the disease evolves rapidly, causing death within weeks or a few months after infection. Little is known on the time-scale of central nervous system invasion by the parasite, although there is suspicion that it takes place shortly after infection occurs.

Diagnosis
Clinical diagnosis
Although pruritus and adenopathy are often observed, fever, headache and joint and muscle pains are common complaints in the early stage of the disease, and neurological symptoms, such as mental alterations, abnormal movements, sensory problems and sleep disturbances, are seen in the second stage after parasites have invaded the central nervous system, there is no single clinical sign or symptom that can be regarded as pathognomonic for sleeping sickness. Therefore, for accurate diagnosis, it is essential to obtain laboratory confirmation of the infection.

Indirect diagnosis
Tests have been developed for the detection of antibodies, circulating antigens or trypanosomal DNA. All are suggestive of infection but, due to lack of sensitivity and specificity, none can be used to ascertain a trypanosomal infection. In mass screening, however, suspicion of infection with *T. gambiense* can be established with the card agglutination trypanosomiasis test (CATT), as it has been shown to be sufficiently sensitive, easy to perform and inexpensive to be applied on a large scale to populations considered at risk for the disease. Suspicion must then be corroborated through parasite detection.

Detection of parasites
Initially, parasites are present at the site of the infecting bite; they rapidly spread to the lymphatic and peripheral blood system. Within days a lymphadenopathy develops and a typical enlargement of the posterior cervical lymph node (Winterbottom's sign) occurs. The nodes are firm, mobile and painless. Parasites can be found by microscopic examination of the lymph node aspirate. Concurrently parasites multiply in the blood. While thin, thick and wet blood films can be used to detect the parasite, concentration methods provide a better

chance of finding trypanosomes. Several concentration methods are available. The most sensitive is probably the miniature anion exchange centrifugation technique (m-AECT), closely followed by the quantitative buffy coat (QBC) technique, initially developed for diagnosing malaria. The capillary tube centrifugation (CTC) technique, while slightly less sensitive, is widely used in the field because of its ease, rapidity of performance and low cost. *In vivo* inoculation and *in vitro* cultures are possible, but they are elaborate and involve costly laboratory procedures.

Determination of the stage of the disease

Treatment of the early and late stages of the disease is different. The second stage requires a drug that crosses the blood–brain barrier, which is associated with the risk of serious complications due to its toxicity. The criteria for advanced-stage infection are based on cerebrospinal fluid (CSF) analysis. Cerebrospinal fluid is considered normal when the leucocyte count is 5 cells mm^{-3} or below, total protein content is 37 mg 100 ml^{-1} or below (measured by a dye-binding protein assay) and trypanosomes are absent (by the double-centrifugation technique). If trypanosomes are present or cells and/or proteins are above the threshold of normality, the patient is recognized to be in the advanced stage.

Transmission

It is generally agreed that there are 31 species and subspecies of tsetse-fly belonging to the genus *Glossina*. Eight species and subspecies are major vectors of sleeping sickness. The limit of *Glossina* distribution is approximately from 14°N (Senegal) and 10°N (Somalia) to 20°S at the northern end of the Kalahari Desert. Some species, such as *G. morsitans*, are found across West Africa to Central and East Africa, whereas others are more restricted in their distribution. For example, *G. palpalis* occurs only in the West African subregion. Maps of the distribution of *Glossina* species have been produced under the auspices of the Inter-African Bureau for Animal Resources of the Organization of African Unity. However, due to drought and deforestation and other environmental changes, the distribution of tsetse-flies fluctuates considerably.

Both male and female *Glossina* are blood-sucking insects. The viviparous female deposits a single larva approximately every 10 days. Tsetse-flies may live for 6 months and take blood meals every 2–3 days. The species and subspecies incriminated in the transmission of the disease belong to two groups, namely the *G. morsitans* group (savanna flies), typically inhabiting savanna woodland and the *G. palpalis* group (riverine and forest flies), occupying secondary forest zones, such as riverine and mangrove forests. A third, the *G. fusca* group (forest flies), is restricted to primary forests, and has not been implicated in the transmission of sleeping sickness.

When trypanosomes in the blood of humans or, in the case of *T. b. rhodesiense*, also from a non-human reservoir host, are sucked up during feeding, they eventually arrive in the fly's stomach. Blood is digested but the *gambiense* and *rhodesiense* trypanosomes are not destroyed but pass into the ectoperitrophic space. Here they multiply and after 3–9 days migrate to infect the proventriculus, from where they pass down the food channel in the proboscis and then up the hypopharynx to invade the fly's salivary glands, become epimastigotes and multiply enormously. Some 15–35 days after an infective blood meal, the tsetse-fly is infective and metacyclic trypanosomes are injected into a vertebrate when the fly feeds. It remains unclear whether there are 'short cuts' to this complicated cycle of development, such as trypanosomes penetrating the stomach and passing into the haemocoel and then migrating directly to the salivary glands.

Treatment

The disease is fatal if untreated but only a very limited number of drugs is available for treatment. No vaccination exists. Pentamidine is currently used for treatment of the early stages of infection due to

T. b. gambiense and suramin for *T. b. rhodesiense*. The organo-arsenical compound melarsoprol is used in the late stage for both forms of infection.

Melarsoprol (Arsobal®)

This drug was introduced in 1949. It is marketed as a 3.6% solution in propylene glycol. It is metabolized to one or several active products, the nature of which is unknown, and has a terminal half-life of 35 h. The mode of action of melarsoprol is unclear. For a long time the affinity of the drug to sulphydryl groups was believed to be responsible for the antitrypanosomal activity. It was shown that especially the pyruvate kinase, which is a key enzyme in African trypanosomes for production of adenosine triphosphate (ATP), was markedly inhibited. Newer investigations have shown that trypanothion, which replaces glutathion in African trypanosomes, forms a stable adduct with melarsen oxide. This complex is an effective inhibitor of trypanothion reductase, leading to disturbance of the redox balance of the parasite. However, this theory was recently questioned and it was suggested that phosphofructokinase, another enzyme of the glycolytic pathway, may be the main drug target.

There is no standardized treatment regimen for the use of melarsoprol; the dosage and duration of therapy differ considerably depending on the country where it is applied (Table 1). The development of all currently used treatment schedules was empirical. Generally melarsoprol treatment consists of several series of three to four consecutive injections, given every 24 h, with an interval of about 1 week between the series. In most schedules the doses increase progressively either during the course of treatment or within the single series. The rest periods between treatment courses have been introduced because of suspicion of arsenic accumulation in body tissues. However, no indications of drug accumulation could be found in elimination studies in rats and kinetic investigations in monkeys and humans. Thus, a treatment schedule for melarsoprol with an abridged duration of only 10 days and 30% less drug has recently

been developed and successfully tested in a large clinical trial. This new protocol is now being evaluated in the context of control operations in different endemic countries.

The major problems associated with melarsoprol therapy are the frequent and often serious adverse events, the relapses and the long duration of treatment. The worst of all adverse events are encephalopathic syndromes, which are clinically characterized by a rapid deterioration of the level of consciousness, seizures or psychotic reactions. In general this complication occurs in 5–10% of the patients. In a Tanzanian hospital the rate of this event was reported as 17.9%, and as 23% in the Bandundu region of DRC. The reaction is fatal for about 10–70% of the patients affected. An immune reaction should be the cause, but the mechanism remains unknown. Other severe adverse reactions reported are polyneuropathies and exfoliative dermatitis (Lyell syndrome was reported by one author at a frequency of 0.8% of the treated cases). Neuropathies may occur in up to 10% of cases and manifest either as a paraesthesia with a 'stocking and glove' distribution or as a motor weakness. Exfoliative dermatitis (bullous eruption) is rather infrequent (1%), and is usually controllable with steroids. Fever, headache, diarrhoea, maculopapular eruptions, pruritus and abdominal and chest pain also occur. The value of prednisolone to protect against encephalopathy was debated for more than 20 years but a recently published large-scale study seems to confirm its usefulness.

Relapses are another major problem of sleeping sickness treatment with melarsoprol. For many decades the frequency reported ranged from 1 to 10%. However, there are recent reports indicating much higher rates of patients not responding to melarsoprol (southern Sudan 19%, northern Uganda 26%, Zaire province of Angola 20%). At present, treatment failures are clinical phenomena with unknown causes. The development of drug-resistant parasites or insufficient drug levels in a crucial body compartment need to be discussed. Reinfections do occur but at a much lower rate.

Table 1. Comparison of a few different schedules for late-stage *T. b. gambiense* sleeping sickness treatment with melarsoprol.

Day of drug application

Schedule	1	2	3	4	5	6	7	8	9	10	11	12	13	14	15	16	17	18	19	20	21	22	23	24	25	26	27	28	29	30	31	32	33	34	35
Schedule used by the National Control Programme in Côte d'Ivoire	P	P		M1	M2	M3	M3										M1	M2	M3	M3										M1	M2	M3	M3		
Schedule used the National Trypanosomiasis Control Programme in Angola	M1	M2	M3	M3										M1	M2	M3	M3										M1	M2	M3	M3					
Schedule used by the Central Bureau for Trypanosomiasis in the DRC	M3	M3	M3											M3	M3	M3											M3	M3	M3						
Schedule used by the National Sleeping Sickness Control Programme in Uganda	Mx	Mx	Mx											Mx	Mx	Mx											Mx	Mx	Mx						
Alternative 10 days schedule under evaluation in different centres	M4	M4	M4	M4	M4	M4	M4	M4	M4	M4																									

P, pentamidine pretreatment 4 mg kg^{-1} body weight (bw); M1, melarsoprol 1.2 mg kg^{-1} bw; M2, 2.4 mg kg^{-1} bw; M3, melarsoprol 3.6 mg kg^{-1} bw (max. 5 ml); Mx, melarsoprol 1st series of 1.8, 2.16, 2.52 mg kg^{-1} bw, 2nd series of 2.52, 2.88, 3.25 mg kg^{-1} bw, 3rd series of 3.6, 3.6, 3.6 mg kg^{-1} bw (max. 5 ml); M4, melarsoprol 2.16 mg kg^{-1} bw (max. 5 ml).

Eflornithine (Ornidy®)

This drug, also called alpha-difluoro-methylornithine (DFMO), was registered by the Food and Drug Administration (FDA) in 1990 for use in *T. b. gambiense* infections and has been described as the miracle drug. It is not effective against *T. b. rhodesiense*. Eflornithine is no longer produced today, but, should production resume, its high cost would become a major obstacle for its extensive use; thus melarsoprol is likely to remain the first-line drug for the next decade. When considering that in some endemic countries the total annual health budget is as low as US$2 per head of population and that eflornithine treatment is approximately US$1000 per patient, it is understandable that such treatment would be out of reach of most African patients and control programmes.

Nifurtimox (Lampit®)

This drug, developed and used for control of Chagas disease (see entry) and not registered for sleeping sickness, has been shown to be effective in the treatment of *T. b. gambiense* sleeping sickness. To date, it has been used, in the absence of eflornithine, exclusively on a compassionate basis for trypanosomiasis cases who do not respond to melarsoprol. In consideration of the considerable increase in the number of melarsoprol-resistant cases, several research projects are examining various drug combinations using melarsoprol, eflornithine and nifurtimox.

Control

In the last few years a resurgence of sleeping sickness has occurred in West and Central Africa, specifically in Angola, Central African Republic, Chad, Congo, Côte d'Ivoire, DRC, Guinea, Sudan, Tanzania and Uganda. In response to this situation an intercountry coordination for surveillance and control has been developed and various approaches have been elaborated to improve surveillance, case finding, treatment and vector control. In November 1995 a WHO Expert Committee on Control and Surveillance of African Trypanosomiasis prepared a compendium of available options and tools to curb the spread of the disease, and underlined the need for urgent action. Considering the technical and economic situation of the countries where sleeping sickness occurs, it is evident that they require assistance to develop their national programmes, establish plans of action and mobilize appropriate resources for implementation of control and surveillance.

Surveillance

Epidemiological surveillance is the continuous and systematic collection, analysis, interpretation and diffusion of public health information. The aim of sleeping sickness surveillance is to assess the epidemiological situation and have the necessary information to implement appropriate actions to prevent and control the disease. It also provides a monitoring tool for programme follow-up. Sleeping sickness surveillance can be passive or active. Depending on the method applied and the tools used, surveillance sensitivity ranges from very low to high. Passive surveillance is fundamentally qualitative. Because clinical signs are so unspecific they cannot be used effectively for surveillance. Use of serology, however, in the existing health infrastructure, will indicate the likeliness of the occurrence of the disease in any given area. Passive surveillance using serology can be loosely interpreted to indicate if there is a risk of 'a lot of sleeping sickness' and, provided the origins of seropositive cases are mapped, the geographical extent of the problem can be estimated. Serology applied actively through surveys, covering a selected percentage of the population in each village, will provide a better insight into the possible occurrence and intensity of sleeping sickness. Coupled with parasitology of seropositive cases, a good assessment can then be made of the prevalence of the disease. Considering the focal nature of trypanosomiasis, large areas must be surveyed to identify foci and their extent. Using vector density as an indicator for sleeping sickness is not appropriate. While the presence of the vector is essential for transmission, the prevalence cannot be associated with the apparent density of the tsetse-fly. Interestingly, epidemics of the *T. b. rhodesiense* form of the disease in East Africa have been associated with a change to peridomestic transmission.

Case finding and treatment

Control options include active case finding and treatment, as well as vector control. Case finding and treatment not only relieve human suffering and reduce the economic burden of families and communities but they decrease the human reservoir, breaking the transmission cycle, and effectively control the disease.

Programme choices for control and surveillance will depend on factors such as epidemiological and environmental conditions, programme structure and organization, coordination of the medical and vector control activities and the human, material and financial resources. Because of the great variability across the numerous known foci of African trypanosomiasis, there is no single strategy that can be advocated. Instead, plans of action must be developed and tailored on an area-to-area basis and staff trained in methods appropriate to their specific control and surveillance needs.

Vector control

A large array of techniques have been developed based on a detailed knowledge of the ecology of the tsetse-fly. Those harmful to the environment have been abandoned. In the past, measures such as culling certain species of game animals in eastern and southern Africa, which were reservoir hosts for *T. b. rhodesiense* infections, were undertaken. Clearance of vegetation and, later, ground and aerial insecticidal spraying of vegetation with residual insecticides to kill resting tsetse-flies were practised. Today these techniques are still used in the control of nagana (see Animal trypanosomiasis), although environmentally these methods are increasingly less acceptable. Since the 1970s research on the response of different *Glossina* species to odours and colours has made it possible to develop alternative and environmentally friendly vector control devices, such as insecticide-impregnated (usually with pyrethroids) traps and screens (targets). Several differently shaped traps (Fig. 3A, B) and screens (Fig. 3C) have been developed to ensure their effectiveness for trapping various species of tsetse-flies.

Preference in vector control approaches is now given to elaborate combinations of techniques. These combinations will include selective insecticidal ground spraying to obtain an initial 'knock-down' of flies, followed by deployment of traps and screens, and possibly achieving localized eradication through using the sterile insect technique (SIT). Such rigorous vector control is justifiable only if compatible with local economics and sustainability of results. Rural development and the enhancement of agriculture may be good reasons to implement vector control activities. However, with sleeping sickness the objective in an epidemic focus is to reduce rapidly and drastically the vector population to a level at which disease transmission is significantly reduced or interrupted. Since vector control is rather costly, areas of application must be strictly delimited to match the extent of disease foci. This can be achieved through surveillance. However, vector control operations must go beyond these borders to limit movements of tsetse-flies into control areas. Control techniques must be chosen according to knowledge of the local environmental and epidemiological conditions and the available human and material resources. If the fly population is not controlled rapidly, it may not be possible to sustain control, owing to lack of funds or loss of motivation in the community.

Conclusion

Sleeping sickness is basically a disease of rural African people and remains a major threat to the health of farmers, ranchers, fishermen and hunters living in sub-Saharan Africa and exposed daily to bites of tsetse-flies. Tourists and visitors may become infected if exposed to an infective fly bite. Although demonstrated in the mid-1960s as being controllable, and despite the availability of new and more effective tools, the ever-deteriorating health services in endemic countries are facing an enormous task to diagnose and treat thousands of patients. Contrary to many other endemic diseases, sleeping sickness epidemics are not self-limiting and, as in the past, if nothing is done, whole areas may soon be abandoned by a population fleeing the dreadful disease and certain death. Concurrently national programmes will have to achieve and sustain a reduction of transmission sufficient to eliminate the disease.

Selected bibliography

Budd, L.T. (ed.) (1999) Human sleeping sickness. In: *DIFID-Funded Tsetse and Trypanosome Research and Development Since 1980*, Vol. 2 – *Economic Analysis*. Department for International Development, pp. 62–65.

Burri, C. (1994) Pharmacological aspects of the trypanocidal drug melarsoprol. A dissertation performed at the Swiss Tropical Institute for the degree of Doctor of Philosophy, University of Basle, 177 pp.

Burri, C, Nkunku, S., Merolle, E., Smith, T., Blum, J. and Brun, R. (2000) Efficacy of new, concise schedule for melarsopol in treatment of sleeping sickness caused by *Trypanosoma brucei gambiense*: a randomised trial. *The Lancet* 355, 1419–1425.

de Raadt, P., Vickerman, K., Smith, D.H., Cattand, P., Molyneux, D.H., Milligan, P.J.M. and Baldry, A.T. (1999) African trypanosomiasis. In: Gilles, H.M. (ed.) *Protozoal Diseases*. Arnold, London, pp. 249–305.

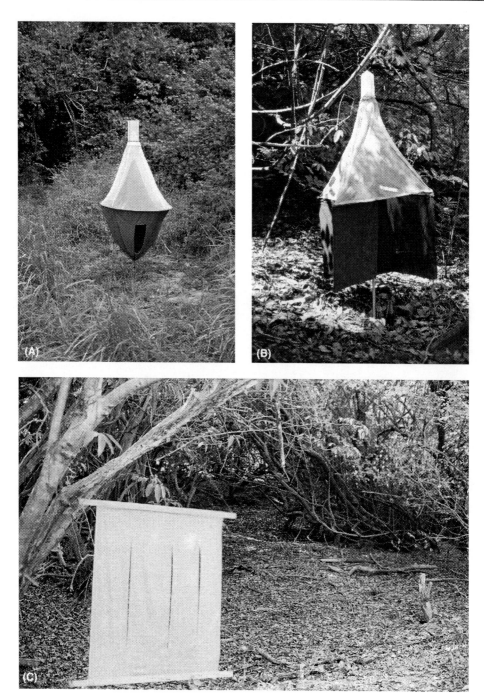

Fig. 3. (A) Biconical trap used to catch *Glossina palpalis* and *G. pallidipes*. (B) Pyramidal trap for trapping the *palpalis* group flies. (C) Pyrethroid-impregnated cloth screen (target) used to attract *G. palpalis* and *G. tachinoides* – the vertical slits are to discourage theft of the material. These traps and screen are used in vector control operations. The screen and lower half of the traps are blue or black. (Fig. 3A courtesy of M.W. Service, 3B and 3C courtesy of A.M. Jordan.)

Dumas, M., Bouteille, B. and Buguet, A. (1999) *Progress in Human African Trypanosomiasis, Sleeping Sickness.* Springer, Paris, 344 pp.

Leak, S.G.A. (1999) *Tsetse Biology and Ecology: Their Role in the Epidemiology and Control of Trypanosomiasis.* CAB International, Wallingford, UK, 568 pp.

World Health Organization (1983) *Trypanosomiasis Control Manual.* WHO, Geneva, 142 pp.

World Health Organization (1998) *Control and Surveillance of African Trypanosomiasis.* Report of a WHO Expert Committee, WHO Technical Report Series 881, WHO, Geneva, 113 pp.

Aino virus

P.S. Mellor

Aino (AINO) virus was originally isolated from mosquitoes in Aino, Nagasaki prefecture, Japan, in 1964.

Distribution

The distribution of Aino virus, along with most of the other four teratogenic Simbu group viruses (Akabane, Douglas, Peaton and Tinaroo) is poorly understood. To date, the virus has been isolated only in Japan and Australia, with specific antibodies also identified in Indonesia, but it is likely to have a much wider distribution, possibly as great as that of Akabane virus (see entry), which includes Australia, southern Asia and Africa.

Aetiological agent

Aino virus is a member of the genus *Bunyavirus*, family Bunyaviridae and is included in the Simbu serogroup with more than 20 other viruses. The virions of these viruses are spherical, enveloped and 90–100 nm in diameter. Four structural proteins have been identified and these surround a genome of three segments of single-stranded RNA (ssRNA).

Clinical signs

All five teratogenic Simbu group viruses are capable of damaging the fetuses of cattle, sheep and possibly goats. Of these, Akabane virus is considered to be the most pathogenic. Aino virus is thought to be less important but when it does cause disease the pathological effects produced are indistinguishable from those induced by Akabane virus. These effects are described in detail in the entry on Akabane virus but are reproduced, in brief, below.

When Akabane virus (and presumably Aino virus) infects serologically naïve, pregnant cattle, sheep or goats, the virus is able to cross the ruminant placenta and replicate in the fetus. The pathological effects of this may be evidenced by abortions, premature births and the birth of young with a range of congenital defects, especially arthrogryposis and hydranencephaly but also including blindness, nystagmus, deafness, dullness, paralysis and incoordination. Adult animals, including the dams of affected young, exhibit no clinical signs of infection.

In Japan, antibodies to Aino virus have been found at low prevalence in serological surveys of humans but no link with human disease has been suggested. However, only the fetuses of pregnant women would be likely to be at risk for this virus and it is not known whether such women were included in the surveys.

Diagnosis

The cause of sporadic cases of arthrogryposis or hydranencephaly is likely to remain undiagnosed. However, when clusters of such cases occur, their presence should suggest a teratogenic virus such as Aino (or other teratogenic Simbu group viruses) as a possible cause. For Aino virus isolation, clinical material should be inoculated into suckling mice by the intracerebral route or into cell culture. The most useful tissues are from aborted fetuses. However, it is unlikely that virus will be isolated from deformed full-term offspring because of neutralizing antibodies formed in the fetus. Virus can be identified by the virus neutralization (VN) test. For diagnosis by serology, the VN test has again proved most useful. Serum samples from the dam and its fetus, or the dam and a presuckling sample from the newborn animal, should be used.

Transmission

Aino virus was first isolated from *Culex tritaeniorhynchus*, and a mixed pool of *Culex pipiens* and *Culex pseudovishnui* in Japan. Subsequently, in Australia, numerous isolations of virus have been made from the biting midge, *Culicoides brevitarsis*. At first sight, therefore, it is difficult to decide whether mosquitoes or biting midges are likely to be the major vectors. However, the related Douglas, Peaton and Tinaroo viruses have been isolated only from *Culicoides*, while Akabane virus has been isolated from five different species of *Culicoides* around the world and has been shown to be transmitted by one of them. Consequently, it is likely that *Culicoides* species are the primary vectors of all five viruses.

Vertebrate hosts

The virus has been isolated only from the blood of healthy cattle in Australia and from an aborted bovine fetus in Japan. However, the host range as inferred by serology includes cattle, sheep, goats, Buffaloes (*Bubalus bulbalis*) and horses.

Evidence for human infection is equivocal. Antibodies to Aino virus have been detected in humans in Fukuoka prefecture, Japan, at a low prevalence (4.7% of 171 sera). However, no antibodies to any Simbu serogroup virus were found in limited surveys of human sera in Australia or in the sera of ten laboratory workers who had been handling the five teratogenic viruses over a 5–10-year period.

Treatment

There is no specific therapy for Aino virus infection.

Prevention and control

The problem with Aino virus and with the other teratogenic Simbu group viruses is that, frequently, the first evidence of their presence in epizootic situations is the birth of deformed young. This usually occurs several months subsequent to infection and after the damage has been done. It also tends to occur after the causative virus has been eliminated by the immune responses of the affected animals. There is thus a certain retrospective element involved in the situation. Nevertheless, control of vectors can be attempted by the elimination of their breeding sites, use of insecticides or housing of susceptible stock during peak vector activity times (dusk to dawn). Also, since the only danger of disease is through the infection of pregnant stock, it may be possible to devise a husbandry programme in which breeding is restricted to those times of the year when the vectors are absent and hence there is no transmission. However, since knowledge concerning the identity and biology of most of the vectors is still inadequate, these measures may be impractical. No vaccines are available or planned for the control of Aino virus infection.

Selected bibliography

Coverdale, O.R., Cybinski, D.H. and St George, T.D. (1978) Congenital abnormalities in calves associated with Akabane virus and Aino virus. *Australian Veterinary Journal* 54, 151–152.

Cybinski, D.H. and St George, T.D. (1978) A survey of antibody to Aino virus in cattle and other species in Australia. *Australian Veterinary Journal* 54, 371–373.

Cybinski, D.H. and Zakrzewski, H. (1983) A dual infection of a bull with Akabane and Aino viruses. *Australian Veterinary Journal* 60, 283.

Doherty, R.L., Carley, J.G., Standfast, H.A., Dyce, A.L. and Snowdon, W.A. (1972) Virus strains isolated from arthropods during an epizootic of bovine ephemeral fever in Queensland. *Australian Veterinary Journal* 48, 81–86.

Fukuyoshi, S., Takehara, Y., Takahashi, K. and Mori, R. (1981) The incidence of antibody to Aino virus in animals and humans in Fukuoka. *Japanese Journal of Medical Science and Biology* 34, 41–47.

Miura, Y., Inaba, Y., Tsuda, T., Tokuhisa, S., Sato, K., Akashi, H. and Matumoto, M. (1982) A survey of antibodies to arthropod-borne viruses in Indonesian cattle. *Japanese Journal of Veterinary Science* 44, 857–863.

St George, T.D. and Standfast, H.A. (1989) Simbu group viruses with teratogenic potential. In: Monath, T.P. (ed.) *The Arboviruses: Epidemiology and Ecology*, Vol IV. CRC Press, Boca Raton, Florida, pp. 145–166.

St George, T.D. and Standfast, H.A. (1994) Diseases caused by Akabane and related Simbu-group viruses. In: Coetzer, J.A.W.,

Thomson, G.R. and Tustin, R.C. (eds) *Infectious Diseases of Livestock with Special Reference to Southern Africa*, Vol. 1. Oxford University Press, Cape Town, pp. 681–687.

Uchinuno, Y., Noda, Y., Ishibashi, K., Nagasue, S., Shirakawa, H., Nagano, M. and Ohe, R. (1998) Isolation of Aino virus from an aborted bovine foetus. *Journal of Veterinary Medical Science* 60, 1139–1140.

Akabane virus

P.S. Mellor

Akabane (AKA) virus was originally isolated from mosquitoes collected in Akabane in Japan in 1959.

Distribution

Akabane virus has a wide distribution and may be regarded as being enzootic in most of Africa, virtually all of Asia (excluding Russia) and Australia.

Aetiological agent

Akabane virus is a member of the genus *Bunyavirus*, family Bunyaviridae, and is included in the Simbu serogroup with more than 20 other viruses. The virion is spherical, enveloped and 90–100 nm in diameter. Four structural proteins have been identified and surround the three segments of single-stranded (ssRNA).

Clinical signs

When AKA virus infects pregnant cattle, sheep or goats the virus is able to replicate in and cross the ruminant placenta, causing a variety of congenital abnormalities in the fetus. The range and severity of these abnormalities is dependent upon the stage of gestation at infection. In adult animals, however, infection is entirely subclinical and in enzootic areas most breeding-age animals will have acquired an active immunity during early life sufficient to prevent the virus from reaching the developing fetus. In these situations the virus exists as a 'silent' infection and no evidence of disease is seen.

The pathogenic effects of AKA virus infection are usually observed only when the virus expands beyond the limits of its enzootic areas to enter zones where most animals are still susceptible when adulthood is reached and are therefore able to be infected during pregnancy. In such situations, an epizootic in cattle, sheep or goats may be noticed by the increased incidence of abortions and premature births in late summer or autumn. This is followed by the birth of calves, lambs or kids with a range of congenital defects, principally arthrogryposis (AG) and hydranencephaly (HE). Young animals with these defects may be stillborn or delivered alive at term. Arthrogryposis is characterized by flexion or extension of various joints, particularly the carpal and tarsal joints, and is seen in approximately 30–50% of affected animals. The birth of some arthrogrypotic animals is associated with dystocia, necessitating embryotomy or caesarean section to save the dam. Young born with HE may survive for several months if hand-reared but they never thrive. Such animals may also show blindness, nystagmus, deafness, dullness, slow suckling, paralysis and incoordination.

Epizootics of AG/HE disease due to AKA virus have been recorded in Japan, Australia, Israel and Turkey, the most severe involving 30,000 calves in Japan and 3000–5000 calves in Australia.

Diagnosis

Sporadic cases of AG/HE due to AKA virus often remain undiagnosed. When a cluster of cases occurs, their presence should suggest a teratogenic virus such as AKA or one of the other closely related Simbu group viruses (Aino, Douglas, Peaton, Tinaroo) as a possible cause. For virus isolation, clinical material should be inoculated into suckling mice by the intracerebral route or into cell culture. The most useful tissues are from aborted fetuses. However, it is unlikely that virus will be isolated from deformed full-term offspring because of neutralizing antibodies formed in the fetus. Virus can be identified by the virus neutralization (VN) test and viral antigens by immuno-fluorescent techniques. For diagnosis by serology, the VN test has proved most useful. Serum samples from the dam and its fetus and a presuckling sample of serum from the affected newborn animal should be used.

Transmission

The virus was first isolated in 1959 in Japan from *Aedes vexans* and *Culex tritaenio-rhynchus* mosquitoes, and then in 1968 it was isolated from the biting midge, *Culicoides brevitarsis*, in Australia. More recently, isolations have been made from *Anopheles funestus* in Kenya, and from *Culicoides* species, such as *C. oxystoma* in Japan, *C. imicola* and *C. milnei* in Zimbabwe, *C. imicola* in Oman, *C. brevitarsis* and *C. wadai* in Australia, and a mixed pool consisting mainly of *C. imicola* in South Africa. The virus has been shown to replicate in *C. brevitarsis* and reaches the salivary glands of infected individuals after 10 days' incubation. The virus also replicates in orally infected *Culicoides variipennis*, by up to 1000-fold, and transmission can occur after 7–10 days' incubation at 25°C. Replication and transmission of the virus have not been demonstrated in any mosquito species. These findings suggest that *Culicoides* species are likely to be the major vectors of AKA virus and that mosquitoes are of lesser importance. Vector midges are able to transmit the virus only by bite; transovarial transmission has not been recorded.

Vertebrate hosts

The virus has been isolated from cattle, sheep and goats. Antibodies have also been detected in horses, pigs, camels (*Camelus* species) and a wide selection of African wildlife, ranging from various species of antelope to Elephant (*Loxodonta africana*) and Giraffe (*Giraffa camelopardalis*).

Treatment

There is no specific therapy for AKA virus infection.

Prevention and control

The problem with AKA virus and with the other teratogenic Simbu group viruses is that, frequently, the first evidence of their presence in epizootic situations is the birth of deformed young. This usually occurs several months subsequent to infection and after the damage has been done. It also tends to occur after the causative virus has been eliminated by the immune responses of the affected animals. There is thus a certain retrospective element involved in the situation. Nevertheless, control of the vectors can be attempted by the elimination of breeding sites, use of insecticides or housing of susceptible stock during peak vector activity times (dusk to dawn). However, since knowledge concerning the identity and biology of most of the vectors is still inadequate, this may be impractical. The main method of prophylaxis is vaccination. Effective, inactivated virus vaccines have been developed and are commercially available in Japan and Australia.

Selected bibliography

Al Busaidy, S., Hamblin, C. and Taylor, W.P. (1987) Neutralising antibodies to Akabane virus in free-living wild animals in Africa. *Tropical Animal Health and Production* 19, 197–202.

Charles, J.A. (1994) Akabane virus. *Veterinary Clinics of North America: Food Animal Practice* 10, 525–546.

Inaba, Y. and Matumoto, M. (1990) Akabane virus. In: Dinter, Z. and Morein, B. (eds) *Virus*

Infections of Ruminants. Elsevier, Amsterdam, pp. 467–480.

Kurogi, H., Inaba, Y., Takahashi, E., Sato, K., Goto, Y., Satoda, K., Omori, T. and Hatakeyama, H. (1978) Development of an inactivated vaccine for Akabane disease. *National Institute Animal Health Quarterly* 18, 97–108.

Matumoto, M. and Inaba, Y. (1980) Akabane disease and Akabane virus. *Kitasato Archives of Experimental Medicine* 53, 1–21.

St George, T.D. and Standfast, H.A. (1994) Diseases caused by Akabane and related Simbu-

group viruses. In: Coetzer, J.A.W., Thomson, G.R. and, Tustin, R.C. (eds) *Infectious Diseases of Livestock with Special Reference to Southern Africa*, Vol. 1. Oxford University Press, Cape Town, pp. 681–687.

St George, T.D., Standfast, H.A. and Cybinski, D.H. (1978) Isolations of Akabane virus from sentinel cattle and *Culicoides brevitarsis*. *Australian Veterinary Journal* 54, 558–561.

Taylor, W.P. and Mellor, P.S. (1994) The distribution of Akabane virus in the Middle East. *Epidemiology and Infection* 113, 175–185.

Alfuy virus

John S. Mackenzie

Alfuy (ALF) virus is a mosquito-borne flavivirus enzootic in northern Australia and possibly in Papua New Guinea. It was first isolated from the serum of a Swamp pheasant (*Centopus phasianinus*) and from *Aedeomyia catasticta* mosquitoes collected at Kowanyama (Mitchell River Mission) in northern Queensland in 1966.

Distribution

Isolations of ALF virus have been reported from Queensland and northern Western Australia, and seroepidemiological results have suggested that it might also extend through parts of New South Wales.

Virus

Alfuy virus is a member of the Japanese encephalitis (see entry) antigenic complex. It was originally classified as a separate member of the group, but in the recent 7th Report of the International Committee for the Taxonomy of Viruses (in Sydney, 1999) it was reclassified as a subtype of Murray Valley encephalitis (see entry) virus.

Clinical symptoms

There has been an unconfirmed report of a mild case of polyarticular disease attributed to ALF virus in Queensland, but no details have been described.

Diagnosis

Diagnosis would be carried out by an immunoglobulin M (IgM) capture enzyme-linked immunosorbent assay (ELISA) or by immunofluorescence, with confirmatory testing by a plaque reduction neutralization test.

Transmission

Alfuy virus has been isolated from *A. catasticta* and *Culex pullus* mosquitoes in Queensland, and from *Culex annulirostris* in Western Australia. However, the role of these species in transmission is not yet known.

Ecology

The vertebrate hosts of ALF virus are believed to be birds, and especially ardeid water-birds. Seroepidemiological studies in New South Wales have suggested that occasional subclinical human infections may occur.

Selected bibliography

Mackenzie, J.S., Lindsay, M.D., Coelen, R.J., Broom, A.K., Hall, R.A. and Smith, D.W. (1994) Arboviruses causing human disease in the Australasian region. *Archives of Virology* 136, 447–467.

American tick-borne typhus *see* **Rocky Mountain spotted fever.**

American trypanosomiasis *see* **Chagas disease.**

Anaplasma species *see* **Anaplasmosis.**

Anaplasmosis

Katherine M. Kocan

Infection of cattle, sheep and wild ruminants with ehrlichial pathogens of the genus *Anaplasma*.

Anaplasmosis, bovine and wild ruminants

Anaplasmosis or gall sickness is a tick-borne disease of cattle, sheep and wild ruminants that is caused by intraerythrocytic parasites of the *genus Anaplasma*, which were first described by Sir Arnold Theiler in South Africa in 1910. *Anaplasma* species were classified within the family *Anaplasmataceae*, order *Rickettsiales*, but recently have been reclassified in the genogroup II of the ehrlichial complex based on comparison of 16S ribosomal RNA (rRNA) gene sequences. *Anaplasma* species were found to be most closely related to *Ehrlichia equi*, *Ehrlichia phagocytophila*, *Ehrlichia platys* and the human granulocytic ehrlichia (HGE). *Anaplasma marginale* and the less virulent *Anaplasma centrale* are parasites of cattle and wild ruminants, while *Anaplasma ovis* infects sheep and goats. Bovine anaplasmosis is endemic in several areas of the USA and is estimated to cause US$300 million loss to cattle production annually. The disease remains a major constraint to cattle production worldwide, along with three other economically important tick-borne diseases of cattle, cowdriosis, theileriosis and babesiosis (see specific entries). The majority of information in this review on anaplasmosis concerns *A. marginale*, which is pathogenic for cattle and is the most economically important species.

Distribution

Anaplasmosis is endemic worldwide in most tropical and subtropical areas of the world, including North and South America, sub-Saharan Africa, Australia, the Caribbean, the former Soviet Union, the Far East and countries bordering the Mediterranean. The distribution of anaplasmosis is similar to that of the tick vectors. The major endemic areas of the USA are the northwestern states and California, the south central states and the south-eastern Gulf states. Isolates from the widely separated geographical areas are antigenically different.

Parasite

Anaplasma species are intracellular ehrlichial haemoparasites that are found within a membrane-bound parasitophorous vacuole in the host cell. *Anaplasma* infection in cattle, sheep and goats has only been described in erythrocytes, in which the *Anaplasma*-containing vacuole, called an 'inclusion' or 'marginal body', contains approximately one to six organisms (Figs 1 and 2). The scientific name is based on staining characteristics and location within the host cell. '*Anaplasma*' refers to the lack of stained cytoplasm, and the species names, *centrale* and *marginale*, refer to the location of the inclusion body in the erythrocyte.

Anaplasma is also found within parasitophorous vacuoles, called colonies, in the tick vectors (Fig. 3). These colonies are considerably larger than the erythrocytic inclusions and each may contain several hundred organisms. Six major surface proteins (MSPs) have been described on erythrocytic-derived *A. marginale* (MSP1 a and b, MSP2, MSP3, MSP4, MSP5). Major surface proteins 1b, 2 and 3 are from multigene families and vary antigenically in persistently infected cattle.

Clinical symptoms

Non-specific resistance *to Anaplasma* infections often occurs in young animals, while older animals may develop mild to severe clinical disease. The clinical signs of anaplasmosis result from varying degrees of anaemia caused by the removal of infected erythrocytes by reticuloendothelial cells. The clinical signs, which include icterus without haemoglobinuria, fever, anaemia,

weakness, anoxia and depression, are observed when approximately 30% of erythrocytes have been removed. Anaemia is apparent by examination of the mucous membranes, which appear pale. Animals may experience respiratory distress and myocardial hypoxia. Nervous symptoms may occur and include unexpected aggressiveness, especially in bulls. Cows that develop acute anaplasmosis during the third trimester of pregnancy may abort and

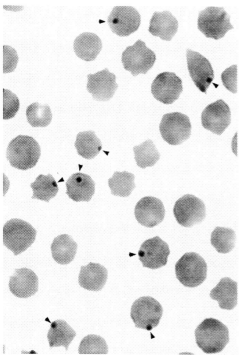

Fig. 1. *Anaplasma marginale* inclusion bodies (arrows) on the margins of bovine erythrocytes in a stained blood smear.

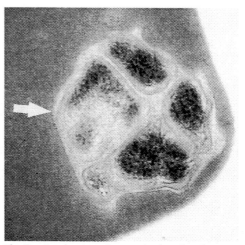

Fig. 2. An electron micrograph of an *Anaplasma marginale* inclusion (arrow) in a bovine erythrocyte. The inclusion body contains four organisms.

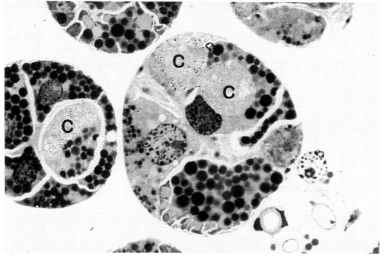

Fig. 3. Tick salivary gland acini that contain three colonies (C) of *Anaplasma marginale*: 1 µm thick plastic section stained with Mallory's stain.

bulls may develop infertility. Cattle that suffer acute anaplasmosis will have noticeable loss of body mass and will take a long period of time to regain condition. Cattle that recover from the initial acute *A. marginale* infection become persistently infected with low levels of organisms. Persistently infected cattle are solidly immune if re-exposed to *A. marginale.*

Diagnosis

A tentative diagnosis of anaplasmosis can be made on the basis of clinical signs. A definitive diagnosis is made by demonstration of anaplasmal inclusion bodies in stained erythrocyte smears, by detection of antibodies by serodiagnostic tests or by molecular tests, including DNA probes or polymerase chain reaction assays. Serodiagnosis is done routinely in most diagnostic laboratories, while molecular assays are currently used mainly as research tools. The complement fixation test (CFT) has long been the approved test for anaplasmosis in the USA, but this test does not consistently identify cattle that are persistent carriers of infection. Also, false-positive reactions occur in CFT tests using guinea-pig complement because of failure to detect all bovine immunoglobulin isotypes. Recently a competitive enzyme-linked immunosorbent assay (cELISA) was developed using MSP5 which was found to be conserved on all *A. marginale* isolates tested, as well as on *A. centrale* and *A. ovis.* The MSP5 was characterized, cloned and expressed and defined by a specific monoclonal antibody that was incorporated into the cELISA. The cELISA has proved to be a sensitive and specific test for bovine anaplasmosis in the USA, was found to be especially useful for identification of persistently infected cattle and will most probably replace the CFT. Similar ELISAs have been tested in many areas of the world and have been found to be effective for serodiagnosis of anaplasmosis.

Transmission

Anaplasma species differ from other tick-borne diseases of cattle because, in addition to cyclical transmission by ticks, transmission can be effected by blood-contaminated fomites or mechanically by biting flies. The major such vectors are tabanids, but stable-flies (*Stomoxys* species), mosquitoes, such as species *of Psorophora* and *Anopheles*, and other Diptera, such as eye-flies (eye-gnats), are also known to be mechanical transmitters of anaplasmosis. Mechanical transmission occurs via any blood-contaminated fomite, including contaminated needles, dehorning saws, nose tongs, tattooing instruments, ear-tagging devices and castration instruments.

Anaplasma marginale is transmitted biologically by ixodid (hard) ticks. Approximately 20 species of ticks have been shown capable of becoming infected and transmitting *A. marginale.* For example, *Boophilus decoloratus* is a vector in Africa and *Boophilus microplus* is an important vector in Australia, while in South Africa *Rhipicephalus simus* is also a vector of *A. marginale.* In the USA transmission is by several tick species, including *Dermacentor andersoni, Dermacentor variabilis* and *Dermacentor albipictus. Rhipicephalus sanguineus* has been shown to be an experimental vector of *A. marginale* but is quite host-specific to dogs. It is also likely that *Dermacentor occidentalis* can vector *A. marginale,* although it does not seem to be a notable vector in the USA.

Transmission of *A. marginale* by ticks occurs after a complex developmental cycle, during which extensive multiplication occurs in several tick tissues. Tick transmission is from stage to stage (trans-stadial) or within a stage (intrastadial) but transovarial transmission from one generation to the next does not occur. Male ticks develop persistent generalized infections, in which many tick cell types become infected with *A. marginale.* Intrastadial transmission by male ticks is believed to be an important mechanism of transmission because male ticks can become infected after a short feeding period on an infected animal, and then can transmit infection during repeated feedings on multiple susceptible cattle. Male ticks, therefore, serve as a reservoir of infection. They readily become infected after feeding on persistently infected cattle and the percentage of infected ticks is related to the parasitaemia during feeding. However, once ticks become infected, the infection rate of individual ticks is similar because of extensive multiplication in tick cells.

Treatment

Tetracyclines (tetracycline hydrochloride, chlortetracycline, oxytetracycline and doxycycline) are the most commonly used drugs for the prevention and treatment of anaplasmosis. Chlortetracycline is usually administered orally, while the others are injected intramuscularly or intravenously. Tetracycline is most effective when administered prior to the onset of parasitaemia. As the parasitaemia increases, infected erythrocytes are rapidly removed by reticuloendothelial cells, which results in anaemia and the related clinical signs. However, by the time clinical symptoms are apparent, the parasitaemia has peaked, rendering tetracycline treatment ineffective. When tetracycline is used as a control strategy and administered to animals as a food or mineral supplement, the drug is effective in reducing parasitaemia and thus clinical disease, providing that individual animals consume an effective dose. Blood transfusion is usually not recommended for an acutely anaemic animal. Large volumes of transfused blood may cause cardiac stress and subsequently heart failure. The period of acute anaemia is usually 24–48 h and animals often have the best chance of recovery when left undisturbed.

Control

The paradox of anaplasmosis control is that persistently infected carrier cattle are solidly immune to reinfection but these carrier cattle serve as the main reservoir hosts of infection for mechanical or biological transmission and thus contribute markedly to the spread of anaplasmosis. Cattle infected with low-level *A. marginale* parasitaemia are often difficult to detect by serodiagnosis. In addition, cattle that are treated with tetracycline, which reduces the number of infected erythrocytes and subsequently reduces antibody titres, may test negative by serological tests.

Control methods for anaplasmosis vary with geographical location and include arthropod control by application of acaricides, administration of antibiotics, premunization with live vaccines, immunization with killed vaccines and maintenance of *Anaplasma*-free herds. Use of control methods is influenced by availability, cost, governmental restrictions and feasibility of application.

Vector control

Arthropod control by application of acaricides can be used for control of both ticks and biting flies but this method is labour-intensive and expensive. Environmental pollution is becoming a more important issue and repeated application of acaricides can result in selection of resistant tick and fly populations and bears the risk of creating a susceptible population of cattle. In areas in which anaplasmosis is endemic, interruption of acaricide application allows susceptible cattle to be at risk of becoming infected and thus may lead to large outbreaks of disease. While tick control is widely practised in Africa, this method is rarely used in the USA, where both ticks and biting flies are often involved in the spread of anaplasmosis.

Chemotherapy

Antibiotic therapy, first tested for control of anaplasmosis beginning in the 1950s, includes the use of tetracycline drugs (tetracycline hydrochloride, chlortetracycline, oxytetracycline and doxycycline), imidocarb and gloxazone. Chemotherapy is directed toward prevention of clinical anaplasmosis and does not prevent cattle from becoming persistently infected with *A. marginale*. In addition, cattle receiving antibiotic therapy may not be cleared of infection. Administration of tetracycline to cattle has been effected by injection, through medicated feed or by incorporation into feed supplements. When added to feed or used as feed supplements, equal doses per bovine are difficult to ensure. Tetracycline is used extensively in some areas of the USA for anaplasmosis control, but rarely in other areas of the world. Tetracycline administration is accompanied by the disadvantage of expense, the requirement of continuous feeding and the risk of selection of *Anaplasma*-resistant organisms, although, to date, resistance of *A. marginale* to antibiotics has not been reported.

Vaccines

Development of long-term immunity by vaccination has been used extensively for control of anaplasmosis throughout most of the world and represents the most effective control measure for anaplasmosis. Vaccination with live or killed vaccines has been directed toward prevention of morbidity and mortality and does not prevent cattle from becoming infected upon challenge exposure. Therefore, immunized cattle can develop persistent field-derived infections and may serve as a reservoir host of *A. marginale* for mechanical or biological transmission. Premunization by infection of cattle with the less pathogenic *A. centrale* has been practised in many areas of the world for over 75 years, including Israel and South Africa. Premunized cattle develop mild to inapparent infections and become persistent carriers, which protects them against clinical anaplasmosis. However, *A. centrale* does not provide effective cross-protection in widely separated geographical areas. Live vaccines are generally not approved for use in the USA. An inactivated (killed) vaccine was first marketed in the USA in the 1960s. The vaccine was effective in preventing clinical anaplasmosis in the south central USA, where geographical isolates were cross-protective. This first vaccine was contaminated with bovine cell membranes, which resulted in neonatal isohaemolytic anaemia in some calves after ingestion of colostrum from immunized dams. Killed vaccines were effective when used in areas where they were cross-protective with endemic anaplasmosis. The extensive purification, dependence upon live animals as an antigen source, requirement for booster immunization and difficulty of standardization has contributed to the expense of producing and using killed vaccines. Subsequent killed vaccines have been purified

to remove host cells, but these vaccines, marketed primarily in the USA, were withdrawn recently and are not available. A cell culture system was developed recently for propagation of *A. marginale* and may serve as a non-bovine source of antigen for development of new and more effective vaccines.

Surveillance and maintenance of disease-free herds

Maintenance of an anaplasmosis-free herd is effective for control of anaplasmosis in areas where anaplasmosis is not endemic. However, serological tests often do not have the sensitivity to detect persistently infected cattle that would enable identification and culling of infected cattle. In the future, molecular diagnosis may be adapted for routine testing of cattle and may allow for reliable detection of infection in persistently infected cattle. Control of anaplasmosis could then be effected by surveillance and removal of persistently infected cattle, which serve as a source of infection for both mechanical and biological transmission of *A. marginale*.

Selected bibliography

Dame, J.B., Mahan, S.M. and Yowell, C.A. (1992) Phylogenetic relationship of *Cowdria ruminantium*, agent of heartwater, to *Anaplasma marginale* and other members of the order Rickettsiales determined on the basis of 16S rRNA sequence. *International Journal of Systematic Bacteriology* 42, 270–274.

Dikmans, G. (1950) The transmission of anaplasmosis. *American Journal of Veterinary Research* 38, 5–16.

Ewing, S.A. (1981) Transmission of *Anaplasma marginale* by arthropods. In: *Proceedings of the 7th National Anaplasmosis Conference, Mississippi State*. College of Veterinary Medicine, Stockville, Mississippi, pp. 395–423.

Knowles, D.P., Perryman, L.E., McElwain, T.F., Kappmeyer, L.S., Stiller, D., Palmer, G.H., Visser, E.S., Hennager, S.G., Davis, W.C. and McGuire, T.C. (1995) Conserved recombinant antigens of *Anaplasma marginale* and *Babesia equi* for serologic diagnosis. *Veterinary Parasitology* 57, 93–96.

Kocan, K.M. (1986) Development of *Anaplasma marginale* in ixodid ticks: coordinated development of a rickettsial organism and its tick host. In: Sauer, J.R. and Hair, J.A. (eds)

Morphology, Physiology and Behavioral Ecology of Ticks. Ellis Horwood, Chichester, UK, pp. 472–505.

Kocan, K.M. (2000) Anaplasmosis control: past, present and future. *Proceedings of the New York Academy of Science* 916, 501–509.

Kocan, K.M., Stiller, D., Goff, W.L., Claypool, P.L., Edwards, W., Ewing, S.A., McGuire, T.C., Hair, J.A. and Barron, S.J. (1992) Development of *Anaplasma marginale* in male *Dermacentor andersoni* transferred from infected to susceptible cattle. *American Journal of Veterinary Research* 53, 499–507.

Palmer, G.H. (1984) *Anaplasma* vaccines. In: Wright, I.G. (ed.) *Veterinary, Protozoan and Hemoparasite Vaccines.* CRC Press, Boca Raton, Florida, pp. 1–29.

Palmer, G.H., Rurangirwa, F.R., Kocan, K.M. and Brown, W.C. (1999) Molecular basis for vaccine development against the ehrlichial pathogen *Anaplasma marginale. Parasitology Today* 15, 281–286.

Stoltsz, W.H. (1993) Bovine anaplasmosis. In: *Current Veterinary Therapy, 3. Food Animal Practice.* W.B. Saunders, Philadelphia, pp. 588–596.

Animal trypanosomiasis

Tudor W. Jones

Animal trypanosomiasis is caused by infection with single-celled, flagellated, extracellular, obligate, blood parasites belonging to the genus *Trypanosoma* (Fig. 1). The disease principally affects domestic livestock in South and Central America, Africa and Asia and is associated with severe production losses, reduced reproductive capability, reduced work output and death. Cattle, buffalo, horses, camels (Camelidae) and pigs are particularly at risk. In Africa, animal trypanosomiasis, often called nagana, is caused by *Trypanosoma vivax, Trypanosoma congolense* or *Trypanosoma brucei brucei.* The disease is found in 37 sub-Saharan countries covering an area of 11 million km² containing 160 million cattle and 260 million sheep and goats with estimated annual production losses of US$5000 million. The animal trypanosomiases are transmitted by a range of blood-sucking insects and the vector–parasite relationships can be highly specific.

Trypanosomes are ingested by the vector during feeding on an infected animal. This is followed, in some trypanosome species, by a period of development in the vector before the parasite is returned to another host during subsequent feeding (cyclical development). Some trypanosome species are transmitted directly between hosts without any development in the vector (mechanical or non-cyclical transmission).

The vector species, the development site in the vector and the route by which infective forms are passed to the vertebrate host are important characteristics of the different trypanosome genera and species (Table 1).

The species of trypanosomes infecting animals range in length from 9 to 100 μm and can be differentiated using a number of morphological criteria (Table 2). All species have a single flagellum, which extends along the length of the organism and is usually joined to the outside of the cell membrane to form an undulating membrane. In some species the flagellum extends beyond the end of the cell body to form a free flagellum. The DNA of trypanosomes is organized into two bodies – a larger single nucleus and a smaller extranuclear body called the kinetoplast, which consists of a network of circular DNA molecules and is the origin of the mitochondrion. Multiplication is by binary fission and there is evidence that genetic exchange takes place between individual organisms, although gamete forms or mating types have not been described.

Taxonomically the trypanosome species infecting animals belong to the order Trypanosomatida (formerly in the Kinetoplastida), family Trypanosomatidae and genus *Trypanosoma.* The genus is divided into two major sections – the Stercoraria and Salivaria – and each section contains a number of subgenera and species. A trinomial

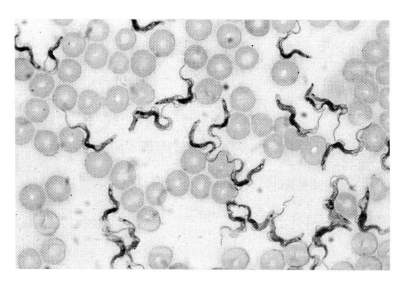

Fig. 1. Trypanosomes (*Trypanosoma evansi*) in the blood of a cow (*Bos taurus*).

system is often used for the nomenclature for trypanosome species, based on genus, (subgenus) and species. In some cases this is extended to include subspecies, e.g. *Trypanosoma* (*Trypanozoon*) *brucei brucei*.

Section Stercoraria

Stercorarian trypanosomes develop in the mid-gut and hind-gut of the vector (posterior station development), and the infective forms (metacyclic trypanosomes) are usually passed out in the vector's faeces immediately after feeding. Trypanosomes then enter the host via the feeding site (contaminative transmission).

The Stercoraria consists of three subgenera – *Megatrypanum*, *Herpetosoma* and *Schizotrypanum*. None of these is of particular importance as an animal pathogen apart from *Schizotrypanum*, which contains the zoonotic *Trypanosoma* (*Schizotrypanum*) *cruzi*, the cause of Chagas disease (see entry) in humans in Central and South America. Dogs and cats can act as reservoir hosts for *T. cruzi* and dogs can develop some of the symptoms associated with human infections, including cardiac lesions.

All trypanosome species of the subgenus *Herpetosoma* infect rodents.

Members of the subgenus *Megatrypanum* are large trypanosomes that infect many hosts, including domestic ruminants,

and are considered to be non-pathogenic. They are transmitted by blood-sucking Diptera; for example, tabanid flies transmit *Trypanosoma theileri* in cattle, while hippoboscids or keds (e.g. *Melophagus ovinus*) are vectors of *Trypanosoma melophagium* in sheep. Most of these trypanosomes are cosmopolitan, with infection rates of up to 100% of animals in some areas.

Section Salivaria

The salivarian trypanosomes are transmitted via the mouthparts of the vector (anterior station development), involving either the proboscis (subgenera *Duttonella* and *Nannomonas*) or salivary glands (subgenera *Trypanozoon* and *Pycnomonas*). These subgenera include species causing severe disease in animals. The salivarian trypanosomes are transmitted by blood-sucking insects during feeding, either after a period of development in the vector (cyclical or biological development) or directly via blood residues on vector mouthparts (non-cyclical or mechanical transmission). Salivarian trypanosome species that undergo cyclical development are transmitted by tsetse-flies (*Glossina* species), while mechanical transmission can be achieved by a range of flies, including tabanid flies (Tabanidae) and stable-flies (*Stomoxys* species).

Table 1. Summary of host and vectors systems for trypanosomes infecting animals.*

Subgenus	Species	Vector		Principal hosts affected
		Species	Development site	
Megatrypanum	T. theileri	Tabanidae	Mid- and hind-gut	Cattle, buffalo, antelope
	T. melophagium	Sheep ked (Melophagus ovinus)	Mid- and hind-gut	Sheep
Duttonella	T. vivax	Glossina species	Labrum, labium, hypopharynx	Cattle, sheep, goats, antelope
		Biting flies	No development, mechanical transfer on proboscis	
	T. uniforme	Glossina species	Labrum, labium, hypopharynx	Cattle, sheep, goats, antelope
Nannomonas	T. congolense	Glossina species	Mid-gut, labrum, hypopharynx	Cattle, sheep, goats, antelope
	T. simiae	Glossina species	Mid-gut, labrum, hypopharynx	Pigs, camels
	T. godfreyi	Glossina species	Mid-gut, labrum, hypopharynx	Pigs
Pycnomonas	T. suis	Glossina species	Mid-gut, salivary glands, hypopharynx	Pigs
Trypanozoon	T. brucei brucei	Glossina species	Mid-gut, salivary glands, hypopharynx	Horses, donkeys, camels, dogs
	T. evansi	Biting flies	No development, mechanical transfer on proboscis	Horses, camels, buffalo, dogs
		Vampire bats (South America)	Blood	

*Trypanosoma brucei rhodesiense and T. b. gambiense are omitted as they do not cause sickness in animals; the animals act only as reservoir hosts.

Table 2. Summary of morphological characteristics of trypanosomes infecting animals as seen in Giemsa-stained blood-smears.

Section:	Stercoraria	Salivaria						
Subgenus:	Megatrypanum	Trypanozoon		Nannomonas		Pycnomonas	Duttonella	
Species:	e.g. *T. theileri*	*T. brucei brucei*	*T. evansi*	*T. congolense* / *T. godfreyi*	*T. simiae*	*T. suis*	*T. vivax*	*T. uniforme*
Nucleus	Central or anterior	Central or posterior	Central	Central	Central	Central	Central	Central
Size	Very large, 60–100 μm	Slender, 23–30 μm; Stumpy, 13–22 μm	Large, 17–30 μm	Small, 9–22 μm	Small, 12–24 μm	Small, 14–16 μm	Medium, 18–26 μm	Small, 12–20 μm
Pleomorphic	No	Yes	No	No	Yes	No	No	No
Free flagellum	Long	Variable	Long	Absent	Absent	Short	Long	Long
Undulating membrane	Prominent	Prominent	Inconspicuous	Inconspicuous	Variable	Inconspicuous	Inconspicuous	Inconspicuous
Shape of posterior end	Fine pointed	Blunt, truncated	Blunt, truncated	Blunt, truncated	Blunt, truncated	Pointed, short	Blunt, rounded	Blunt, rounded
Kinetoplast position	Marginal, far from posterior end	Subterminal	Subterminal	Subterminal	Subterminal	Subterminal	Terminal	Terminal
Size	Large	Small	Small	Medium	Medium	Small	Large	Large

Tsetse-transmitted trypanosomes

The relationship between the tsetse-transmitted trypanosomes and the vector is highly specific, which effectively limits their distribution to that of the tsetse-fly – principally areas of Central and southern Africa between 15°N and 29°S. Most of these trypanosomes can be transmitted by a range of *Glossina* species depending on the habitat – *G. morsitans* (savanna areas), *G. palpalis* (river and lake areas), G. fusca (forest areas). Tsetse-transmitted trypanosome species can usually infect a range of animal species, but cattle (Fig. 2) and horses are usually more severely affected than small ruminants such as sheep and goats. However, pigs can be severely affected by certain species of trypanosome. Exotic breeds of livestock are often more severely affected than indigenous breeds, which frequently show a degree of resistance to the effects of infection (trypanotolerance). Animals are often infected with more than one species of trypanosome and the common name given to the disease associated with animal trypanosomiasis is nagana, which usually relates to infection with trypanosomes *per se*, rather than infection with a particular species.

Trypanosome species can be differentiated using morphological features, such as their length, characteristics of the flagellum, position of subcellular organelles, such as the nucleus and kinetoplast, and their development site in the vector (Tables 1 and 2). However, species and subspecies usually consist of a number of morphologically similar populations (strains or stocks) that have different properties, such as pathogenicity, host range and drug sensitivity. These populations can usually be differentiated only by using molecular or biochemical criteria.

Parasites

The salivarian trypanosomes are divided into four subgenera – *Duttonella, Nannomonas, Trypanozoon* and *Pycnomonas* – which differ in their morphology (Table 1) and their developmental behaviour in the vector.

Subgenus Duttonella

This subgenus consists of two species *T. (D.) vivax* and *T. (D.) uniforme*.

TRYPANOSOMA (DUTTONELLA) VIVAX (NAGANA)

Distribution. Found in Africa and also in South America. It is thought to have been introduced into Latin America in the late 19th century in cattle exported from Africa.

Morphology. Parasites have a characteristically rapid movement in fresh blood; they are principally monomorphic, with an

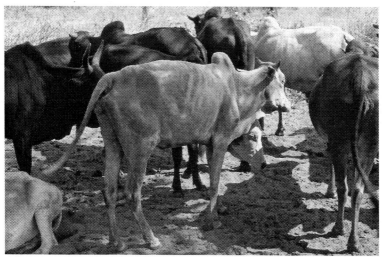

Fig. 2. A sick zebu cow (infected with trypanosomes) among healthy ones (courtesy of A.M. Jordan).

overall length of 18–26 μm including the free flagellum. The kinetoplast is large and found close to the posterior end of the parasite, which appears swollen, making the trypanosome appear club-shaped.

Pathogenicity. The principal hosts affected by *T. vivax* in Africa and Latin America are cattle, horses, sheep and goats, with cattle being most severely affected (Fig. 2). Although principally a blood parasite, *T. vivax* can be found in other body tissues, particularly the lymphatic system. *Trypanosoma vivax* can also affect the anterior chambers of the eyes, leading to severe conjunctivitis. Acute infections with some strains of *T. vivax* can lead to extensive haemorrhages beneath the skin, often leading to death within a few days of the onset of symptoms. The haemorrhagic form of *T. vivax* is found more frequently in West Africa than in East or Central Africa. Sheep and goats often recover from *T. vivax* infection, while horses usually develop chronic infections. Pigs and dogs are refractory to infection with *T. vivax*.

Transmission. In Africa *T. vivax* is transmitted by a range of *Glossina* species, with development restricted to the proboscis of the fly; the salivary glands are not involved. In Latin America transmission is considered to be effected by a range of blood-sucking flies, principally tabanid flies.

TRYPANOSOMA (DUTTONELLA) UNIFORME

Distribution. This species is uncommon, being found only in cattle, sheep and goats in certain areas of Central and East Africa.

Morphology and pathogenicity. Parasites are morphologically similar to *T. vivax* but shorter, measuring only 12–20 μm. *Trypanosoma uniforme* has a development cycle in *Glossina* species similar to that of *T. vivax*. Infection usually becomes chronic.

Subgenus Nannomonas

This consists of three species, namely *T. (N.) congolense*, *T. (N.) simiae* and *T. (N.) godfreyi*, which are morphologically similar but can be differentiated by their behaviour in the vertebrate host and by certain biochemical and molecular criteria. Initial development takes place in the gut of the tsetse-fly and the trypanosomes eventually move forward to colonize the proboscis, and in the hypopharynx they transform into the infective metacyclic forms, which are introduced into the vertebrate host during feeding.

TRYPANOSOMA (NANNOMONAS) CONGOLENSE (NAGANA)

Distribution. East and Central Africa.

Morphology. Parasites move slowly in fresh blood related to their lack of free flagellum and poorly developed undulating membrane. They are principally monomorphic but with considerable variation in length (9–22 μm). A medium-sized kinetoplast is found close to the posterior margin.

Pathogenicity. *Trypanosoma congolense* can infect cattle, horses, dogs, sheep, goats and pigs. It is the principal cause of severe trypanosomiasis in cattle in East and Central Africa, where it manifests itself as the characteristic wasting disease associated with animal trypanosomiasis. In areas of high challenge *T. congolense* can lead to death in sheep and goats, with reduction in productivity in areas of low challenge. The disease is more acute in horses than in cattle, often resulting in swelling of the genitalia, which can interfere with reproduction; or in death. Infections in dogs produce a wasting disease and a severe anaemia, with exotic breeds at greater risk than local breeds. *Trypanosoma congolense* infection in pigs is not as severe as in ruminants but can disrupt growth rates.

Transmission. Vectors are species of *Glossina*, such as *G. morsitans* and *G. fusca*.

TRYPANOSOMA (NANNOMONAS) SIMIAE

Distribution. Widely distributed throughout Africa.

Morphology. Parasites are pleomorphic, with three morphological forms in the blood: (i) long stout forms, which usually make up the majority; these have a free flagellum and a well-developed undulating membrane; (ii) long slender forms, with a less prominent undulating membrane and a free flagellum present in some individuals; and (iii) short forms, which are similar to *T. congolense*.

Pathogenicity. This parasite is the most important trypanosome species affecting domestic pigs, usually resulting in an acute infection that is invariably fatal, but it can also cause severe disease in camels. *Trypanosoma simiae* infections in pigs are characterized by fever and inappetence, with death often taking place within hours. Warthogs (*Phacochoerus aethiopicus*) and Bushpigs (*Potamochoerus porcus*) act as asymptomatic carriers.

Transmission. The parasites are transmitted cyclically by *Glossina* species, especially *G. morsitans* and *G. fusca*, but also mechanically by other blood-sucking flies within piggeries.

TRYPANOSOMA (NANNOMONAS) GODFREYI
Distribution. East and Central Africa.

Morphology. The parasites are morphologically similar to *T. congolense* but biochemically and genetically different from this species and the other member of the subgenus (*T. simiae*). This species infects pigs in East and Central Africa, producing a chronic infection.

Transmission. This species is transmitted by *Glossina brevipalpis* and *G. morsitans*.

Subgenus Trypanozoon

This subgenus consists of the three subspecies of *T.* (*T.*) *brucei*, and one other species *T.* (*T.*) *evansi*. Two of the subspecies, *T. brucei rhodesiense* and *T. brucei gambiense* are the cause of African human trypanosomiasis (see entry). The remaining subspecies, *T.* (*T.*) *brucei brucei*, and *T.* (*T.*) *evansi* infect only animals. Both *T. b. rhodesiense* and *T. b. gambiense* can also infect animals, which can act as reservoir hosts for African human trypanosomiasis. All species, other than *T. evansi*, undergo cyclical development in *Glossina* species.

Trypanosoma evansi is transmitted mechanically by haematophagous flies, such as tabanids and stable-flies (*Stomoxys* species), and also by Vampire bats (*Desmodus rotundus*) in South America.

TRYPANOSOMA (TRYPANOZOON) BRUCEI BRUCEI (NAGANA)
Distribution. Widely distributed in sub-Saharan Africa.

Morphology. The parasites are moderately active in fresh blood and show marked polymorphism during the course of infection, with three morphological forms: (i) long slender forms, 22–30 μm in length, with a long free flagellum and a prominent undulating membrane; (ii) short stumpy forms, 13–22 μm in length, with a conspicuous undulating membrane but often without a free flagellum; in some individuals the nucleus is found towards the posterior of the cell; and (iii) intermediate forms, with a free flagellum and a conspicuous undulating membrane; they are intermediate in length between the long slender and short stumpy forms.

Pathogenicity. Parasites infect horses, dogs, sheep, goats, cattle and pigs but they are most important in horses where they often result in severe disease and usually death. Dogs can also be severely affected, involving the eyes and central nervous system, leading to behaviour changes. Infection in sheep and goats can result in death. Cattle are the least likely of domesticated animals to be clinically affected, though a high proportion of cattle may be infected in endemic areas.

Transmission. Transmitted by a range of *Glossina* species, where the trypanosomes develop initially in the gut of the fly, they then invade the salivary glands, with the infective metacyclic forms entering the vertebrate host with the tsetse-fly's saliva during feeding.

TRYPANOSOMA (TRYPANOZOON) EVANSI (SURRA)
Distribution. Widely distributed in Asia, Central and South America, Africa and in

parts of the Commonwealth of Independent States (CIS).

Morphology. *Trypanosoma evansi* is considered to have evolved from *T. b. brucei* in Camel (*Camelus dromedarius*) populations away from tsetse-infested areas. Morphologically it is indistinguishable from the long slender form of *T. b. brucei* but is both biochemically and genetically different.

Populations sometimes develop in which the kinetoplast does not stain with Romanovsky-type stains (dyskinetoplastic strains).

Pathogenicity. This is the most widely distributed trypanosome, affecting animals in Latin America, North Africa and Asia. Infects camels, Water buffalo (*Bubalus bubalis*), cattle, horses and dogs. It causes a wasting disease generally known as surra, but also as el debab, guifar, dioufar, tahaga or doukane. In Latin America it is known as murrina, caderas disease, derrengadera or tristeza. Infections in dogs and horses are usually rapidly fatal, with death occurring within a few weeks. Cattle, sheep and goats are less severely affected but can act as reservoir hosts. In Asia, Water buffalo can be severely affected, especially if trypanosome-naïve animals are moved into endemic areas.

Transmission. The infection is transmitted in the absence of tsetse-flies, probably mechanically by blood-sucking flies, such as tabanids and *Stomoxys* species. There is also transmission by Vampire bats (*D. rotundus*) in South America.

Subgenus Pycnomonas
Distribution. Principally in Central Africa, such as Burundi and Zaïre, but also in Tanzania.

Morphology and pathogenicity. There is just one species, *Trypanosoma* (*Pycnomonas*) *suis*, a monomorphic trypanosome of pigs, usually resulting in a chronic infection in adult pigs characterized by fever and progressive weakness. In young pigs it often results in acute disease and death.

Transmission. The vectors are *G. brevipalpis* and *G. vanhoofi*.

Clinical signs of animal trypanosomiasis

Trypanosome infections can result in the development of lesions in many of the major body systems, leading to a range of symptoms that can be confused with other infections. General symptoms include intermittent bouts of fever, anaemia, oedema, splenomegaly, polyadenitis, nervous disorders with hind-limb paresis, pica, eye disorders, emaciation, cachexia and death.

Anaemia, the principal pathological effect of animal trypanosomiasis, is characterized by a severe reduction in the host's erythrocyte mass. In the early stages of infection anaemia is haemolytic from increased red cell destruction by host phagocytes, resulting from the presence of large numbers of trypanosomes, immunological reactions, fever and disseminated intravascular coagulation. Later stages are characterized by continuing erythrocyte destruction, impairment of the haemopoietic system, reduced parasite density and reduced erythropoiesis. The final phase is characterized by haemosiderosis and irreversible damage to bone marrow function. Death can occur at any stage of infection, usually due to congestive heart failure brought on by anaemia and myocardial damage. In some cases, evidence of damage to the central nervous system is seen as posterior paralysis in the later stages of infection. The impact of trypanosome infection on individual animals, however, depends on a combination of parasite and host factors, with considerable differences between host species, breeds and individual animals.

Diagnosis of animal trypanosomiasis

The principal tests used for the diagnosis of trypanosome infection are as follows.

Parasitological (direct) methods

BLOOD FILM ANALYSIS This is simple to carry out but is the least sensitive method because of the small volume of blood that can be examined. Trypanosomes are detected by microscopy in wet-film preparations from fresh blood based on their characteristic movement, or in fixed dried blood smears stained with Romanovsky-type stains, such as Giemsa's or Leishman's stain. Stained smears of lymph fluid are sometimes used if *T. vivax* infection is suspected.

CONCENTRATION METHODS These enable a larger volume of blood to be examined than can be examined with blood films. Most methods are based on differential centrifugation of blood to separate the host's blood cells from trypanosomes, which collect at the leucocyte–plasma interface. This separation is usually carried out in glass capillary tubes using a haematocrit centrifuge (micro-haematocrit centrifugation technique). Trypanosomes are identified either by microscopal examination of the leucocyte–plasma interface directly through the capillary wall or by examination of the interface region as wet films using dark-ground illumination (buffy coat method).

Other concentration methods involve the selective lysis of host cells using detergents, or the removal of host cells by adsorption on to anion exchange resins, such as diethyl aminoethyl cellulose (mini-ion exchange centrifugation technique).

EXPANSION (CULTURE) METHODS Expansion methods are not used for the routine diagnosis of animal trypanosomiasis due to lack of suitable culture systems and due to cost. Some trypanosome species (*T. brucei, T. congolense, T. evansi*) can be expanded in laboratory rodents. Xenodiagnosis is restricted to the diagnosis of human *Trypanosoma cruzi* infections (see Chagas disease).

Indirect methods

Indirect diagnostic methods are based on the detection of host antibody to trypanosomes in serum (serodiagnosis), trypanosome components circulating in the blood (circulating antigen methods) or trypanosome DNA in blood (molecular methods).

ANTIBODY DETECTION METHODS Trypanosome infections elicit a strong humoral immune response from the host, which can be used as an indicator of infection. A large number of diagnostic tests based on the detection of antibody to trypanosomes have been developed which are based on the specificity of the antigen–antibody bond and physico-chemical properties of antibody molecules and antigen–antibody complexes. Antigens used for these tests usually consist either of whole trypanosomes (agglutination test, fluorescent antibody staining technique) or soluble extracts of trypanosomes (indirect haemagglutination test, complement fixation test, enzyme-linked immunosorbent assay (ELISA)). The interpretation of results from antibody detection assays is complicated by the presence of antigens that are common to all trypanosome species, making differential diagnosis difficult in areas where more than one trypanosome species is present. Trypanosome antibodies also persist in animals for many months after infection even when infections have been eliminated by drug treatment, thus making it difficult to distinguish between active and past infections.

AGGLUTINATION TESTS These use either intact trypanosomes or fixed and stained trypanosomes (card agglutination test for trypanosomes (CATT)) as antigen, which forms visible clumps in the presence of trypanosome antibody. Soluble extracts can also be coated onto carrier systems, such as erythrocytes (indirect haemagglutination test), or inert particles, such as latex (latex agglutination test) or polystyrene, which clump together in the presence of trypanosome antibody.

COMPLEMENT FIXATION TESTS These are carried out with soluble extracts of trypanosomes as antigen and are based on the ability of antigen–antibody complexes to reduce the amount of free complement in the medium, which can then be measured using an erythrocyte–anti-erythrocyte indicator system. Complement fixation tests can be difficult to carry out with serum samples from ruminants, because of poor fixation of complement by their antibodies and the presence of anticomplementary factors in their serum.

LABELLED ANTIBODY TECHNIQUES Techniques such as the indirect fluorescent antibody

(IFA) test and ELISA are extensively used as diagnostic tests for trypanosome infections. The assays are based on the binding of anti-gen–antibody complex to a second anti-host species antibody that has been labelled with either a fluorochrome (IFA) or an enzyme (ELISA), which is often referred to as a con-jugate. In each case the presence of the label is taken as an indication that binding of host antibody to the antigen has taken place.

In the case of IFA whole trypanosomes, either intact or air-dried on glass microscope slides, are used as antigen preparations. In the presence of antibody the trypanosomes fluoresce as a result of the binding of the fluorochrome-labelled conjugate (second antibody) to host antibody bound, in turn, to the trypanosomes. The fluorescence can be seen using a fluorescence microscope. In the case of ELISA, soluble trypanosome antigen preparations are bound to a solid support, such as polystyrene, which combines with trypanosome-specific antibody. The pres-ence of bound antibody can then be detected using a range of secondary systems, includ-ing second antibody preparations labelled with enzymes such as horseradish per-oxidase and alkaline phosphatase, labelled biotin–avidin systems or label–antilabel sys-tems such as peroxidase–anti-peroxidase.

Detection of trypanosome components

ANTIGEN-CAPTURE ASSAYS A polyclonal or monoclonal antibody preparation to one or more trypanosome antigens is used to capture any target antigen molecule present in host blood. The binding of the target molecule to the antibody is then detected, using another antibody preparation to the target molecule that has been labelled with an appropriate indicator system, such an enzyme or biotin. An antigen-capture latex agglutination test has also been developed by coating latex particles with the capture antibody. The particles agglutinate in the presence of the target antigen.

DETECTION OF TRYPANOSOME DNA The poly-merase chain reaction (PCR) assay can be used to amplify small amounts of DNA from intact trypanosomes or from disintegrated trypanosomes circulating in the blood or dried onto filter paper, using short oligo-nucleotide primer sequences in the presence of a polymerase enzyme. This amplified DNA can then be detected by gel electrophoresis.

Control of animal trypanosomes

The control of animal trypanosomosis depends principally on the use of vector reduction techniques, the administration of chemical compounds with trypanocidal properties, or a combination of both. The severity of the disease can be reduced through the use of tolerant breeds (trypano-tolerance), such as the West African N'dama cattle (Fig. 3)

Vector reduction methods

In the case of the tsetse-transmitted animal trypanosomes, vector reduction methods can be used to reduce the intensity of trypanosome challenge. Tsetse populations can be controlled through the application of insecticides, such as the pyrethroids, delta-methrin, cypermethrin, lamdacyhalothrin or the organochlorine insecticide endo-sulphan, delivered by aerial or ground spraying, often as ultra-low-volume (ULV) applications. Control is often by sequential applications (up to five sprayings). Insecti-cides are directed at vegetation on which tsetse-flies rest (Fig. 4) when they are not host-seeking. Applications are best made during the dry season so that rain does not wash the deposit from foliage and when there is minimum vegetative growth, which would otherwise provide unsprayed resting sites. Cattle can be treated with insecticides, such as with 'pour-on' preparations of organophosphates or pyrethroids, together with an adjuvant oil that assists in rapidly spreading the insecticide over most of the animal. Insecticide-impregnated ear tags or collars have also been used to reduce tsetse-flies feeding on cattle.

Visual attraction traps, such as biconical or monoconical ones (Fig. 5), can sometimes prove effective in catching both riverine vectors, such as G. palpalis and Glossina tachinoides, and the more widely dispersed G. morsitans and Glossina

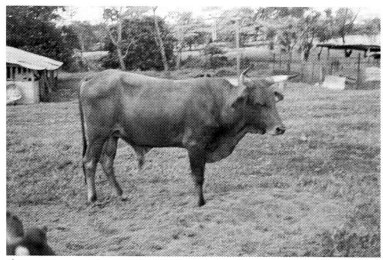

Fig. 3. A trypanotolerant N'dama bull (courtesy of Centre for Tropical Veterinary Medicine).

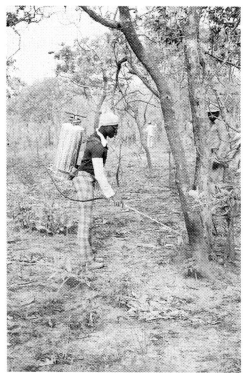

Fig. 4. Insecticidal spraying of the bases of trees and other vegetation to kill tsetse-flies when they rest on such sites (courtesy of A.M. Jordan).

pallidipes. Traps are often sprayed with residual insecticides to kill those flies resting on the traps but which are unlikely to enter them. A simpler idea is to use targets, such as dark blue screen cloths impregnated with insecticides (Fig. 6) to kill flies attracted to them; no attempt is made to trap them. Occasionally targets have incorporated electric grids that kill flies on impact.

Currently, there are no reported cases of insecticide resistance being developed in tsetse-flies.

Sterile insect techniques (SIT), involving the release of many male flies sterilized by radiation, have sometimes been used as a means of eliminating residual populations remaining after control using other methods, such as insecticidal ones. However, logistic and financial problems can be prohibitive with many SIT programmes. Environmental management, such as partial (discriminative, selective) bush clearing, which involves removing selected woody vegetation known to comprise favoured tsetse resting sites, can be used to make areas less hospitable for tsetse-flies, or to create breaks between grazing areas and forest reservoir areas.

With non-tsetse-transmitted animal trypanosomiasis, vector control is difficult to implement because the precise vector species for these parasites have often not been clearly identified or their behaviour studied in any detail. Moreover, some infections can be transmitted by a wide range of biting flies,

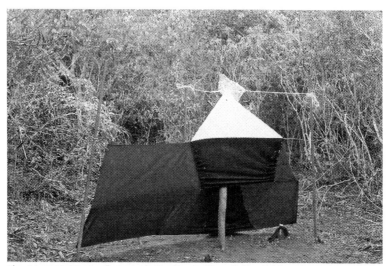

Fig. 5.   A Ngu tsetse-fly trap, devised by R. Dransfield, and used in the control of animal trypanosomiasis in Kenya (courtesy of A.M. Jordan).

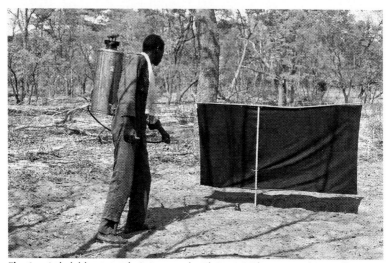

Fig. 6.   A dark blue target being sprayed with insecticide to control tsetse-fly vectors of animal trypanosomiasis in Africa (courtesy of A.M. Jordan).

such as tabanids and stable-flies, whose biologies differ substantially.

Drug treatment

The use of trypanocidal drugs is an important component of most control regimens for animal trypanosomiasis. However, the number of chemical compounds available for the control of animal trypanosomiasis is limited to formulations of five chemical classes (Table 3). The choice of drug is determined by the species of trypanosome in an area, the host species, the kind of control required and the local availability of drugs. The appearance of drug-resistant populations is common in areas where particular compounds have been in use for a long time and cross-resistance is often encountered between compounds with a similar chemical structure.

Treatment of animal trypanosomiasis can be either curative or prophylactic.

Table 3. Properties of drugs used for the control of animal trypanosomiasis.

General name	Chemical class	Curative use		Prophylactic use			Comments
		Dose rate	Route	Dose rate	Route	Protective period	
Isometamidium	Phenanthridium	0.25 mg kg^{-1}	i.m.	0.5–1.0 mg kg^{-1}	i.m.	2–4 months	Possible side-effects in camels
Homidium chloride	Phenanthridium	1.0 mg kg^{-1}	i.m.	–	–	–	Possible severe local reactions in horses
Homidium bromide	Phenanthridium						
Diminazine aceturate	Aromatic amidine	3.5 mg kg^{-1}	s.c. or i.m.	–	–	–	Toxic for camels
Suramin	Naphthalene derivative	10 mg kg^{-1}	i.v.	–	–	–	No activity against *T. vivax* or *T. congolense*
Quinapyramine sulphate	Quinoline derivative	5 mg kg^{-1}	s.c.	–	–	–	
Quinapyramine Pro salt (sulphate and chloride)	Quinoline derivative	–	–	7.4 mg kg^{-1}	s.c.	2–3 months	
Melarsenoxide cysteamine	Arsenical	0.25 mg kg^{-1}	i.m.	–	–	–	*T. evansi* infections in camels

i.m., intramuscular; i.v., intravenous; s.c., subcutaneous.

Curative drugs have little or no residual activity in the host and are used when the incidence of trypanosome challenge is low or intermittent. Prophylactic treatment is used when animals are subjected to a constant trypanosome challenge. Curative treatments are usually administered to individual animals in response to signs of clinical trypanosomiasis, while prophylactic drugs are usually administered to herds on a regular basis.

Vaccination against animal trypanosomiasis
Trypanosomes are able to prevent elimination of an infection by the host immune response by changing the composition of their surface antigen throughout the course of infection. This phenomenon is known as antigenic variation. New variants are produced at 2–3-day intervals by complex rearrangements of the trypanosome genetic material and each trypanosome infection is considered to have the potential to produce several thousand different antigenic types (variant antigen types) during the course of an infection. Apart from enabling the parasite to survive in the host, antigenic variation frustrates attempts to develop an effective vaccine against trypanosome infection as protective immunity is directed against individual antigenic types. Antibodies produced to one antigen type are, therefore, not effective against any other antigenic type.

Selected bibliography

Budd, L.T. (ed.) (1999) *DIFID-Funded Tsetse and Trypanosome Research and Development Since 1980*, Vol. 1 *Scientific Review*, 325 pp., Vol. 2 *Economic Analysis*, 120 pp., Vol. 3 *Summary of Projects*, 123 pp. Department for International Development, London.

Hide, G., Mottram, J.C., Coombs, G.H. and Holmes, P.H. (eds) (1997) *Trypanosomiasis and Leishmaniasis: Biology and Control.* CAB International, Wallingford, UK, 384 pp.

Hoare, C.A. (1972) *The Trypanosomes of Mammals: a Zoological Monograph.* Blackwell Scientific Publications, Oxford, 749 pp.

Lumsden, W.H.R. and Evans, D.A. (eds) (1979) *Biology of the Kinetoplastida*, Vol. 1, 563 pp., Vol. 2, 738 pp. Academic Press, London.

Molyneux, D.H. and Ashford, R.W. (1983) *The Biology of* Trypanosoma *and* Leishmania *Parasites of Man and Domestic Animals.* Taylor & Francis, London, 294 pp.

Mulligan, H.W. (ed.) (1970) *The African Trypanosomiases.* George Allen & Unwin, London, 950 pp.

Stephens, L.E. (1986) *Trypanosomiasis: a Veterinary Perspective.* Pergamon Press, Oxford, 551 pp.

Taylor, K.A. and Mertens, B. (1999) Immune response of cattle infected with African trypanosomes. *Memorias do Instituto Oswaldo Cruz* 94, 239–244.

Trail, J.C.M., d'Ieteren, G.D.M. and Murray, M. (1991) Practical aspects of developing genetic resistance to trypanosomiasis. In: Owen, J.B. and Axford, R.F.E. (eds) *Breeding for Disease Resistance in Farm Animals.* CAB International, Wallingford, UK, pp. 224–234.

Anthrax

Daniel C. Dragon

Infection of humans and other mammals with the bacterium *Bacillus anthracis*. The infection is global in its distribution, occurring from the tropics to the Arctic. An estimated 20,000 people and 1,000,000 animals are infected yearly, mostly in developing countries or in regions where there has been a breakdown in veterinary services.

Distribution

Sub-Sahelian Africa and central Asia and adjoining regions are the most severely affected parts of the world. The disease is endemic to south-west Texas and regions of northern Canada. Endemic regions are observed in all South American countries and the disease is a serious problem throughout Central America and Africa. In

Europe and Asia Minor, most cases occur within a belt running from central Spain through Greece and Turkey to Pakistan.

Bacterium

Bacillus anthracis is an aerobic Gram-positive rod. Central to its maintenance in a region is its ability to form metabolically dormant endospores, which may remain viable for over 60 years. The spores are resistant to desiccation, temperature and pH extremes, ultraviolet irradiation and a wide variety of deleterious reagents.

Clinical symptoms

In humans the disease is classified by the route of infection. Cutaneous anthrax accounts for 95–99% of human cases. The spores gain entry via small cuts, abrasions or insect bites. Two to 5 days after exposure classic black eschars and oedema develop at the affected site, accompanied by malaise and fever. Seven to 10 days after onset 80% of cases spontaneously resolve. Intestinal anthrax results from ingestion of spore-contaminated meat. Nausea, vomiting, anorexia and fever develop and are followed by abdominal pain, haematemesis and occasionally bloody diarrhoea. The disease may then progress to a generalized toxaemia, shock, cyanosis and death in 50% of cases. Inhalation anthrax occurs when the spores gain access to the lungs. At the onset of illness symptomology is mild, resembling a common upper respiratory tract infection. After several days the patient exhibits a sudden onset of acute dyspnoea, diaphoresis and cyanosis, with death occurring within 24 h in most cases.

In animals, especially herbivores, the disease is usually rapidly fatal. In extremely sensitive species, such as Impala (*Aepyceros melampus*) the disease manifests as a severe peracute septicaemia, with death occurring in less than 24 h. In other herbivores, such as cattle and North American bison (*Bison bison*), a haemorrhagic septicaemia develops, including severe congestion, multiple petechial haemorrhages, cyanosis, poorly clotting blood and pronounced splenomegaly. Carnivores typically develop localized lesions with no or later-onset septicaemia. The lesions are of variable severity and are usually localized on the face or in the oral cavity.

Diagnosis

Isolation *of B. anthracis* provides the standard for confirmation of anthrax. Direct sampling of suspect cutaneous lesions is recommended. Samples should be obtained before therapy is initiated as vegetative cells are rapidly eliminated by antibiotics. With suspected animal cases a blood sample is best; however, the microbe may also be recovered from nasal and anal swabs, oedematous swellings or peripheral blood from an ear or tail. Detection of the components of the anthrax toxin is also diagnostic. This may be accomplished with various monoclonal and polyclonal sera against the components in immunoassays using blood or tissue specimens or cultured organisms.

Transmission

The vast majority of human cases are contracted directly from infected carcasses or the handling of contaminated products from morbid animals. Transmission of anthrax spores has been demonstrated with a wide variety of tabanid and mosquito species, and with stable-flies (*Stomoxys* species), but insects are not believed to play a major role in epizootics. Successful ingestion of infective doses of the microbe by biting insects occurs only within a limited period a few hours before death, when a large-scale bacteraemia develops, and a few hours after death, before the vegetative cells are destroyed by the putrefactive process.

Although domestic animal outbreaks of the disease may be traced to contaminated feed or nutrient supplements, in most cases the source of the spores remains unknown. Water may concentrate spores to infectious levels and may transport them to areas where they have a greater chance of contact with a susceptible animal. Similarly, excavations may uncover spores left during previous outbreaks and allow them to infect new hosts. Ants, earthworms and some coprophagous and necrophagous beetles (e.g. Dermestidae, see Beetles) have been implicated in transferring spores from buried carcasses back to the surface but their contribution to the initiation of outbreaks remains speculative. Recently it was demonstrated that blow-flies (Calliphoridae) can spread the disease from grazing to browsing herbivores during active outbreaks. The blow-flies feed on the carcasses of grazers which contract the spores from the soil with their grass diet. When disturbed the flies fly from the carcass and alight on nearby foliage, where they deposit spores in their faeces and vomit. Later browsing herbivore species eat the soiled leaves and contract anthrax. House-flies (*Musca domestica*) have been suspected of mechanically spreading anthrax, but there is little or no proof that they actually spread infections.

Treatment

The drugs of choice for treatment are erythromycin and tetracycline, which are given for 5–7 days and are almost 100% effective against cutaneous anthrax. Antibiotic treatment is also effective against intestinal anthrax, although, because it is a more systemic infection, mortality is still 25% with treatment. Antibiotics are only effective against vegetative cells, not the spores. Spores can remain in the alveolar spaces of the lungs for extended periods of time following inhalation. Because of this, it has been found effective to use vaccination in conjunction with antibiotic treatment when dealing with inhalation anthrax. The antibiotic eliminates any *B. anthracis* that germinate in the body prior to the development of immunity, which then provides protection once the antibiotic treatment is discontinued. Although antibiotic treatment is also effective in animal cases of anthrax, it is impractical with large or wild herds.

Control

Vaccines are available for personnel potentially at risk of contracting the disease and for domestic animals in endemic regions. During outbreaks in domestic animals the affected herd is quarantined and vaccinated, and infected carcasses are burned or buried to minimize environmental contamination from scavengers rending the carcasses. With wild herds quarantine and vaccination are impossible and control is limited to surveillance and rapid disposal of carcasses.

Selected bibliography

Braack, L.E. and de Vos, V. (1990) Feeding habits and flight range of blow-flies (*Chrysomyia* spp.) in relation to anthrax transmission in the Kruger National Park, South Africa. *Onderstepoort Journal of Veterinary Research* 57, 141–142.

Bradaric, N. and Punda-Polic, V. (1992) Cutaneous anthrax due to penicillin-resistant *Bacillus anthracis* transmitted by an insect bite. *The Lancet* 340, 306–307.

Dixon, T.C., Meselson, M., Guillemin, J. and Hanna, P.C. (1999) Anthrax. *New England Journal of Medicine* 341, 815–826.

Turell, M.J. and Knudson, G.B. (1987) Mechanical transmission of *Bacillus anthracis* by stable flies (*Stomoxys calcitrans*) and mosquitoes (*Aedes aegypti* and *Aedes taeniorhynchus*). *Infection and Immunity* 55, 1859–1861.

Arboviruses

C.A. Hart

Most of the infections listed in this book are caused by a special category of viruses (see entry) termed arboviruses. The word arbovirus is derived from <u>ar</u>thropod-<u>bo</u>rne <u>vi</u>rus – that is, a virus biologically transmitted by haematophagous arthropods, such as mosquitoes or ticks, biting vertebrate hosts. The virus replicates in the vector and, following a particular migration route, such as passing to the vector's stomach during ingestion of a blood meal, it then migrates to the salivary glands. In the vertebrate host arboviruses usually produce viraemia. Other viruses can be mechanically transmitted by arthropods but involve no replication or long-term survival in the vector, such as fleas and mosquitoes transmitting myxoma viruses causing myxomatosis in rabbits; these are not arboviruses. The term arbovirus has no taxonomic significance, merely describing the mode of transmission of viruses of many families, subfamilies and genera.

Nearly all arboviruses are zoonotic; that is, they are primarily infections of vertebrates other than humans. However, a few appear to involve only humans. Certain birds and rodents are termed maintenance or reservoir hosts because they provide a mechanism for the long-term survival of viruses. In addition to serving as reservoir hosts of virus in a particular geographical area, some maintenance hosts can carry infections into new areas, even to different continents (e.g. West Nile in New York in 1999 and 2000).

Maintenance hosts often show no signs of illness. Ticks, which can live for many years, are sometimes also regarded as maintenance hosts. Other animals, pigs in the case of Japanese encephalitis virus, are amplifying hosts because they produce very high-titre viraemias in their blood, often for relatively long periods. This ensures that a potential vector ingests large numbers of viruses, thus greatly enhancing its likelihood of becoming infected. Viraemias of low titre and short duration are less likely to be infectious for vectors.

The most important arboviruses are in the families Togaviridae (only genus *Alphavirus*), Flaviviridae (only genus *Flavivirus*), Bunyaviridae (members of the genera *Bunyavirus*, *Nairovirus*, *Phlebovirus* and a number of unassigned viruses), Reoviridae (genera *Orbivirus* and *Coltivirus*) and Rhabdoviridae (genera *Ephemerovirus* and *Vesiculovirus*). Other viruses have been isolated from arthropods but they are not arboviruses.

With the exception of African swine fever (a DNA virus) and a very few other viruses, all arboviruses are RNA viruses. Of the 504 arboviruses listed in the 1985 international catalogue of arboviruses, 115 are considered to be definitely arboviruses, 92 are probably arboviruses, 265 are possible arboviruses and the remaining 32 most probably are not true arboviruses. Of the arboviruses, some 100 infect humans and about 40 infect livestock. The greatest number of arboviruses belong to the family Bunyaviridae (*c.* 250 species), but the most important economically are in the families Flaviviridae (*c.* 67 species) and the Togaviridae (*c.* 26 species). Families containing the most well-known viruses are as follows:

Togaviridae

Enveloped (50–70 nm), single-stranded, positive-sense RNA viruses with an icosahedral nucleocapsid (e.g. eastern equine encephalitis, western equine encephalitis, Venezuelan equine encephalitis, Ross River, Semliki Forest, Sindbis viruses).

Flaviviridae

Enveloped (45 nm), single-stranded, positive-sense RNA viruses with icosahedral symmetry (e.g. mosquito-borne viruses, such as dengue, Japanese encephalitis, yellow fever, St Louis encephalitis and West Nile, and tick-borne viruses, such as louping ill, Kyasanur Forest disease, tick-borne encephalitis and Powassan viruses).

Bunyaviridae

Enveloped (80–120 nm), single-stranded, trisegmented, negative-sense RNA viruses with icosahedral symmetry (e.g. genus *Bunyavirus*: Bunyamwera, Akabane, Oropouche, Germiston and La Crosse viruses; genus *Phlebovirus*: Phlebotomus fever and Rift Valley fever viruses and the Uukuniemi group; and genus *Nairovirus*: Crimean–Congo haemorrhagic fever, Nairobi sheep disease and Dugbe viruses).

Reoviridae

Unenveloped (70 nm), multiply segmented, double-stranded RNA viruses with spherical symmetry (e.g. genus *Orbivirus*: bluetongue, African horse sickness viruses; genus *Coltivirus*: Colorado tick fever virus).

Rhabdoviridae

Enveloped (usually 50–100 nm), bullet- or rod-shaped viruses with a negative-sense, linear RNA genome (e.g. genus *Ephemerovirus*: bovine ephemeral fever viruses; genus *Vesiculovirus*: vesicular stomatitis viruses).

Asfaviridae

Enveloped (175–215 nm), double-stranded, DNA viruses with icosahedral symmetry. The only member is African swine fever, formerly classified with the Iridoviridae.

Only the more important or scientifically more interesting arboviruses are considered in this encyclopedia.

Selected bibliography

Fields, B.N., Knipe, D.M. and Howley, P.M. (eds) (1996) *Fields Virology*, 3rd edn, Vol. 1, pp. 1–1504, Vol. 2, pp. 1505–2950. Lippincott-Raven, Philadelphia.

Karabatsos, N. (ed.) (1985) *International Catalogue of Arboviruses Including Certain Other Viruses of Vertebrates*, 3rd edn. American Society of Tropical Medicine and Hygiene, San Antonio, Texas, 1147 pp.

Monath, T.P. (ed.) (1988) *The Arboviruses: Epidemiology and Ecology*, Vol. I, introductory chapters, 329 pp. In the following volumes viruses are listed alphabetically: Vol. II, African horse sickness to dengue, 272 pp.; Vol. III, eastern encephalomyelitis to o'nyong nyong, 234 pp.; Vol. IV, Oropouche to Venezuelan equine encephalomyelitis, 243 pp.; Vol. V, Vesicular stomatitis to yellow fever, 241 pp. CRC Press, Boca Raton, Florida.

Murphy, F.A., Fauquet, C.M., Bishop, D.H.L., Ghabrial, S.A., Jarvis, A.W., Martelli, G.P., Mayo, M.A. and Summers, M.D. (eds) (1995) Sixth report of the International Committee on Taxonomy of Viruses. *Archives of Virology*, Suppl. 10, 586 pp.

Porterfield, J.S. (ed.) (1980) *Andrewes' Viruses of Vertebrates*. Baillière-Tindall, London, 457 pp.

Saluzzo, J.F. and Dodet, B. (eds) (1997) *Factors in the Emergence of Arbovirus Diseases*. Elsevier, London, 286 pp.

Webster, R.G. and Granoff, A. (eds) (1998) *Encyclopedia of Virology*. Academic Press, London, 1997 pp.

Astrakan fever *see* **Tick-borne typhuses.**

Avian borreliosis

Klaus Kurtenbach and Stefanie M. Schäfer

Avian borreliosis, or avian spirochaetosis, historically refers to infection of domestic birds with *Borrelia anserina*. However, various other species of the genus *Borrelia* are now known to infect avian hosts, such as *B. burgdorferi* sensu stricto or *B. garinii*, the causative agents of Lyme borreliosis (see entry) in humans.

Distribution

Borrelia anserina is distributed worldwide and is of economic importance in breeding domestic poultry, such as turkeys, Pheasants (*Tragopan satyra*) and chickens. Although largely under control in industrialized countries, it remains an important avian pathogen in the tropics.

Aetiological agent

Like other spirochaetes of the genus *Borrelia*, *B. anserina* has an ultrastructure which is unique amongst eubacteria. The 0.20–025 μm wide cells are helically shaped, with a length of 9–21 μm. Their wavelength of 1.7 μm is shorter than that found for Lyme borreliosis spirochaetes. An outer surface membrane consisting of lipoproteins encases the protoplasmic cylinder, in which up to eight flagella are inserted. These periplasmic flagellae, which confer motility, are ultrastructurally and chemically similar to external flagellae of other eubacteria.

Borrelia anserina used to be perpetuated through experimental birds or embryonated chicken eggs. The development of modified Barbour–Stoenner–Kelly (BSK) medium to culture *B. burgdorferi* sensu lato and relapsing fever spirochaetes now allows the *in vitro* propagation of *B. anserina*. However, infectivity of *B. anserina* for chickens is lost after a few *in vitro* passages. Murinization of *B. anserina* has proved to be impossible.

Phylogeny and taxonomy

Traditionally, many *Borrelia* species have been delineated and named using Linnaean binomials based on the tick species by which they are transmitted. *Borrelia anserina* comprises *Borrelia* strains that are associated with soft (argasid) ticks of the genus *Argas*. Phylogenetic analysis of the flagellin genes has placed *B. anserina* in a cluster together with American relapsing fever spirochaetes, such as *Borrelia hermsii*. Phylogeny based on the 16S ribosomal RNA (rRNA) sequences, however, indicates that *B. anserina* constitutes a cluster separate from the relapsing fever spirochaetes (see Tick-borne relapsing fever).

Clinical signs and pathology

Avian spirochaetosis is acute and characterized by fever, cyanosis of the head and diarrhoea. Mortality is normally high in domestic chickens; however, it varies with the *B. anserina* strain, as well as the race and age of the host. Peak spirochaetaemia in susceptible, experimentally infected chickens is recorded 72–96 h after infection, followed by progressive enlargement of spleen, extensive erythrophagocytosis in various organs and extravascular haemolysis. As with other species of the genus *Borrelia*, no defined pathogenicity factors have yet been found, but it has been suggested that immune mechanisms, involving solubilized antigens, may underlie pathogenicity. Lipoproteins ranging between 20 and 22 kDa have recently been identified as possible determinants of the pathogenic potential of *B. anserina*. These belong to the family of 20 kDa outer surface proteins (Osps) found in many *Borrelia* species, comprising the small variable membrane proteins (Vmps)

of relapsing fever spirochaetes and the OspC of *B. burgdorferi* sensu lato.

Diagnosis

Diagnosis of acute avian spirochaetosis in domestic chicken populations mainly relies on the recognition of clinical symptoms, such as greenish diarrhoea, and on direct microscopical detection of the spirochaetes in blood smears stained by Giemsa.

Transmission

Transmission cycles involve mainly domestic birds and soft (argasid) ticks, and outbreaks of the disease among domestic fowl are still frequent in many parts of the tropics. *Argas persicus* and *Argas sanchezi* are among the most important vector species. Although wild fowl and perhaps other avian species are susceptible to *B. anserina*, the precise roles wildlife plays in the global spread of this pathogen are unknown.

Prevention and control

Prevention of avian spirochaetosis is based on antibiotics and the application of acaricides in order to control tick infestations. No vaccine exists because of the strain-specific nature of immunity.

Selected bibliography

DaMassa, A.J. and Adler, H.E. (1979) Avian spirochetosis: natural transmission by *Argas* (*Persicargas*) *sanchezi* (Ixodoidea: Argasidae) and existence of different serologic and immunologic types of *Borrelia anserina* in the United States. *American Journal of Veterinary Research* 40, 154–157.

Fukunaga, M., Okada, K., Nakao, M., Konishi, T. and Sato, Y. (1996) Phylogenetic analysis of *Borrelia* species based on flagellin gene sequences and its application for molecular typing of Lyme disease borreliae. *International Journal of Systematic Bacteriology* 46, 89–905.

Hovind-Hougen, K. (1995) A morphological characterization of *Borrelia anserina*. *Microbiology* 141, 79–83.

Lad, P.L. and Soni, J.L. (1982) Soluble spirochaete antigen–antibody immune complex in plasma of *Borrelia anserina*-infected chickens.

Indian Journal of Animal Science 53, 583–541.

Marti-Ras, N., Lascola, B., Postic, D., Cutler, S.J., Rodhain, F., Baranton, G. and Raoult, D. (1996) Phylogenesis of relapsing fever *Borrelia* spp. *International Journal of Systematic Bacteriology* 46, 859–865.

Rao, M.L.V. and Soni, J.L. (1986) Preliminary studies on murinization of *Borrelia anserina*.

Indian Journal of Animal Science 56, 1187–1189.

Sambri, V., Marangoni, A., Olmo, A., Storni, E., Montagnani, M., Fabri, M. and Cevenini, R. (1999) Specific antibodies reactive with the 22-kilodalton major outer surface protein of *Borrelia anserina* Ni-NL protect chicks from infection. *Infection and Immuniy* 67, 2633–2637.

Avian malarias *see* Malaria, avian.

Babesia species *see* **Babesiosis**.

Babesiosis

Gerrit Uilenberg

Distribution

Babesiosis of domesticated animals is a group of diseases, caused by different pathogenic agents, occurring from temperate to tropical regions. It is particularly important in tropical and subtropical areas, but may cause losses even in temperate areas, particularly in traditional production systems.

Parasite

Babesiosis is caused by intra-erythrocytic protozoan parasites of the genus *Babesia*, belonging to the class Apicomplexa (= Sporozoa). They are members of the family Babesiidae, tick-borne parasites which live and multiply as 'piroplasms' in the red cells of the vertebrate host. These piroplasms do not contain pigment (as do the erythrocytic stages of *Plasmodium*), and in this respect resemble the related Theileriidae (main genus *Theileria*). A fundamental difference between *Babesia* and *Theileria* (see Theilerioses) is the absence in the former of multiplication by schizogony, which *Theileria* undergoes in lymphocytes or other cells, preceding the erythrocytic stage. Some parasites formerly classified in the genus *Babesia* have thus been assigned to *Theileria* after their extra-erythrocytic schizogony and other relevant differences with *Babesia* were discovered. An example is *Theileria equi*, until recent years considered to be a *Babesia*. Another difference with the Theileriidae is that the multiplication of the piroplasm, by budding, usually results in two daughter parasites, against four in *Theileria*; this is not, however, an absolute rule. The cycle of *Babesia* in the invertebrate (tick) host is also different from that of *Theileria*. In both cases the piroplasms apparently form gametocytes and zygotes in the gut of the tick, but in the case of *Babesia* the zygotes multiply and penetrate as 'vermicules' into numerous tick organs, including the ovaries, so that there is transovarial transmission to ticks of the next generation, contrary to what happens in *Theileria*. Infections by *Babesia* are known to occur in all groups of mammals, including humans, and even in some other vertebrates.

Transmission

It is usually the female tick that becomes infected by ingesting parasites with the blood meal. New hosts are infected with sporozoites in the saliva of ticks of the next generation, larvae, nymphs and/or adults. The sporozoites are the end result of sporogony in the salivary glands, infected by vermicules. Maturation of the sporozoites is stimulated by feeding, and therefore transmission does not occur immediately upon fixation of the tick on the host, so that its early removal may prevent transmission. Certain *Babesia* species may maintain themselves in several generations of ticks, even without new infections (this is in particular well known of *Babesia ovis*).

Epidemiology

One of the important aspects of babesiosis is the fact that animals remain long-term carriers of the parasite after recovery, and as long as the parasite exists in their organism reinfections will not cause disease. In circumstances where tick vectors are sufficiently numerous to cause frequent reinfections, the immune status of the animals persists indefinitely. Other extremely important points include tolerance or resistance (the animals are not refractory to infection, but tolerate its effects rather well). Young animals possess an age-linked tolerance to the clinical effect of infection and breeds in endemic areas have acquired innate tolerance (genetic resistance), the effect of natural selection. These points have been particularly well studied in cattle babesiosis in tropical countries (due to *Babesia bigemina* and/or *Babesia bovis*), where it is possible to attain a state of *endemic stability*. In stable endemic areas the number of ticks is sufficient to infect all young calves, which do not suffer unduly from the effects, particularly if they belong to a breed with innate tolerance, and the immunity thus acquired is maintained by frequent reinfections.

It should be pointed out that some of the statements made in this entry are rather simplistic, in order not to make it too long and complicated. For example, the existence of antigenically different strains of *Babesia* will not be dealt with, nor will the the fact that various immunodepressive factors may occasionally be responsible for a breakdown of the balance between host and parasite and cause relapses. Another point that will not be gone into is the fact that a 'sterile immunity' may persist for some time after the carrier state is lost.

Babesiosis of various animal species is briefly discussed below, with remarks on aspects specific to each species. Epidemiology, symptoms, pathology, diagnosis, chemotherapy and prophylaxis are presented in general terms. Human babesiosis is also briefly mentioned, but babesiosis of some domestic animals (such as cats and pigs) is not included; although this may be locally of some importance, its worldwide impact is not great. Table 1 shows the species discussed, with vectors and distribution.

Bovine babesiosis

The main species of *Babesia* of cattle in the tropics and subtropics are *B. bigemina* and *B. bovis*, with *Boophilus* species as the main tick vectors. Both *Babesia* species are transmitted by *Boophilus microplus* and *Boophilus annulatus*, but *Boophilus decoloratus* is a vector of *B. bigemina* only; the vector role of *Boophilus geigyi* is not yet well established. The most important *Babesia* species in temperate Europe is *B. divergens*, which has also been found in North Africa. It is transmitted by the tick *Ixodes ricinus*. *Babesia major*, another species in Europe, is a much milder infection; vectors are species of *Haemaphysalis*, *H. punctata* in western Europe. *Babesia ovata* is a closely related

Table 1.   Selected *Babesia* species of some domestic animals.

Domestic host	Main vector genus	Distribution
Cattle		
B. bigemina	*Boophilus*	Tropical and subtropical areas of all continents
B. bovis	*Boophilus*	Tropical and subtropical areas of all continents*
B. divergens	*Ixodes*	Europe, North Africa
B. major	*Haemaphysalis*	Europe
Small ruminants		
B. motasi	*Haemaphysalis*	Africa, Asia, Europe
B. ovis	*Rhipicephalus*	Africa, Asia, Europe
Horses (and other equines)[†]		
B. caballi	*Dermacentor, Hyalomma, Rhipicephalus*	Africa, America, Asia, Europe
Dogs		
B. canis	*Dermacentor, Haemaphysalis, Rhipicephalus*	All continents[‡]
B. gibsoni	*Haemaphysalis, Rhipicephalus*	Africa, America, Asia, Europe

Babesia bovis is less widespread in tropical Africa; the most common *Boophilus* species in that region, *B. decoloratus*, is not a vector of *B. bovis* (but is of *B. bigemina*).

[†] *Theileria equi*, transferred from genus *Babesia*, is not included in this list, but is mentioned in the text.

[‡] The species *B. canis* consists of three different but morphologically similar parasites; the one transmitted by *Dermacentor* ticks occurs in Europe and probably parts of Asia, that transmitted by *Haemaphysalis* is African and the parasite transmitted by *Rhipicephalus* occurs on all continents.

species in Japan, also transmitted by *Haemaphysalis* ticks. *Babesia bigemina* is large (Fig. 1), *B. major* is slightly smaller and *B. bovis* and *B. divergens* are much smaller. Most of the piroplasms of the last-mentioned species are situated at the periphery of the red cell (Fig. 2). Red cells infected by *B. bovis* are concentrated in the capillaries of the internal organs, such as the cerebral cortex (Fig. 3), while they are usually scanty in the peripheral circulation. An early name for the disease due to *B. bigemina* is 'Texas fever', as it was first described in Texas. *Babesia bovis* is particularly pathogenic for European cattle (*Bos taurus*), much less so for zebu cattle (*Bos indicus*) and indigenous African and Middle East taurine cattle.

Babesiosis of sheep and goats

The main species described so far are *Babesia motasi*, which is large and transmitted by *Haemaphysalis punctata*, and *B. ovis*, small round parasites, situated usually at the periphery of the red cell. The latter is transmitted by *Rhipicephalus bursa*. The taxonomy and even the geographical distribution of babesial parasites of small ruminants are not quite settled. Isolates of *B. motasi* from north-western Europe are far milder clinically than those from the Mediterranean basin, and there are serological differences as well. Babesial parasites of small ruminants in tropical countries do not always have the classical morphology of *B. motasi* or *B. ovis*. On the

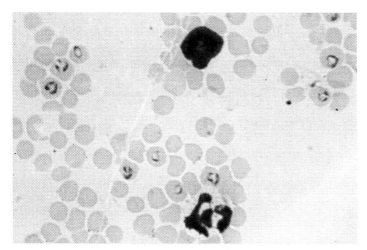

Fig. 1. *Babesia bigemina* in a bovine blood smear.

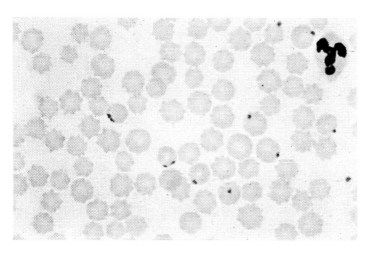

Fig. 2. *Babesia divergens* in a bovine blood smear.

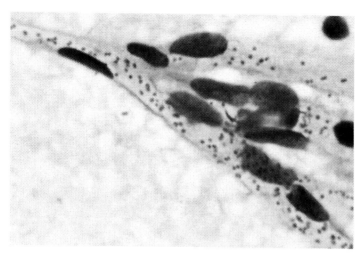

Fig. 3. Cerebral capillary filled with red cells infected with *Babesia bovis*.

whole *B. ovis* is a more important parasite than *B. motasi*, and generally sheep are more susceptible to the clinical effects of babesial infections than goats.

Equine babesiosis

Babesia caballi and *Theileria equi* generally have the same tick vectors, belonging to the genera *Dermacentor, Hyalomma* and *Rhipicephalus*; therefore equine babesiosis and theileriosis are usually discussed together. The term 'equine piroplasmosis' covers both, piroplasmosis being the old name for diseases in which piroplasms are found in red cells. These diseases may be important in their own right, but they are also an important obstacle to international movement of horses and other equines, as several countries require that all equines be tested for antibodies to both parasites before allowing their importation, thus affecting not only trade, but also international equestrian sporting events. It is relatively easy to sterilize horses from *B. caballi* by administering high and repeated doses of certain babesicides, so that after a certain time the antibody titres will drop below the detection threshold, but getting rid of *T. equi* is far more problematic, if not impossible.

Canine babesiosis

Canine babesiosis occurs on all continents. Although all large parasites of dogs are usually called *Babesia canis*, they actually belong to three different subspecies or perhaps even species, transmitted by different tick vectors. The common dog tick, *Rhipicephalus sanguineus*, is the main vector of the cosmopolitan parasite *B. canis vogeli*, which causes a comparatively mild disease. The European *B. canis canis*, transmitted by *Dermacentor* ticks, such as *D. reticulatus*, is far more pathogenic, while the African *B. canis rossi*, which has ticks of the *Haemaphysalis leachi* group as its vectors, is the most virulent of the three. As it is impossible to distinguish morphologically between the three parasites, they are usually just called *B. canis*.

Besides these large parasites, there is a small species, *Babesia gibsoni* which may cause a fatal disease. It is common in Asia and Africa, where it appears to be transmitted by *Haemaphysalis* as well as *Rhipicephalus* ticks. Although cases have been recorded where the parasite has been contracted in the USA and in Europe, apparently transmitted by the common dog tick, *R. sanguineus*, most cases, in European countries at least, are observed in dogs imported from endemic areas of Asia or Africa. Recent molecular studies have shown that the name *B. gibsoni* has been applied to two or more very different parasites of dogs, which resemble each other morphologically.

Human babesiosis

Babesia divergens of cattle in Europe causes babesiosis in humans without a spleen, while intact individuals are apparently refractory to infection. Such cases are sporadic, but usually fatal.

It was later discovered that *Babesia microti* (or at least what is called *B. microti* in the USA) of rodents can infect human beings, even those with an intact spleen. The disease is serious in individuals without a spleen, but much milder in intact people. It should be added that schizogony has been described in *B. microti* infections and, as division in the red cell results in four daughter parasites, the rodent parasite may well be much nearer to *Theileria* than to *Babesia*. Other babesial parasites which infect humans have also been discovered; animals are always the source of the infection.

Symptomatology and pathology

The classical signs of babesiosis are fever, haemoglobinuria and anaemia, followed by icterus, but all these signs are not always present; it depends on the stage of the infection, the *Babesia* species and the individual case. After having divided, the parasites break out of their host cell, the erythrocyte, and haemoglobin is liberated into the blood plasma. When the haemoglobin reaches a critical level, it is excreted in the urine, causing haemoglobinuria or 'red-water'; thus red-water fever is a common name for babesiosis. (The colour of the urine may be brown, depending on the proportion of haemoglobin converted into methaemoglobin.) The urine foams, because of the high protein content. It is important to distinguish between haemoglobinuria and haematuria, which results from bleeding; if in doubt, the difference can be demonstrated by centrifuging a urine sample, as in the case of haematuria there will be blood cells in the sediment. When many infected red cells are destroyed, anaemia develops, which is associated with the usual regenerative blood picture (normoblasts, Howell–Jolly bodies, reticulocytes, anisocytosis, poikilocytosis, etc.). Some of the haemoglobin is changed in the liver into bilirubin – hence the development of icterus after some time.

Pathological post-mortem findings are also explained by the pathogenesis. The carcass is anaemic, often icteric, and the urine bladder may contain reddish or brownish urine. The spleen is usually enlarged and the liver congested, with a distended biliary bladder. In some cases of bovine babesiosis due to *B. bovis* there are central nervous symptoms. Infected cells tend to stick together in the capillaries of internal organs and prevent a normal blood flow and, when this occurs extensively in the cerebral cortex, central nervous symptoms are observed. Similar nervous signs are also seen sometimes in canine babesiosis.

Diagnosis

It is probably good to point out straight away the important difference between 'infection by *Babesia*' and 'babesiosis', the latter meaning disease caused by *Babesia* infections.

Serological tests are actually the only ones allowed to detect carrier horses, and are generally useful for detecting past infections in all animal species. Such tests may also be useful for helping in the diagnosis of atypical chronic cases of canine babesiosis, but in general the diagnosis of babesiosis, i.e. the disease, depends on the presence of clinical signs, associated with the detection of parasites in blood smears. Diagnosis is rather easy when all the classical symptoms are present (fever, anaemia, haemoglobinuria, icterus). Many other infections may be the cause of each of these separate symptoms; all of them are not always present in babesiosis and their appearance also depends on the stage of the disease. When in doubt, a blood smear made at the right moment, fixed with methanol and stained with Giemsa (or fast stains such as Diff-Quik), will confirm the clinical diagnosis. However, a negative result does not always exclude babesiosis, because the parasites are often scanty after the first peak (and usually throughout in the case of *B. bovis*). Signs of anaemia (regenerative changes in the blood picture) may be of help.

For research purposes there are specific tests, based on molecular techniques such as nucleic acid probes and the polymerase chain reaction, which are able to accurately identify various species and even subtypes.

Prevention and control
Tick control

Babesiosis is a vector-borne disease; it is therefore logical to think of breaking the cycle by controlling the tick vectors. However, some ticks, such as the European *Ixodes ricinus*, vector of *B. divergens*, can complete their life cycle on several wild as well as domestic animal species, and controlling the tick on the target host species will not affect this permanent and inaccessible reservoir of infection. Furthermore, intensive tick control is expensive and cost–benefit is often negative, while intensive use of acaricides inevitably leads to acaricide resistance and also constitutes a public health problem because of residues in animal products. In certain conditions, and particularly in cattle in tropical countries, it is preferable to try to attain endemic stability, in which all cattle are infected early in life, when they are least susceptible to the effects of the infection. This means that tick control, often necessary because of the direct effects of large numbers of ticks, should not be so intensive that the state of endemic stability is disrupted; at the same time the onset of acaricide resistance in ticks is delayed when the intervals between applications are longer.

In certain conditions it may be possible to avoid contact with ticks by taking a few simple measures, such as keeping cattle on zero grazing – that is, in stables. Also, cattle often come into contact with *I. ricinus* on the edge of forests or shrub vegetation and hedges; this tick species needs the protection of a vegetational layer and will not survive on pastures with short grass. A buffer zone between the pasture and surrounding vegetation may therefore be of help.

In short-haired dogs it is certainly good practice to inspect the animal daily and remove all ticks that are encountered, but it is far easier and more effective to use good tick collars. These are made of synthetic material impregnated with an acaricide; the active ingredient is slowly released and diffuses over the skin. Many of the collars sold against fleas are not reliable against ticks. No collar can be relied upon entirely to prevent tick-borne diseases (babesiosis,

ehrlichiosis, Lyme disease, etc.). Relatively reliable collars are those containing an amidine, amitraz (which, however, is not active against fleas!) or pyrethroids, such as deltamethrin or flumethrin, in combination with the carbamate insecticide, propoxur.

For the last few years, there have been commercialized vaccines against the important tropical cattle tick *Boophilus microplus*, vector of *B. bigemina* and *B. bovis* (and also of bovine anaplasmosis). These vaccines are based on an antigen of the intestine of the tick, produced by recombinant techniques. The vaccinated animals develop antibodies against the antigen, and ticks which ingest these are affected by the destruction of their intestinal cells containing the antigen. These vaccines also act against the related tick *Boophilus annulatus*. As they are based on antibody levels, they have to be administered at intervals of 6 months or so. They are unlikely to constitute the ultimate answer to the problem of ticks and tick-borne diseases, but appear to be very promising as part of integrated control. The approach appears to be less promising for ticks which are not so specific for their host.

Immunization

Another approach to preventing clinical babesiosis is to immunize against the infection. This has been done for many decades by the 'infection and treatment' method and, with very few exceptions, is still the only method available. *Babesia* parasites are injected with blood from an infected animal and, where necessary, the reaction is treated with a specific babesicide, which in endemic areas should suppress the clinical reaction but not eliminate the parasite entirely. The method is mainly used against tropical babesiosis of cattle. Treatment is not often needed, as parasites of low pathogenicity are used. There are various problems associated with this method, a major one being the fact that blood containing live organisms may, and often does, contain unwanted pathogens. There are examples of bovine leucosis or anaplasmosis having been disseminated in this way. For these reasons, the infective material is usually produced by government laboratories; private industry is not keen to become involved.

Vaccines

There is one inactivated vaccine commercially available, against European canine babesiosis (*B. canis canis*), based on soluble antigens from *in vitro* cultures of the parasite. No such vaccine against babesiosis of other animals is currently available.

For many years various research teams have been trying to develop modern inactivated vaccines against babesiosis, based on molecular biology and/or genetic engineering. So far, none of these efforts has gone beyond an experimental stage, but future progress is to be expected, at least for those target species where the financial aspects are promising for private industry (e.g. valuable horses, pet animals).

Chemoprophylaxis

This is yet another way of preventing babesiosis, by administering a long-acting anti-babesial drug, such as imidocarb dipropionate, to animals which are then exposed to natural infection, in the hope that clinical signs will be mitigated and immunity will be installed. There are conflicting reports on the efficacy of this method. It probably depends on the frequency of natural infections, as it is of course imperative that an infection occurs while the drug level in the blood is sufficiently high.

Treatment

Finally, there is the curative treatment of individual cases of babesiosis, as a last resort but sometimes the only one if no effective method of prophylaxis can be applied. It should be realized that the number of available babesicidal drugs is very small. A number of drugs have been withdrawn from the market, which is generally too small to greatly interest the pharmaceutical industry. Rather than submit existing drugs to expensive tests as required by the newer safety regulations, they have been abandoned. The main drugs still available are summarized in Table 2; no new one has appeared for over 30 years! Additional supportive treatment may be essential in advanced stages of the disease with severe anaemia or nervous symptoms.

Selected bibliography

Bock, R.E., Kingston, T.G. and de Vos, A.J. (1999) Effect of breed of cattle on transmission rate and innate resistance to infection with *Babesia bovis* and *B. bigemina* transmitted by *Boophilus microplus*. *Australian Veterinary Journal* 77, 461–464.

Callow, L.L., Dalgiesh, R.J. and de Vos, A.J. (1997) Development of effective living vaccines against bovine babesiosis – the longest field trial. *International Journal of Parasitology* 27, 747–767.

FAO (1984) *Ticks and Tick-borne Disease Control. A Practical Field Manual.* Vol. I. *Tick Control,* pp. 1–299, Vol. II. *Tick-borne Disease Control,* pp. 300–621. Food and Agriculture Organization, Rome.

Table 2. Anti-babesial drugs*.

Common name	Some trade name(s)	Dosage and route	Comments
Imidocarb dipropionate	Imizol, Carbesia	1–3 mg kg^{-1} (3–6 in dogs), s.c. or i.m.	Residual effect (also prophylactic); in many countries restricted to animals, not used for human consumption
Phenamidine isethionate	Pirvedine	10 mg kg^{-1}, s.c. or i.m	Still used in dogs
Diminazene aceturate	Berenil, Ganaseg	3.5–5 mg kg^{-1}, i.m.	Not available in all countries
Quinuronium sulphate	Acaprine	1 mg kg^{-1}, s.c.	Still used against *B. ovis* infection in a few countries

*Dosage rates differ according to toxicity for individual animal species and efficacy against various *Babesia* species.

Friedhoff, K.T. and Soulé, C. (1996) An account of equine babesioses. *Revue Scientifique et Technique de l'Office International des Epizooties* 15, 1191–1201.

L'Hostis, M., Chauvin, A., Valentin, A., Marchand, A. and Gorenflot, A. (1995) Large-scale survey of bovine babesiosis due to *Babesia divergens* in France. *Veterinary Record* 136, 36–38.

Mahoney, D.F. (1994) The development of control methods for tick fevers of cattle in Australia. *Australian Veterinary Journal* 71, 283–289.

Mehlhorn, H. and Schein, E. (1984) The piroplasms: life cycles and sexual stages. *Advances in Parasitology* 23, 37–103.

Persing, D.H. and Conrad, P.A. (1995) Babesiosis – new insights from phylogenetic analysis. *Infectious Agents and Disease – Reviews Issues and Commentary* 4, 182–195.

Uilenberg, G. (1995) International collaborative research: significance of tick-borne haemoparastic diseases to world animals. *Veterinary Parasitology* 57, 19–41.

Yeruham, I., Hadani, A. and Galker, F. (1998) Some epizootiological and clinical aspects of ovine babesiosis caused by *Babesia ovis* – a review. *Veterinary Parasitology* 74, 153–163.

Bacillus anthracis see **Anthrax**.

Bacteria

C.A. Hart

Bacteria are prokaryotes – that is, they have no internal organelles, such as lysosomes or mitochondria (indeed, it is thought that mitochondria have evolved from primitive intracellular bacteria), nor do they have a nucleus. Most bacteria have a single loop of double-stranded DNA as a chromosome, although some, such as spirochaetes or *Burkholderia*, have several replicons, which can be linear or loops. Most are free-living but some, such as *Rickettsia*, *Ehrlichia* and *Chlamydia* species, are obligate intracellular pathogens.

Originally bacteria were classified by phenotypic characteristics, but more recently sequencing of 16S ribosomal RNA genes has been adopted. Phenotypic characteristics employed include the nature of the bacterial cell wall and presence or absence of spores. Gram-positive bacteria have only one cell membrane but a thicker cell wall, whereas Gram-negative bacteria have two cell membranes, and some bacteria, such as *Mycoplasma*, have no cell wall. Spores are tough structures that allow bacteria such as *Bacillus anthracis* (see Anthrax) or *Clostridia* to survive desiccation or heat. Other characteristics are atmospheric growth conditions (anaerobes will only grow in the absence of oxygen), bacterial shape (spheres: cocci; rods: bacilli; bent: *Vibrio* and *Campylobacter*; spiral: *Borrelia*, *Treponema*, *Leptospira*) and metabolic requirements.

Arthropods may be mechanical or biological vectors of bacteria. *Salmonella*, and *Shigella*, causing gastroenteritis, and *Chlamydia trachomatis*, causing trachoma, are transmitted mechanically by flies such as house-flies (*Musca domestica*), but there is no replication in the vector. In contrast, *Yersinia pestis* (plague), *Francisella tularensis* (tularaemia), *Ehrlichia chaffeensis* (monocytic ehrlichiosis) and *Rickettsia* species (e.g. spotted fever group of typhuses) replicate in their arthropod vectors and are biologically transmitted by them. Finally, some bacteria are employed as biopesticides – for example, *Bacillus thuringiensis* subspecies *israelensis* (*B. thuringensis* serotype H-14) and *Bacillus sphaericus*, both of which have been used to kill larvae of disease vectors, such as mosquitoes and simuliid black-flies.

Selected bibliography

Kreig, N.R. and Holt, J.G. (eds) (1984) *Bergey's Manual of Systematic Bacteriology*, 8th edn, Vol. 1, pp. 1–944. Vol. 2: Sneath, P.H.A., Mair, N.S., Sharpe, M.E. and Holt, J.G. (eds) (1986) pp. 965–1599. Vol. 3: Staley, J.J., Bryant, M.P., Pfennig, N. and Holt, J.G. (eds)

(1989) pp. 1601–2298. Vol. 4: Wiliams, S.T., Sharpe, M.E. and Holt, J.G. (eds) (1989)

Williams and Wilkins, Baltimore, Maryland, pp. 2299–2648.

***Balantium coli* *see* Cockroaches.**

Bancroftian filariasis

M.B. Nathan

Infection of humans with the filarial worm *Wuchereria bancrofti.* Together with *Brugia malayi* and *Brugia timori* (see Brugian filariasis), collectively referred to as human lymphatic filariasis because the adult worms live in the lymphatic system; otherwise known as elephantiasis due to the disfiguring enlargement of the limbs and thickening of the skin associated with chronic infection.

Distribution

Of an estimated 120 million human lymphatic filarial infections, approximately 90% are caused by *W. bancrofti.* They are found in over 70 humid, tropical and subtropical countries (Fig. 1). One-third of bancroftian filariasis infections are in India.

Other endemic countries in Asia include Bangladesh, Nepal, Sri Lanka, Maldives, Indonesia, the countries of the Mekong region (Laos, Cambodia, Vietnam, Thailand and Myanmar) and China, where the distribution has been greatly diminished by control measures. Bancroftian filariasis also occurs in Papua New Guinea and the Philippines. The nocturnal periodic form is by far the commonest, but a diurnal subperiodic form of the parasite occurs mainly in, but is not limited to, the eastern Pacific islands, including New Caledonia, Fiji, French Polynesia, Samoa, Tuvalu and the Cook Islands. A nocturnal subperiodic form exists in Thailand.

Another one-third of infections are found in Africa. The disease occurs in the

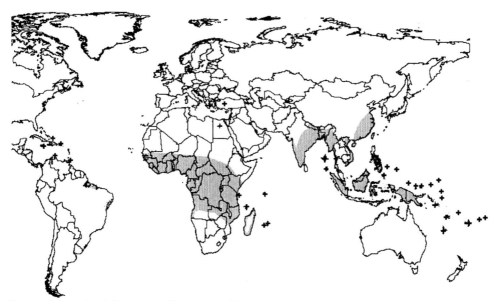

Fig. 1. Geographical distribution of bancroftian filariasis; crosses (+) denote very small foci, mainly on small islands.

Nile Delta area of Egypt, while south of the Sahara it is highly endemic in the coastal areas of Kenya, Tanzania, Zanzibar and Madagascar and in other areas of West and Central Africa.

Distribution in the Neotropics is limited to Haiti, Dominican Republic and coastal areas of Guyana and Brazil. Localized, low-level transmission may still persist in Trinidad and Tobago, Costa Rica and Suriname.

Parasite

Adult male (approximately 40 mm) and female (80–100 mm) *W. bancrofti* worms live in the lymphatic system within or adjacent to lymph nodes. Six months to a year after infection and fertilization, females begin to release large numbers of embryos, or microfilariae, each about 250 μm long and 'sheathed' in the egg membrane. Adult females live 4–6 years and produce millions of microfilariae, which actively migrate to the bloodstream, where they circulate for up to 2 years. They may also appear in hydrocoel fluid and in chylous urine. No further larval development occurs, until or unless the microfilariae are ingested by an intermediate mosquito host during blood-feeding.

Clinical symptoms

There is a wide range of clinical manifestations, with some geographical variance. More than 50% of people with microfilaraemia are clinically asymptomatic, even though they have hidden damage to their lymphatic or renal systems. Some individuals with microfilariae remain asymptomatic for years; others develop clinical disease while microfilariae continue to circulate or after the microfilariae have disappeared from the bloodstream. Clinical incubation is most commonly 8–16 months but can be considerably longer. Acute manifestations include recurrent and irregular 'filarial' fevers and general malaise, often associated with lymphadenitis and lymphangitis. Such attacks can last for up to 2 weeks and may recur several times a year. In males lymphangitis may be localized in the genitals.

Chronic disease typically develops 10–15 years after onset of the first acute attack but can occur much earlier. It is caused, at least in part, by lymphatic dysfunction, which frequently manifests as hydrocoel (Fig. 2), lymphoedema, elephantiasis (Fig. 3) and chyluria, the incidence and severity of which tend to increase with age. Hydrocoel typically presents as a swelling caused by accumulation of usually clear, straw-coloured fluid, sometimes containing microfilariae, within the membrane (tunica vaginalis) that surrounds each of the testicles. Other genital manifestations include inflammatory swelling of the spermatic cord and lymphoedematous thickening of the scrotal skin.

Elephantiasis begins as recurrent episodes of lymphoedema and leads to gradual loss of skin elasticity and fibrosis of the subcutaneous tissues, resulting from blockage of the lymphatics. The leg or legs are most commonly affected, either from the thigh or from the knee. However, the scrotum, arm(s), penis, vulva and breast(s) may also be affected. Bacterial and fungal infections of the skin are frequently associated with elephantiasis and play a major role in the

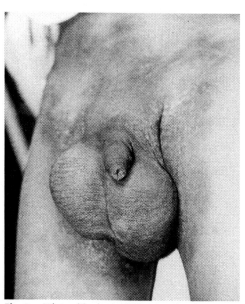

Fig. 2. Bilateral hydrocoel associated with *Wuchereria bancrofti* infection (courtesy of Eric Ottesen).

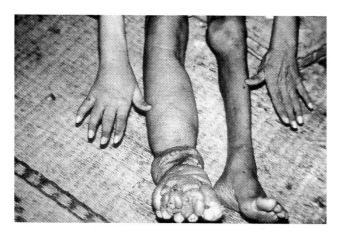

Fig. 3. Elephantiasis of the right leg and lymphoedema of the right hand in a patient infected with *Wuchereria bancrofti* (courtesy of Rifky Faris).

progression of disease and the frequency and severity of clinical symptoms. Chyluria, the excretion of 'milky urine' containing lymph and dietary lipids and proteins in the urinary tract, occurs in a minority of patients and is sometimes associated with haematuria. Occult filariasis, in which microfilariae cannot be found in the blood, is due to a hypersensitivity to microfilarial antigens. One manifestation of this immunological response is tropical pulmonary eosinophilia, a syndrome that is more common in males than females, and in which classical clinical manifestations are absent. It occurs particularly in endemic areas of the Indian subcontinent and South-East Asia, causing nocturnal paroxysmal cough, impaired lung function and chronic lung disease.

Chronic filarial disease imposes psychological, social and economic burdens on affected individuals, as well as physical suffering and disability. Persons with *hydrocoel*, lymphoedema and elephantiasis are often stigmatized and become isolated in their communities. Their ability to work may be compromised, leading to dependence on others for care and financial support. It has been estimated that, in India alone, over US$1000 million of productivity is lost every year as a consequence of infection.

Diagnosis

Detection and identification of microfilariae in the blood are widely used in situations where newly developed circulating filarial antigen tests are unavailable. Except in countries with diurnal subperiodic forms, microfilariae appear in the peripheral blood at night (nocturnal periodicity) and the optimal time for drawing samples is between 2200 h and 0200 h, which is extremely difficult under field conditions. Each method has its own advantages and disadvantages. However, the most commonly used method is to prepare and microscopically examine a Giemsa-stained thick blood film obtained by finger-prick. An alternative procedure is the counting-chamber method, in which a similar amount of anticoagulated capillary blood is lysed in water and examined under a microscope for motile microfilariae.

Increased sensitivity can be achieved by examining larger amounts of blood obtained by venepuncture. One such method is Knott's concentration, in which 1 ml of blood is shaken with 9 ml of distilled water and 1 ml of 40% formalin, centrifuged and the sediment examined as a wet or stained preparation under a microscope. Another, more efficient, method is by membrane filtration and involves the passage of up to 10 ml of anticoagulated blood through a polycarbonate filter with 3–5 µm pore size. Pre-filtered water and then air are passed through the filter, which is subsequently placed on a microscope slide, dried, stained with Giemsa and examined in clear mounting medium under a coverslip.

In some areas where the only microfilariae present are nocturnally periodic *W. bancrofti*, the diethylcarbamazine (DEC) provocative test has been used. This entails the oral daytime administration of 2–8 mg kg^{-1} body weight of DEC, which results in the subsequent appearance of microfilariae in the peripheral circulation. Finger-prick blood is usually taken and examined about 30 min after administration of the provocative dose. Because of severe host reactions to the dead or dying micro-filariae, this test should not be used in areas where there are infections with *Onchocerca volvulus* or *Loa loa* (see entries on Oncho-cerciasis and Loiasis).

A recent breakthrough in diagnosis is based on detection of circulating filarial antigens and has important implications for monitoring the effectiveness of treatment and control programmes. All individuals with microfilaraemia, as well as a proportion of those with clinical manifestations but with no circulating microfilariae, have detectable circulating antigen. Such tests are very sensitive and specific, require only finger-prick blood, which can be drawn at any time, and are available as commercial kits, one of which is in the form of a 'card test'.

Transmission

The vectors are anopheline and culicine mosquitoes; a list of the principal species is shown in Table 1. The nocturnal periodicity of the parasite throughout much of its distribution is such that the microfilariae are at their greatest concentration in the peripheral blood during the night, when the majority of vectors feed most avidly and the likelihood of ingesting microfilariae from capillary blood is greatest. Globally the most widespread and important vector is *Culex quinquefasciatus*, a circumtropical and mainly urban or peri-urban species that breeds prolifically in polluted water and feeds at night (see culicines under entry on Mosquitoes).

Some important anopheline vectors of malaria are also major vectors of *W. bancrofti*, particularly in more rural parts of Africa and elsewhere, e.g. *Anopheles gambiae* and *Anopheles funestus* in Africa, *Anopheles subpictus* in rural Indonesia and *Anopheles balabacensis* in Malaysia. In West Africa, *C. quinquefasciatus* is evidently a poor vector of anopheline-adapted strains of the parasite. Similarly, in parts of India anophelines are refractory to *C. quin-quefasciatus*-adapted strains of the parasite.

In the endemic Polynesian islands, the principal vectors are species within the *Aedes scutellaris* group. Here the parasite is diurnally subperiodic, in adaptation to the daytime or crepuscular biting behaviour of these mosquitoes. In a localized forest situation in west Thailand, a nocturnally subperi-odic strain of the parasite is transmitted by mosquitoes of the *Ochlerotatus[1] niveus* group.

The majority of mosquito species are refractory to *W. bancrofti*. If there is uptake during blood-feeding, microfilariae may be lethally damaged by the cibarial and pharyngeal armatures. In the stomach, rapid coagulation of the blood may inhibit their movement and penetration through the peritrophic membrane and gut wall; or after migration through the stomach wall they may be encapsulated and killed in the haemocoel or in the flight muscles. The

Table 1. Summary of the principal mosquito vectors of *Wuchereria bancrofti*.

Parasite strains	Geographical distribution	Vectors
Nocturnal periodic	Tropics, except Polynesia	*Culex quinquefasciatus*
	Tropics, except Polynesia	*Anopheles* species
	New Guinea	*Mansonia uniformis*
	China	*Ochlerotatus togoi*
	Philippines	*Ochlerotatus poicilius*
Diurnal subperiodic	Polynesia	*Aedes polynesiensis*
	Fiji	*Aedes pseudoscutellaris*
Nocturnal subperiodic	New Caledonia	*Ochlerotatus vigilax*
	Thailand	*Aedes niveus* group

physiological bases of such phenomena are not well understood. Even in vector species, some losses attributable to these mechanisms also occur. However, within hours of entering the mid-gut, surviving microfilariae lose their sheaths, penetrate the stomach wall and enter the thoracic muscles, where they metamorphose into sausage-shaped, first-stage larvae. Over a period of 10–14 days they moult twice and rapidly elongate into third-stage, infective larvae (1.2–1.6 mm long and 18–23 μm in diameter). Morphological features of the infective larva, in particular the shape and position of the three caudal papillae, aid in identification of the parasite in the intermediate mosquito host. The mature larvae leave the thoracic muscles and may be found in other parts of the body cavity, including the head and proboscis. During blood-feeding, larvae leave the proboscis and enter the skin via the puncture wound. Surviving larvae find their way into the lymphatics and thence to a site within or adjacent to a lymph node, where they develop to maturity and mate.

Intensity of transmission, expressed as the annual transmission potential (ATP), varies according to local epidemiology and the vector species involved. The ATP is the estimated number of infective larvae to which a person is exposed over a 1-year period. This in turn is derived from: (i) the annual biting rate (ABR), estimated from 24-h human bait landing catches conducted at regular intervals throughout a 12-month period; (ii) the proportion of mosquitoes which harbour infective (third-stage) larvae, determined by microscopic dissection; and (iii) the mean density of infective larvae per biting mosquito. Monitoring changes of the ATP using standardized methods can provide a useful measure of the impact of control measures on transmission, although human bait mosquito collection techniques are used less frequently than in the past, not least for practical and ethical reasons. The use of polymerase chain reaction (PCR) methods to detect species-specific parasite DNA in mosquitoes appears to offer some promise as an alternative to the slow and laborious dissection of mosquitoes for the study of filariasis transmission.

Treatment

For treatment of the infection in individual patients, single or repeated courses of DEC are given, usually at 6–8 mg kg^{-1} day^{-1} for 12 days, though recent data suggest that a single day of treatment (6–8 mg kg^{-1}) is as effective as the 12-day regimen. Such regimens are not invariably effective in eliminating infection, and DEC is not safe in patients with onchocerciasis or loiasis. Alternative drugs are ivermectin, which does not appear to kill the adult worms but effectively reduces microfilaraemia, and albendazole, which kills the adult worms but must be given daily for 2–3 weeks.

For affected individuals, managing the consequences of debilitating infection is often a main concern. Recognition that much of the pathology results from bacterial and fungal infection of tissues with compromised lymphatic function has led to significant advances in treatment. Simple, rigorous hygiene interventions can provide symptomatic relief and prevent both acute inflammatory episodes and further disease progression. These include the treatment of lymphoedema and elephantiasis with soap and water, applying antiseptic creams to small wounds and abrasions, raising the affected limb(s) at night, keeping the nails clean, bandaging and exercise, and the use of footwear. Systemic antibiotics may be needed to treat bacterial cellulitis. New surgical techniques and better management of lesions can improve the prospects for males with hydrocoel and other forms of genital damage.

Prevention and control

There is no animal reservoir host of *W. bancrofti*. Prevention and control can be achieved either by reducing contact between humans and infective vectors or by treating humans to reduce or eliminate microfilariae circulating in the bloodstream.

Vector control

In some tropical and subtropical areas, infrastructure development, particularly the provision of reliable water supplies and improved solid and liquid waste management, have contributed to a decline in densities of *C. quinquefasciatus* and a spontaneous reduction and even interruption of transmission, e.g. in Japan and the Caribbean islands of Barbados and Puerto Rico. In contrast, in many other areas, rapid unplanned urbanization, with inadequate sanitation systems, has led to the proliferation of polluted water bodies and high densities of *C. quinquefasciatus* and to the geographical expansion, intensified transmission or reappearance of bancroftian filariasis in areas where transmission had ceased.

In some areas where spraying the interior walls and ceiling/roof with residual insecticides has been conducted for malaria control (see Malaria, human) and in which the targeted anopheline vector is also a vector of lymphatic filariasis, there has been a reduction or cessation of transmission of the latter parasite, e.g. in the Solomon Islands. Similarly, in other geographical areas, indoor residual spraying for malaria control has had a beneficial effect on transmission of filarial parasites by mosquito genera other than *Anopheles*. The availability and proper use of insecticide-treated mosquito nets (usually with pyrethroid insecticides, such as permethrin) for individual protection against malaria vectors appears to offer additional prospects for reducing filariasis transmission involving nocturnal vectors. However, the extent to which pyrethroid resistance might reduce the efficacy of such measures has not been adequately explored, particularly in situations where *C. quinquefasciatus* is the main vector.

Insecticidal control of adult *Aedes* vectors is difficult given their general exophily and diurnal feeding behaviour. Similar considerations pertain to some *Mansonia* species, whereas other, endophagic, nocturnal species are more amenable to methods used for the control of adults of malaria vectors.

The application of larvicides to control the vectors in their aquatic stages, including chemical insecticides, insect growth regulators and bacterial larvicides (e.g. *Bacillus thuringiensis* subsp. *israelensis*), can also reduce adult mosquito populations in areas where the larval habitats are restricted. However, alone, these and other vector control methods have rarely been successful in controlling lymphatic filariasis, due, in large part, to the long lifespan of the adult worms and the difficulty of sustaining intensive vector control measures for such lengthy periods.

In local circumstances, notably in some townships of Zanzibar in the United Republic of Tanzania, where pit latrines are the major larval habitat of *C. quinquefasciatus*, several years of vector control have been achieved through application of expanded polystyrene beads to the pits. A floating layer of beads on the water surface forms an inert, permanent physical barrier which prevents gravid female mosquitoes from depositing their eggs. In combination with mass chemotherapy using DEC, transmission was greatly reduced in one township.

Treating the human host

Control programmes usually afford priority to chemotherapy interventions, intended to reduce microfilaria rates to levels at which transmission will cease. Successful mass or selective chemotherapy campaigns have been conducted in several countries using various DEC regimens, e.g. China, Suriname and Brazil. However, following cessation of treatment, there can be a reversal of gains in situations where there is continued presence of large vector populations and low-level parasitaemias. In recent years, two-drug treatment regimens, using albendazole and either ivermectin or DEC, have been developed. They are administered in a single dose given once yearly and have proved extremely effective in eliminating microfilariae. Their development led to a global initiative, launched by the World Health Organization in 1998, to eliminate lymphatic filariasis as a public health problem by the year 2020. The strategy for most countries will entail yearly mass treatments for 4–6 years of all 'at risk' populations in order to decrease microfilariae, interrupt transmission and thereby prevent infection. An alternative intervention is to use common table or cooking salt fortified with DEC in the endemic area for 1 year. At the same time, to alleviate the suffering caused by the disease, community education programmes will be carried out to promote the benefits of intensive and appropriate hygiene practices. A global partnership, which has been established to develop and implement the plans, involves ministries of health of the endemic countries, international organizations and development agencies, the private sector, non-governmental organizations and academia.

Note
1   *Ochlerotatus* was formerly a subgenus of *Aedes.*

Selected bibliography
King, C.L. and Freedman, D.O. (2000) Filariasis. In: Strickland, G.T. (ed.) *Hunter's Tropical Medicine,* 8th edn. W.B. Saunders, Philadelphia, pp. 740–753.

Nutman, T.B. (ed.) (2000) *Lymphatic Filariasis.* Tropical Medicine: Science and Practice, Vol. 1, Imperial College, London, 292 pp.

Ottesen, E.A., Duke, B.O.L., Karam, M. and Behbehani, K. (1997) Strategies and tools for the control/elimination of lymphatic filariasis. *Bulletin of the World Health Organization* 75, 491–503.

Sasa, M. (1976) *Human Filariasis. A Global Survey of Epidemiology and Control.* University Park Press, Tokyo, 819 pp.

Webber, R.H. (1979) Eradication of *Wuchereria bancrofti* infection through vector control. *Transactions of the Royal Society of Tropical Medicine and Hygiene* 73, 722–724.

Weil, G.J., Lammie, P.J. and Weiss, N. (1997) The ICT filarial test: a rapid-format antigen test for diagnosis of bancroftian filariasis. *Parasitology Today* 13, 401–404.

White, G.B. (1989) Lymphatic filariasis. In: World Health Organization (ed.) *Geographical Distribution of Arthropod-borne Diseases and Their Principal Vectors.* WHO/VBC/89.967, WHO, Geneva, pp. 23–34.

World Health Organization (1992) *Lymphatic Filariasis: the Disease and its Control.* Technical Report Series 821, 1–71.

Bangkok haemorrhagic disease *see* **Leucocytozoonosis.**

Barmah Forest virus disease

John S. Mackenzie

Infections of humans with Barmah Forest virus

Barmah Forest (BF) virus is the aetiological agent of an epidemic polyarthritic disease, known as Barmah Forest virus disease. It accounts for about 10% of cases of epidemic polyarthritis-like illness in Australia, and is thus the second most common arboviral disease in Australia. There are about 700 cases on average reported each year. The virus was first isolated from *Culex annulirostris* mosquitoes trapped in 1974 from the Barmah Forest of northern Victoria. At about the same time, a second isolate was obtained from *C. annulirostris* collected in south-west Queensland, and was initially called Murweh virus. Although early isolations in the mid-1970s were obtained from various mosquito species across a wide geographical area, including Victoria,

Queensland and the Northern Territory, BF virus was not associated with human infection until 1986, or with human disease until 1988. The first recognized epidemic of Barmah Forest disease occurred at Nhulunbuy in the Northern Territory in 1992 concurrently with an epidemic of Ross River (RR) virus (see entry), a closely related virus.

Distribution
Barmah Forest virus is found in all mainland states of Australia. There has been no evidence of the virus in offshore islands or in Papua New Guinea. Virus isolations have been made from a number of mosquito species and there has been a single report of isolation from *Culicoides marksi* from the Northern Territory near Darwin. There is evidence that the virus has only recently emerged in Western Australia; the virus

was first detected in 1989 in the north of the State, but it did not spread or cause apparent disease until a small epidemic in 1993–1994, and it then spread the following year into the south-west of the State. The mechanism of this spread is unknown.

Virus

Barmah Forest virus is an alphavirus with a positive single-stranded RNA genome of 11,488 nucleotides (prototype strain). Sequence studies show that it is related most closely to RR and Semliki Forest viruses (see entries), but on antigenic grounds it is placed as the sole member of a serological group. The BF virus envelope protein E2 is unique among sequenced alphaviruses in having no N-linked glycosylation sites.

Clinical symptoms and pathogenesis

Barmah Forest virus disease is an epidemic polyarthritis-like disease similar to that described for RR virus, a related Australian alphavirus, and indeed cannot be distinguished from it on clinical grounds. Barmah Forest virus disease has been reported in people in all age groups from 5 to 75 years. After an incubation period that is believed to be from 7 to 9 days in most cases, the clinical disease develops, characterized by arthritis, arthralgia, myalgia, fatigue, fever and rash. The rash appears to be relatively common, and its incidence has varied between just over 50% in one outbreak to 100% in another. Most patients present with a florid, erythematous, maculopapular rash covering about 75% of the body surface and, although it can last for 3–21 days, most commonly it lasts for about 4 days. The rash can be vesicular in about 10% of patients. Joint involvement is seen in most patients (69–86%), but only about 30% of cases report stiffness and swelling. The joints most commonly involved are the knees, wrists, ankles and metacarpophalangeal and interphalangeal joints of the fingers, but the elbows, toes, tarsal joints, vertebral joints, shoulders and hips can be involved. The signs of involvement can vary from restricted movement to prominent swelling and tenderness. There is less information

on chronicity of symptoms; there is anecdotal evidence that joint symptoms can last for at least 6 months. In one outbreak, 10% of cases had joint tenderness at 6 months, whereas in another up to 45% of patients had not fully recovered after a year.

No studies have been carried out to investigate the pathogenesis of BF virus disease.

Diagnosis

Laboratory diagnostic tests have only been available relatively recently, and it is probable that the incidence of BF virus infections is significantly under-reported. Laboratory diagnoses are made on the basis of serological tests, and are usually done by detection of immunoglobulin M (IgM) antibody. Frequently, only single specimens are sent for diagnosis and, as IgM antibody is believed to persist for several months, such diagnoses can only be considered presumptive. False-positive IgM responses have been a problem with first-generation commercial kits, so that tests with such kits should be considered negative if IgG antibody is absent. Antibody responses to BF virus appear to be slow and, in one outbreak, IgG antibody was not detected in most cases until 28 days after presentation with a rash. Virus isolation is not normally attempted. It is seldom effective, is technically demanding and labour-intensive and is only possible from seronegative patients. If early samples fail to show IgG antibodies, collecting a late-convalescent serum sample at least 4 weeks after onset of symptoms is recommended.

Transmission

The vertebrate hosts of BF virus are believed to be mammals, including marsupials, although the involvement of birds cannot be ruled out. Seroepidemiological studies have shown that the prevalence of antibodies is quite low in a number of marsupial species, and lower than found for the related RR virus. Barmah Forest virus has been isolated from a range of mosquito species, although the ability for most of them to transmit the virus is less certain. In coastal areas, two salt-marsh-breeding species,

Ochlerotatus[1] *vigilax* and *Ochlerotatus camptorhynchus*, are major vectors of BF virus. In inland rural areas and probably some urban areas, the major vector is *C. annulirostris*. Elsewhere, temporary ground-pool-breeding species, such as *Ochlerotatus bancroftianus*, *Ochlerotatus normanensis* and *Ochlerotatus pseudonormanensis*, are probably involved in transmission cycles, and *Coquillettidia linealis* is believed to be involved in urban areas.

Epidemiology and ecology

Most cases of BF virus disease are sporadic rather than epidemic, and the majority of cases are reported from Queensland. The first outbreak of BF virus disease occurred at Nhulunbuy in the Northern Territory during the summer of 1991–1992. This was followed by a smaller epidemic in Western Australia in 1993–1994. The largest epidemic to be reported occurred in the south coast area of New South Wales in 1994–1995, with 135 cases. Some outbreaks have been concurrent with RR virus, but, although both viruses share vectors and vertebrate hosts, this does not always occur.

Molecular epidemiological studies have shown limited sequence diversity between virus isolates from different geographical areas and/or collected in different years, but all strains sequenced are within a single topotype. This finding is a little surprising given the vertebrate hosts of the virus, all of which are sedentary. Thus the involvement of avian species or bats as additional vertebrate hosts of the virus cannot be ruled out.

Treatment

No specific treatment is available.

Prevention and control

Prevention has been largely directed at behavioural changes, with local warnings disseminated when epidemic activity is predicted. These warnings suggest the use of personal protection by applying insect repellents and wearing tops with long sleeves and long trousers at dusk and dawn. Adult mosquito control using insecticides is rarely used because of the difficulty in applying such agents effectively in most settings, and also because of environmental concerns. Larvicides have been employed successfully in certain habitats close to human habitation. Runnelling and improved drainage have been important in decreasing mosquito breeding in salt-marsh habitats.

Note

[1] *Ochlerotatus* was formerly a subgenus of *Aedes*.

Selected bibliography

Doggett, S.L., Russell, R.C., Clancy, J., Haniotis, J. and Cloonan, M.J. (1999) Barmah Forest virus epidemic on the south coast of New South Wales, Australia, 1994–1995: viruses, vectors, human cases, and environmental factors. *Journal of Medical Entomology* 36, 861–868.

Flexman, J.P., Smith, D.W., Mackenzie, J.S., Fraser, R.E., Bass, S., Hueston, L., Lindsay, M.D.A. and Cunningham, A.L. (1998) A comparison of the diseases caused by Ross River virus and Barmah Forest virus. *Medical Journal of Australia* 169, 159–163.

Lee, E., Stocks, C., Lobigs, M., Hislop, A., Straub, J., Marshall, I., Weir, R. and Dalgarno, L. (1997) Nucleotide sequence of the Barmah Forest genome. *Virology* 227, 509–514.

Mackenzie J.S. and Smith, D.W. (1996) Mosquito-borne viruses and epidemic polyarthritis. *Medical Journal of Australia* 164, 90–93.

Mackenzie, J.S., Lindsay, M.D., Coelen, R.J., Broom, A.K., Hall, R.A. and Smith, D.W. (1994) Arboviruses causing human disease in the Australasian region. *Archives of Virology* 136, 447–467.

Poidinger, M., Roy, S., Hall, R., Turley, P., Scherret, J., Lindsay, M., Broom, A., Burgess, G. and Mackenzie, J. (1997) Genetic stability among temporally and geographically diverse isolates of Barmah Forest virus. *American Journal of Tropical Medicine and Hygiene* 57, 230–234.

Russell, R.C. (1998) Vectors vs. humans in Australia – who is on top down under? An update on vector-borne disease and research on vectors in Australia. *Journal of Vector Ecology* 23, 1–46.

Bartonella bacilliformis *see* **Carrión's disease.**

Bartonella henselae *see* **Bartonella quintana** and **Bartonella henselae,** *and* **Cat-scratch disease**.

Bartonella quintana and Bartonella henselae

Karim E. Hechemy and Burt E. Anderson

Bartonellosis

The infections described here are due to former members of the genus *Rochalimaea* that were merged in 1993 with the genus *Bartonella*. They are to be distinguished from human bartonellosis, *Bartonella bacilliformis*, which causes Carrión's disease (see entry), also known as Oroya fever, which is endemic in the highlands of the Andes in South America.

The new members of the *Bartonella* are the epitome of the rationale for studying emerging infections and re-emerging infections. *Bartonella quintana*, the agent of trench fever, which all but disappeared after the First World War (1914–1918), has re-emerged as one of the agents of bacillary angiomatosis and bacillary peliosis in human immunodeficiency virus (HIV)-infected patients and patients with trench fever that have been identified recently. A new *Bartonella* agent, *Bartonella henselae*, was described in 1992 and subsequently associated with the above syndromes, and was shown to be the primary agent of cat-scratch disease (see entry). In addition, *B. henselae, B. quintana* and a third species, *Bartonella elizabethae*, have been implicated in causing endocarditis. A number of additional species have been isolated from a variety of different rodents, feline species, cattle and other animals. However, currently none of these species is thought to be a common human pathogen.

Nomenclature

Gene sequence data of 16S ribosomal RNA (rRNA) and DNA hybridization data revealed high levels of relatedness between *B. bacilliformis* and members of the former genus *Rochalimaea*, namely, *B. quintana*, *Bartonella vinsonii* and *B. henselae* (Table 1). The removal of these species from the

genus *Rochalimaea*, named after H. da Rocha-Lima in 1917, into the genus *Bartonella*, named after A.L. Barton in 1909, is because of the precedence of the *Bartonella* taxon. Both 16S rRNA gene sequencing and, to a lesser extent, DNA hybridization data have been used extensively to establish species and define phylogenetic relationships within the genus *Bartonella*.

Bacteria

Members of the genus *Bartonella* resemble members of the genus *Rickettsia* in morphology and staining. They are piliated, non-flagellated (except for *Bartonella clarridgeiae* and *B. bacilliformis*), short rods, 0.3–0.5 to 1.0–1.7 μm in size and frequently slightly curved. They are Gram-negative, and in the Giménez stain procedure *Bartonella* species retain the basic fuchsin dye. They are aerobic organisms that are both fastidious and relatively slow growers. They are cultivated in axenic media, unlike *Rickettsia* species, which are obligate intracellular organisms. They are also co-cultivated in cell culture, where they may be found in large intracellular aggregates contained within a vacuole or on the cell surface of several different types of eukaryotic cells. Succinate, pyruvate, glutamine or glutamate, but not glucose, serve as a source of

Table 1. Per cent identity of the 16S rRNA gene from the major human pathogens of the genus *Bartonella*. Full-length sequences were aligned for maximum identity. *Bartonella vinsonii* subspecies *vinsonii* is shown for reference.

	B. henselae (Bh)	B. quintana (Bq)	B. bacilliformis (Bb)	B. vinsonii (Bv)
Bh	–	98.7	98.2	99.3
Bq		–	98.1	99.0
Bb			–	98.6
Bv				–

energy. The biochemical characteristics are negative for catalase, oxidase, nitrate reduction, indole and urease, and the bacterium produces acid from carbohydrates. Cellular fatty content in *Bartonella* species is mainly $C_{18:1}$ and $C_{16:0}$. The main fatty acids in *B. quintana* and in *B. henselae* are $C_{16:0}$ and $C_{18:1}$, respectively.

Isolation procedures

All members of the genus can be grown on enriched bacteriological media containing blood or amino acids, yeast extract and fetal bovine serum or haematin in 5–10% CO_2 at 35–37°C (except *B. bacilliformis,* which grows best at 25–28°C). The bacterium can also be isolated by cell culture. *Bartonella* species are susceptible to antimicrobial agents *in vitro*; hence collection of blood should be made prior to the initiation of antimicrobial therapy. Suitable specimens include blood, pus or homogenized tissue suspension, inoculated on to blood agar plates or co-cultivated with endothelial cell culture. The agar plates are incubated for as long as 3–4 weeks, when small, translucent colonies appear on the plate. In tissue culture, elongated pleomorphic organisms are observed within 72 h. The microorganisms are checked for morphological and staining properties and confirmed by direct immunofluorescence, using fluorescent-conjugated specific antibodies. The presence *of Bartonella* species can also be identified in isolated colonies, in co-cultivated cultures and directly in tissue specimens, lesions, pus or blood by nucleic acid amplification methods coupled with sequence analysis of the amplification product, or by hybridization with a specific probe.

Laboratory diagnosis

Because of the difficulty and the time needed to grow the organism from patient specimens, determination of antibodies to *Bartonella* infections has become the test of choice for laboratory diagnosis. Both enzyme immunoassay (EIA) and indirect fluorescent antibody (IFA) tests are available, although the latter has been more thoroughly evaluated. It is often difficult to speciate the specific causative bartonella

agent because of the substantial cross-reactivity, both qualitative and quantitative, observed when reacting a patient's serum with various *Bartonella* species. The sensitivity of the serological modalities is 85–95%. When available, the sensitivity and specificity of a formatted polymerase chain reaction (PCR) test for routine testing of specimens can approach 100%.

Trench fever

Distribution

Trench fever was first recognized in the First World War (1914–1918) as a febrile illness of up to 6 days' duration. It was considered the most common disease that afflicted the soldiers on both sides of the war. It disappeared after the First World War and reappeared in the armies of the eastern front during the Second World War (1939–1945). The disease disappeared again after the Second World War and then reappeared in homeless people in North America and Europe. Trench fever has also been reported from Mexico and North Africa.

Clinical symptoms

Trench fever is distinguished by an array of self-limiting clinical symptoms. The incubation period of trench fever varies from 5 to 30 days. Clinical manifestations are variable. There may be uninterrupted fever for from 2 to 6 weeks. Alternatively, the patient can undergo single or multiple bouts of fever lasting 5 days each, giving rise to the name *B. quintana*. With the fever, the patient may experience episodes of chills. Other symptoms are headache, malaise, myalgias and bone pain. A macular rash similar to the typhoid fever rash may develop.

Transmission

The disease is caused by *B. quintana*. The vector is the human body louse, *Pediculus humanus,* and the host/reservoir is both the human and the body louse. Pathogens ingested by the louse with a blood meal attach to the walls of the gut, where they multiply, but do not penetrate the cells, as do typhus rickettsiae, and so are not injurious to the louse. The disease is spread through crushing lice or by the faeces coming into contact with mucous membranes or skin abrasions. The bacteria can remain viable in louse faeces for many months. Once infected, the louse continuously excretes the bacterium with the faeces. Transovarial infection does not occur. Between epidemics, little is known about the prevalence of the bacterium in nature.

Treatment

Treatment regimens have not been established because very few cases of trench fever have been described in the literature since the discovery of antibiotics. Based on *in vitro* sensitivity studies, tetracyclines are likely to be the drugs of choice.

Bacillary angiomatosis (BA)/Bacillary peliosis hepatitis (BPH)

Both syndromes are a reactive vascular proliferation due to infection with either *B. henselae*, the more predominant of the two bacteria, or *B. quintana*. Human-to-human transmission has not been observed, and the reservoir hosts appear to be cats and their fleas. Bacillary angiomatosis can affect almost all organs. The lesions can be few or several and have a vascular appearance. They range from skin-coloured to deep red-purple, with a surface that can be smooth or ulcerated, often with a collarette of scale. The extent of the lesions is a function of the patient's immune status. In immunocompromised patients the number and extent of the lesions are significantly higher than in patients with no underlying disease. The clinical diagnosis of these lesions is difficult because they can be mistaken for Kaposi's sarcoma. Diagnosis can only be ascertained after histopathological examination to detect the presence of the bacterium.

Bacillary peliosis hepatitis (BPH) is a disorder with a hallmark that is a unique vascular lesion associated with hepatomegaly or splenomegaly. It can cause elevated transaminase, with normal or slightly elevated bilirubin. The condition may cause catastrophic intra-abdominal haemorrhage.

Endocarditis

The spectrum of human bartonella infections now includes endocarditis. Because the bartonellas are slow growers, diagnostic laboratories are advised to prolong the incubation times of cultures of blood and tissues from patients with suspected endocarditis. This is especially true in the case of a failure to isolate an alternative causative organism from tissues that are normally sterile. *Bartonella quintana*, *B. henselae* and *B. elizabethae* have all been associated with endocarditis.

Treatment

Patients, especially HIV patients with vascular lesions, should be treated with a prolonged course of antibiotics to avoid relapses. The antibiotics are of the cycline series, such as tetracycline, doxycycline or minocycline, or a macrolide antibiotic, such as erythromycin. The treatment may be extended to the lifetime of the patient. The antibiotics should be given by injection for 4–8 weeks, followed by extended oral therapy.

Control

The vectors of trench fever (*B. bartonella*), body lice, can be controlled by applying 10% DDT powder between the body and underclothes of louse-infested people. If DDT-resistant lice are present, other insecticides that have very low dermal toxicities can be used. Clothing impregnated with pyrethroid insecticides can keep people free of lice for many months.

Conclusions on *Bartonella* infections

The spectrum of disease attributed to members of the genus *Bartonella* has not yet been completely defined. A role for these bacteria in endocarditis, as possible triggers of 'autoimmune' disorders and as the aetiological agent of fever of unknown origin should be further explored. Likewise, the role of *B. quintana*, *B. henselae* and *B. bacilliformis* in human disease has been firmly established; however, the role of many other *Bartonella* species in causing human disease is probably currently under-appreciated. Considering the ubiquitous nature of the reservoir hosts of these agents (i.e. cats, rodents), the potential to cause disease in humans and companion animals remains large.

Selected bibliography

Anderson, B.E. and Neuman, M.A. (1997) The genus *Bartonella* as emerging human pathogens. *Clinical Microbiology Reviews* 10, 203–219.

Brenner, D.J., O'Connor, S.P., Winkler, H.H. and Steigerwalt, A.G. (1993) Proposals to unify the genera *Bartonella* and *Rochalimaea*, with descriptions *of Bartonella quintana* comb. nov., *Bartonella vinsonii* comb. nov., *Bartonella henselae* comb. nov., and *Bartonella elizabethae* comb. nov., and to remove the family *Bartonellaceae* from the order *Rickettsiales. International Journal of Systematic Bacteriology* 43, 777–786.

Brouqui, P., Lascola, B., Roux, V. and Raoult, D. (1999) Chronic *Bartonella quintana* bacteremia in homeless patients. *New England Journal of Medicine* 340, 184–189.

Dehio, C., Meyer, M., Berger, T.G., Schwarz, J.H. and Lanz, C. (1997) Interactions of *Bartonella henselae* with endothelial cells results in bacterial aggregation on the cell surface and the subsequent engulfment and internalisation of the bacterial aggregate by a unique structure, the invasome. *Journal of Cell Science* 110, 2141–2154.

Jackson, L.A. and Spach, D.H. (1996) Emergence of *Bartonella quintana* infection among homeless persons. *Emerging Infectious Diseases* 2, 141–144.

Koehler, J.E., Quinn, F.D., Berger, T.G, LeBoit, P.E. and Tappero, J.W. (1992) Isolation of *Rochalimaea* species from cutaneous and osseous lesions of bacillary angiomatosis. *New England Journal of Medicine* 327, 1625–1631.

Bartonella bacilliformis see **Carrión's disease.**

Bartonella henselae see **Cat-scratch disease** *and Bartonella quintana* **and** *Bartonella henselae.*

Bartonellosis *see* **Carrión's disease**, **Cat-scratch disease** *and Bartonella quintana* **and** *Bartonella henselae.*

Beetles (Coleoptera)

M.W. Service

There are more than 400,000 species of beetles and the Coleoptera comprise the largest order of the insects. They are found in all regions of the world except the polar areas.

Biology

Beetles are minute (0.5 mm long) to very large (120 mm long) in size. They are robust and heavily sclerotized, with the fore-wings modified to form the elytra, which cover the hind-wings. The elytra of *Lytta vesicatoria*, the so-called 'Spanish fly', contains the blistering agent cantharadin. Most beetles are terrestrial but a few are aquatic. The eggs hatch into larvae, usually having legs, and the larvae develop into pupae and eventually into adults.

Diseases

Generally, beetles are of very minor medical or veterinary importance. However, some coprophagous and necrophagous beetles, such as species of *Dermestes*, *Anthrenus* and *Attagenus* (Fig. 1) in the family Dermestidae, have been suspected of spreading spores of anthrax (*Bacillus anthracis*) mechanically. Other species, belonging to the Silphidae, have also been recorded in the transmission of anthrax.

Control

There are no effective control measures for beetles transmitting anthrax.

Selected bibliography

Thédoridès, J. (1950) The parasitological, medical and veterinary importance of Coleoptera. *Acta Tropica* 7, 48–60.

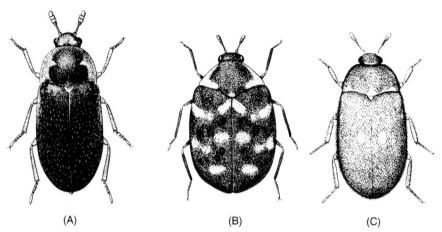

Fig. 1.   Adult beetles. (A) *Demestes* species; (B) *Anthrenus* species; (C) *Attagenus* species. (From *Common Insect Pests of Stored Products*, British Museum (Natural History), London, 1989.)

Biliary fever *see* **Theilerioses.**

Biphasic milk fever *see* **Tick-borne encephalitis.**

Biting house-flies *see* **Stable-flies.**

Biting midges (Ceratopogonidae)

M.W. Service

Biting midges (midges, punkies, no see-ums) have an almost worldwide distribution. Unfortunately, they are sometimes called sand-flies, a term that should be restricted to phlebotomine sand-flies (see entry). There are about 5000 species of biting midges in over 120 genera, the most important from the medical and veterinary aspects being the genus *Culicoides*, which has over 1200 species.

Biology

Eggs are laid on the surface of wet soil, mud, decaying leaf litter, manure, semi-rotting vegetation, in tree holes or on objects near or partially submerged in water. Some vector species (*Culicoides grahamii*, *Culicoides milnei* group) lay their eggs in the cut stumps of banana plants. Eggs hatch within 2–9 days, but a few temperate species overwinter as eggs. Larvae occur in freshwater or salt-water marshy areas, in wet, boggy and semi-waterlogged ground, manure, banana stumps, etc. There are four larval instars. The mature larva is whitish, except for a blackish head, and is cylindrical, legless and nematode-like (Fig. 1). In warm countries larval development is completed within 2–4 weeks, but in temperate regions many species overwinter as larvae. The pupal period is 3–10 days. The life cycle (Fig. 1) from egg to adult emergence can be 20–40 or more days.

Only female adults take blood meals, which can be from humans or a wide range of mammals and birds. Biting can occur at any time; most species are mainly active in the evening and early part of the night, but *C. grahamii* bites mainly in the morning. Most biting occurs out of doors but *C. grahamii* and the *C. milnei* group will enter houses to feed. Adults are weak fliers, dispersing only a few hundred metres from their larval habitats, unless they become wind-borne.

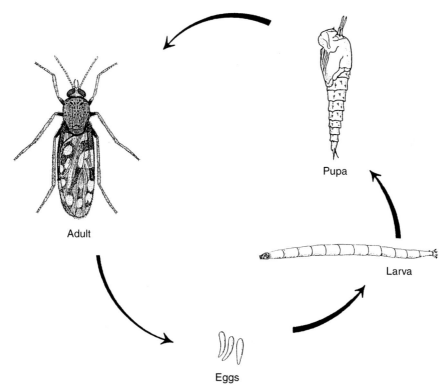

Fig. 1. Life cycle of a typical biting midge (*Culicoides* species) (modified from M.W. Service (2000) *Medical Entomology for Students*, Cambridge University Press, Cambridge).

Diseases

Biting midges are more important as vectors of veterinary than of human infections. Various *Culicoides* species transmit filarial worms, causing bovine and equine onchocerciasis, arboviruses, causing diseases such as African horse sickness, Aino, Akbane and bluetongue, bovine ephemeral disease, epizootic haemorrhagic disease and Issyk-Kul virus disease, and protozoans, such as *Haemoproteus nettionis*, *Haemoproteus meleagradis* and sometimes *Leucocytozoon* species. Biting midges also transmit to humans Oropouche virus and filarial infections, such as *Mansonella perstans*, *Mansonella streptocerca* and, in Central and South America, *Mansonella ozzardi*. (See entries on all these infections.) *Forcipomyia townesvillensis* has been reported as transmitting filarial parasites, causing bovine onchocerciasis.

Control

Some personal protection may be obtained by applying insect repellents to the skin and the use at night of insecticide-impregnated bed nets, the holes in which need to be smaller than in many mosquito-nets, otherwise midges will squeeze through. Ultra-low-volume (ULV) applications of insecticides may kill adults resting in vegetation but the effects are short-lived. Animal quarters, such as stables, can also be sprayed with residual insecticides to minimize contact between midges and hosts. Although elimination of larval habitats, such as by drainage or filling in, can eradicate breeding, this is costly, laborious and often impractical. Sometimes semi-aquatic habitats, such as muddy areas, can be flooded to ensure that the soil is never exposed, thus destroying suitable larval habitats. Insecticidal spraying the diffuse and often extensive larval habitats is often impractical and environmentally unacceptable.

Selected bibliography

Kettle, D.S. (1977) Biology and bionomics of blood-sucking ceratopogonids. *Annual Review of Entomology* 22, 33–51.

Mellor, P., Boorman, J. and Baylis, M. (2000) *Culicoides* biting midges: their role as arbovirus vectors. *Annual Review of Entomology* 45, 307–340.

Reynolds, D.G. and Vidot, A. (1978) Chemical control of *Leptoconops spinisofrons* in the Seychelles. *Pest Articles and News Summaries* 24, 19–26.

Black-flies (Simuliidae)

M.W. Service

Simuliid black-flies (buffalo gnats, sand-flies, reed smuts) have an almost worldwide distribution. There are some 1720 species in 26 genera.

Biology

Eggs are brown or blackish and are laid in sticky masses or strings, usually either attached to submerged objects, such as stones, rocks or vegetation, or deposited in bottom sediment of flowing waters. Some species, however, such as *Simulium ochraceum*, scatter their eggs over flowing water while flying over it. Breeding places range from small trickles of water to large fast-flowing rivers. Eggs usually hatch within a few days. There are normally seven larval instars. Larvae do not swim but are sedentary for long periods, attaching themselves to submerged vegetation, rocks or stones, except for a few phoretic species (e.g. *Simulium neavei*) that attach themselves to the bodies of mayflies (Ephemeroptera) or crabs and prawns (Crustacea). Larval development can be as short as 6–12 days, but in some species larval duration may extend over several months. The mature larva spins a slipper-shaped cocoon, which is firmly attached to rocks or vegetation, and then pupates within this protective cocoon (Fig. 1). After usually 2–6 days an adult emerges from the pupa, floats to the water surface and eventually flies away. The life cycle (Fig. 1) from egg to adult emergence can be just 26–63 days, but is sometimes considerably longer. Adult females normally live for about 3–4 weeks.

Only female black-flies bite and are consequently disease vectors. Feeding occurs during the day on warm-blooded vertebrates. Some species prefer feeding on mammals, including humans, while others feed almost exclusively on birds. Their bites may cause severe allergic reactions in humans and animals. After feeding, blood-engorged females rest in a variety of natural outdoor sites until the blood meal has been digested and the resultant gravid female is ready to oviposit. Adults often fly just a few hundred metres, but they not infrequently fly 15–30 km, and a few species have been transported 250–600 km on prevailing winds.

Diseases

The most important vector species belong to the genus *Simulium*, although certain veterinary parasites are transmitted by species of *Austrosimulium*, *Prosimulium* and *Cnephia*. Black-flies are vectors to humans of filarial worms causing onchocerciasis (*Onchocerca volvulus*) and mansonelliasis (*Mansonella ozzardi*). They are of veterinary importance because they transmit filarial worms causing bovine and equine onchocerciasis (*Onchocerca* species), *Leucocytozoon* parasites to poultry, occasionally the virus causing vesicular stomatitis to livestock, and the filarial parasite *Splendidofilaria fallisensis* to ducks, and a few other veterinary infections. They also transmit several other filarial and protozoon parasites to wildlife.

Control

The application of insect repellents may give some degree of personal protection

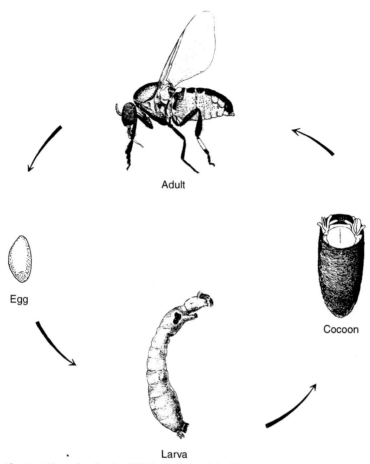

Adult

Egg

Cocoon

Larva

Fig. 1. Life cycle of a simuliid black-fly (modified from M.W. Service (2000) *Medical Entomology for Students,* Cambridge University Press, Cambridge).

from bites of black-flies, but is not usually very effective. Control is almost exclusively based on killing the larvae, such as by repeatedly dosing their aquatic breeding sites with insecticides, mainly with organophosphates, such as temephos (Abate). If insecticide resistance develops, the microbial insecticide consisting of *Bacillus thuringiensis* subsp. *israelensis* can be used in larval breeding places (see Onchocerciasis, human).

Selected bibliography

Crosskey, R.W. (1990) *The Natural History of Blackflies.* John Wiley & Sons, Chichester, UK, 711 pp.

Crosskey, R.W. (1999) *First Update to the Taxonomic and Geographical Inventory of World Blackflies (Diptera: Simuliidae).* The Natural History Museum, London, 10 pp.

Crosskey, R.W. and Howard, T.M. (1997) *A New Taxonomic and Geographical Inventory of World Blackflies (Diptera: Simuliidae).* The Natural History Museum, London, 144 pp.

Blow-flies *see* **Flies**.

Bluebottles *see* **Flies**.

Bluetongue virus

P.S. Mellor

Bluetongue (BT) virus causes a non-contagious, infectious, insect-borne disease of wild and domestic ruminants, particularly sheep. Bluetongue, the disease, was first described in South Africa in the late 18th century, subsequent to the introduction of Merino sheep into the Cape Colony. However, since that time the virus has spread widely throughout much of the world and now affects ruminants on six continents, causing losses in terms of disease and trade estimated at US$3000 million year^{-1}. For these reasons BT virus has been allocated by the Office International des Epizooties (OIE) List A status (that is, communicable diseases which have the potential for very rapid spread, irrespective of national borders, which are of serious socio-economic or public health consequence and which are of major importance in the international trade of livestock or livestock products).

Distribution

The global distribution of BT virus lies approximately between latitudes 35°S and 40°N, although in parts of western North America and northern China it may extend up to almost 50°N. Within these areas the virus has a virtually worldwide distribution, being found in North, Central and South America, Africa, the Middle East, the Indian subcontinent, China, South-East Asia and Australia. Bluetongue virus has also at times made excursions into Europe (Spain and Portugal 1956–1960, and Spain 2000, Greece 1979 and 1998–2000, European Turkey 1998–2000, Italy 2000, France 2000 and Bulgaria 1999), although it has not been able to establish itself permanently in that continent. Nevertheless, the 1956–1960 epizootic in Spain and Portugal resulted in the deaths of almost 180,000 sheep and is the most severe outbreak of bluetongue on record. As a general rule BT virus can be considered as infecting ruminant livestock in all countries lying in the tropics and subtropics. Additionally, several countries that are close to the subtropics, such as the USA have enzootically infected livestock. It is also the case that those countries whose territory spans a wide range of latitudes (e.g. USA and Australia) frequently include large geographical areas where BT virus activity is apparently absent.

Aetiological agent

Bluetongue virus is the type species of the genus *Orbivirus* in the family Reoviridae. Complete virions have a diameter of about 80 nm and possess a double-layered capsid. The diffuse outer layer, comprising two proteins, can be removed, enzymatically or by manipulating the salt concentration and pH, to reveal a highly structured core particle. The core particle has a diameter of about 54 nm, consists of 32 ring-like capsomeres arranged in icosahedral symmetry and contains five proteins. The name of the genus is derived from this structure (*orbis* = ring in Latin). The capsomeres are in fact tubular structures and consist of smaller structural units arranged in regular hexagonal and pentagonal patterns. The double-stranded RNA (dsRNA) genome consists of ten segments that vary in size from 0.5 kDa to 2.7 kDa and function as genes (i.e. they are translated individually into functional viral proteins). Genome segments are labelled 1–10 in descending order of size, whereas the viral polypeptides are divided into structural proteins (VP1–VP7) and non-structural proteins (NS1–NS3). Two of the viral proteins, VP2 and VP5, form the diffuse outer capsid layer and are responsible for the induction of serotype-specific neutralizing antibodies in the vertebrate hosts. At present 24 distinct serotypes of the virus have been recognized. However, all of these are to a greater or lesser degree related to one another, as evidenced by cross-reactions in neutralization tests, cross-protection in *in vivo* challenge infections and the development of heterotypic antibodies in infected ruminants. It has been suggested that these relationships may have an evolutionary basis.

Bluetongue virus is relatively heat-resistant and is stable at 20°C, 4°C and –70°C, but is labile at –20°C. It is partially resistant to lipid solvents but is rapidly inactivated at pH levels below 6.5.

Clinical signs

Although BT virus infects many species of animal, clinical signs are generally associated with sheep and hence most descriptions of disease apply to this species. Clinical disease in sheep is dependent upon the breed, the virus type or strain and interactions with the environment. In extent it can vary from a subclinical infection, through fever, to severe clinical disease, including death. Generally speaking, it is the fine-wool and mutton breeds that suffer the most severely. The first clinical sign is a rise in temperature and the animal may appear depressed. This is followed by hyperaemia of the oral cavity and swelling of the mucous membranes, leading to oedema of the lips, tongue and muzzle. The animal may also be anorexic. There is lachrymation, a serous nasal discharge becoming mucopurulent, excessive salivation and conjunctivitis. At a later stage there may be necrosis of the epithelium of the nose and mouth with excoriation. Oedema may extend to the ears and brisket, and there may be wool-break. The feet are often affected with coronitis and laminitis, leading to lameness. The animal may kneel on its hocks or may be reluctant to stand at all. Torticollis may occur in some sheep. In pregnant ewes, abortion or mummification of the fetus may occur and at term deformed or weak lambs may be born. Paradoxically, cyanosis of the tongue, from which coloration the disease derives its common name (i.e. bluetongue), is rarely seen.

Certain wild ruminants, such as the North American White-tailed deer (*Odocoileus virginianus*), the Pronghorn antelope (*Antilocapra americana*) and the American bighorn sheep (*Ovis canadensis*) may also develop severe clinical blue-tongue similar to that seen in domesticated sheep.

In cattle, BT virus infection is usually inapparent. Where clinical disease does occur, bluetongue is seen as a transient fever followed by hyperaemia and erosions of the nose, buccal and lingual mucosa and, rarely, the teats. Affected cattle salivate excessively and may walk with a stiff gait. The skin of the nose appears mottled and dark and has been described as 'burnt muzzle', and may slough off. Fewer than 1% of infected cattle show signs of bluetongue, and there is mounting evidence that the expression of clinical disease is due to an immunoglobulin E (IgE)-mediated hypersensitivity reaction induced by previous exposure to BT or related viruses.

Bluetongue in goats is rarely seen and when it does occur is usually mild.

Pathology and post-mortem findings

The post-mortem appearance of an animal that has died of BT virus (usually a sheep) is not spectacular and is usually remarkable only for the absence of pathognomonic lesions. The lesions seen, by and large, relate to the severity of damage caused to the microvascular system, which results in vascular permeability with consequent oedema, haemorrhage, thrombosis, ischaemia and necrosis of a wide range of tissues, including those of the digestive tract, muscular system, cardiovascular system and respiratory system. Haemorrhages in the tunica media at the base of the pulmonary artery have been described as being pathognomonic for BT virus infection, but these lesions can be difficult to see and have also been recorded in a number of other infections of sheep (Rift Valley fever, heartwater (see entries) and pulpy kidney disease). In sheep, most deaths apparently occur as a result of secondary (broncholobular) pneumonia, which is frequently associated with the inspiration of vomit due to partial paralysis of the musculature of the oesophagus.

Diagnosis

A presumptive diagnosis of bluetongue in affected sheep, based on the clinical signs and lesions, can frequently be made. However, in most other ruminant species and, indeed, in many sheep, BT virus infection will usually be subclinical and laboratory confirmation, either by virus isolation or identification or by serology, is required. The following samples are likely to be required:

1. Blood for virus isolation; collected as early as possible from febrile animals into anticoagulants, such as heparin or ethylenediamine tetra-acetic acid (EDTA) and kept cool (4°C) but not frozen.*

2. Tissues for virus isolation (or antigen detection by enzyme-linked immunosorbent assay (ELISA) or polymerase chain reaction (PCR)). Spleen and lymph nodes are preferred. These tissues should be collected at autopsy and should be kept and transported to the reference laboratory at 4°C.

3. Serum for serological tests. Preferably paired samples should be taken 14–28 days apart and should be kept frozen at –20°C.

Confirmation of BT virus infection is by one or more of the following:

1. Identification of the virus directly from submitted samples by group-specific, antigen-detection ELISA or by PCR-based assays.

2. Isolation of infectious virus in suckling mice or embryonating hens' eggs followed by adaptation to cell culture and identification first by the group-specific agar gel immunodiffusion (AGID) test or antigen-detection ELISA, and then the serotype-specific, virus-neutralization or reverse-transcription (RT)-PCR tests.

3. Identification of BT virus-specific antibodies by the group-specific, antibody-detection ELISA, AGID and complement fixation (CF) tests, or by the serotype-specific virus-neutralization test.

Transmission

Bluetongue virus is transmitted between its ruminant hosts almost entirely via the bites of certain species of *Culicoides* biting midge, which act as true biological vectors. In consequence, its world distribution is restricted to areas where vector species of

midge occur, and transmission is limited to those times of the year when adult vectors are active. In epizootic areas this usually means during the late summer and autumn since this is when vector abundance is highest. Midges become infected with BT virus when feeding upon viraemic ruminants and are able to support virus replication by up to 10,000-fold. Infected midges become competent to transmit after the virus has reached and replicated in the salivary glands, which takes about 6–8 days at 25°C but progressively longer as ambient temperature falls. Once infected, a vector remains infected for life and can transmit virus at each and every blood meal. A single midge bite is sufficient to infect a susceptible ruminant host. However, transovarial or vertical transmission of BT virus through the vectors does not seem to occur.

In the Americas the most important *Culicoides* vector species of midge are *C. variipennis* (North America) and *C. insignis* (mainly Central and South America). In Africa the vector is *C. imicola* and possibly *C. bolitinos,* while in southern Europe it is *C. imicola* and possibly *C. obsoletus.* In Australia, *C. brevitarsis, C. fulvus, C. wadai* and *C. actoni* are the most significant vectors, while across much of Asia *C. imicola* is involved in transmission in addition to these four species. In each of these geographical areas other species may also from time to time play a lesser role in transmission.

In general, *Culicoides* species have a flight range of a few kilometres or less. However, in common with many other groups of flying insects, they have the capacity to be transported as aerial plankton over much greater distances. Indeed, the introduction of the BT virus vector *C. wadai* into northern Australia in 1971 may have been a wind-borne introduction from Indonesia, where it is common. In this context, a considerable body of evidence exists to suggest that the extension of BT virus into new areas may sometimes be due to long-range dispersal of infected vector *Culicoides* carried on the prevailing winds.

In addition to transmission via vector species of *Culicoides,* BT virus may occasionally be transmitted directly in semen collected during the viraemic phase of the disease. Consequently, shipment of ruminant semen from BT virus-infected countries to BT virus-free regions is strictly controlled and detailed protocols exist that must be complied with to ensure safety. Similarly, protocols also exist to ensure that embryo transfer from infected dams does not result in virus transmission to the recipients, although the perceived risk is lower than when transferring semen. Transplacental transmission has been recorded but is not considered to be an important mechanism for viral maintenance.

Vertebrate hosts

Bluetongue virus has a very wide host range and probably all species of ruminant are susceptible to infection. However, the outcome of infection can vary greatly between different species and breeds, as well as among individuals of the same species. In certain breeds of sheep and some species of deer the outcome can be severe and often fatal, while in most other species of ruminant infection is usually inapparent. In fact, the degree of clinical disease seems to be dependent upon the breed and species of animal, the serotype or strain of virus and certain ill-defined interactions with the environment (e.g. sheep that are stressed or subject to high levels of solar radiation are reputed to develop more severe lesions than those not so treated).

It is possible that, historically, the primary BT virus cycle involved species of African antelope and *Culicoides* biting midges. With the agricultural development of large parts of Africa and with the introduction of BT virus into countries outside that continent, the traditional role of wild game animals has been largely taken over by cattle. The virus now seems to be maintained in a midge–cattle cycle and, once a certain level of infection is attained, it spills over to initiate a secondary cycle in sheep. This generally occurs in late summer or autumn when vector midge populations are at a maximum.

Incubation period and viraemia

Upon introduction into a ruminant host BT virus first replicates in the local lymph nodes and thereafter in other lymph nodes, blood-forming organs and the endothelial cells lining capillaries and small blood-vessels. In most animals viraemia is first detected from about 3–6 days post-infection, depending upon the infecting dose and route of infection. Viraemia in sheep usually lasts for 6–10 days and rarely persists for longer than 14 days, although a maximum time of 54 days has been reported. A peak titre of around 10^6 tissue culture infective dose for 50% $(TCID)_{50}$ of virus per ml may be reached. In cattle, viraemia may peak at a similar level to sheep but tends to have a longer duration (7–28 days) and occasionally may extend for as long as 100 days. The maximum duration of viraemia in other ruminant species (domestic goats, Blesbok or Bontebok (*Damaliscus pygargus*), White-tailed deer (*Odocoileus virginianus*), Elk (*Cervus elaphus*), Arabian gazelle (*Gazella* species), Swamp (= Water) buffalo (*Bubalus bubalis*) seems to vary from 10 to 50 days.

While in the blood system it is thought that most BT virus is sequestered in immunologically privileged sites, primarily in the membranes of circulating erythrocytes and to a lesser extent the cells of the buffy coat, and is thus protected from the effects of humoral antibody. In consequence, virus and antibody may coexist in the circulatory system and virus is likely to persist until the 'infected' erythrocytes are eventually removed. Since the half-life of bovine erythrocytes has been estimated at 120 days, isolation of BT virus from bovine blood for up to 100 days post-infection, as reported above, is consistent with this theory.

Treatment

Apart from supportive treatment there is no specific therapy for bluetongue. Affected animals should be nursed carefully, placed in sheds or stables and protected from extremes of temperature and direct solar radiation. Small amounts of soft green food should be given during the stage when buccal lesions make feeding painful. Secondary bacterial infections can be controlled by antibiotic therapy. During convalescence ruminal activity should be maintained or induced and this should reduce the time until restoration of full health.

Prevention and control

Importation of ruminants and their germ-plasms from known infected areas to virus-free zones should be restricted. If importation of animals is permitted, they should be quarantined in insect-proof accommodation prior to movement for a period of time sufficient to ensure that any viraemia has ended. Germ-plasms should only be imported if it can be confirmed that the donor animals were uninfected at the time that the samples were taken.

Following an outbreak of bluetongue in a country or zone that has previously been free of the disease, attempts should be made to limit further transmission of the virus and to achieve eradication as quickly as possible. It is important that control measures be implemented as soon as a suspected diagnosis of bluetongue as been made and without waiting for the diagnosis to be confirmed. In epizootic situations the following measures should be taken:

- Delineate the area of infection, taking into consideration topographical features, such as mountain ranges and wide stretches of water.
- Prevent the movement of all ruminants within, into and out of the infected area.
- Ruminants should be moved to high pastures or, if possible, housed in insect-proof buildings, particularly during the period from dusk to dawn, the major activity time for the *Culicoides* vectors. The use of insect repellents inside buildings and on animals may enhance protection from vector bites.
- Vector abatement measures should be implemented, e.g. insecticide treatment in and around animal holdings and of suspect *Culicoides* breeding sites, elimination of breeding sites through improved water management and waste disposal (see Biting midges).
- Daily clinical examination of all susceptible sheep to detect infected

animals as early as possible. Animals with an on-going infection should be slaughtered or housed in insect-proof buildings to prevent access by vectors and further spread of the virus.[1]
- Susceptible sheep may be vaccinated, immediately, with polyvalent vaccines until the causative virus has been serotyped and the relevant monovalent vaccine has become available. All vaccinated animals should be identified.[2]
- The virus serotype responsible for the outbreak should be determined as soon as possible and a suitable monovalent vaccine produced and administered to sheep.
- The OIE should be notified immediately of all cases of disease. In enzootic situations and in regions where bluetongue outbreaks occur almost every year, regular annual vaccination of sheep with live, attenuated polyvalent vaccines, effective against all known local serotypes of BT virus, is recommended. However, sheep vaccinated during early pregnancy may abort or give birth to malformed lambs.

Notes

[*]   While in circulation, most BT virus is sequestered in immunologically privileged sites in the erythrocyte membranes and as such is protected against the effects of humoral antibody. Virus and antibody, therefore, may coexist in the circulatory system. Consequently, blood and tissue samples collected for virus isolation should be kept cool but must not be frozen; otherwise upon defrosting the erythrocytes will lyse and the released virus may be neutralized by serum antibody. Washing protocols have been devised to remove antibody from non-lysed blood prior to virus isolation procedures.

[1]   Though sheep may exhibit clinical bluetongue, most other ruminant species, including cattle and goats, usually display only subclinical infections. These other ruminant species are likely, therefore, to provide a covert source of virus for vector midges, enabling the virus transmission cycle to persist.

[2]   The only BT virus vaccines available contain live, attenuated viruses. They are usually available in pentavalent form. Monovalent vaccines can be produced to special order but may take several months to deliver. These factors can be a

cause for disquiet since the possibility of reversion always exists with live virus vaccines, and many authorities, therefore, are reluctant to potentially introduce into their ecosystems five viruses only one of which may be already present. Furthermore, all existing BT virus vaccines are designed to protect sheep from clinical disease. There are no data available to assess their efficacy in preventing the field virus from continuing to cycle, covertly, through cattle, goats and other ruminant species.

Selected bibliography

Barber, T.L. and Jochim, M.M. (1985) *Bluetongue and Related Orbiviruses.* Alan R. Liss, New York, 746 pp.

Campbell, C.H. and Grubman, M.J. (1985) Current knowledge on the biochemistry and immunology of bluetongue. In: Pandey, R. (ed.) *Progress in Veterinary Microbiology and Immunology* 1, 58–79.

Erasmus, B.J. (1990) Bluetongue virus. In: Dinter, Z. and Morein, B. (eds) *Virus Infections of Ruminants.* Elsevier, Amsterdam, pp. 227–237.

Gibbs, E.P.J. and Greiner, E.C. (1988) Bluetongue and epizootic hemorrhagic disease. In: Monath, T.P. (ed.) *The Arboviruses: Epidemiology and Ecology,* Vol. II. CRC Press, Boca Raton, Florida, pp. 39–70.

Howell, P.G. (1963) Bluetongue. In: *Emerging Diseases of Animals.* Agricultural Studies, Food and Agriculture Organization, Rome, pp. 111–153.

Meiswinkel, R., Nevill, E.M. and Venter, G.J. (1994) Vectors: *Culicoides* spp. In: Coetzer, J.A.W., Thomson, G.R. and Tustin, R.C. (eds) *Infectious Diseases of Livestock with Special Reference to Southern Africa,* Vol. 1. Oxford University Press, Cape Town, pp. 68–89.

Mellor, P.S. and Boorman, J. (1995) The transmission and geographical spread of African horse sickness and bluetongue viruses. *Annals of Tropical Medicine and Parasitology* 89, 1–15.

Roy, P. and Gorman, B.M. (1990) *Bluetongue Viruses.* Current Topics in Microbiology and Immunology 162, Springer-Verlag, Berlin, 200 pp.

Verwoerd, D.W. and Erasmus, B.J. (1994) Bluetongue. In: Coetzer, J.A.W., Thomson, G.R. and Tustin, R.C. (eds) *Infectious Diseases of Livestock with Special Reference to Southern Africa,* Vol. 1. Oxford University Press, Cape Town, pp. 443–456.

Walton, T.E. and Osburn, B.I. (1992) *Bluetongue, African Horse Sickness and Related Orbiviruses.* CRC Press, Boca Raton, Florida, 1042 pp.

Borrelia anserina see **Avian borreliosis.**

Borrelia burgdorferi see **Lyme borreliosis.**

Borrelia duttonii see **Tick-borne relapsing fever.**

Borrelia recurrentis see **Louse-borne relapsing fever.**

Borrelia theileri

Ronald D. Smith

Borrelia theileri is a relatively non-pathogenic member of the genus *Borrelia* that is transmitted by several species of ixodid (hard) ticks. It is most commonly reported from cattle, but may also infect a number of other domestic and wild vertebrate hosts. Its importance lies in its widespread geographical distribution and possibility of being confused with more pathogenic members of the genus.

Geographical and host distribution
Naturally occurring *B. theileri* infections are most commonly reported in cattle, but tick-borne infections have been induced in sheep, horses and deer. Two other species

of *Borrelia* infect cattle: *B. burgdorferi* and *B. coriaceae*. Since the geographical ranges of vector ticks and vertebrate hosts for *B. theileri*, *B. burgdorferi* and *B. coriaceae* overlap, species distinctions are important.

Borrelia theileri has been reported from the African, Australasian and American continents, reflecting the geographical distribution of its tick vectors, *Boophilus microplus*, *Boophilus annulatus*, *Boophilus decoloratus* and *Rhipicephalus evertsi*. As ticks which transmit *B. theileri* may also be vectors for bovine babesiae, the presence of *B. theileri* in Giemsa-stained blood smears is often an incidental finding during studies on bovine babesiosis (see Babesiosis).

Parasite

Borrelia theileri is classified in the family Spirochaetaceae and the bacterial order Spirochaetales. Other pathogenic spirochaetes in the family include *Treponema* and *Leptospira*. As a group the borreliae are more pleomorphic than leptospires and treponemes. The borreliae contain loose coils whose wave amplitudes may vary considerably, even within the same organism. Replicating borreliae elongate and then divide by transverse fission to form two daughter cells. Dividing cells are longer, more linear and thinner than non-dividing forms. Borreliae stain well with aniline dyes such as the Romanowsky-type stains used in routine blood smears. Giemsa's stain is most commonly used. *Borrelia theileri* is weakly Gram-negative, but the bacterial DNA is readily visible using acridine orange staining and ultraviolet illumination.

Bovine blood forms of *B. theileri* (Fig. 1) are generally shorter and thicker and show less evidence of active division than tick tissue or haemolymph forms (Fig. 2), but lengths of all forms vary considerably. *Borrelia theileri* in Giemsa-stained bovine blood smears consist of populations of post- and pre-division forms in approximately a 2:1 ratio. The relative proportions of these two populations will affect estimates of the mean length of the parasite in cattle and ticks. As a result, inconsistent descriptions of the morphology and dimensions of *B. theileri* have occurred. Reports of mean lengths of 20–30 μm for bovine blood forms are erroneous and are actually based on maximum lengths of *B. theileri* reported by earlier authors. The mean length of blood forms has been reported as 10.2–13 μm (range of individual spirochaetes 6–19.5 μm), with approximately five spirals per spirochaete. The mean length for tick haemolymph forms is 14.8–15.4 μm (range 8.3–32 μm), with approximately seven spirals per spirochaete. Tick tissue forms tend to be longer than haemolymph forms, with a mean length of 17.7 μm (range 8–28 μm). Tissue stages

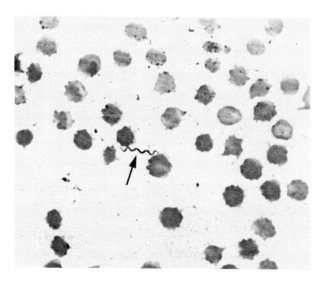

Fig. 1. *Borrelia theileri* (arrowed) in a bovine blood smear. Giemsa-stained. (Source: Smith, R.D. and Rogers, A.B. (1998) *Borrelia theileri*: a review. *Journal of Spirochetal and Tick-borne Diseases* 5, 63–68. With permission.)

are too pleomorphic for meaningful assessment of spiral counts.

Within a given spirochaete the diameter is relatively constant (0.1–0.3 μm depending on stage of division) except for a gradual tapering to a point near the poles. Wave amplitude within and between organisms is too variable to permit meaningful measurements. Wave amplitudes of less than 0.25 μm are common in the long, thin dividing forms (Fig. 2). In contrast, the short non-dividing forms (Fig. 1) may exhibit wave amplitudes up to 1.25 μm in the centre, which decrease to less than 0.5 μm near the poles.

The borrelial surface structure consists of an outer surface layer, an outer membrane and a cytoplasmic membrane. Periplasmic flagella are located between the outer and cytoplasmic membranes. Synonyms for these structures are axial fibrils, periplasmic fibrils and endoflagella. Periplasmic flagella originate near the poles of the spirochaete and course towards the middle of its length, where they overlap. The number of flagella varies between species and also within species. Most borreliae have flagella ranging in number from 16 to 30. From 5 to 10 flagella have been observed in cross-sections of *B. theileri*, suggesting that five flagella originate from each of the poles and intersect in the middle of the organism. However, organisms may occasionally contain up to 14–16 flagella. Membrane blebs, or gemmae, can also be seen in negative stains of *B. theileri*.

When wet mounts of infected bovine blood, tick tissues or short-term cultures are observed by dark-field or phase-contrast microscopy, *B. theileri* display translation (linear propulsion) fore and aft, flexion and rotational motility, similar to those of other borreliae. Free-swimming organisms propel themselves linearly or curvilinearly, or may remain stationary while undergoing rapid gyrations. Periods of activity may alternate with periods of quiescence. Spirochaetes often have one end embedded in a cell or piece of tissue while the free ends undergo gyrations to varying degrees.

In vitro *cultivation*

Short-term primary cultures of *B. theileri* established from infected *Boophilus microplus* ovaries have been used to obtain relatively pure suspensions of organisms for use as antigen in indirect fluorescent antibody testing. The culture medium was modified from that used to maintain *Borrelia recurrentis* (the louse-borne relapsing fever spirochaete) *in vitro*. Active *B. theileri* were observed in the culture for 6 weeks post-inoculation. Viable organisms were observed in association with tick ovarian tissue. One end of most spirochaetes was embedded in tissue while the free end gyrated rapidly. Sometimes clusters of spirochaetes were seen in the absence of tick tissue. Free-swimming individual borreliae were occasionally observed. Spirochaetes exhibited translational (linear) motility, flexion and corkscrew rotation. Replication of *B. theileri* led to high concentrations of organisms over the first few weeks *in vitro*. Large clusters containing hundreds to thousands

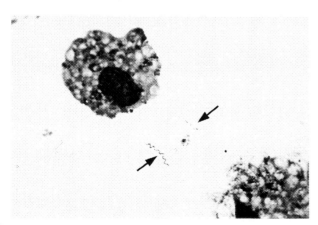

Fig. 2. Two morphological forms of *Borrelia theileri* (arrowed) in the haemolymph of an ovipositing *Boophilus microplus* female. (Source: Smith, R., Brener, J., Osorno, M. and Ristic, M. (1978) Pathobiology of *Borrelia theileri* in the tropical cattle tick *Boophilus microplus. Journal of Invertebrate Pathology* 32, 182–190. With permission).

of borreliae were seen in the first few weeks. In subsequent weeks the number of active organisms diminished.

Clinical signs

Bovine borreliosis due to *B. theileri* is benign in most cases, even in highly susceptible splenectomized calves. Parasitaemia is first detectable in Giemsa-stained thin blood smears from 2 to 4 weeks after exposure to infected ticks, but lasts only a few days. During the parasitaemic phase infected cattle may exhibit mild temperature elevations, lethargy, reductions in packed cell volume and possibly haematuria. Clinical signs, when present, usually last only a few days and are followed by uneventful recovery. Infections persist indefinitely, during which parasite recrudescences, characterized by spirochaetaemia with no outward signs of illness, may occur.

Diagnosis

Borrelia theileri may be very difficult to find in thin blood smears, even during peak parasitaemia. Five or more minutes may be required to locate one parasite. Ticks appear to be susceptible to infection during all stages of bovine parasitaemia, and may be the best indicator of bovine infection (xenodiagnosis). Although *B. theileri* causes a relatively mild disease in cattle, infections could potentially be misdiagnosed as being the more pathogenic *B. burgdorferi* or *B. coriaceae*.

Immunological response

An antibody response to tick-borne *B. theileri* infection is first detectable 3 weeks after tick-borne exposure of calves. The antibody titre then rises rapidly and persists at high levels through at least 10 weeks post-exposure. Anti-*B. theileri* antibodies cross-react with *B. burgdorferi* and *B. coricaeae* whole-cell antigens in indirect fluorescent antibody tests. Serological cross-reactivity among these species is probably due, in part, to a shared, genus-specific 39–41 kDa flagellar antigen. The *B. burgdorferi*-specific outer surface protein A (OspA) antigen does not appear to be present on either *B. theileri* or *B. coriaceae*.

Transmission

Most studies of *B. theileri* in ticks have focused on the one-host cattle tick, *Boophilus microplus*. Replication of *B. theileri* appears to occur at a higher rate in *B. microplus* ticks than in bovine blood, as masses of replicating *B. theileri* are readily found in association with tick haemocytes (Fig. 3). Spirochaetes have also been observed in close association with tick ovaries and in oviposited eggs, but they are relatively rare. Despite extensive invasion of and replication in tick tissues, *B. theileri* appears to be non-pathogenic for the tick.

Only the nymphal and adult stages of *Boophilus microplus* transmit the spirochaete to cattle, despite the fact that transovarial infection occurs and borreliae can be found in larvae within 72 h after being placed on calves. It may be that too few spirochaetes arrive in the larval salivary glands to effect transmission. Tick-borne infections with *B. theileri* have also been established in sheep, horses and deer under experimental conditions. *Borrelia theileri* can also be transmitted by injecting fresh whole blood from borrelaemic into naïve cattle.

Treatment and control

Therapeutic or sterilizing treatments for *B. theileri* have not been reported, probably because of the non-pathogenic nature of infection. Presumably antibiotics that are used to treat other borreliae would be effective against *B. theileri* as well. Co-infection with *B. theileri* could interfere with the interpretation of studies of other borreliae or haemoparasites in tick vectors or their bovine hosts. In this situation a system to assure freedom from *B. theileri* infection is desirable. Tick colonies can be freed of infection through systemic examination and segregation of uninfected ovipositing females. The process may have to be repeated for several tick generations before a borrelia-free colony emerges. Progeny of these ticks will not transmit infection to cattle, and subsequent generations will remain free of infection. However, because of the non-pathogenic nature of *B. theileri* infections, systematic screening of subsequent tick generations is required to assure

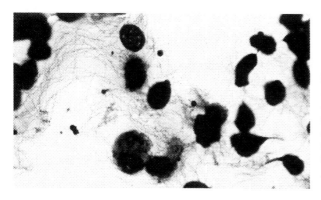

Fig. 3. *Borrelia theileri* in *Boophilus microplus* haemolymph. Note close association with haemocytes and many long thin forms suggestive of active replication. Giemsa-stained. (Source: Smith, R.D. and Rogers, A.B. (1998) *Borrelia theileri*: a review. *Journal of Spirochetal and Tick-borne Diseases* 5, 63–68. With permission.)

that bovine and tick hosts remain free of infection.

Selected bibliography

Anon. (1994) Group 1. The spirochetes. In: Holt, J.G., Krieg, N.R., Sneath, P.H.A., Staley, J.T. and Williams, S.T. (eds) *Bergey's Manual of Determinative Bacteriology,* 9th edn. Williams & Wilkins, Baltimore, Maryland, pp. 27–37.

Kelly, R. (1984) Genus IV. *Borrelia,* Swellengrebel 1907. In: Krieg, N.R. and Holt, J.G. (eds) *Bergey's Manual of Systemic Bacteriology,* Vol. 1. Williams & Wilkins, Baltimore, Maryland, pp. 57–62.

Rogers, A.B. (1992) Morphology, short-term cultivation, and serodiagnosis of *Borrelia theileri.* MS thesis, Department of Veterinary Pathobiology, University of Illinois, Urbana, 64 pp.

Smith, R.D. and Rogers, A.B. (1998) *Borrelia theileri*: a review. *Journal of Spirochetal and Tick-borne Diseases* 5, 63–68.

Smith, R., Brener, J., Osorno, M. and Ristic, M. (1978) Pathobiology of *Borrelia theileri* in the tropical cattle tick *Boophilus microplus. Journal of Invertebrate Pathology* 32, 182–190.

Smith, R.D., Miranpuri, G.S., Adams, J.H. and Ahrens, E.H. (1985) *Borrelia theileri*: isolation from ticks (*Boophilus microplus*) and tick-borne transmission between splenectomized calves. *American Journal of Veterinary Research* 46, 1396–1398.

Borreliosis *see* **Avian borreliosis** *and named* Borrelia *species.*

Boutonneuse fever *see* **Tick-borne typhuses**.

Bovine ephemeral fever

P.S. Mellor

Bovine ephemeral fever is an arthropod-borne disease of cattle and Water buffalo (*Bubalus bubalis*) caused by bovine ephemeral fever (BEF) virus, a member of the family Rhabdoviridae. The disease was first recognized as a distinct entity in 1906 in Zimbabwe, although written accounts alluding to the disease can be traced back as far as 1867. The disease has had a variety of common names, including 3-day-sickness, stiff sickness, bovine epizootic fever, lazy man's disease and dengue of cattle. However, the term 'ephemeral fever', coined near the beginning of the 20th century, is by far the most widely used name.

Distribution

Bovine ephemeral fever virus occurs in virtually all of Africa, the Middle East, Asia (south of the former USSR) and Australasia (excluding Papua New Guinea and New Zealand). The limits of occurrence in countries that are partially free, such as Japan, China and Australia, are determined by climate through its effects on the insect vectors. Europe and the Americas are free from infection.

Aetiological agent

The genome of BEF virus is a negative-sense single-stranded RNA (ssRNA) virus belonging to the family Rhabdoviridae. It has five structural and no non-structural proteins. In preparations of the virus three different particle shapes may be seen. Their approximate diameter is 73 nm, which is close to the usual diameter of 70 nm given for animal rhabdoviruses. The longest virions are bullet-shaped with a length of approximately 183 nm, having parallel sides and a precisely coiled helical nucleocapsid. Particles also occur that have a truncated bullet shape, while others appear as blunt cones. The length of the shorter particles varies from 70 to 140 nm. These shorter virions are considered to be defective and to cause interference with the growth of BEF virus in tissue culture, sometimes making isolation via this system uncertain. Surprisingly, BEF virus seems to grow very poorly, or not at all, in cell lines of bovine origin, though it grows well in cell lines of other origins, such as baby hamster kidney (BHK) and African green monkey cells (VERO) and in cells from the mosquito *Aedes albopictus.*

Bovine ephemeral fever virus is very sensitive to lipid solvents and is inactivated at pH levels below 5 or above 10. The virus therefore survives poorly outside its vertebrate or invertebrate hosts and is rapidly inactivated by the high concentrations of lactic acid which develop in the muscles of cattle after death. Consequently, fomites, bodily discharges and tissues play no part in the transmission of the virus.

For many years BEF virus was considered to be unrelated to other rhabdoviruses. However, strong antigenic similarities have recently been shown with Kimberley, Berrimah, Malakal, Puchong and Adelaide River viruses, and all six viruses have now been grouped together within the genus *Ephemerovirus*. Consequently, any virus isolated from a suspect case of bovine ephemeral fever must now be identified by the virus neutralization (VN) test with antiserum to BEF virus itself, and not simply by complement fixation, enzyme-linked immunosorbent assay (ELISA) or immunofluorescence techniques, which are merely ephemerovirus group-specific assays.

Clinical signs

Clinical disease has been recorded only in cattle and Water buffalo (*B. bubalis*). In these animals the severity of disease can vary widely from virtually imperceptible clinical signs to death. In general, disease tends to be more severe in adult cattle than in young animals, in fat animals than in lean animals, in heavy bulls than in light steers and in high-lactating cattle than in dry cows. Typically, in a herd of cattle, one or several animals will show signs about a week ahead of the main wave of disease and the passage of the virus through the herd may take 2–4 weeks, or longer, if the herd is large. The clinical course of disease can be divided into four main phases: onset of fever, period of disability, recovery and sequelae.

Onset of fever

Onset is sudden and the fever may reach a peak of 40–42°C within a few hours. Pyrexia may be biphasic, triphasic or even, occasionally, multiphasic. Concurrently, slight changes in behaviour or stance may also be seen and milk production may drop. This phase may last for half a day.

Period of disability

This phase may be of 1–2 days' duration. The first peak of pyrexia has passed but the rectal temperature may still be elevated. The most characteristic signs are severe depression, a 'tucked-up' appearance, anorexia, general muscle stiffness and lameness, with or without joint swelling. There may also be ocular and nasal discharge and excessive salivation. The animal usually remains standing but may adopt sternal recumbency although still able to rise if forced to do so. Milk production may have virtually ceased and the quality of the remaining milk will be reduced. The heart and respiratory rates are increased. Dry rales progressing to moist rales may be detected in the lungs. Superimposed on these signs may be others that are associated with hypocalcaemia, such as muscular fibrillation, an uncoordinated gait, inability to rise, ruminal stasis, constipation, loss of swallowing reflex and refusal to drink. In severe cases the animal may lapse into lateral recumbency with bloat and further reflex loss, progressing to coma and death.

Recovery

In the majority of cases recovery occurs after 1–2 days of disability and can be gradual or dramatic. Death ensues in less than 2% of uncomplicated cases but can occur during the acute disease or at the stage when most animals are recovering uneventfully.

Sequelae

Except for cows in late lactation, milk yield increases steadily after recovery but only to 80–90% of pre-illness levels. Complications may also occur and are manifested by pneumonia, mastitis, hindquarters paralysis, abnormal gait, abortion in late pregnancy and temporary (up to 6 months) infertility in bulls. Pulmonary and subcutaneous emphysema are rare occurrences. In general, animals with clinical signs of bovine ephemeral fever that are forced to exercise or are subject to any other form of climatic or physical stress are more likely to die or suffer complications than animals not so treated.

Pathology and post-mortem findings

Bovine ephemeral fever is an inflammatory disease: serofibrinous polysinovitis, polyarthritis, polytendovaginitis, cellulitis and focal necrosis of skeletal muscles are the most common pathological lesions. These lesions vary in severity, being barely discernible in some animals and very marked in others. The lesions in both joints and muscles are more severe in the limbs on which the animal was limping. A generalized oedema of lymph nodes is invariably present and the lungs may also show patchy oedema.

Microscopically there are inflammatory changes in the small blood-vessels in a range of organs and these are considered to be the fundamental histopathological lesions though they are not pathognomonic of bovine ephemeral fever.

The lesions observed in an animal dying of bovine ephemeral fever depend on the stage of disease at which it dies. If death occurs early, a fibrinous exudate is found in the serous cavities of the thorax, abdomen and joints and fibrin plaques may be found on virtually all articular surfaces. If death occurs late in the course of disease, the effects of dehydration may be apparent, as many sick animals exhibit aversion to water. Abortion can occur if cows experience disease very late in pregnancy. However, the virus does not appear to cross the placenta or affect the fertility of the female.

Diagnosis

A presumptive diagnosis of bovine ephemeral fever is possible based on the sudden onset of febrile disease in late summer, lasting from 2 to 5 days, with spontaneous recovery, affecting cattle in areas where BEF virus is known to occur. The clinical signs of oropharyngeal secretions, joint pains and stiffness are also of value.

A confirmatory diagnosis can be obtained by carrying out differential leucocyte counts on blood smears. If there is no neutrophilia with at least 30% of immature forms, the animal does not have bovine ephemeral fever. However, the test is not pathognomonic since certain other generalized infections may have a similar effect. Confirmation of bovine ephemeral fever can also be obtained by isolation of the causative virus, from whole blood samples, in cultures of BHK cells, VERO cells or *A. albopictus* cells, or by the intracerebral inoculation of suckling mice and then identification by the VN test. The VN test must be used to ensure differentiation between BEF virus and the other ephemeroviruses that may be present and which are considered to be non-pathogenic. Serological confirmation of BEF virus may be obtained by the demonstration of a fourfold rise in specific neutralizing antibody titre between paired sera collected

2–3 weeks apart. However, animals that have been exposed to one of the other ephemeroviruses may already have low titres of neutralizing antibodies to BEF virus and so may exhibit an anamnestic response on infection, possibly causing antibody titres to plateau by the time that the first serum sample is taken.

Transmission

Although no arthropods have yet been shown to transmit BEF virus, the epidemiological evidence that the virus is transmitted by one or more species of flying insect is overwhelming. Such evidence includes the overall pattern of outbreaks, the fact that bovine ephemeral fever epizootics occur in summer and autumn and have a strong association with recent rainfall, and that in temperate regions outbreaks terminate abruptly with the onset of winter (frosts). Also, in many regions northwards and southwards spread of the virus seems to be limited by latitude rather than by quarantine, topography or the lack of suitable vertebrate hosts. These patterns are all compatible with those of vector-borne diseases.

In the field, BEF virus has been isolated from a pool of *Culicoides* species (*C. kingi, C. nivosus, C. bedfordi, C. imicola, C. cornutus*) in Kenya, from *C. imicola* and *C. coarctatus* in Zimbabwe, from *C. brevitarsis* in Australia, and from a mixed pool of culicine mosquitoes (mainly *Culex orbostinensis, Verrallina* (formerly *Aedes*) *carmenti, Uranotaenia nivipes* and *Uranotaenia albescens*) and from *Anopheles bancrofti* in Australia. All of these isolations were made from insects free from the overt remains of a blood meal and therefore are unlikely to represent mere incidental contaminations. Furthermore, the virus has been shown to replicate in the mosquito *Culex annulirostris* and in *Culicoides marksi* and *C. brevitarsis*, when these insects were fed upon mixtures of blood and virus in the laboratory. Nevertheless, despite this wide range of insects as potential vectors, there must also be other species involved, as the areas of the world where BEF virus occurs extend well beyond the distribution of the species so far implicated. Clearly much work remains to be carried out before the relative significance of mosquitoes and *Culicoides* as vectors of BEF virus is fully understood, and before the major vector species in the different parts of the world are identified.

Vertebrate hosts

Bovine ephemeral fever virus infects and can cause disease in cattle (*Bos taurus, Bos indicus, Bos javanicus*) and Water buffalo (*Bubalus bubalis*). Antibodies have also been detected in a range of free-living ruminant species in Africa, Australia and Asia (African buffalo (*Syncerus caffer*), Waterbuck (*Kobus ellipsiprymnus*), Wildebeest (*Connochaetes taurinus*), Hartebeest (*Alcelaphus buselaphus*), Red deer (*Cervus elaphus*), Chital or Spotted deer (*Axis axis*), Rusa or Timor deer (*Cervus timorensis*)) but attempts to isolate virus from these species have been uniformly unsuccessful. It is not yet known whether some of these other vertebrate species can act as 'symptomless' reservoir hosts of BEF virus, or whether the detection of antibodies is merely incidental. Sheep and domestic ruminant species, other than cattle and Water buffalo, appear to be insusceptible to BEF virus, though the virus has been passaged experimentally through sheep.

Incubation period and viraemia

The natural incubation period in cattle is unknown but is suspected to be of some 4–8 days' duration, which is consistent with the 3–10 days which has been recorded after experimental inoculation of the virus. Viraemia in experimentally infected cattle usually lasts for about 4–5 days, commencing the day before fever and terminating 1–2 days after clinical recovery. Very occasionally viraemia may extend for as long as 13 days after infection but there is no long-term persistence. In the circulation, the virus appears to be primarily associated with the white cell fraction of the blood and has been demonstrated in neutrophils.

Treatment

Unlike most other viral diseases, early treatment of the clinical effects of bovine ephemeral fever can significantly ameliorate the effects of disease. The first principle is to rest the sick animal, preferably for at least a week. The second is to give nothing by mouth unless the swallowing reflex has been observed to be functional. In general, treatment is directed towards the generalized inflammation and the depression of serum calcium. Inflammation can be treated with phenylbutazone given intramuscularly 8-hourly for periods of up to 3 days. Treatment with calcium borogluconate (intravenously or subcutaneously) is beneficial when signs of hypocalcaemia are present. Supplementary antibiotic treatment to control secondary infection and rehydration with isotonic fluids in cases of dehydration may also be warranted. Prospects for prognosis depend upon the time of intervention and the duration of the illness.

Prevention and control

Live attenuated vaccines with adjuvants have been produced in South Africa, Japan and Australia. These vaccines have been shown to protect against experimental challenge with virulent virus. In Japan, a killed virus vaccine has also been used to boost the initial immunity produced by a live virus vaccine.

In enzootic areas it is important to vaccinate cattle, particularly dairy and feedlot herds and valuable breeding stock, to preclude production losses caused by bovine ephemeral fever. Vaccination, therefore, should be carried out in spring to ensure a high level of immunity during the ensuing summer and autumn when vector arthropods are likely to be most abundant and hence virus challenge most intense. In calves younger than 6 months of age, maternally derived antibody may interfere with the response to vaccine.

The arthropod vectors of BEF virus have not all been identified, neither has the relative importance of *Culicoides* biting midges and mosquitoes been properly assessed, so at present the efficacy of any vector control programme is likely to be uncertain.

Selected bibliography

Calisher, C.H., Karabatsos, N., Zeller, N., Digoutte, J.-P., Tesh, R.B., Shope, R.E., Travassos da Rosa, A.P.A. and St George, T.D. (1989) Antigenic relationships among rhabdoviruses from vertebrates and hematophagous arthropods. *Intervirology* 30, 241–257.

Davies, F.G. and Walker, A.R. (1974) The isolation of ephemeral fever virus from cattle and *Culicoides* midges in Kenya. *Veterinary Record* 95, 63–64.

Kay, B.H., Carley, J.G. and Filippich, C. (1975) The multiplication of Queensland and New Guinean arboviruses in *Culex annulirostris* (Skuse) and *Aedes vigilax* (Skuse) (Diptera: Culicidae). *Journal of Medical Entomology* 12, 279–283.

Murphy, F.A., Gibbs, E.P.J., Horzinek, M.C. and Studdert, M.J. (1999) Bovine ephemeral fever. In: *Veterinary Virology,* 3rd edn. Academic Press, London, pp. 441–442.

Nandi, S. and Negi, B.S. (1999) Bovine ephemeral fever: a review. *Comparative Immunology, Microbiology and Infectious Diseases* 22, 81–91.

St George, T.D. (1990) Bovine ephemeral fever virus. In: Dinter, Z. and Morein, B. (eds) *Virus Infections of Ruminants.* Elsevier, Amsterdam, pp. 405–415.

St George, T.D. (1994) Bovine ephemeral fever. In: Coetzer, J.A.W., Thomson, G.R. and Tustin, R.C. (eds) *Infectious Diseases of Livestock with Special Reference to Southern Africa,* Vol. 1. Oxford University Press, Cape Town, pp. 553–562.

St George, T.D. and Standfast, H.A. (1988) Bovine ephemeral fever. In: Monath, T.P. (ed.) *The Arboviruses: Epidemiology and Ecology,* Vol. II. CRC Press, Boca Raton, Florida, pp. 71–86.

Standfast, H.A., St George, T.D. and Dyce, A.C. (1976) The isolation of ephemeral fever virus from mosquitoes in Australia. *Australian Veterinary Journal* 52, 242.

Theodoridis, A., Boshoff, S.E.T. and Botha, M.J. (1973) Studies on the development of a vaccine against bovine ephemeral fever. *Onderstepoort Veterinary Journal* 40, 77–82.

Theodoridis, A., Giesecke, W.H. and Du Toit, I.J. (1973) Effects of ephemeral fever on milk production and reproduction. *Onderstepoort Veterinary Journal* 40, 83–91.

Bovine epizootic fever *see* **Bovine ephemeral fever.**

Brugian filariasis

M.B. Nathan

Infection of humans with the filarial worms *Brugia malayi* and *Brugia timori*. Together with *Wuchereria bancrofti* (see Bancroftian filariasis), they are collectively referred to as lymphatic filariasis.

Distribution

Brugia malayi occurs only in south and east Asia (Fig. 1) and accounts for about 10% of lymphatic filariasis infections worldwide. In India it is mostly restricted to Kerala State but foci have also been reported from Orissa, Assam, Madhya Pradesh, Andra Pradesh and Tamil Nadu. Elsewhere it is found in widely varying degrees of endemicity in Sri Lanka, Thailand, Malaysia, Indonesia, Philippines, Vietnam and Korea. Since the early 1980s, China has reported a dramatic decline in transmission of lymphatic filariasis (*B. malayi* and *W. bancrofti*)

as a result of the efforts of the national control programme. A nocturnally periodic strain, the most prevalent form, in which microfilariae appear in the peripheral blood at night, and a nocturnally subperiodic strain, in which the microfilariae also circulate in the peripheral blood during the daytime, have adapted to the diel biting behaviour of the local vector mosquitoes. The latter is less common and is found mainly in Malaysia, in Indonesia in west Sumatra and northern and eastern Sumatra, and in south-east and east Kalimantan. Leaf monkeys (*Presbytis* species) and Macaques (*Macaca* species), zoonotic reservoir hosts of subperiodic *B. malayi*, are abundant on these islands in localities where the human infection occurs.

Brugia timori, recognized as a new species in 1965, is confined to Flores, Timor and

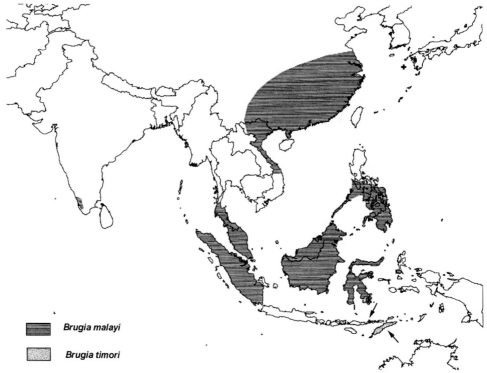

Brugia malayi

Brugia timori

Fig. 1.   Geographical distribution of *Brugia malayi* and *Brugia timori*.

lowland areas of small neighbouring islands east of Java. It is nocturnally periodic. No animal reservoir host has been identified.

Parasites

Adult worms of both *Brugia* species live in the lymphatics of the reservoir host and have an essentially similar development and life cycle to those of *W. bancrofti* (see Bancroftian filariasis). Adult female *B. malayi* are morphologically similar to those of *W. bancrofti* but are usually smaller (43–55 mm long, 130–170 µm in breadth). Male worms vary in length from 14–23 mm and are approximately 70 µm in breadth. The copulatory spicules and caudal papillae distinguish them from *W. bancrofti* males. The sheathed microfilariae are 200–275 µm long and 4–7 µm wide. Adult *B. timori* females (27 mm × 72 µm) and males (17 mm × 72 µm) are smaller than those of *B. malayi*.

Clinical symptoms

As with bancroftian filariasis, brugian filariasis causes a wide range of clinical manifestations, which often differ from one endemic area to another. Recurring lymphadenitis and lymphangitis of the limbs, with fever and chills, are major signs which occur with greater frequency than with *W. bancrofti*. Most commonly involved are the inguinal and axillary nodes and their afferent lymphatics. In Indonesia, and to a lesser extent in Malaysia and Thailand, superficial lymphatic abscesses may form with consequent scarring. Hydrocoel and other genital involvement is only rarely associated with brugian filariasis. Characteristic sites of elephantiasis are the leg(s) but, unlike bancroftian filariasis, swelling usually occurs only below the knee(s) or, less commonly, the arm(s) below the elbow(s). The swelling is usually a soft pitting oedema and is seldom accompanied by verrucous changes to the skin.

Diagnosis

See entry on bancroftian filariasis for parasitological diagnosis. No antigen detection test is currently available for brugian filariasis.

Transmission

A list of the principal vectors of brugian filariasis is shown in Table 1. Many endemic areas with nocturnally periodic *B. malayi* are open swamp habitats, where transmission is mainly by *Mansonia uniformis* and other related species, and ricefield habitats, where *Anopheles* species, including *A. barbirostris*, are common vectors. *Ochlerotatus*[1] *togoi,* a vector which breeds in rock pools near the littoral zone, is also a vector in some areas. The nocturnally subperiodic strains occur mostly in villages in or near swamps, where vectors of the *Mansonia bonneae/dives* group breed in high densities; *Coquillettidia crassipes* is a secondary vector.

Anopheles barbirostris is the only known vector of *B. timori.*

Whereas nocturnally periodic *B. malayi* is found almost exclusively in humans, nocturnally subperiodic *B. malayi* has species of *Macaca,* and *Presbytis* monkeys as important zoonotic reservoir hosts. Infection also

Table 1. Summary of the principal mosquito vectors of *Brugia malayi* and *Brugia timori*

Parasite strains	Geographical distribution	Vectors
Brugia malayi		
Nocturnal periodic	South and east Asia	*Anopheles* species
		Mansonia uniformis
		Mansonia annulata
		Mansonia annulifera
Nocturnal subperiodic	Malaysia, Indonesia	*Mansonia bonneae*
	Thailand, Philippines	*Mansonia dives*
		Mansonia annulata
		Mansonia uniformis
Brugia timori		
Nocturnal periodic	Timor, Flores, Alor, Sumba, Roti, Savu	*Anopheles barbirostris*

occurs naturally in certain wild carnivores. Domestic cats and dogs are also susceptible hosts but their importance as reservoir hosts of infection has not been determined.

Treatment
See entry on bancroftian filariasis for treatment.

Prevention and control
Prevention and control measures are essentially similar to those for *W. bancrofti* (see Bancroftian filariasis for more details), involving treatment of humans to reduce or eliminate microfilariae circulating in the bloodstream and reducing contact between humans and infective vectors. However, the aquatic stages of *Mansonia* mosquitoes are unusual in that they obtain their oxygen not at the water surface, but by piercing and drawing it from the roots of floating vegetation, such as *Pistia*, *Eichhornia* and *Salvinia*, as well as from some rooted plants. Through removal of the host plants of these vectors from ponds, canals and ditches, either physically or with herbicides, the distribution and prevalence of *B. malayi* has been reduced in parts of south Asia.

In forest and forest-fringe settlements where monkeys are important zoonotic reservoir hosts of nocturnally subperiodic *B. malayi*, control efforts have been relatively unsuccessful, probably because parasites from monkeys are transferred to the treated human population by the mosquito vectors. In some situations, the forest area bordering communities has been cleared in efforts to increase the separation of zoonotic and human hosts but the extent to which this has proved effective is not clear.

Note
[1]   *Ochlerotatus* was formerly a subgenus of *Aedes*.

Selected bibliography
Dennis, D.T., Partono, F. and Purnomo, Atmosoedjono, S. and Saroso, J.S. (1976) Timor filariasis: epidemiologic and clinical features in a defined community. *American Journal of Tropical Medicine and Hygiene* 25, 797–802.

Michael, E. and Bundy, D.A.P. (1997) Global mapping of lymphatic filariasis. *Parasitology Today* 13, 472–476.

Nutman, T.B. (ed.) (2000) *Lymphatic Filariasis.* Tropical Medicine: Science and Practice, Vol. 1. Imperial College, London, 292 pp.

Wharton, R.H. (1962) The biology of *Mansonia* mosquitoes in relation to the transmission of filariasis in Malaya. *Bulletin of the Institute of Medical Research of the Federation of Malaysia* 11, 1–114.

Buffalo disease *see* **Theilerioses.**

Bunyamwera virus

Michèle Bouloy

Bunyamwera (BUN) virus is an African virus isolated by K.C. Smithburn and colleagues in Uganda in 1943 from mosquitoes collected for yellow fever studies. In 1973, when the genus *Bunyavirus* and the Bunyaviridae family were created, BUN virus became the type species. This virus causes only minor diseases in humans but is the ninth most frequent arbovirus infecting humans in Africa, after chickungunya, Sindbis, yellow fever, West Nile, Wesselsbron, Zika, Semliki Forest (see entries) and Uganda S viruses.

Human infections
Distribution
Bunyamwera virus circulates in many regions of Africa but, with the exception of Egypt, where a low prevalence was observed, it has never been found in North Africa. It is endemic in Uganda, Tanzania and Mozambique, and in South Africa antibody prevalence is relatively high in northern Natal. A low prevalence of BUN antibodies has been reported in Madagascar. However, the highest seroprevalence is observed in Central Africa, where 100% of the adult population

inhabiting the rain forest of the Democratic Republic of Congo was found seropositive. In West Africa, the Guinean population has a relatively high prevalence.

Serological studies seem to indicate that virus activity is associated with rivers and riverine forests in Nigeria and Republic of Central Africa.

Virus

Studies on the structure of BUN virus, the molecular organization of its genome and its replication have largely contributed to a better understanding of this group of viruses.

Structure

Like every member of the family, the particle is roughly spherical, with a 90–100 nm diameter and composed of a lipid envelope with an outer surface covered with two glycoproteins G1 (115 kDa) and G2 (38 kDa). The lipid envelope is derived from the cellular site of maturation which, for most of the viruses of this family, occurs in the Golgi complex. The inner structures consist in three circular nucleocapsids containing the large (L), medium (M) or small (S) single-stranded RNA genome segment, the nucleoprotein N (19 kDa) and a few copies of the L protein (259 kDa), the RNA-dependent RNA polymerase.

The viral genome has been analysed: the S, M and L segments are, respectively, 961 nucleotides, 4458 nucleotides and 6875 nucleotides long, making the complete genetic information contained within 12,294 nucleotides. A characteristic feature of viruses of the *Bunyavirus* genus is the fact that the genome segments possess 5′ eight terminal consensus nucleotides UCAUCACA . . . which are complementary to the 3′ terminal sequences and form panhandle structures.

The genome organization is of negative polarity. Every step of the viral cycle occurs in the cytoplasm. During transcription, three subgenomic messenger RNA. (mRNAs) are synthesized. These lack poly-A at their 3′ ends and are slighly shorter than their corresponding templates. Moreover, these mRNAs possess a 5′ methylated cap and 10–18 additional non-viral nucleotides derived from cellular RNAs, which are used to initiate the mRNA synthesis with a cap-snatching mechanism, like influenza virus. Translation of these mRNAs leads to the expression of the four structural proteins and two non-structural proteins, called NSs and NSm as they are coded by the S and M segments, respectively. The M segment mRNA synthesizes a polypeptide precursor, which is cleaved co-translationally and generates, in this order, the envelope glycoprotein G1, the NSm protein (16 kDa) and the glycoprotein G2. To simplify the nomenclature, it was proposed to designate the glycoproteins G_N and G_C, as this indicates the position within the polypeptide precursor. The NSm protein, the role of which is not known, localizes to perinuclear regions, suggesting that, like the structural proteins, it is present in the Golgi complex and may participate in the assembly of the virus. The NSs protein is expressed from a bicistronic mRNA: the first open-reading frame (ORF) codes for the N protein (233 amino acids) and the second one, overlapping the N ORF in a different frame, codes for the NSs (101 amino acids, 11 kDa). Recently, A. Bridgen and R.M. Elliott have established a system for reverse genetics and generated a BUN virus mutant lacking NSs. This mutant virus grows in tissue culture and mice but has a reduced pathogenicity and is impaired in its ability to shut off host cell protein synthesis. This methodology, applied for the first time to a virus of this family, was very helpful in determining the role of NSs as an interferon antagonist.

Evolution

Like other viruses with a segmented genome, BUN virus can exchange the different segments of its genome and generate reassortants in dually infected hosts. Reassortants between Bunyamwera and Maguari, Batai or Northway were obtained in cell cultures. It is of note that, although reassortment between closely related viruses of the same genus and serogroup appears to be property of this family, some viruses of the BUN serogroup, such as Main Drain and Northway, two bunyaviruses circulating in

North America, were not able to exchange their genetic material. No genetic exchange was observed between BUN and viruses of the California serogroup.

Sequences of the S segment of several viruses of the BUN, California and Simbu serogroups were analysed and the data confirmed the earlier classification into three groups obtained by complement fixation tests. However, relationships among viruses of the BUN serogroup, established by complement fixation and neutralization tests, were not always in accordance. Since neutralization tests assay the glycoproteins and the M segment, sequencing of the M segment of these viruses (only two, BUN and Germiston, have been published) would be of value to decipher possible reassortment between ancestral viruses.

Although within the BUN serogroup, the N proteins share more than 62% homology and more than 40% between serogroups, little conservation is observed within the NSs proteins and it is very difficult to find homology between similar proteins of viruses in different genera. Some insight into the evolutionary relationships within this family was obtained by analysis of the L proteins of representative members of the different genera. The polymerase module of the L proteins of the Bunyaviridae were aligned together with those of Arenaviridae and Orthomyxoviridae, and the phylogenetic tree (Fig. 1) indicates that the Bunyaviridae sequences form two clusters, one containing bunyaviruses, hantaviruses and tospoviruses and the other containing phleboviruses and nairoviruses. This strongly suggests the existence of different origins within the family.

Clinical symptoms

Bunyamwera virus infection results in mild symptoms, such as fever, headache, joint pains and rash, and affects children particularly. In some cases, visual disturbances and vertigo are observed. However, recovery is fast (less than 7 days). Immunodeficient patients can suffer from a severe encephalitis.

Diagnosis

Like all arboviruses, BUN virus infections can be diagnosed by isolating the virus from the blood, serum or plasma, since infection leads generally to a viraemia lasting for 1–2 days after the onset of the illness. Several methods are used for virus isolation: intracerebral inoculation of suckling mice, which develop paralysis and die rapidly, and inoculation of cell cultures. In the latter case, monkey kidney (VERO), baby hamster

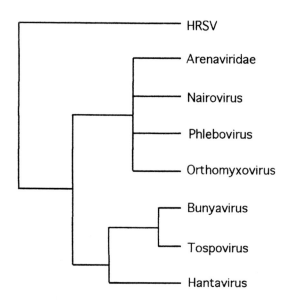

Fig. 1. Maximum parsimony consensus tree constructed using the Phylip package. Only the genus- and family-level branches are shown. HRSV: human respiratory syncytial virus, which served as an outgroup. (Adapted from Marriott, A.C. and Nuttall, P.A. (1996) *Journal of General Virology* 77, 1775–1780.)

kidney (BHK-21), *Aedes albopictus* mosquito (C6/36) or *Aedes pseudoscutellaris* mosquito (AP 61) cell lines are widely utilized.

The most recent methods for serological diagnosis involve complement fixation, neutralization, inhibition of haemagglutination or enzyme-linked immunosorbent assays (ELISA), or immunofluorescence tests. More recently, detection of immunoglobulin M (IgM) antibodies has been introduced in the battery of tests to diagnose a recent infection. Because of the serological cross-reactivity among members of the Bunyaviridae family, a collection of viruses and reference sera are necessary for an unambiguous answer.

As molecular diagnosis has been developed for many viruses, reverse-transcription polymerase chain reaction (RT-PCR), with appropriate primers can be used to detect the genome of BUN virus and other bunyaviruses.

Transmission

Although *Aedes* species appear to play a major role for transmission of BUN virus, isolations have been performed from two other genera of mosquitoes, *Mansonia* and *Culex*. In South Africa, many strains were isolated from *Aedes circumluteolus*.

Bunyamwera virus has been shown to replicate after intrathoracic inoculation of *Aedes* species, such as *A. vexans* and *A. aegypti*, and of *Ochlerotatus*[1] *canadensis*, *O. triseriatus*, *Psorophora ferox*, *Culex pipiens* and *Anopheles quadrimaculatus*. Oral infection and transmission were demonstrated after experimental infection of *A. aegypti* with BUN virus. The virus also replicates in C6/36 (*A. albopictus*) mosquito cell lines, but, in contrast to the situation observed in mammalian cells, which die rapidly after infection, no cytopathic effect was observed and persistently infected cell lines could be established. Persistence is accompanied by the generation of viruses with variable genetic and phenotypic properties. If a similar accumulation of mutations takes place in a mosquito known to generate reassortants, the vector would appear to be a host favouring viral evolution.

Animal infections

Bunyamwera virus has never been isolated from naturally infected vertebrates but experiments showing that wild African rodents replicate the virus and develop viraemia suggest that they may be natural hosts involved in the viral transmission cycle. Neutralizing antibodies against BUN virus have been found in domestic cattle.

Treatment and control

No vaccine or treatment against this virus is curently available, but, in the absence of large epizootics or epidemics, there is not a strong need when compared with other diseases caused by members of the family.

Note

[1] *Ochlerotatus* was formerly a subgenus of *Aedes*.

Selected bibliography

Elliott, R.M. (1996) *The Bunyaviridae*. Plenum Press, New York, 360 pp.

Gonzalez, J.P. and Georges, A.-J. (1986) Bunyaviral fevers: Bunyamwera, Ilesha, Germiston, Bwamba and Tataguine. In: Monath, T.P. (ed.) *The Arboviruses: Epidemiology and Ecology*, Vol. II. CRC Press, Boca Raton, Florida, pp. 87–98.

Gonzalez-Scarano F. and Nathanson, N. (1990) Bunyaviruses. In: Fields, B.N. and Knipe, D.M. (eds) *Virology*, 2nd edn., Vol. 1. Raven Press, New York, pp. 1195–1228.

Smithburn, K.C., Haddow, A.J. and Mahaffy, A.F. (1946) A neurotropic virus isolated from *Aedes* mosquitoes caught in the Semliki Forest. *American Journal of Tropical Medicine and Hygiene* 26, 189–208.

Bwamba and Pongola viruses

Richard M. Kinney

Mosquito-borne infection of humans and other mammals in countries of sub-Saharan Africa with viruses of the Bwamba serogroup, genus *Bunyavirus*, family Bunyaviridae.

Distribution

Bwamba (BWA) and Pongola (PGA) viruses are widely distributed in countries of sub-Saharan Africa. Geographical distribution has been confirmed by BWA and/or PGA virus isolations from humans or mosquitoes in Uganda, Ethiopia, Côte d'Ivoire, South Africa, Senegal, Kenya, Central African Republic, Mozambique and Nigeria. Based on serosurveys for the presence of BWA virus group-specific antibodies in humans and animals, countries of suspected virus distribution include Tanzania, Botswana, Angola and Namibia. Many people in sub-Saharan Africa become infected with BWA serogroup viruses. Human serosurveys have identified high prevalence of neutralizing antibodies against BWA virus or PGA virus in both children and adults in a number of these countries. Bwamba virus group-specific antibodies have been identified in up to 44% of individuals tested in Uganda and up to 74% in various populations in Nigeria. In one study, PGA virus-specific antibody prevalence in humans was measured at 80% along the east coast of the Simbu Pan, Natal, region of South Africa, and 2.6% in the interior Transvaal region of this country.

Virus

The Bunyaviridae family contains over 250 viruses, most of which are organized into 41 serogroups and five genera (*Bunyavirus, Phlebovirus, Hantavirus, Nairovirus,* and *Tospovirus*) by cross-complement fixation tests (genus) and cross-neutralization and cross-haemagglutination inhibition tests (group). Bunyaviruses contain a single-stranded, negative-sense, tripartite RNA genome consisting of large, medium and small RNA segments, which encode the large viral RNA polymerase, glycoproteins G1 and G2 and the nucleocapsid protein, respectively. The viruses replicate in the cytoplasm and mature by budding through the Golgi apparatus of infected cells. Conserved, shared antigenic determinants of the capsid protein elicit complement-fixing antibodies. The glycoproteins, which are present in a host-derived lipid membrane surrounding the nucleocapsid, elicit neutralizing and haemagglutination-inhibiting antibodies that permit differentiation of closely related viruses within serogroups. Serological testing has been the method of choice for identification of unidentified isolates. However, genetic analyses of genomic nucleotide sequences can be expected to complement serological identification in the near future.

The BWA serogroup is one of 16 antigenic groups assigned to the genus *Bunyavirus*. The BWA serogroup currently contains only two viruses, BWA and PGA, which appear to be closely related. Bwamba virus (prototype strain M 459) was first isolated in 1937 from mice inoculated with sera from non-resident febrile patients who became infected while working on a new road in a forested area north-west of the Ruwenzori range of mountains in Bwamba county, Western Province of Uganda. Pongola virus (prototype strain SAAR 1) was isolated in 1955 from a pool of *Aedes circumluteolus* mosquitoes collected near Lake Simbu and the Pongola River in Natal, South Africa.

Clinical symptoms

Bwamba virus causes a mild febrile illness in humans of all ages. An incubation period of less than 2 weeks' duration can only be estimated. When infection is evident, the onset is sudden and moderately severe with fever, slow pulse, severe frontal headache, backache in the lumbar or cervical regions, general body aches and moderate weakness.

A furred tongue with bright red margins and tip and transitory albuminuria, but not haematuria, have been noted. A rash has not been observed. Fever generally lasts for 2–5 days, headache and backache for another 2–3 days. Convalescence is rapid, complete and without sequelae. No fatal cases have been reported. Intracranial inoculation of BWA virus in Rhesus monkeys (*Macaca mulatta*) results in transient, mild fever and the development of neutralizing antibodies.

Diagnosis

Virus isolation can be performed in a variety of cell lines or in laboratory mice. Mice are highly susceptible to both BWA and PGA viruses administered by the intracranial route. Following such treatment, 4-week-old and younger mice suffer 100% mortality, with average survival times of 3–5 days. Paralysis of the hindquarters is sometimes, but not generally, observed. Adult mice are not susceptible to either virus following peripheral inoculation.

Complement fixation, haemagglutination inhibition and neutralization tests have been employed in the serodiagnosis of BWA group viruses and infections. Bwamba and Pongola viruses appear to be closely related and may be genetic variants of the same virus. However, certain inconsistencies have been apparent in attempts to differentiate isolates of these two viruses or to differentiate immune sera resulting from infections with these viruses. Sera positive for BWA virus by haemagglutination inhibition testing are often negative for BWA virus, but positive for PGA virus in virus neutralization tests. Many human sera neutralize one of the BWA serogroup viruses but not the other. In one study, monkeys immunized with BWA virus developed antibodies that neutralized both BWA and PGA viruses, while those immunized with PGA virus produced PGA virus-specific neutralizing antibodies. Twelve strains isolated in Nigeria and first identified as BWA virus by complement fixation and neutralization tests were later identified as PGA virus by agar-gel diffusion and immunoelectrophoretic techniques.

Bwamba and Pongola viruses appear to co-circulate in Nigeria and Kenya. It has been hypothesized that the antigenic structure of these viruses is unstable or variable, depending on their recent passage history in nature. This idea is supported by the finding that most BWA serogroup viruses that have been isolated from mosquitoes have been identified as PGA virus, while human isolates have generally been identified as BWA virus. In agar-gel diffusion tests, one strain (NY-45) of BWA virus, which was isolated from a child in Kenya, exhibited a line of identity with PGA antiserum after passage of the virus in *Mansonia uniformis* or *Anopheles gambiae* mosquitoes, but not after mouse brain passage only. Antigenicity may be influenced by viral mutations or differences in viral maturation, such as variable glycosylation of envelope glycoproteins, in different host cells. Further study of the antigenicity of these closely related viruses following passage in different hosts would be useful. Serodiagnostic tests for BWA group viruses should include both BWA and PGA viruses or antigens. Neutralization tests should be performed by the serum-dilution plaque-reduction method. Characterization by nucleotide sequence analyses of the glycoprotein genes would undoubtedly shed considerable light on the genetic relationship between BWA and PGA viruses.

Transmission

Bwamba and Pongola viruses are probably not highly infectious for humans. They are arthropod-borne viruses transmitted by a wide variety of mosquitoes, including species of *Aedes, Mansonia, Culex* and *Anopheles*. *Aedes circumluteolus*, which feeds on large mammals in the bush, has been shown to transmit PGA virus experimentally and is probably significantly involved in the natural transmission of BWA group viruses in South Africa, Nigeria and elsewhere. Isolations have been made from *M. uniformis/Mansonia africana* in Uganda, Kenya, South Africa, Ethiopia, Central African Republic, Mozambique and Nigeria; from *Anopheles,* including *A. coustani* and *A. gambiae,* in Uganda, Kenya, Côte d'Ivoire, Nigeria and Senegal;

and from *Aedes* species, including *A. vittatus*, *A. tarsalis* and *A. fowleri*, in Senegal, Côte d'Ivoire and Central African Republic. Pongola virus has been isolated from *Culex zombaensis* in Kenya.

Virus activity is lowest during the late dry season and peaks during the rainy season when there are large mosquito populations.

Neutralizing antibodies against BWA virus have been found in wild monkeys, and in cattle, sheep, goats and donkeys.

Treatment

There is no specific treatment for Bwamba fever. Standard passive treatment includes bedrest, maintenance of fluids and treatment to reduce aches.

Control

Insect repellents, such as diethyltoluamide (DEET), can offer effective personal protection against mosquito bites. Repellents that contain greater than 20–30% concentrations of DEET may be toxic for children. Insecticidal fogging or spraying can result in temporary and localized control, and application of larvicides to standing water may be effective, but when mosquitoes are not found around habitations this approach is impractical. Protection against night-biting vectors, such as anophelines and *Mansonia* species, can be obtained through use of mosquito bed nets impregnated with pyrethroid insecticides such as permethrin or deltamethrin.

Selected bibliography

Bishop, D.H.L. (1990) *Bunyaviridae* and their replication. Part I: *Bunyaviridae*. In: Fields, B.N., Knipe, D.M., Chanock, R.M., Hirsch, M.S., Melnick, J.L., Monath, T.P. and Roizman, B. (eds) *Fields Virology*, 2nd edn, Vol. 1. Raven Press, New York, pp. 1155–1173.

Johnson, B.K., Chanas, A.C., Squires, E.J., Shockley, P., Simpson, D.I.H. and Smith, D.H. (1978) The isolation of a Bwamba virus variant from man in western Kenya. *Journal of Medical Virology* 2, 15–20.

Karabatsos, N. (ed.) (1985) *International Catalogue of Arboviruses, Including Certain Other Viruses of Vertebrates*, 3rd edn. The Subcommittee on Information Exchange of the American Committee on Arthropod-Borne Viruses, American Society of Tropical Medicine and Hygiene, San Antonio, Texas. 1147 pp.

Kokernot, R.H., Smithburn, K.C. and Weinbren, M.P. (1956) Neutralizing antibodies to arthropod-borne viruses in human beings and animals in the Union of South Africa. *Journal of Immunology* 77, 313–323.

Kokernot, R.H., Smithburn, K.C., Weinbren, M.P. and de Meillon, B. (1957) Studies on arthropod-borne viruses of Tongaland. VI. Isolation of Pongola virus from *Aedes (Banksinella) circumluteolus* Theo. *South African Journal of Medical Sciences* 22, 81–92.

Lennette, E.H. and Koprowski, H. (1944) Influence of age on the susceptibility of mice to infection with certain neurotropic viruses. *Journal of Immunology* 49, 175–191.

McIntosh, B.M., Jupp, P.G. and de Sousa, J. (1972) Further isolations of arboviruses from mosquitoes collected in Tongaland, South Africa, 1960–1968. *Journal of Medical Entomology* 9, 155–159.

Smithburn, K.C., Mahaffy, A.F. and Paul, J.H. (1941) Bwamba fever and its causative virus. *American Journal of Tropical Medicine and Hygiene* 21, 75–90.

Tomori, O. and Fabiyi, A. (1976) Differentiation of Bwamba and Pongola viruses by agar-gel diffusion and immunoelectrophoretic techniques. *American Journal of Tropical Medicine and Hygiene* 25, 489–493.

Tomori, O., Monath, T.P., Lee, V., Fagbami, A. and Fabiyi, A. (1974) Bwamba virus infection: a sero-survey of vertebrates in five ecological zones in Nigeria. *Transactions of the Royal Society of Tropical Medicine and Hygiene* 68, 461–465.

Cache Valley virus

Paul R. Grimstad

Cache Valley (CV) virus (family Bunya-viridae, genus *Bunyavirus*, Bunyamwera serogroup) has been recognized only recently as a potentially serious vertebrate pathogen in North America, with transmission primarily between several mosquito species and larger ungulates. The death of a previously healthy adult male associated with a mid-autumn (1995) onset of primary Cache Valley encephalitis, serological evidence of additional human central nervous system (CNS) disease in the USA, sero-surveys showing widespread human and ungulate infection and linkage to a range of reproductive problems in domestic animals and possibly humans mark CV virus as a newly recognized 'emerging' teratogenic and neuropathogenic virus. No other North American arbovirus has been linked to both fatal CNS disease and overt vertebrate tera-togenicity; CV virus may be more important as a domestic animal and human teratogen than as the agent of CNS disease.

The disease
No name has been given to the few clinically recognized human CNS cases; however, it is most appropriately called 'Cache Valley virus encephalitis' or alternatively 'Cache Valley encephalitis', rather than invoking the serogroup name, 'Bunyamwera encephalitis'.

Distribution
Cache Valley virus is distributed throughout parts of Canada, most of the USA and into northern Mexico (one Jamaican isolate). Fort Sherman virus from Panama and Tlacotalpan virus from Mexico, considered a subtype and variant of CV virus, respectively, may be more representative of the CV-like viruses circulating south of the USA. Cache Valley virus was first isolated in 1956 from *Culiseta inornata* mosquitoes collected in Utah's Cache Valley; almost 400 CV virus isolates came from 29 additional mosquito species in the next three decades (data summarized in Calisher *et al.*, 1986). Isolates have also come from large ungulates, such as Caribou (*Rangifer tarandus terraenovae*), White-tailed deer (*Odocoileus virginianus*), horses and sheep, and from the one fatal human case. Cache Valley virus may not be a single virus species *per se*. Studies using cross-neutralization tests with a number of isolates have suggested multiple subtypes; recent work has demonstrated that the broad range of CV virus isolates represents a viral species complex, including several antigenically distinct forms.

The virus
Cache Valley is an enveloped virus whose genome is composed of three single-stranded, negative-sense RNA segments. The large (L) segment of related bunya-viruses is approximately 6800 bases in length and encodes a probable viral polymerase. The middle (M) CV virus segment has a 4463-nucleotide sequence. In bunya-viruses, this segment encodes two glyco-proteins, G1 and G2, plus a non-structural protein; G1 functions in vertebrate cell infection, while G2 appears critical for mosquito infection. Cache Valley virus's G1 glycoprotein consists of 958 amino acids and five glycosylation sites, two of which are unique to CV virus when compared with Fort Sherman and Tlacotalpan viruses. The third and shortest (S) segment encodes for the nucleocapsid and a second non-structural protein.

Nucleotide sequences are conserved within the genus.

Clinical symptoms and record of infection
In the USA, inapparent human infection is well documented from retrospective sero-surveys, in which anti-CV virus antibody prevalence ranged from 3% in residents of southern Illinois to a mean of 7% among

residents of 22 Indiana counties, and 19% in coastal Virginia residents. An Indiana study, using almost 2000 cord bloods from live births at one regional hospital, found a 2.9% specific antibody prevalence against CV virus, with an overall bunyavirus sero-positive rate of 8.4%. The range of clinical CNS symptoms associated with human CV virus infection is unknown because only a single fatality attributed to CV virus infection has been reported. The annual (ende-mic) clinical : subclinical case ratio is also unknown, as no public or private medical laboratories routinely include Cache Valley in differential diagnoses. Febrile illness may be the norm; in Africa, 'Bunyamwera fever' has been described and other BUN serogroup viruses, including Fort Sherman, are associated with febrile illness. Sero-surveys of cattle, dogs, goats, horses, sheep and pigs have found many with neutraliz-ing (N) antibodies, suggesting frequent infection. Antibody prevalence is higher in larger domestic animals, as with wildlife; CV virus seroprevalence in Indiana and Michigan cattle and horses was similar to that of White-tailed deer (i.e. 50–75%). More than 82% of East Coast (USA) dairy cattle and 95% of horses had neutralizing antibody.

The most significant isolations of CV virus from a domestic animal occurred in Texas in 1987, when it was recovered from aborted sheep; neutralizing antibody against CV virus was detected in all ewes that lost lambs. These results came from the investi-gation of an epizootic of birth defects (arthro-gryposis with hydranencephaly, i.e. AGH syndrome, spontaneous abortion, stillbirth) occurring in that sheep flock. Subsequent inoculation of sheep and follow-up studies proved that CV virus was a teratogen of sheep and cattle.

Reports of epizootics and other out-breaks of musculoskeletal and CNS defects in sheep linked to CV virus through sero-logies and virus isolations suggest that its teratogenicity is of considerable veterinary importance. A 1995 study of 500 human sera noted a significant correlation between maternal infection in the first trimester of pregnancy, seroconversion to CV virus and their infants presenting with macrocephaly. In ungulate studies, the critical period is also the first trimester. Antibody prevalence in wild ungulates and especially White-tailed deer suggests that they are important CV virus hosts, with neutralizing antibody prevalence reaching 100%. One serosurvey of deer in the greater Minneapolis–St Paul metropolitan area (Minnesota, USA) showed a 91% antibody prevalence rate; in that study essentially every deer was seroposi-tive against either CV virus or Jamestown Canyon virus (see entry) or both. Sero-positive rates are considerably lower when smaller wildlife are sampled. Only 6.1% (5/82) of eastern Cottontail rabbits (*Sylvilagus floridanus*) had N antibody in northern Indiana regions where high human and domestic animal N antibody prevalence against CV virus prevailed.

Diagnosis

In contrast to the major arboviral encepha-litides in North America, complement fixation (CF), haemagglutination inhibition (HI) or enzyme-linked immunosorbent assay (ELISA) kits or reagents are not widely available for routine serological diagnosis of CV virus infection. Antibody neutralizing viral infectivity has generally been meas-ured because CF and HI assays are group-specific and do not allow for accurate iden-tification of closely related Bunyamwera (BUN) serogroup viruses. Virtually all human infections have been typed using viral neutralization tests (NT), especially in serosurveys. Use of NT is essential, given the overlapping geographical range of some of the North American BUN serogroup viruses. Cache Valley virus isolation has primarily been accomplished using green monkey kidney (VERO) cells and/or suck-ling mice. During investigations of arbo-virus outbreaks other than CV virus, a variety of mosquito species have yielded multiple CV virus isolations. During inves-tigations of the 1980 eastern equine enceph-alitis (EEE) virus (see entry) epizootic in Michigan (USA), 54 of the 60 CV virus iso-lates were from the mosquito *Coquillettidia perturbans*. This mosquito was targeted because of its regional association with EEE virus. In the fatal human case, CV virus was isolated at the Special Pathogens Branch, Centers for Disease Control and Prevention (CDC), Atlanta, due to the persistence of those workers in identifying the agent, and because of the fortuitous sample submission due to the severity of the patient's illness. The likelihood is high that CV virus isolates, from both invertebrates and vertebrates, especially human, have been missed in the past.

Transmission

Multiple mosquito species are probably involved in regional CV virus transmission cycles. The combined geographical ranges of four species, *Anopheles quadrimaculatus* and *Anopheles punctipennis* (the sources of 32.5% of all CV virus isolates), *Coquillettidia perturbans* and *Culiseta inornata*, completely overlap the broad range of CV virus and may well represent the primary vectors. These four mosquitoes (the sources of 58% of all CV virus isolates) feed preferentially on large mammals and, less commonly, or rarely, on small mammals. The majority of CV virus isolates have occurred from collections made in the latter part of July into late October, suggesting greater involvement of late-season vectors, especially the two anophelines. Vector competence trials have shown that *A. punctipennis*, *A. quadrimaculatus*, *C. perturbans*, *C. inornata*, *Ochlerotatus*[1] *sollicitans*, *Ochlerotatus taeniorhynchus* and *Aedes vexans* are all capable of oral transmission of this virus, although at lower levels.

Since a single geographical CV virus cycle has yet to be elucidated, it is hypothesized that CV virus is transmitted primarily in the latter half of the summer into early autumn by anophelines, and perhaps other mosquito species, to a wide range of larger ungulates. Infection of captive White-tailed deer (Michigan, USA) occurred after mid-August in multiple years when the only mosquitoes feeding on large ungulates at the site were *A. quadrimaculatus* and *A. punctipennis*.

Local veterinarians have anecdotal records of AGH syndrome outbreaks in sheep during the local season when peak anopheline populations occurred. Cache Valley virus may overwinter in blood-fed anophelines as no spring isolation from other mosquito species has been obtained prior to the emergence of overwintering anophelines (see also Jamestown Canyon virus). This hypothesis does not preclude the possibility of CV virus overwintering transovarially in culicine species, as occurs with other bunyaviruses. Alternatively, late spring and early summer isolations from aedine mosquitoes in the northern half of the USA could result from their merely probing viraemic ungulates and not from their role as biological vectors. Since populations of species that are competent in one region may not be competent in a different geographical region, extensive vector and host competence studies are essential to elucidate the role that each species from which CV virus has been isolated may play in the overall North American transmission cycles.

Treatment

The clinical treatment of a CNS case associated with CV virus infection would be similar to that for any other arboviral neuropathogen; symptoms (high fever, seizures, coma) are treated until recovery occurs. There have been no studies utilizing antiviral drugs to treat CV virus infection, nor is there likely to be a vaccine produced, given the current lack of interest in associating this and other bunyaviruses with clinical disease in domestic animals and humans.

Control

Efforts to control the probable primary vectors of CV virus in North America would probably be ineffective, given their basic biology, the range of different breeding sites and the environmental impact of markedly affecting the *A. quadrimaculatus*, *A. punctipennis* and perhaps the *C. perturbans* and *C. inornata* populations. Timely public education remains the key.

Note

[1] *Ochlerotatus* was formerly a subgenus of *Aedes*.

Selected bibliography

Blackmore, C.G.M., Blackmore, M.S. and Grimstad, P.R. (1998) Role of *Anopheles quadrimaculatus* and *Coquillettidia perturbans* (Diptera: Culicidae) in the transmission cycle of Cache Valley virus (*Bunyaviridae: Bunyavirus*) in the Midwest, U.S.A. *Journal of Medical Entomology* 35, 660–664.

Brockus, C.L. and Grimstad, P.R. (1999) Sequence analysis of the medium (M) segment of Cache Valley virus, with comparison to other *Bunyaviridae*. *Virus Genes* 19, 73–83.

Calisher, C.H. and Karabatsos, N. (1988) Arbovirus serogroups: definition and geographic distribution. In: Monath, T.P. (ed.) *The Arboviruses: Epidemiology and Ecology*, Vol. I. CRC Press, Boca Raton, Florida, pp. 19–57.

Calisher, C.H. and Sever, J.L. (1995) Are North American Bunyamwera serogroup viruses etiologic agents of human congenital defects of the central nervous system? *Emerging Infectious Diseases* 1, 147–151.

Calisher, C.H., Francy, D.B., Smith, G.C., Muth, D.J., Lazuick, J.S., Karabatsos, N., Jakob, W.L. and McLean, R.G. (1986) Distribution of Bunyamwera serogroup viruses in North America, 1956–1984. *American Journal of Tropical Medicine and Hygiene* 35, 429–443.

Chung, S.I., Livingston, C.W., Edwards, J.F., Crandell, R.W., Shope, R.E., Shelton, M.J. and Collisson, E.W. (1990) Evidence that Cache Valley virus induces congenital malformations in sheep. *Veterinary Microbiology* 21, 297–307.

Hardy, J.L. (1994) Arboviral zoonoses of North America. In: Beran, G.W. (ed.) *Handbook of Zoonoses Section B: Viral*, 2nd edn. CRC Press, Boca Raton, Florida, pp. 185–200.

Nowicki, W.L. (1995) Bunyavirus infections and the associated immune response and birth defects. PhD dissertation, University of Notre Dame, Notre Dame, Indiana, 135 pp.

Sexton, D.J., Rollin, P.E., Breitschwerdt, E.B., Corey, G.R., Meyers, S.A., Dumais, M.R., Bowen, M.D., Goldsmith, C.S., Zaki, S.R., Nichol, S.T., Peters, C.J. and Ksiazek, T.G. (1997) Life-threatening Cache Valley virus infection. *New England Journal of Medicine* 336, 547–549.

California group viruses *see* **Jamestown Canyon, Keystone, La Crosse** *and* **San Angelo viruses.**

Canine hepatozoonosis *see* **Hepatozoonosis, canine.**

Carrión's Disease

Richard J. Birtles

Carrión's disease, or bartonellosis, is a biphasic disease, caused by the Gram-negative bacterium *Bartonella bacilliformis*, which affects inhabitants of the Andean cordillera in South America. Infection manifests either as a haemolytic anaemia (Oroya fever) or as a benign eruptive syndrome characterized by blood-filled angiogenic skin lesions (verruga peruana). Although the infectious nature of the disease was not confirmed until the beginning of the 20th century, recognition of verruga peruana as a disease entity predates Christopher Columbus. That the two phases of the disease were indeed caused by the same aetiological agent was demonstrated by the foolhardy exploits of a Peruvian medical student, Daniel Carrión, from whom the disease takes its name. Carrión inoculated himself with fluid drawn from a skin lesion of a verruga peruana patient and subsequently succumbed to Oroya fever. Although the clinical course of Carrión's illness was unexpected, his death was not. Oroya fever is estimated to be fatal in over 80% of untreated patients. The name Oroya fever was coined following a severe epidemic that killed 7000 immigrant labourers working on the railway between Lima and La Oroya, Peru, in 1871.

Distribution

Although Carrión's disease has been reported along the length of the Andes between Colombia and northern Chile, the vast majority of cases are Peruvian. An endemic zone for the disease exists on the western slopes of the mountains in the centre of the country, between Cajamarca in the north and Huancavelica in the south, with most cases occurring in the communities living between 1000 and 3000 m altitude. The endemic zone has long been considered as being limited to the area inhabited by the phlebotomine sand-fly, *Lutzomyia verrucarum*, which was identified in the 1930s as the most likely vector of Carrión's disease and has remained the leading contender ever since. Foci of Carrión's disease have recently been encountered in regions of Peru where the disease was previously unknown, such as Cusco in the Andean Sierra and the area around Chachapoyas (Amazonas) in the north of the country.

Aetiological agent

Bartonella species are facultative intracellular haemotrophic bacteria whose natural life cycles require a warm-blooded host (see also *Bartonella quintana* and *Bartonella henselae*, and Cat-scratch disease). *Bartonella bacilliformis* possesses an unremarkable morphology of a small Gramnegative bacterium, although the presence of polar flagella differentiates it from most other members of the genus.

Clinical symptoms

Acute bartonellosis (Oroya fever) is classically considered as a severe haemolytic anaemia accompanied by high fever, chills and headache. The syndrome is characterized by rapid onset and progression, leading to rheumatic pain, lymphadenopathy and neurological dysfunction. Immunosuppression renders patients especially prone to secondary infections, most often with *Salmonella* species. It appears to be these complications, as much as the direct effects of Carrión's disease, that lead to profound illness, coma and death. However, this severe progression occurs mainly in visitors to endemic areas or in inhabitants of places where new foci of the disease emerge. In contrast, most cases occurring among the population of endemic areas (especially among children) appear to be of a much milder nature. Anaemia may or may not be apparent, whereas severe headaches, joint aches, fever and malaise are common.

Verruga peruana is manifested by multiple blood-filled skin lesions that result from angioproliferation of the subdermal vasculature. The form and number of lesions can vary. Newly formed lesions are friable but older forms are more robust. Although often disfiguring, the verrugas are self-limiting and gradually disappear. Classical descriptions suggest that verruga peruana follows weeks after Oroya fever, but this is not necessarily accurate. Some Oroya fever sufferers never develop verruga peruana whereas, for other people, the appearance of verrugas may be the first indication of Carrión's disease. Alternatively, patients may develop verrugas many years after recovering from Oroya fever.

Pathogenicity

The biphasic nature of Carrión's disease results from tropism for both erythrocytes and (micro)vascular endothelial cells. The ability of *Bartonella* species to invade erythrocytes is unique among bacteria, but only a handful of virulence factors associated with this process have been identified. Notably, flagella appear to play a significant role in erythrocyte interaction and an invasion-potentiating two-gene locus has been identified. Perhaps the most remarkable virulence trait of *B. bacilliformis* is its ability to induce proliferation of vascular endothelial cells. This ability appears to be mediated by a protein factor released by the bacteria. As yet this factor remains virtually uncharacterized, although rigorous efforts to do so are in progress.

Diagnosis

The examination of peripheral blood smears has long been used to confirm cases of Oroya fever. On Giemsa staining, bartonellae appear as coccobacillary forms within erythrocytes. However, this method is relatively insensitive, especially if the anaemia is mild. Polymerase chain reaction (PCR)-based methods for the detection of *B. bacilliformis* have been developed and, in a reference laboratory setting, have proved reliable and sensitive. Cultivation of *B. bacilliformis* from infected blood is also possible, usually using a blood-rich agar (other media have also proved useful). However, long incubation times compromise the usefulness of this approach. Histopathological diagnosis is the most often employed method for the diagnosis of verruga peruana, although visualization of the bacteria is problematic and diagnosis often relies on the observation of non-specific pathologies such as angioblastic proliferation. Serological assays have been described and some have performed well in evaluations. However, such assays are of little use for acute-phase diagnosis, and the relevance of titres, especially if an asymptomatic carrier state exists, is uncertain.

Transmission and epidemiology

For most of the *Bartonella* species, a non-human mammalian reservoir host has been implicated, but for *B. bacilliformis* and *B. quintana* humans are thought to be the principal reservoir host. Attempts to identify non-human hosts by screening bloods from animals inhabiting areas of Peru where Carrión's disease is endemic yielded several *Bartonella* species, but not *B. bacilliformis*. However, two recent epidemiological investigations found the risk of disease increased when animals were housed inside the home or when sick chickens and Guinea-pigs (*Cavia porcellus*) were reported. Evidence for a human reservoir host is derived from the relatively frequent reports of isolation of *B. bacilliformis* from asymptomatic individuals (many of whom had previously suffered from Oroya fever). Indeed, some surveys have indicated that as many as 10% of inhabitants of endemic areas may be carriers of the bacterium. However, a recent study of 243 children in southern Ecuador failed to identify any asymptomatic infections despite Carrión's disease being present in the region for at least the last 15 years.

Although the phlebotomine sand-fly, *L. verrucarum*, is still considered the principal vector of Carrión's disease, this species is absent from many of the areas where new foci of the disease have emerged. Other *Lutzomyia* species may act as vectors under these circumstances. Nothing is known about the mechanism of transmission, or whether the bacterium interacts with the vector in any way.

Treatment

Appropriate antibiotic therapy reduces mortality among Oroya fever patients to less than 10%. Although many antibiotics are effective against *B. bacilliformis*, it is the usefulness of chloramphenicol against secondary infections due to salmonellae that has made it the drug of choice.

Control

There are no realistic control measures to prevent infection, although sleeping under a sand-fly net and the use of insect repellents may reduce the biting of potential vectors, such as phlebotomine sand-flies.

Selected bibliography

Ellis, B.A., Rotz, L.D., Leake, J.A.D., Samalvides, F., Bernable, J., Ventura, G., Padilla, C., Villaseca, P., Beati, L., Regnery, R., Childs, J.E., Olsen, J.G. and Carrillo, C.P. (1999) An outbreak of acute bartonellosis (Oroya fever) in the Urubamba region of Peru. *American Journal of Tropical Medicine and Hygiene* 61, 344–349.

Garcia, F.U., Wojta, J., Broadley, K.N., Davidson, J.M. and Hoover, R.L. (1990) *Bartonella bacilliformis* stimulates endothelial cells *in vitro* and is angiogenic *in vivo*. *American Journal of Pathology* 136, 1125–1135.

Gray, G.C., Johnson, A.A., Thornton, S.A., Smith, W.A., Knobloch, J., Kelley, P.W., Escudero, L.O., Huayda, M.A. and Wignall, F.S. (1990) An epidemic of Oroya fever in the Peruvian Andes. *American Journal of Tropical Medicine and Hygiene* 42, 215–221.

Herrer, A. (1990) *Epidemiologia de la verruga peruana*. Gonzales-Mugaburu, Lima, Peru, 120 pp.

Ihler, G.M. (1996) *Bartonella bacilliformis*: dangerous pathogen slowly emerging from deep background. *FEMS Microbiology Letters* 144, 1–11.

Mitchell, S.J. and Minnick, M.F. (1995) Characterisation of a two-gene locus from *Bartonella bacilliformis* associated with the ability to invade human erythrocytes. *Infection and Immunity* 63, 1552–1562.

Cat-scratch disease and other related *Bartonella* infections

Bruno B. Chomel and Chao-chin Chang

Cat-scratch disease

Cat-scratch disease (CSD), first clinically identified in humans in the 1930s, was described in 1950 in France. However, it was only in the early 1990s that the appropriate aetiological agent, *Bartonella henselae*, was identified. It was an indirect and unexpected consequence of the acquired immune deficiency syndrome (AIDS) epidemic, as this bacterium was also identified as the cause of bacillary angiomatosis in immunocompromised individuals. Bacillary angiomatosis is a potentially deadly vascular proliferative infection of the skin, bone and other organs associated with the presence of clumps of bacteria. Cat-scratch disease in humans is typically a benign, subacute regional lymphadenopathy resulting from dermal inoculation of the causative agent. Domestic cats are the major source of human infection and represent the main reservoir of the organism. The cat flea, *Ctenocephalides felis*, is the main vector of transmission from cat to cat.

Distribution

Cat-scratch fever has a worldwide distribution, especially in warm and humid countries. There is, however, a prevalence gradient from the south to north, at least for the northern hemisphere.

Aetiological agent

The bacterial origin of this disease was demonstrated in 1983 by the presence of bacilli in histological sections after silver staining (Warthin–Starry staining). In 1988, a pleiomorphic Gram-negative bacterium was isolated from the lymph node of an infected individual and named *Afipia felis*. It was regarded as the aetiological agent of CSD for a few years. However, the isolation, identification by polymerase chain reaction (PCR) or the presence of *B. henselae*-specific antibodies, and the lack of *Afipia felis* antibodies or organisms from CSD patients, either by isolation or by PCR, led

to the exclusion of this bacterium as the aetiological factor for CSD. Furthermore, only *Bartonella* DNA was identified in dermal tests that were used for CSD diagnosis. Based on serological evidence, two human cases of CSD have been associated with infection by *Bartonella clarridgeiae*, a flagellated organism first isolated from domestic cats, which represent the natural reservoir host.

Clinical symptoms

In humans, 1–3 weeks elapse between the scratch or bite and the appearance of clinical signs. Usually, patients develop a small skin lesion at the inoculation site within 3–10 days after the scratch. Within 3 weeks, a unilateral, painful lymphadenopathy develops, usually in the epitrochlea, axillary, cervical or inguinal lymph nodes, and persists for a few weeks to several months. Suppuration and atypical or systemic manifestations, including encephalitis, may occur in 15% of the cases. Furthermore, the clinical spectrum of symptoms associated with *B. henselae* infection has expanded in recent years to include fever of unknown origin, endocarditis and haemolytic anaemia.

Diagnosis

Since 1992, serological tests and techniques to isolate, or to identify by PCR, the presence of the bacteria have been developed. The most common test is the detection of specific antibodies by immunofluorescence assay (with a titre $\geq 1 : 64$ for positive individuals). Isolation by blood culture often leads to false-negative results, and is classically substituted by PCR from a lymph node biopsy, or PCR on an ethylenediamine tetraacetic acid (EDTA) blood sample. Two serotypes of *B. henselae* have been identified, with possible negative results for one or the other. Similarly, cross-reactivity for *B. clarridgeiae* and *B. henselae* in humans may be limited.

Epidemiology and transmission

There were an estimated 22,000 individuals with CSD in the USA in 1992, of whom 2000 required hospitalization. It is also estimated that 2000 CSD cases occur annually in The Netherlands. Cat-scratch disease occurs in immunocompetent patients of all ages, with more than half of the cases being less than 20 years of age. It is the most common cause of chronic benign adenopathy in children and young adults. More than 90% of the cases have a history of some contact with cats, and 57–85% of patients recall being scratched by a cat. In a case–control study, cases were more likely than healthy cat-owning controls to have at least one kitten ≤ 12 months of age, to have been scratched or bitten by a kitten, to have at least one kitten with fleas and to have found a tick on their own body.

Human infection usually results from a cat scratch. It has been suggested that cats inoculate infective faeces from fleas (*C. felis*) with their claws during scratching. In at least one instance, human infection was associated with flea exposure. Two human cases of CSD have also been associated with tick bites.

Domestic cats are the main reservoir host of *B. henselae* and *B. clarridgeiae* and transmission of infection from cat to cat has only been successful in the presence of infected fleas. Up to 40% of stray and free-roaming cats have been found to be bacteraemic with *B. henselae*. In Europe and in the Philippines, up to one-third of the cats were *B. clarridgeiae*-bacteraemic, whereas in North America and Japan *B. clarridgeiae* prevalence was approximately 10%. Co-infection in cats with both species has also been reported.

Treatment

Most individuals with CSD experience mild illness and require minimal treatment. Antibiotics may be recommended in severe forms and in immunocompromised individuals. Ciprofloxacin, rifampin or gentamycin have been suggested, as well as azithromycin. In immunocompromised individuals, doxycycline and erythromycin are the antibiotics of choice.

Other related *Bartonella* infections

Besides the well-known infections caused by *Bartonella bacilliformis*, causing Carrión's disease (see entry) and veruga peruana, transmitted by phlebotomine sand-flies in the Andes, and by *Bartonella quintana* causing trench fever (see *Bartonella quintana* and *Bartonella henselae*), transmitted by human body lice (*Pediculus humanus*), several new *Bartonella* species or subspecies have been recently associated with human or animal diseases or infections.

Several *Bartonella* species, which have rodent reservoir hosts, have been found to cause human endocarditis (*B. elizabethae*), myocarditis (*B. washoensis*), neuroretinitis (*B. grahamii*) or high fever with neurological symptoms (*B. vinsonii* subsp. *arupensis*). Unfortunately, in no instances, were the sources and vectors of infection identified. More recently, a human case of endocarditis caused by *B. vinsonii* subsp. *berkhoffii* has been reported from Europe. Similarly, no source of infection or vector was identified.

In domestic animals, *Bartonella* have also been isolated from dogs suffering from endocarditis (*B. vinsonii* subsp. *berkhoffii*) or peliosis hepatis (*B. henselae*). For dogs infected with *B. vinsonii* subsp. *berkhoffii*, tick transmission has been suggested, based on epidemiological evidence. *Bartonella koehlerae* has been isolated from two cats from northern California and *B. weissii* has been isolated from cats in Utah and Illinois, USA. In cattle, we isolated a new *Bartonella* species, *B. bovis*, closely related to *B. weissii*, and its transmission is likely to be tick-borne.

Several *Bartonella* species have also been isolated from wildlife, including many rodent species (*B. taylorii*, *B. doshiae*, *B. tribocorum*, *B. birtlesii*), rabbits (*B. alsatica*) and carnivores such as Coyotes (*Canis latrans*) and Gray foxes (*Urocyon cinereoargenteus*) which are infected with *B. vinsonii* subsp. *berkhoffii*; and there is as yet an unidentified *Bartonella*, close to *B. weissii*, infection in wild Mule deer[1] (*Odocoileus hemionus*) and Elk (*Cervus elaphus*).

Note

[1] Mule deer and Black-tailed deer are usually considered to be the same species.

Selected bibliography

Birtles, R.J., Harrison, T.G., Saunders, N.A. and Molyneux, D.H. (1995) Proposals to unify the genera *Grahamella* and *Bartonella*, with descriptions of *Bartonella talpae* comb. nov., *Bartonella peromysci* comb. nov., and three new species, *Bartonella grahamii* sp. nov., *Bartonella taylorii* sp. nov., and *Bartonella doshiae* sp. nov. *International Journal of Systematic Bacteriology* 45, 1–8.

Breitschwerdt, E.B., Kordick, D.L., Malarkey, D.E., Keene, B., Hadfield, T.L. and Wilson, K. (1995) Endocarditis in a dog due to infection with a novel *Bartonella* subspecies. *Journal of Clinical Microbiology* 33, 154–160.

Chang, C.C., Chomel, B.B., Kasten, R.W., Heller, R., Kocan, K.M., Ueno, H., Yamamoto, K., Bleich, V.C., Pierce, B.M., Gonzales, B.J., Swift, P.K., Boyce, W.M., Jang, S.S., Boulouis, H.J. and Piemont, Y. (2000) *Bartonella* spp. isolated from wild and domestic ruminants in North America. *Emerging Infectious Diseases* 6, 306–311.

Chomel, B.B. (2000) Cat-scratch disease. *Revue Scientifique et Technique de l' Office International des Epizooties* 19, 136–150.

Chomel, B.B., Kasten, R.W., Floyd-Hawkins, K.A., Chi, B., Yamamoto, K., Roberts-Wilson, J., Gurfield, A.N., Abbott, R.C., Pedersen, N.C. and Koehler, J.E. (1996) Experimental transmission of *Bartonella henselae* by the cat flea. *Journal of Clinical Microbiology* 34, 1952–1956.

Drancourt, M., Birtles, R., Chaumentin, G., Vandenesch, F., Etienne, J. and Raoult, D. (1996) New serotype of *Bartonella henselae* in endocarditis and cat-scratch disease. *The Lancet* 347, 441–443.

Flexman, J.P., Lavis, N.J., Kay, I.D., Watson, M., Metcalf, C. and Pearman, J.W. (1995) *Bartonella henselae* is a causative agent of cat scratch disease in Australia. *Journal of Infection* 31, 241–245.

Foil, L., Andress, E., Freeland, R.L., Roy, A.F., Rutledge, R, Triche, P.C. and O'Reilly, K.L. (1998) Experimental infection of domestic cats with *Bartonella henselae* by inoculation of *Ctenocephalides felis* (Siphonaptera: Pulicidae) feces. *Journal of Medical Entomology* 35, 625–628.

Heller, R., Kubina, M., Mariet, P., Riegel, P., Delacour, G., Dehio, C., Lamarque, F., Kasten, R., Boulouis, H.J., Monteil, H., Chomel, B.

and Piemont, Y. (1999) *Bartonella alsatica* sp. nov., a new *Bartonella* species isolated from the blood of wild rabbits. *International Journal of Systematic Bacteriology* 49, 283–288.

Higgins, J.A., Radulovic, S., Jaworski, D.C. and Azad, A.F. (1996) Acquisition of the cat scratch disease agent *Bartonella henselae* by cat fleas (Siphonaptera: Pulicidae). *Journal of Medical Entomology* 33, 490–495.

Jacomo, V., and Raoult, D. (2000) Human infections caused by *Bartonella* spp. Part 1. and Part 2. *Clinical Microbiology Newsletter* 22, 1–5, 9–13.

Kerkhoff, F.T., Bergmans, A.M.C., Van der Zee, A. and Rothova, A. (1999) Demonstration of *Bartonella grahamii* DNA in ocular fluids of a patient with neuroretinitis. *Journal of Clinical Microbiology* 37, 4034–4038.

Kitchell, B.E., Fan, T.M., Kordick, D., Breitschwerdt, E.B., Wollenberg, G. and Lichtensteiger, C.A. (2000) Peliosis hepatis in a dog infected with *Bartonella henselae*. *Journal of the American Veterinary Medical Association* 216, 519–523.

Koehler, J.E., Glaser, C.A. and Tappero, J.W. (1994) *Rochalimaea henselae* infection – a new zoonosis with the domestic cat as reservoir. *Journal of the American Medical Association* 271, 531–535.

Kordick, D.L., Hilyard, E.J., Hadfield, T.L., Wilson, K.H., Steigerwalt, A.G., Brenner, D.J. and Breitschwerdt, E.B. (1997) *Bartonella clarridgeiae*, a newly recognized zoonotic pathogen causing inoculation papules, fever, and lymphadenopathy (cat scratch disease). *Journal of Clinical Microbiology* 35, 1813–1818.

Lucey, D., Dolan, M.J., Moss, C.W., Garcia, M., Hollis, D.G. and Wegner, S. (1992) Relapsing illness due to *Rochalimaea henselae* in immunocompetent hosts: implication for therapy and new epidemiological associations. *Clinical Infectious Diseases* 14, 683–688.

Pappalardo, B.L., Correa, M.T., York, C.C., Peat, C.Y. and Breitschwerdt, E.B. (1997) Epidemiologic evaluation of the risk factors associated with exposure and seroreactivity to *Bartonella vinsonii* in dogs. *American Journal of Veterinary Research* 58, 467–471.

Regnery, R.L., Anderson, B.E., Clarridge, J.E., Rodriguez-Barradas, M.C., Jones, D.C. and Carr J.H. (1992) Characterization of a novel *Rochalimaea* species, *R. henselae* sp. nov., isolated from blood of afebrile, human immunodeficiency virus-positive patient. *Journal of Clinical Microbiology* 30, 265–274.

Roux, V., Eykyn, S.J., Willy, S. and D. Raoult, D. (2000) Report of *Bartonella vinsonii* subspecies *berkhoffii* as an agent of afebrile blood culture negative endocarditis in man. *Journal of Clinical Microbiology* 38, 1698–1700.

Welch, D.F., Carroll, K.C., Hofmeister, E.K., Persing, D.H., Robinson, D.A., Steigerwalt, A.G. and Brenner, D.J. (1999) Isolation of a new subspecies, *Bartonella vinsonii* subsp. *arupensis*, from a cattle rancher: identity with isolates found in conjunction with *Borrelia burgdorferi* and *Babesia microti* among naturally infected mice. *Journal of Clinical Microbiology* 37, 2598–2601.

Zangwill, K.M., Hamilton, D.H., Perkins, B.A., Regnery, R.L., Plikaytis, B.D., Hadler, J.L., Cartter, M.L. and Wenger, J.D. (1993) Cat scratch disease in Connecticut. Epidemiology, risk factors, and evaluation of a new diagnostic test. *New England Journal of Medicine* 329, 8–13.

Cattle-tick fever *see* **Babesiosis.**

Central European encephalitis *see* **Tick-borne encephalitis.**

Ceratopogonidae *see* **Biting midges.**

Cerebrospinal nematodiasis *see* **Setariosis.**

Chagas disease, human

C.J. Schofield

Chagas disease (also known as American trypanosomiasis) is a protozoon infection in humans named after the Brazilian clinician Carlos Justiniano das Chagas, who first described the disease in 1909. Chagas also determined the infectious agent and worked out most of its life cycle, including recognition of its insect vectors and some reservoir hosts. In Latin America, 16–18 million people were estimated to be infected in 1990, with about 100 million considered at risk, and the World Bank ranked Chagas disease as the most serious parasitic infection of the Americas in terms of its social and economic impact. Since then, transmission has been substantially reduced, following extensive vector control programmes.

Distribution

As a zoonotic infection of small mammals and marsupials, *Trypanosoma cruzi* occurs throughout the Americas from the Great Lakes of North America to southern Patagonia. Human infection is primarily among poorer rural communities of Latin America, living in houses infested with the insect vectors – large blood-sucking bugs of the subfamily Triatominae. However, about 10% of parasite transmission occurs through blood transfusion from infected donors, so that increasing numbers of infected people are recorded from cities, including some cases outside the Americas. Cases of congenital (transplacental) transmission from infected mothers living outside the Americas have also been recorded.

Parasite

Trypanosoma cruzi is a flagellated protozoan, typically about 8–15 μm long, characterized by a large DNA-containing kinetoplast at the base of the flagellum. It undergoes transformation and division in mammalian cells, particularly those of smooth muscle and cardiac muscle, eventually rupturing these cells to allow escape of the parasites and infection of further cells. Some of the parasites escape to the peripheral bloodstream, where they may be taken up by feeding triatomine bugs. These parasites transform and multiply in the bug's gut, and may be shed in the bug's faecal droplets when it next feeds.

Clinical symptoms

Human infection with *T. cruzi* proceeds through two phases, acute and chronic, either or both of which may be with or without clinical symptoms. There may be a characteristic lesion at the portal of entry, known as a chagoma, and, if the portal of entry was the optic mucosa, there may be a highly characteristic unilateral ocular oedema, known as Romaña's sign. Following a brief incubation period, the acute phase of infection typically lasts about 2–4 weeks. During this time the parasites are circulating in the peripheral bloodstream and progressively invading cells of various tissues, particularly heart muscle. There may be a patent parasitaemia, but not always. Acute-phase symptoms may include fever, malaise, hepatomegaly and splenomegaly, lymphadenopathy, meningoencephalitis and acute or diffuse myocarditis, but many acute cases are undetected. Mortality during the acute phase is estimated to be 5–15% (mainly among younger children), depending on the strain of parasite and state of the patient.

Immune response to the circulating parasites increases during the acute phase of infection, gradually clearing the bloodstream of parasites. Bloodstream parasites are thus rare during the chronic phase of infection, although there may be a reactivation of the acute phase if the patient becomes immunocompromised (e.g. through human immunodeficiency virus (HIV) infection or the use of immunosuppressants). Generally, the chronic phase is without symptoms, but 20–30% of chronic-phase patients may eventually develop clinical symptoms as a result of progressive tissue destruction over a period of several years. The most frequent symptoms involve progressive destruction of muscle and nervous tissue of the heart, leading to arrhythmias, atrial fibrillation, conduction problems and insufficiency. Patients may feel tired and present peripheral cold oedemas due to chronic cardiac insufficiency, which may be the direct cause of death. Severe lesions may also result in aneurisms of the cardiac wall, causing sudden death (*morte subita*), often following unaccustomed exercise. Parasite strains that most usually circulate in the Southern Cone countries of Latin America also show some tropisms for intestinal tissues, causing destruction of the digestive autonomous nervous plexus, leading to intestinal 'mega-syndromes' (gross dilatations of parts of the intestinal tract). Most common are mega-oesophagus, which can lead to difficulties in swallowing (*mal de engasgo*), and mega-colon, which can lead to failure in stool transit and consequent faecaloma. More generalized nervous system disorders have been reported, but now seem less frequent.

Trypanosoma cruzi is a common infection of marsupials, armadillos (*Dasypus* species), rodents and other small mammals in Latin America, although clinical disease due to the infection is rarely seen in such animals. Birds and reptiles are refractory to the infection (the parasite is killed through complement-mediated lysis in bird blood). Large domestic mammals, such as cows, pigs and horses, are rarely infected (probably because they have little contact with infected bugs, and the parasite may have difficulty in penetrating the skin). Goats are more frequently infected, probably because goat corrals often have heavy infestations of triatomine bugs. Domestic dogs and cats are readily infected, and often show clinical symptoms similar to those described for humans.

Diagnosis

Acute chagasic infection can be suspected in patients complaining of fever who are residents of endemic rural areas of Latin America, especially if a possible chagoma is apparent and/or the patient's abode is known to be infested with triatomine bugs. Romaña's sign (unilateral ocular oedema) is strongly diagnostic. During the acute phase, parasites may be seen in fresh blood films (e.g. from finger-prick blood) or thin films stained with Giemsa, but not always. Serological diagnosis can be made in late acute infections and in chronic infections, using enzyme-linked immunosorbent assay (ELISA), indirect haemagglutination (IHA) and/or indirect fluorescent antibody (IFA) tests, but it is recommended that at least two serological tests be carried out for confirmation. Parasitological diagnosis can be confirmed by haemoculture and/or xeno-diagnosis (feeding uninfected triatomine bugs on the patient and then examining the bug's faecal material for parasites some 20–30 days later).

Transmission

Over 80% of transmission of *T. cruzi* to humans is by the insect vectors, large blood-sucking bugs of the subfamily Triatominae (see Triatomine bugs). Well over 100 species of Triatominae have been described from the Americas, but the majority are of sylvatic habit and rarely come into contact with people. Important vector species are those that have adapted to living in human dwellings (Fig. 1), particularly *Triatoma infestans* in the Southern Cone countries, *Triatoma brasiliensis* and *Panstrongylus megistus* in north-eastern Brazil, and *Rhodnius prolixus* and *Triatoma dimidiata* in the Andean Pact countries and parts of Central America. Domestic species gener-ally feed at night when their potential hosts are asleep. Both sexes and all five nymphal stages of triatomine bugs feed on vertebrate blood and can become infected if feeding on an infected host. Once infected, bugs

remain so for life and infection rates of 50% or more among domestic bug populations are not uncommon. Ingested parasites pass to the mid-gut and rectum of the bug, where they transform and multiply, with infective trypomastigote forms subsequently passed out with the bug's faecal droplets. Efficient vectors are those that defecate during the act of feeding, so that the infected faecal droplets are passed out directly on to the host. Parasites in the bug's faeces may be able to penetrate the host skin, especially if abraded. More usually, the host will rub the bitten area and then touch the eye, nose or mouth, allowing the parasites to pass readily through the mucosal mem-branes. Parasites are not transmitted by the bite of the insects, and transmission by the faecal route is relatively inefficient. It has been statistically estimated that on average over 1000 contacts with infected bugs are required to result in a new human infection, but in heavily infested houses people may be receiving over 25 bites per night so that transmission during the first year of life becomes highly probable.

Trypanosoma cruzi can also be trans-mitted by blood transfusion from infected donors or by transfusion of infected blood products, with a transmission efficiency

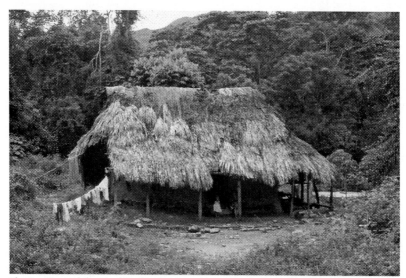

Fig. 1. Typical thatched-roof house in rural Trujillo, Venezuela, infested with *Rhodnius prolixus*.

variously estimated between 20 and 40%. Organ transplants from infected donors (especially kidney transplants) can also result in transmission, even if the donor is pretreated with trypanocidal drugs. Congenital transplacental transmission is also recorded, although this is usually in less than 2% of births to infected mothers. Oral-route transmission is highly efficient, but of infrequent occurrence; it may involve eating undercooked meat or blood from infected mammals (particularly opossums (*Didelphis* species) and armadillos (*Dasypus* species)) or from food or drink contaminated with infected bug faeces. It seems likely, however, that oral-route transmission is the usual transmission method among wild mammals, by eating infected bugs, and this may also be common among domestic cats and dogs. Several cases of accidental transmission of *T. cruzi* among laboratory workers have been recorded (usually by accidental finger-pricking with contaminated syringes).

Treatment

Two drugs are available for specific treatment of acute infections – nifurtimox (Lampit® from Bayer) and benznidazole (Rochagan® or Radanil® from Hoffman La Roche). In both cases the drugs must be given over extended periods, at dosages that are close to their therapeutic limits, so that toxic side-effects are common. For treatment of acute infections in adults, nifurtimox is given at 10–12 mg kg^{-1} day^{-1} divided into three spaced doses per day after meals, for up to 60 days. Benznidazol is given at 5–7 mg kg^{-1} day^{-1} in two or three spaced doses before meals, for up to 60 days. Children seem to have better tolerance and can be given higher doses, up to 15 mg kg^{-1} day^{-1} for nifurtimox and up to 10 mg kg^{-1} day^{-1} for benznidazol. In all cases, early initiation of treatment is more likely to result in cure, and for accidental laboratory infections, where treatment is begun within 24 h of the presumed infection, the treatment schedule can be reduced to 10–12 days. This is important because toxic side-effects generally begin from the eighth day onwards.

Chronic infections are more difficult to treat successfully, and large-scale treatment is not usually recommended for chronically infected adults because of the low likelihood of cure and high likelihood of side-effects. In children, however, treatment is now being recommended even in chronic infections because of their higher tolerance to the treatment and improved likelihood of at least limiting the progression of chronic lesions. For chronically infected adults, non-specific symptomatic treatment may include vasodilators and antiarrythmic drugs, such as amiodarone, although advanced cardiac arrythmias may require pacemaker implants. Mega-syndromes can sometimes be corrected by surgical intervention.

Control

The primary concept in Chagas disease control is to halt transmission by eliminating domestic vector populations and by improved screening of blood donors to reduce the risk of transfusional transmission. Serological screening of blood donors to reject those infected with *T. cruzi* (and other blood-borne infections, such as HIV, hepatitis and syphilis) is now carried out routinely by many Latin American countries, with a consequent reduction in the likelihood of transfusional transmission. In some rural clinics, blood for transfusion is treated for 24 h with 0.4% gentian violet, which will clear the blood parasites but results in a transient bluish colour for the recipient. Regrettably, however, donor screening for *T. cruzi* is not yet carried out in all countries of the Americas.

Vector control is carried out by large-scale spraying of infested premises with residual formulations of synthetic pyrethroid insecticides – mainly with deltamethrin, cyfluthrin, lambdacyhalothrin or cypermethrin (Fig. 2). The initial spraying is followed up by programmes of community-based vigilance (to report any residual infestations), with selective respraying where necessary. Large-scale control of domestic vector populations can be highly effective, as shown by campaigns against *R. prolixus* in Venezuela during the 1960s and against *T. infestans* in Brazil and Argentina during the 1970s–1980s.

The problem was that treated premises remain susceptible to reinfestation by bugs carried in from untreated foci. This problem has been addressed by very large-scale regional campaigns designed to eliminate all domestic foci of the primary vector species. The first of these campaigns, known as the Southern Cone Initiative, was formally launched in 1991 by Argentina, Bolivia, Brazil, Chile, Paraguay and Uruguay, joined in 1996 by Peru. These countries encompass the entire geographical range of *T. infestans,* and the campaign to eliminate all domestic populations of this species has already been highly successful, especially in Brazil, Chile, Argentina and Uruguay, where *T. infestans* is now extremely rare and transmission rates have been drastically reduced. Ongoing campaigns in north-eastern Brazil are also controlling domestic infestations of *T. brasiliensis* and *P. megistus.* Based on the Southern Cone experience, two further regional initiatives were formally launched in 1997 for the Andean Pact countries (mainly involving Colombia, Ecuador and Venezuela) and Central America (mainly involving Guatemala, El Salvador, Honduras and Nicaragua). For these countries the main vector targets are *R. prolixus* and *T. dimidiata.*

Where vector control has been successfully carried out, even in the absence of other measures, it has been found that the likelihood of transfusional and congenital transmission has also declined, possibly because reinfection has been stopped, thus reducing the frequency of bloodstream parasites in patients already infected with *T. cruzi.*

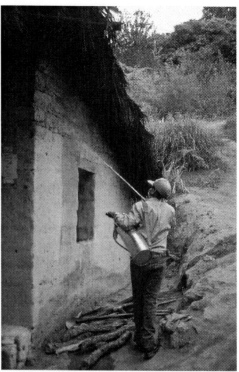

Fig. 2.   Spraying a pyrethroid insecticide (cyfluthrin wettable powder) to eliminate *Triatoma dimidiata* and *Rhodnius prolixus* from a bug-infested house in Madriz, Nicaragua. Spraying also eliminates scorpions and provides transient control of cockroaches, house-flies, fleas and mosquitoes, which are also a nuisance in the house.

Dias, J.C.P. and Schofield, C.J. (1998) Controle da transmissão transfusional da doença de Chagas na Iniciativa do Cone Sul. *Revista da Sociedade Brasileira de Medicina Tropical* 31, 373–383.
Schofield, C.J. and Dias, J.C.P. (1998) The Southern Cone Initiative against Chagas disease. *Advances in Parasitology* 42, 1–27.
Schofield, C.J. and Dujardin, J.P. (1997) Chagas disease vector control in Central America. *Parasitology Today* 13, 141–144.

Selected bibliography

Dias, J.C.P. and Coura, J.R. (1997) *Clinica e Terapêutica da Doença de Chagas.* Editora FIOCRUZ, Rio de Janeiro, 486 pp.

Chigger-borne rickettsiosis *see* **Scrub typhus.**

Chiggers *see* **Mites.**

Chikungunya virus

Jack Woodall

An infection of humans and other primates. Chikungunya (CHIK) virus was first isolated from serum collected from a patient during an outbreak of dengue-like illness in the former Tanganyika, East Africa, in 1953. A second outbreak occurred in South Africa in 1956, and the virus has since been recovered from other outbreaks in Africa and Asia. Huge epidemics, some lasting for years, others sweeping through a city and infecting the whole population within a few months, have been recorded. The name means 'that which bends up' in the language of the people of the Makonde plateau, Newala Province, which is what the people there called the first recognized epidemic. It is a descriptor, not a place name like most other arboviral names, so it does not begin with a capital letter (cf. dengue, yellow fever).

Distribution

Chikungunya virus is found in sub-Saharan Africa from Senegal across to Ethiopia and south to Angola, Zimbabwe, Mozambique and South Africa. It is also found in India, Sri Lanka and tropical South-East Asia – Cambodia, Indonesia, Malaysia, Myanmar, Philippines, Thailand and Vietnam. Antibody surveys have shown that 20–90% of a given population may be immune to it. Haemagglutination-inhibiting (HI) antibodies have been detected in 15% of 83 sera tested in the former USSR, but these could have been due to infection with a cross-reacting alphavirus.

Domestic animals

Only one of 183 zebu cattle tested in the Central African Republic had enzyme-linked immunosorbent assay (ELISA) antibody to CHIK virus, and only 4/370 domestic animals in South Africa had neutralizing antibodies; 5/220 domestic animals in Nigeria, 171/755 in Thailand and 11/112 horses in Indonesia were seropositive by haemagglutination inhibition (HI). But, in the absence of any virus isolation from livestock, these results may only indicate cross-reactions with another alphavirus, and CHIK virus has not been associated with disease in livestock anywhere.

Virus

An RNA virus, family Togaviridae, genus *Alphavirus*, which includes the viruses of eastern equine encephalitis, western equine encephalitis and Venezuelan equine encephalitis, Getah, Ross River, Semliki Forest, Sindbis (see entries), Sagiyama and others. By electron microscopy the virion diameter is 42–59 nm. The nucleocapsid is surrounded by a lipid envelope derived from host cell membrane during budding, containing two distinct glycoproteins.

The genome contains about 12,000 nucleotides arranged as single, non-segmented positive-sense strands of RNA. The genomes are polyadenylated at the 3′ end and capped with 7-methylguanosine at the 5′ end. Subgenomic messenger RNA (mRNA) (26S RNA) is formed during replication and contains about 4100 nucleotides, the sequence of which is identical to the 3′ terminal third of the genomic RNA. This RNA is also polyadenylated and capped and is the template for the four viral structural proteins; the 49S RNA non-structural region serves as the template for four non-structural proteins and the capsid. The genome can accept mutations in the conserved regions without destroying biological activity; only sequences at the 3′ and 5′ termini are essential for amplification and packaging. Where the non-structural and structural genes meet, 19 nucleotides upstream from the beginning of the 26S RNA sequence and five downstream from it are needed for production of 26S RNA. The non-structural proteins of alphaviruses are more conserved than the structural proteins.

The virus forms plaques and causes cytopathic effects in vertebrate cell cultures (HeLa (named after a patient), VERO, LLC-MK2, baby hamster kidney (BHK-21), chick and duck embryo) and invertebrate cultures (C6/36 from *Aedes albopictus* mosquitoes). These cells can be used as substrates for ELISA or for tests to detect neutralizing antibodies to the virus.

Alphaviruses have common antigenic determinants, as shown by many serological tests, including HI, complement-fixation (CF), ELISA and immunofluorescence. They have been classified into six antigenic complexes: (i) eastern equine encephalitis; (ii) Middelburg; (iii) Ndumu; (iv) Semliki Forest; (v) Venezuelan equine encephalitis; and (vi) western equine encephalitis. Chikungunya virus has several varieties and two subtypes: CHIK and o'nyong-nyong (ONN) (see entries). Getah virus has three subtypes: Getah, Sagiyama and Bebaru, and Mayaro virus has two: Mayaro and Una. (See entries on all of these except for Ndumu, Sagiyama and Una.) Phylogenetic trees indicate that CHIK virus originated in Africa, and that Asian strains are most closely related to strains from East and South Africa, which are in their turn distinguishable from those from West Africa.

Field strains of the virus are non-pathogenic to adult mice but are pathogenic for suckling and weanling mice inoculated intracranially. Humans, newly hatched chickens, laboratory mice and other rodents, such as the White-tailed mouse (*Mystromys albicaudatus*), African vervet monkeys (*Chlorocebus aethiops*[1]) and Asian Rhesus monkeys (*Macaca mulatta*), Chacma baboon (*Papio ursinus*), African prosimians, such as the Lesser galago (*Galago senegalensis*), and bats (species of *Tadarida*, *Pipistrellus* and *Scotophilus*) are susceptible to the virus and develop high-titre viraemias, without necessarily causing any symptoms.

Clinical symptoms

Chikungunya virus infection can be symptomless; two infections without any clinically recognized disease occurred in laboratory technicians in Nigeria. When symptoms do appear, the incubation period is normally 2–3 days (range 1–12 days), followed by sudden onset of fever, severe chills, arthralgia, leucopenia and often a rash. Biphasic fevers occur, contributing to

difficulty in distinguishing CHIK virus infection clinically from malaria (see entry). Severe polyarthralgia commences at or soon after onset of fever and chills, predominantly affecting the small joints of the hands, wrists, ankles and feet (distinguishing it from dengue, which usually attacks the elbows and knees), but it moves around and may affect more than one joint at a time. Generalized myalgia is also common. Arthralgias usually resolve within a week but may persist for weeks, months or even years. More than 10% of patients with chikungunya disease develop chronic joint symptoms.

Headache, photophobia, conjunctival inflammation, retro-orbital pain, anorexia, nausea, vomiting and abdominal pains occur but are not usually severe or pathognomonic. The rash is maculopapular and ranges from mild to extensive; it is often confused with the rash caused by dengue viruses, and mixed epidemics of chikungunya and dengue have been recorded. The rash has been seen from as early as the day of onset to as late as the tenth day after onset; however, it usually appears at the time the fever abates and lasts 1–5 days. Severe arthralgia is the symptom most indicative of chikungunya illness. Lympadenitis occurs, but is much less marked than in o'nyong-nyong infection. Petechiae may be present, but haemorrhagic manifestations are unusual. However, in infants and young children infected with the virus, haemorrhagic manifestations have been seen, followed by the rare fatality. A mixed epidemic due to the CHIK virus and yellow fever was seen in Senegal in 1996. The occurrence of focal seizures, repeated seizures and convulsions in adults suggests that CHIK virus may on occasion directly involve the brain.

Diagnosis

Because of serological cross-reactions with other alphaviruses, virus isolation is the standard for laboratory diagnosis. Alphaviruses can be distinguished one from another by use of virus-specific or strain-specific monoclonal antibodies employed in HI, neutralization, ELISA and other tests. Both antigenic and biological variation have been detected between strains of CHIK virus from widely different geographical areas. African and Asian strains of CHIK virus can be distinguished by using kinetic haemagglutination inhibition tests or by the use of monoclonal antibodies in any of various tests, including ELISA.

Antibody to CHIK virus cross-reacts in immunoglobulin M (IgM)-capture ELISA tests with heterologous alphaviruses, but is most reactive with other viruses of the same antigenic complex. Immunoglobulin M antibody from patients with chikungunya disease have highest titres to CHIK virus, lower titres to ONN and Mayaro viruses (which are in the same complex), and even lower to, for example, eastern equine encephalitis virus (which is not in the same complex). Immunoglobulin M antibody peaks 3–5 weeks after onset of illness and persists for about 2 months. Immunoglobulin G antibody also appears relatively soon after onset but, unlike IgM, persists for many months or years after the illness. Immunoglobulin M antibody inhibits haemagglutination by the virus, immunofluoresces and neutralizes it; IgG antibody reacts in these tests and in CF tests as well. Thus, IgM ELISA is the diagnostic test of choice for determining recent infections (if confirmed by neutralization tests) and may be applied to single serum samples in some instances. The presence of IgG antibody to any of these viruses is simply an indication of past infection and, without demonstration of a significant (fourfold or greater) increase or decrease between paired acute-phase and convalescent-phase serum samples, cannot be used to implicate the virus in the aetiology of the illness; the usefulness of IgG assays is limited because of cross-reactivity.

Transmission

The virus is transmitted between vertebrate hosts by mosquitoes; aerosol transmission has been recorded in the laboratory. Human infections with CHIK virus occur primarily in the rainy season when mosquito populations peak. In tropical Africa the virus has been isolated from many species of mosquitoes, including many *Aedes* species, such as *A. aegypti*, *A. africanus*, *A. cordillieri*, *A. furcifer*, *A. luteocephalus*, *A. opok* and *A. taylori*, and *Mansonia africana*. Transmission has been obtained in the laboratory for many of these. The evidence is that the principal vectors in Africa are the sylvan mosquitoes *A. furcifer* and *A. africanus*. In Asia the vectors are probably urban *A. aegypti* and various species of *Culex*, as isolations have been made from them. The Asian mosquito *A. albopictus* may also be a vector, since after experimental infection it transmitted the virus by bite, and also transmitted it transovarially in the laboratory (but only when co-infected with microfilariae, and then only to the F1, but not the F2, generation).

Humans develop high-titre viraemias and the peridomestic *A. aegypti* transmits the virus to humans in both urban and village settings. Chikungunya virus has been isolated from an African vervet monkey (*C. aethiops*) and a Baboon (*Papio hamadryas*) in Senegal, indicating that non-human primates are the primary vertebrate hosts in Africa, with spread to humans occurring under favourable conditions. But in Asia the virus is maintained in a human-to-human cycle through *A. aegypti* mosquitoes.

A single isolate was obtained from 100,000 ixodid (hard) ticks collected and processed in the Republic of Guinea between 1978 and 1991, and which yielded multiple isolates of 12 other viruses; a single isolate was also obtained from *Ornithodoros sonrai* ticks in Senegal. This suggests that ticks are not important vectors of this virus, and, in fact, the isolates could have come from an undigested blood meal in the tick's gut rather than from infection of the tick.

Although experimentally infected Asian monkeys (*Macaca* species) develop high-titre viraemia, they do not appear to serve as the principal reservoir host of the virus there, as they do in Africa. Antibody to the virus has been detected in Chimpanzees (*Pan troglodytes*) and in various species of monkeys; there has been one isolate from a bird, the Golden sparrow (*Auripasser luteus*), and two from bats (*Scotophilus* species), both in West Africa.

Treatment

Since there is no specific antiviral drug, treatment consists primarily of supportive therapy. Symptoms respond partially to non-steroidal anti-inflammatory drugs, haemorrhagic cases require whole blood and platelet transfusions.

Control

Prevention of infection involves reducing contact between humans and mosquitoes by avoidance behaviour and mosquito control operations. Clothing that covers arms and legs, insect repellents on exposed skin, staying indoors in mosquito-screened houses after dark and using bed nets, preferably insecticide-impregnated, are all effective. Larviciding, done by hand or by spraying insecticides from backpacks, and adulticiding, by spraying insecticides from trucks or planes, can temporarily interrupt transmission. Community education and media publicity are essential to engage the general public in cleaning up the environment to get rid of mosquito breeding places. Providing piped water and proper sewage disposal and managing irrigation systems have all been successfully used to reduce vector populations.

The widespread prevalence of CHIK virus in both Africa and South-East Asia and of competent vectors for the virus (*A. albopictus*, *A. aegypti*) in the USA and focally through a substantial portion of the Americas, and a human population completely susceptible to these viruses, together with the isolation of the virus from travellers arriving in North America sick with CHIK virus infection, suggest that a vaccine would be useful. A live, attenuated vaccine has been developed by the US military and is being tested in humans. It has been found that it greatly diminishes the response to subsequent Venezuelan equine encephalitis (VEE) (see entry) vaccination and, conversely, that the VEE vaccine greatly diminishes the response to subsequent CHIK vaccination. This could indicate that a CHIK vaccine might cross-protect against the closely related o'nyong-nyong and Mayaro viruses (see entries), and that VEE vaccination could provide some protection against CHIK virus infection.

Note

[1] Formerly in the genus *Cercopithecus*.

Selected bibliography

Calisher, C.H., Shope, R.E., Brandt, W., Casals, J., Karabatsos, N., Murphy, F.A., Tesh, R.B. and Wiebe, M.E. (1980) Proposed antigenic classification of registered arboviruses I. *Togaviridae, Alphavirus. Intervirology* 14, 229–232.

Jupp, P.G. and McIntosh, B.M. (1988) Chikungunya virus disease. In: Monath, T.P. (ed.) *The Arboviruses: Epidemiology and Ecology*, Vol. II. CRC Press, Boca Raton, Florida, pp. 137–157.

McClain, D.J., Pittman, P.R., Ramsburg, H.H., Nelson, G.O., Rossi, C.A., Mangiafico, J.A., Schmaljohn, A.L. and Malinoski, F.J. (1998) Immunologic interference from sequential administration of live attenuated alphavirus vaccines. *Journal of Infectious Diseases* 177, 634–641.

Peters, C.J. and Dalrymple, J.M. (1990) Alphaviruses. In: Fields, B.N. and Knipe, D.M. (eds) *Virology*, Vol. 1, 2nd edn. Raven Press, New York, 713–761

Pile, J.C, Henchal, E.A., Christopher, G.W., Steele, K.E. and Pavlin, J.A. (1999) Chikungunya in a North American traveler. *Journal of Travel Medicine* 6, 137–139.

Powers, A.M., Brault, A.C., Tesh, R.B. and Weaver, S.C. (2000) Re-emergence of chikungunya and o'nyong-nyong viruses: evidence for distinct geographical lineages and distant evolutionary relationships. *Journal of General Virology* 81, 471–479.

Ross, R.W. (1956) The Newala epidemic III. The virus: isolation, pathogenic properties and relationship to the epidemic. *Journal of Hygiene* 54, 177–191.

Sarkar, J.K., Chatterjee, S.N., Chakravarti, S.K. and Mitra, A.C. (1965) Chikungunya virus infection with haemorrhagic manifestations. *Indian Journal of Medical Research* 53, 921–925.

Thaikruea, L., Charearnsook, O., Reanphumkarnkit, S., Dissomboon, P., Phonjan, R., Ratchbud, S., Kounsang, Y. and Buranapiyawong, D. (1997) Chikungunya in Thailand: a re-emerging disease? *Southeast Asian Journal of Tropical Medicine and Public Health* 28, 359–364.

Theiler, M. and Downs, W.G. (1973) *The Arthropod-borne Viruses of Vertebrates.* Yale University Press, New Haven, Connecticut, 578 pp.

Cholera *see* **Flies.**

Chrysops **species** *see* **Horse-flies.**

Cimicidae

M.W. Service

The Cimicidae are a well-defined family of blood-sucking bugs, containing almost 100 species, the best known of which are the bedbugs (*Cimex lectularius* and *Cimex hemipterus*). However, bedbugs are not vectors of any of the infections in this encyclopedia, but the swallow bug, *Oeciacus vicarius*, is a vector of the Bijou Bridge subtype of Venezuelan equine encephalitis. This bug has a Nearctic and western Palaearctic distribution.

Adults of *O. vicarius* are flattened dorsoventrally, brown in colour and about 5 mm long and lack wings. The life cycle consists of eggs, followed by five nymphal stages, all of which blood-feed on swallows or sometimes on other birds, and finally the adults. The bugs do not migrate with the swallows during winter and many die, but some, mainly adults, overwinter in a semi-dormant state in cracks and crevices of their nests; occasionally they may attach to other species of birds and blood-feed. Very occasionally, *O. vicarius* bites humans but they cannot mature their eggs on a diet of human blood.

Selected bibliography

Ryckman, R.E., Bentley, D.G. and Archbold, E.F. (1981) The Cimicidae of the Americas and Oceanic Islands, a checklist and bibliography. *Bulletin of the Society of Vector Ecologists* 6, 93–142.

Usinger, R.L. (1966) *Monograph of the Cimicidae (Hemiptera–Heteroptera).* Thomas Say Foundation, Vol. 7. Entomological Society of America, Baltimore, Maryland, 585 pp.

Clegs *see* **Horse-flies.**

Cockroaches (Blattaria)

M.W. Service

There are about 4000 species of cockroaches (roaches, steam-bugs, black-beetles), of which some 50 species have become domestic pests. They have an almost worldwide distribution, but tend to be more numerous in warm climates. The most important vectors of disease pathogens to humans and animals are the German cockroach (*Blatella germanica*), the American cockroach (*Periplaneta americana*) and the Oriental cockroach (*Blatta orientalis*).

Biology

Eggs are laid encased in a brown bean-shaped capsule called an ootheca (Fig. 1), which commonly contains 24–50 eggs. Female cockroaches are often seen running around with an ootheca protruding from the abdomen. Small pale miniature editions of the adults, called nymphs, hatch from the eggs after 1–3 months, the time depending mainly on temperature. Nymphs are wingless. There are usually six nymphal instars, although in *P. americana* there can be 13; older nymphs are progressively darker and resemble more closely the adults. Duration of the nymphal stages depends on temperature, abundance of food and species, but can vary from about 3 months to 2 years. The fore-wings, called tegmina, are brown and rather leathery and fold over one another to protect the hind-wings (Fig. 1); there are no elytra (see Beetles).

Cockroaches like warmth and during the day hide in almost any dark place, ranging from under tables and in cupboards to cesspools, underground sewers and drains; they become very active at night. They can be very common in kitchens, bakeries, hospitals and restaurants, where nymphs and adults feed on discarded foods. They are voracious and omnivorous feeders, consuming dried blood, sputum, excreta and almost any vegetable or animal matter. They frequently disgorge partially digested meals and deposit their excreta on food. Adults can live for many months.

Diseases
Because of their insanitary habits, cockroaches have long been suspected of mechanically transmitting a great variety of pathogens and parasites to humans and, to a lesser extent, to animals. Although many pathogens can be isolated from the body and legs of cockroaches and their excreta, there is usually insufficient evidence that they can actually result in infections, especially when such pathogens are easily spread directly from person to person without the aid of cockroaches. Consequently, it is difficult to prove that cockroaches are the prime cause of any disease outbreak. Nevertheless, cockroaches are known to carry pathogenic viruses, such as those responsible for poliomyelitis and hepatitis; bacteria, such as *Escherichia coli*, *Staphylococcus aureus*, *Klebsiella pneumoniae*, *Shigella dysenteriae*, *Salmonella typhi*, *Salmonella typhimurium* and other species; and protozoans, such as *Entamoeba histolytica*, *Toxoplasma gondii*, *Trichomonas hominis*, *Giardia intestinalis* and *Balantium coli*.

In addition, cockroaches have been incriminated in triggering various respiratory infections, including asthma.

Control
Ensuring food is covered and not left out overnight may help reduce contamination with pathogens from cockroaches. However, the main method of alleviating disease risks is to destroy the cockroach population. Residual insecticides, such as the organophosphates and pyrethroids, or insect growth regulators (IGRs) can be sprayed in kitchens and other places harbouring cockroaches. Alternatively, various very simple attractant traps, baited with food or pheromones, can be employed to catch and/or kill cockroaches.

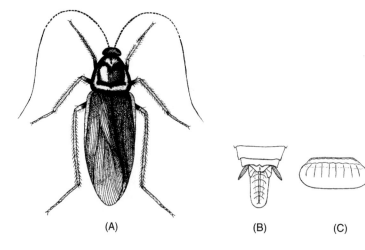

Fig. 1. (A) Adult cockroach (*Periplaneta americana*); (B) ootheca (egg capsule) protruding from abdomen of *Blatta germanica*; (C) typical ootheca. (Modified from M.W. Service (2000) *Medical Entomology for Students*, Cambridge University Press, Cambridge.)

(A)   (B)   (C)

Selected bibliography

Burgess, N.R.H. and Chetwyn, K.N. (1981) Association of cockroaches with an outbreak of dysentery. *Transactions of the Royal Society of Tropical Medicine and Hygiene* 75, 332–333.

Cochran, D.G. (1982) V. Cockroaches: biology and control. WHO/VBC/82,856, World Health Organization mimeographed document, Geneva, 53 pp.

Cornwell, P.B. (1968) *The Cockroach*, Vol. 1. *A Laboratory Insect and an Industrial Pest.* Hutchinson, London, 391 pp.

Cornwell, P.B. (1976) *The Cockroach*, Vol. 2. *Insecticides and Cockroach Control.* Associated Business Programmes, London, 557 pp.

LeGuyader, A., Rivault, C. and Chaperon, J. (1989) Microbial organisms carried by brown-banded cockroaches in relation to their spatial distribution in a hospital. *Epidemiology and Infection* 102, 485–492.

Roth, L.M. and Willis, E.R. (1957) The medical and veterinary importance of cockroaches. *Smithsonian Miscellaneous Collections* 134, 1–147.

Roth, L.M. and Willis, E.R. (1960) The biotic associations of cockroaches. *Smithsonian Miscellaneous Collections* 141, 1–470.

Schal, C. and Hamilton, R.L. (1990) Integrated suppression of synanthropic cockroaches. *Annual Review of Entomology* 35, 521–551.

Colorado tick fever

Charles H. Calisher

In the mid-19th century, settlers in and visitors to the Rocky Mountain region of North America mentioned 'mountain fever' as a cause of morbidity and occasional mortality. 'Mountain fever' was probably any of a number of illnesses, including typhoid fever, Rocky Mountain spotted fever, Colorado tick fever and other febrile illnesses. The subsequent association of fever, chills, headache, myalgia and arthralgia with onset in spring and summer in the Rocky Mountain region suggested a connection between the illness and transmission by ticks. L. Florio and co-workers isolated Colorado tick fever (CTF) virus from humans and from *Dermacentor andersoni* ('the wood tick') and demonstrated that this virus is the aetiological agent of the disease. When the maintenance cycle of CTF virus in natural foci in Colorado and Montana was better understood, it was apparent that the virus and probably the disease were more widespread than first recognized.

Distribution

The distribution of CTF virus roughly approximates that of its vector tick, *D. andersoni*. It has been isolated from humans, ticks or both in Colorado, Utah, Montana, California, Wyoming, Idaho, Oregon, South Dakota, Washington, New Mexico and Nevada, and also in southern Alberta and British Columbia, Canada. Many of these areas are vacation destinations, frequented during the tick season (spring and early summer) by large numbers of tourists. Colorado tick fever virus has been isolated from humans vacationing in or travelling through these states and physicians should be aware of the possibility of Colorado tick fever in febrile patients returning from these regions.

Aetiological agent

Colorado tick fever virus has been placed in the family Reoviridae (genus *Coltivirus*). It is an RNA virus, so that genotypic and phenotypic variations among isolates are common. Nine genera and one proposed genus comprise the family Reoviridae. More than 138 viruses have been arranged in the genera *Aquareovirus*, *Coltivirus*, *Cypovirus*, *Fijivirus*, *Orthoreovirus*, *Orbivirus*, *Oryzovirus*, *Phytoreovirus* and *Rotavirus* or in the proposed genus of plant reoviruses. All members of the family are composed of ten to 12 segments of double-stranded RNA, six to ten proteins and carbohydrate. Members of this virus family replicate in cytoplasm and genetic recombination occurs very efficiently by genome segment reassortment. Colorado tick fever virus is the prototype member of the genus *Coltivirus* (from <u>Co</u>lorado <u>ti</u>ck fever <u>virus</u>), established because it has 12 RNA segments, compared with ten in members of the genus *Orbivirus*, in which it had been placed originally. Also, the surface capsomeric structure of the core particles differs from that of the orbiviruses. The coltiviruses are spherical particles 80 nm in diameter, with two outer capsid shells and a core with no projections. They are labile at pH 3 and are scarcely sensitive to lipid solvents (as opposed to most other arboviruses, which are extremely sensitive to lipid solvents). Replication occurs in cytoplasmic viroplasms; during morphogenesis regularly structured filaments and tubules form.

Viruses with genomes consisting of 12 segments of double-stranded RNA were isolated from mosquitoes collected in Indonesia. It is thought that these isolates represent two new genotypes and they have been placed in the genus *Coltivirus*. In addition, viruses isolated from adult *Ixodes ricinus* ticks and *Ixodes ventalloi* larvae in Germany and France are members of this genus. Comparisons of numerous strains of CTF virus from ticks, humans and other mammals by neutralization, hybridization and polyacrylamide gel electrophoresis indicated that, although multiple genotypes and some antigenic variations exist and therefore reassortment of gene segments must occur, most of the 12 genes were highly conserved over the 33-year period represented.

Clinical symptoms

Classically, symptoms of Colorado tick fever appear abruptly, with initial features of high fever, chills, joint and muscle pains, severe headache, ocular pain, conjunctival injection, nausea and occasional vomiting. Fever, headache, lumbar pains, aching in the extremities and anorexia may continue for a few days more; the spleen and liver may be palpable. A transitory petechial or maculopapular rash is seen in a minority of patients. The biphasic character of Colorado tick fever is exemplified by defervescence for a few days followed by a relapse of 2–3 days. A small proportion of patients complain of more severe illness, including extended prostration, anorexia, continuing

fatigue and convalescence for several or more weeks. A more severe picture is occasionally seen in children, who may have haemorrhagic manifestations, ranging from more pronounced rash to disseminated intravascular coagulopathy and gastrointestinal bleeding. Central nervous system involvement, including aseptic meningitis and encephalitis, has been seen in severely affected children. Rarely, adult orchitis, pericarditis, hepatitis and symptoms mimicking myocardial infarction have been reported. Because few fatalities have been associated with CTF virus infection, little information on human pathological changes is available.

Diagnosis

The incubation period of Colorado tick fever is <1 to 19 days (average about 4 days), possibly dependent on the dose of CTF virus the patient receives from the infecting tick.

Antibody to CTF virus is not detected until 1–2 weeks after the onset of illness. A remarkable finding in both humans and experimental animals is prolonged viraemia, which may last for several months, a phenomenon advantageous for diagnosis. Early in the disease, virus can be isolated from both serum and blood clots with about the same frequency, but later it is more easily isolated from blood clots. Because there are no pathognomonic profiles, no specific symptom or array of signs and symptoms, no physical findings, laboratory abnormality, radiographic or electroencephalographic features that can be used to define Colorado tick fever, a differential diagnosis on clinical grounds can be very difficult. However, a thorough knowledge of illness caused by CTF virus, of the epidemiological aspects of the natural cycles of CTF virus and of the patient should enable an attentive clinician to make a rational differential diagnosis.

Numerous serological surveys have demonstrated that human populations in endemic areas have low, moderate or high prevalence of antibody to CTF virus. Thus, detecting antibody to CTF virus cannot be taken as absolute evidence of an association of the current illness with that virus but antibody to CTF virus is certainly evidence of infection with that virus.

A history of tick exposure, knowledge of a patient being fed on by ticks (90% of patients recall having had an attached tick or having seen a tick crawling on their body or clothing) or early clinical signs and symptoms may provide preliminary evidence that the patient has Colorado tick fever or Rocky Mountain spotted fever. However, the characteristics of the rash and the progression of the illness, as well as the presence of leucocytosis, distinguish Rocky Mountain spotted fever from Colorado tick fever. Other diseases with which Colorado tick fever might be confused are tick-borne tularaemia, relapsing fever and acute rheumatic fever. Differential diagnosis of these infections is important because Colorado tick fever is not treatable with antibiotics.

Geographical distribution, principal arthropod vector and vertebrate hosts of CTF virus have been well established for many years, and yet this disease continues to be under-recognized and under-reported. For example, only 441 cases of Colorado tick fever occurred between 1985 and 1989 in the states that had active Colorado tick fever surveillance programmes, namely Colorado, Montana, Utah, Wyoming, California, and Idaho. An analysis of 606 Colorado tick fever cases by age and sex, revealed: 11.6% were 0–9 years of age, 16.4% 10–19 years, 23% 20–29 years, 12.7% 30–39 years, 12.8% 40–49 years, 9.6% 50–59 years, 10.9% 60–69 years and 3.0% > 70 years of age. In all, 71.5% of cases were in males and 28.5% in females. The excess number of cases in males and people aged 20–29 years is probably indicative of more time spent in outdoor activities. The primary risk factor for acquiring Colorado tick fever is exposure to infected *D. andersoni* ticks in CTF virus-endemic areas.

Whole blood and serum, taken for virus isolation attempts, should be processed immediately or placed on dry ice (–70°C) or otherwise suitably frozen until they can be tested. Serological conversion from a negative or low titre to a positive or high titre is most often used for confirmatory diagnosis. Because a person can be infected and seroconvert to a virus without becoming ill, identifying CTF virus isolated from the patient is a more dependable basis for laboratory confirmation. Because CTF virus replicates in erythrocytes this virus is sequestered from the quenching effect of antibody and can be isolated for an extended period; and the probability of obtaining a CTF virus isolate from patient blood is high. When an isolate is obtained, various methods are available for its identification.

Electron microscopy can be used at an early stage of virus identification, allowing placement of the isolate into a particular virus family and thus greatly facilitating or making unnecessary subsequent characterization (determination of size, species of nucleic acid, ether or sodium deoxycholate sensitivity, pH stability and spectrum of animal or cell culture sensitivity). Detection of viral antigen by immunofluorescence has been a standard assay for many years; detection and identification of CTF virus RNA by polymerase chain reaction has recently become available and holds many advantages for diagnosis, surveillance and research. Virus antigen or nucleic acid is either detected directly in the infected specimen or after amplification in laboratory animals, vertebrate cell cultures (VERO, LLC-MK2, baby hamster kidney (BHK-21)), or live ticks inoculated with material suspected to contain CTF virus.

Direct immunofluorescence with antibody to CTF virus is used to detect CTF virus antigen in cell cultures infected with the virus; indirect immunofluorescence also uses polyclonal antibodies but requires the additional use of anti-species antibody. Nevertheless, the latter is a more widely used test because of its flexibility. Enzyme-linked immunosorbent assay (ELISA) depends on reactions between viral antigens and antibodies to them (for example, those prepared in mice) and then uses an enzyme-labelled reporter antibody (continuing the example, anti-mouse) to demonstrate those reactions.

For rapidly determining virus identity, group-specific and complex-specific antibodies to CTF virus are available from arbovirus reference centres and from various research laboratories. For final identification, an antiserum is also prepared against the isolate and cross-tested against reference antigens and viruses of the serogroup to which the isolate belongs. Ultimate definitive determination of genotypic variation can only be done by fingerprint (gene sequencing) or footprint (protein sequencing) genomic analyses.

Infection with CTF virus leads to production of immunoglobulin M (IgM), IgG and, probably, IgA antibodies. These can be detected by ELISA, immunofluorescence, neutralization, complement fixation or any of a great variety of other assays.

Immunoglobulin M antibody to CTF virus does not cross-react with antibody to any other North American virus, so that detecting such antibody, even in a single serum, can be considered presumptive evidence of recent infection with that virus. However, IgM antibody to CTF virus is not detected until 1–2 weeks after the onset of illness and may persist for some weeks or months. Immunoglobulin G antibody to CTF virus appears relatively soon after onset but, unlike IgM, persists for many months or years after the illness or may persist for life.

Because IgG antibody to CTF virus persists, detecting IgG antibody to CTF virus in a serum sample from an acutely ill, a convalescing or a recovered patient cannot alone be used as evidence of current infection with that virus. Detecting IgM antibody to a given virus in a serum sample from an acutely ill, a convalescing or a recovered patient is at least provisional evidence of infection with that virus.

The IgM antibody-capture ELISA (MAC-ELISA) is the serodiagnostic test of choice for determining recent human infections with CTF virus. The MAC-ELISA has the distinct advantage of being able to provide the clinician with relevant results within a matter of hours, rather than days or weeks as with most other techniques. Nevertheless, whereas it might be acceptable to consider MAC-ELISA-positive sera as presumptive evidence of recent infection during such a situation, in all such instances supportive epidemiological information must be obtained and attempts made to obtain additional serum specimens.

A serologically *confirmed* infection with CTF virus requires demonstration of significant (fourfold or greater) increase or decrease in antibody titre between paired acute-phase and convalescent-phase serum samples collected days to weeks apart. A serologically *presumptive* infection is one in which only an acute-phase serum is available, but that serum contains IgM antibody to CTF virus and it is negative or shows only very low titre to CTF virus by other assays, including those for IgG antibody; often, collecting and testing another serum later in the illness reveal antibody of sufficient titre to allow shifting the 'presumptive' designation to 'confirmed'. Whereas IgM antibody usually begins to decline a few weeks or a few months after onset of illness, a minority of patients have prolonged IgM antibody responses, somewhat limiting the value of these assays as a measure of very recent infection. Thus the presence of IgM class antibody in a patient with an illness clinically compatible with Colorado tick fever is, in itself, not confirmatory of such an infection.

Antibody, assistance in preparing such antibodies, antigens, viruses and additional information can be obtained from any of the World Health Organization Centres for Arbovirus Reference and Research. The World Reference Centre is at the University of Texas, Medical Branch, Galveston, Texas; the reference centre for the Americas is at the Centers for Disease Control and Prevention (CDC), Fort Collins, Colorado.

Transmission

Colorado tick fever virus is transmitted exclusively by ticks in North America. Infection of ticks by CTF virus appears to be lifelong, with no observable pathological changes or untoward effects on the tick.

Many factors help to determine the effectiveness of a vertebrate as a CTF virus reservoir host. Among those of greatest importance are the presence of a high-titre viraemia of duration adequate to infect a critical number of ticks, attractiveness to the tick and a continuing availability of additional non-immune individuals. Humans are dead-end or tangential hosts for tick-borne viruses and do not play a significant role in the maintenance and dissemination of CTF virus.

The vertebrate host spectrum varies for each virus; generally, particular species of smaller vertebrates with high population replacement rates, such as birds or rodents, serve as hosts, but larger mammals can be involved.

Colorado tick fever virus is transovarially (adult female→egg) and transtadially (larva→nymph→adult) transmitted in *D. andersoni* ticks. The virus has also been isolated occasionally from some other *Dermacentor* species, as well as from ticks in other genera. In a detailed study of CTF virus and Colorado tick fever in Rocky Mountain National Park, Colorado, increased CTF virus activity was detected at sites with south-facing slopes, open stands of Ponderosa pine and shrubs on dry, rocky surfaces, and these landscape characteristics were determined to be fundamental in maintaining the virus. These specific ecological characteristics were vital to tick populations, as they comprised specific habitats for the small mammals on which the ticks depend for both blood meals and shelter. Mammals involved in the natural cycle of CTF virus include the Golden-mantled ground squirrel (*Spermophilus lateralis*), Porcupine (*Erithizon dorsatum*), Least chipmunk (*Tamias minimus*), Deer mouse (*Peromyscus maniculatus*) and Bushy-tailed woodrat (*Neotoma cinerea*).

The biological transmission cycle of CTF virus can be conceived of as beginning with an uninfected, susceptible and competent tick taking a blood meal from an infected vertebrate. If there is no 'mesenteronal escape barrier' (a not yet understood mechanism that prevents virus from moving from infected gut tissue to other tissues), ingested virus then replicates in the tick's mid-gut and is disseminated to other tissues.

Treatment

There is no specific antiviral therapy for Colorado tick fever. Therapeutic efforts are directed towards managing symptoms, such as reducing fever and relieving headache. Because CTF virus is not transmitted from person to person, containment barriers are not necessary, but care should be taken in handling tissues and body fluids because they may contain virus, and laboratory infections can occur. Vaccines for pre-exposure prophylaxis are not available for Colorado tick fever. Prevention (education) is the best defence. People should be aware of CTF virus in their home areas and in the areas they visit and learn to avoid contact with suspected vectors during the transmission season.

Control

Potential vector control measures include spraying or fogging insecticides (larvicides and adulticides) from the air or by ground equipment, and reducing or altering habitats (source reduction). These measures should be supplemented by surveillance programmes intended to provide early warning of virus activity. However, no such methods have been applied to the control of ticks that carry CTF virus because of the impossibly monumental effort this would require.

Selected bibliography

Becker, F.E. (1930) Tick-borne infections in Colorado. II. A survey of occurrence of infections transmitted by the wood tick. *Colorado Medicine* 27, 87–95.

Bodkin, D.K. and Knudson, D.L. (1987) Genetic relatedness of Colorado tick fever virus isolates by RNA–RNA blot hybridization. *Journal of General Virology* 68, 1199–1204.

Borden, E.C., Shope, R.E. and Murphy, F.A. (1971) Physicochemical and morphological relationships of some arthropod-borne viruses to bluetongue virus – a new taxonomic group. Physicochemical and serological studies. *Journal of General Virology* 13, 261–271.

Bowen, G.S. (1989) Colorado tick fever. In: Monath, T.P. (ed.) *The Arboviruses: Epidemiology and Ecology*, Vol. II. CRC Press, Boca Raton, Florida, pp. 159–176.

Brown, S.E., Miller, B.R., McLean, R.G. and Knudson, D.L. (1989) Co-circulation of multiple Colorado tick fever virus genotypes. *American Journal of Tropical Medicine and Hygiene* 40, 94–101.

Calisher, C.H., Poland, J.D., Calisher, S.B. and Warmoth, L.A. (1985) Diagnosis of Colorado tick fever virus infection by enzyme immunoassays for immunoglobulin M and G antibodies. *Journal of Clinical Microbiology* 22, 84–88.

Florio, L. and Miller, M.S. (1948) Epidemiology of Colorado tick fever. *American Journal of Public Health* 38, 211–213.

Florio, L., Stewart, M.D. and Mugrage, E.R. (1950) Colorado tick fever. Isolation of the virus from *Dermacentor andersoni* in nature and a laboratory study of the transmission of the virus in the tick. *Journal of Immunology* 64, 257–263.

Karabatsos, N., Poland, J.D., Emmons, R.W., Mathews, J.H., Wolff, K.L. and Calisher, C.H. (1987) Antigenic variants of Colorado tick fever virus. *Journal of General Virology* 68, 1463–469.

Knudson, D.L. and Monath, T.P. (1990) Orbiviruses. In: Fields, B.N. and Knipe, D.M. (eds) *Virology*, Vol. 2, 2nd edn. Raven Press, New York, pp. 1405–1433.

McLean, R.G., Shriner, R.B., Pokorny, K.S. and Bowen, G.S. (1989) The ecology of Colorado tick fever in Rocky Mountain National Park in 1974. III. Habitats supporting the virus. *American Journal of Tropical Medicine and Hygiene* 40, 86–93.

Oshiro, L.S., Dondero, D.V., Emmons, R.W. and Lennette, E.H. (1978) The development of Colorado tick fever virus within cells of the haemopoietic system. *Journal of General Virology* 39, 73–79.

Cone-nose bugs *see* **Triatomine bugs.**

Conjunctivitis *see* **Eye-flies and Flies.**

Cornybacteriun pyogenes see **Mastitis.**

Corridor disease *see* **Theilerioses.**

Cowdria ruminantium see **Heartwater.**

Cowdriosis *see* **Heartwater.**

Coxiella burneti see **Q fever.**

Crimean–Congo haemorrhagic fever

P.A. Nuttall

Disease of humans caused by Crimean–Congo haemorrhagic fever (CCHF) virus.

Crimean–Congo haemorrhagic fever, human

The name derives from the separate regions in Asia and Africa where severe and often fatal human cases of haemorrhagic disease and fever were recognized in the 1940s and 1950s. Virus isolates from the two regions are antigenically indistinguishable. The disease came to people's attention in the Crimea when about 200 military personnel became ill while helping peasants to harvest grain. Russian scientists, led by Professor M.P. Chumakov, isolated the virus from human patients and from ticks. The same virus was isolated by C. Courtoise in 1956 from a 13-year-old patient in the Belgian Congo (Democratic Republic of Congo). However, Crimean–Congo haemorrhagic fever has a much longer history, with the first record in the early 12th century. Although ticks transmit CCHF virus to a wide variety of animal species, the severe disease only affects humans. Cattle, sheep and small mammals, such as hares (*Lepus* species) may develop mild fever following infection. The disease in humans is comparatively rare but a cause for concern because of high mortality and transmission through contact with patients. Handling the virus requires the highest degree of laboratory containment.

Distribution

Second only to dengue viruses (see entry) as the most widely distributed medically important arthropod-borne virus. Recorded in Africa, the Middle East, Europe and Asia (Fig. 1); see under Epidemiology below for a more detailed account. The virus distribution largely corresponds with the distribution of *Hyalomma* species of ticks that occur in semi-desert, steppe, savannah and foothill biotopes. Exceptions are the deciduous forests of Moldavia, where *Hyalomma* has been replaced by *Ixodes ricinus* and *Dermacentor* and *Rhipicephalus* species, and in Madagascar, where *Hyalomma* ticks do not occur and where CCHF virus has been isolated from *Boophilus microplus*. Environmental changes associated with wartime neglect of agricultural land or conversion of flood plains and marshy deltas to farmland, significantly increase the prevalence of CCHF virus. In temperate regions CCHF virus enzootic foci occur in areas of warm summers and relatively mild winters. *Hyalomma marginatum*, the primary tick vector in Eurasia, cannot survive monthly mean winter temperatures below −20°C.

Virus

Crimean–Congo haemorrhagic fever virus is the type species of the *Nairovirus* genus in the virus family, Bunyaviridae. The genus is named after Nairobi sheep disease virus (see entry), a tick-borne relative of CCHF virus that causes disease in sheep and goats. All nairoviruses infect vertebrates (mammals and/or birds) and most of them are transmitted by ticks.

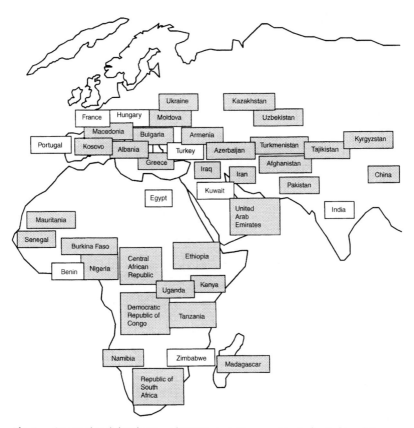

Fig. 1.   Geographical distribution of CCHF virus. For countries indicated in white boxes, evidence is based solely on antibody detection in humans and/or other animals.

Viewed using an electron microscope, CCHF virus appears spherical, approximately 100 nm in diameter (buoyant density, 1.17 g ml⁻¹), with a dense core (capsid) surrounded by a lipid envelope, through which protrude spikes, 5–10 nm in length. The viral genome is segmented, comprising three circular, single strands of negative-sense RNA. All three genomic RNA segments have a unique 3′ end sequence of 3′-AGAG-(A/U)UUCU. The small (S) segment (approx. 1.7 kb) has a single open-reading frame encoding the nucleocapsid (N) protein. In contrast, the medium (M) segment (approx. 5.0 kb) encodes a large polyprotein, which is processed into the two surface glycoproteins, G1 and G2, and several non-structural proteins. The large (L) segment encodes a single L protein of approximately 460 kDa, which is probably the viral polymerase.

Virus infection of cells is probably through receptor-mediated endocytosis, followed by fusion of the viral envelope with endosomal membranes. Monoclonal antibodies directed against G1 (but not against the N protein) neutralize viral infectivity, suggesting an important role for G1 in the infection process. All stages of viral replication occur in the cell cytoplasm, although comparatively little is known of these events. As the viral RNA is negative-sense, the first step in replication is the transcription of the incoming genomic RNA into viral complementary RNA. The transcriptase has not been identified. Viral messenger RNA (mRNA) has host-derived primer sequences, indicating a 'cap-snatching' mRNA priming mechanism, as found with influenza viruses. Virion assembly occurs in the Golgi complex. Nucleocapsids acquire their outer envelope by budding into the Golgi lumen. Virions are then transported to the cell membrane and released from the infected cell by exocytosis.

Clinical symptoms

Disease severity appears similar wherever Crimean–Congo haemorrhagic fever occurs. Clinical signs of the disease follow an incubation period of 1–7 days but this may be longer when infection is by contagion rather than by tick feeding. The disease is characterized by a sudden onset with severe headache, dizziness, neck pain and stiffness and photophobia. Fever with chills occurs at about the same time. Patients rapidly develop general myalgia and malaise, with intense leg and back pains. By the second to fourth day of illness, patients may have a flushed appearance. In severe cases, a petechial rash appears on the trunk and limbs by the third to sixth day of illness (Fig. 2). Internal and external bleeding are common, although sometimes a tendency to haemorrhage is apparent only from the oozing of blood from injection or venepuncture sites. Severely ill patients may show hepato-renal and pulmonary failure from about

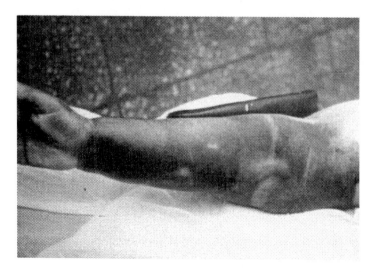

Fig. 2. Haemorrhagic rash on the arm of a CCHF patient (courtesy of D.S. Ellis and the Tropical Medicine Resource, The Wellcome Trust, London).

day 5 onwards, and become progressively drowsy, stuporous and comatose. Deaths generally occur on the 5th to 14th day of illness. Recovery from Crimean–Congo haemorrhagic fever begins on day 9 or 10 with the abatement of the rash and a general improvement, although convalescence may continue for a month or longer.

Pathogenicity

Pathogenesis resulting from an infection of CCHF virus is poorly understood. As an arthropod-transmitted virus, it probably undergoes local replication in the skin site of infected tick feeding. In humans, the virus then probably spreads via blood and/or lymph, infecting organs (such as the liver) that are major sites of replication. Capillary fragility is a feature of CCHF virus, suggesting infection of endothelium. Circulating immune complexes may form, which, together with complement activation, would contribute to damage to the capillary bed and to renal and pulmonary failure. Endothelial damage would account for the characteristic rash and contribute to haemostatic failure by stimulating platelet aggregation and degranulation, with consequent activation of the intrinsic coagulation cascade.

Complete autopsies are seldom performed on patients who die from Crimean–Congo haemorrhagic fever. Examination is often confined to blood changes and liver biopsies. Disseminated intravascular coagulopathy is probably an early event, the severity of which predicts a fatal outcome. Liver lesions vary from disseminated necrotic foci to massive necrosis. Necrotic hepatocytes appear as acidophilic, amorphous masses and there is little or no inflammatory response.

Diagnosis

Early diagnosis is essential because infection can be transmitted by contagion. Clinical symptoms and exposure details provide the first indicators – for example, if patients from endemic regions have been in contact with or bitten by ticks or exposed to fresh blood or other tissues of livestock or human patients. A characteristic symptom is the sudden onset of a severe influenza-like illness. The disease is easier to recognize once a rash appears and there are haemorrhagic signs. Laboratory diagnosis is based on virus isolation from serum or plasma taken early in the disease or demonstration of an immune response in samples taken later. Isolation is by intracerebral inoculation of day-old mice with blood from patients or by inoculation of patient samples into African green monkey kidney (VERO) cells. The virus is only weakly cytopathic in cell culture and is detected by immunofluorescent antibody tests. Although not as sensitive as mouse inoculation, virus isolation in cell culture is more rapid, taking 1–5 days compared with 5–8 days in mice. More recently, the polymerase chain reaction (PCR) has been used to detect CCHF viral RNA in patient tissues. Antibodies to CCHF virus are detectable by indirect immunofluorescence assay from about day 7 of illness, and are present in the sera of survivors by day 9 at the latest. Immunoglobulin M (IgM) antibody levels decline and become undetectable by the fourth month after infection. Immunoglobulin G levels may also begin to decline at this time but remain detectable for at least 5 years. Recent or current infection is confirmed by demonstrating seroconversion, an equal or greater than fourfold increase in antibody in paired serum samples or IgM antibody in a single specimen. Patients who succumb rarely develop an antibody response, and the diagnosis is confirmed by virus isolation from serum or liver specimens taken after death.

Differential diagnosis should consider tick-borne typhus (*Rickettsia conorii* infection, known as tick-bite fever; see Tick-borne typhuses), which responds to broad-spectrum antibiotics. Other infections presenting as haemorrhagic disease include bacterial septicaemias and viral haemorrhagic fevers. In Africa, the latter include Marburg disease, Ebola fever and Lassa fever, none of which is tick-borne. Haemorrhagic fever with renal syndrome is more widespread and caused by rodent-borne hantaviruses (see Haemorrhagic fever with renal syndrome). Mosquito-borne yellow fever and dengue viruses (see entries) are

capable of causing fatal haemorrhagic
diseases in humans.

Transmission

Vectors are ixodid (hard) ticks (Fig. 3).
Although CCHF virus has been isolated
from at least 31 different tick species and
subspecies (including two argasid (soft)
species), the primary vectors are *Hyalomma*
species, particularly *H. marginatum marginatum*, *H. marginatum rufipes* (the African
representative of the *H. marginatum* complex), and *H. anatolicum anatolicum*. All
three species are two-host ticks: immature
stages (larvae and nymphs) feed on the
same individual host before dropping off to
moult to the adult stage which then feeds on
a second host. Both immature stages and
adults of *H. a. anatolicum* feed on domesticated mammals, whereas *H. m. marginatum*
and *H. m. rufipes* immature stages and
adults feed on dissimilar hosts: immature
stages on birds, hares (*Lepus* species) and
hedgehogs (*Erinaceus* and *Hemiechinus*
species), and adults on cattle and other
large mammals (Fig. 4). Adult ticks successfully attack humans, only being detected
after a few days of feeding when they
become enlarged with blood. It is unlikely
that humans contribute to the transmission
cycle. Hares (*Lepus* species), hedgehogs
(*Erinaceus* and *Hemiechinus* species) and
cattle are probably important amplifying
hosts. Feeding on viraemic animals may
provide the source of infection for ticks.
However, screening domestic and wild vertebrates for CCHF viraemia has often failed
to identify viraemic host species that maintain the viral enzootic cycle. Transmission
from infected to uninfected ticks feeding
together on non-viraemic hosts provides an
alternative route. This route exploits the
pharmacological properties of tick saliva
that promote virus transmission. Sheep and
ground-feeding birds, such as Hornbills
(*Tockus erythrorhynchus*) and Ostriches
(*Struthio camelus*), may act as non-viraemic
hosts. Otherwise birds play an important
role in disseminating ticks, particularly
those of the *H. marginatum* complex. Virus
can be transmitted sexually, from infected
male to uninfected female ticks during

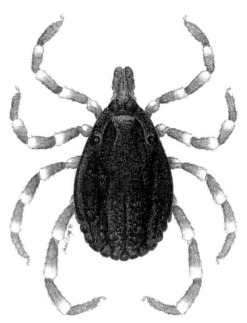

Fig. 3.   Adult female *Hyalomma* tick (artwork by
André Olwage, copyright Oxford University Press).

mating (venereal transmission), and transovarially, from infected females to their
offspring. The epidemiological significance
of vertical (transovarial) transmission is
unknown. However, it could provide an
important amplification mechanism if virus
is transmitted from infected to uninfected
larvae co-feeding on the same host. Virus
survival in infected ticks and the ability
of *Hyalomma* species to survive at least
800 days without a blood meal indicate that
ticks act as virus reservoirs. Direct transmission through contact with infected blood
and body fluids and, possibly, crushed ticks
is an important route of human infections.

Epidemiology

The disease in humans has been recorded in
Africa (Mauritania, Burkina Faso, Central
African Republic, Democratic Republic of
Congo, Tanzania, Uganda, Namibia, Repub-
lic of South Africa), the Middle East (Iraq,
United Arab Emirates), Europe (Bulgaria,
Albania, Macedonia, Kosovo, Moldavia)
and Asia (Russia, Ukraine, Kyrgyzstan,
Tajikistan, Uzbekistan, Kazakhstan, Turk-
menistan, Armenia, Pakistan, western

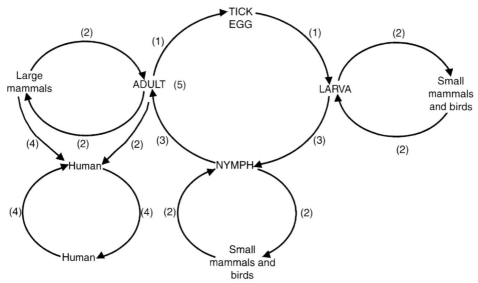

Fig. 4. Routes of CCHF virus transmission. (1) Vertical (transovarial) transmission from infected adult tick to offspring; (2) horizontal transmission from infected tick to uninfected vertebrate host or from infected vertebrate host to uninfected tick during tick blood-feeding; (3) trans-stadial persistence during moulting from one tick stage to the next stage; (4) direct transmission from infected human or non-human to uninfected human by contagion; (5) sexual transmission from infected male to uninfected female tick.

China). In addition, the virus has been isolated from ticks collected in Greece, Senegal, Nigeria, Madagascar, Kenya, Uganda, Ethiopia, Afghanistan, Iran and Azerbaijan, although there have been no records of human disease in these countries. There is limited evidence of infections in France, Portugal, Turkey, India, Hungary, Kuwait, Benin, Zimbabwe and Egypt, based on antibody detection in humans and/or other animals.

Enzootic foci have often been recognized only after unpredictable and sudden occurrences of human Crimean–Congo haemorrhagic fever cases. For example, Crimean–Congo haemorrhagic fever was not recognized in South Africa until 1981, when a child was bitten by a *Hyalomma* tick in the western Transvaal. Subsequent serosurveys of livestock and wild vertebrates revealed that CCHF virus was present long before its presence was first recognized. New enzootic foci may arise following dispersal of infected ticks carried by birds and livestock. Despite the lack of systematic surveillance for CCHF virus, morbidity data reveal a characteristic

pattern of sporadic occurrence and widely scattered cases, both spatially and temporally. In the Rostov region of the Ukraine, the reported morbidity rate was 13.5/100,000 persons between 1963 and 1969, whereas only a few cases were registered during 1970–1971, and none in 1972–1973. Mortality rates average 30%, but higher rates have been reported, particularly when infection has been by contagion.

In Eurasia, transmission appears during early spring until late autumn, with human cases peaking in June to August. In milder climates where ticks remain active, transmission probably occurs throughout the year. Agricultural practices, particularly involving livestock, are important risk factors for human Crimean–Congo haemorrhagic fever cases acquired from tick-borne infections.

Treatment

Antiviral therapy may be effective in treating CCHF viral infections if given early in the course of disease. Promising results were obtained in a trial of the chemotherapeutic drug, ribavirin. However, as human cases generally occur in less developed parts of the world, the availability of such treatment is limited. Treatment of the symptoms is the usual course of action, and consists of supportive and replacement therapy with blood products. Immune-plasma therapy has been used extensively when available.

Control

Acaricide treatment of livestock and controlling the numbers of hares are effective in reducing the population of infected ticks and hence the risk of infection. However, tick control is impractical in many regions of the world where *Hyalomma* ticks are most prevalent. Clothing impregnated with pyrethroid acaricides can give some protection against tick bites. Wearing gloves and limiting exposure of naked skin to fresh blood and other tissues of animals are practical control measures that should be undertaken by veterinarians, slaughter workers and others involved with potentially infected livestock, and by medical staff treating patients.

Inactivated virus vaccines prepared from infected newborn mouse brain have been used successfully in humans in the former USSR and Bulgaria. Commercial vaccines are not available.

Selected bibliography

Hoogstraal, H. (1979) The epidemiology of tick-borne Crimean-Congo haemorrhagic fever in Asia, Europe and Africa. *Journal of Medical Entomology* 15, 307–417.

Linthicum, K.J. and Bailey, C.L. (1994) Ecology of Crimean-Congo haemorrhagic fever. In: Sonenshine, D.E. and Mather, T.N. (eds) *Ecological Dynamics of Tick-Borne Zoonoses.* Oxford University Press, New York, pp. 392–437.

Marriott, A.C. and Nuttall, P.A. (1996) Nairoviruses. In: Elliott, R.M. (ed.) *The Bunyaviridae.* Plenum Press, New York, pp. 91–104.

Swanepoel, R. (1994) Crimean–Congo haemorrhagic fever. In: Coetzer, J.A.W., Thomson, G.R. and R.C. Tustin, R.C. (eds) *Infectious Diseases of Livestock*, Vol. 1. Oxford University Press, Cape Town, pp. 723–729.

Watts, D.M., Ksiazek, T.G., Linthicum, K.J. and Hoogstraal, H. (1988) Crimean–Congo haemorrhagic fever. In: Monath, T.P. (ed.) *The Arboviruses: Epidemiology and Ecology*, Vol. II. CRC Press, Boca Raton, Florida, pp. 177–222.

Crimean tick-borne typhus *see* **Tick-borne typhuses.**

Culicoides **see Biting midges.**

Deer-flies *see* **Horse-flies.**

Deer-fly fever *see* **Tularaemia.**

Dengue

Vincent Deubel and Bernadette Murgue

Dengue is caused by any one of four viruses vectored mainly by the mosquito *Aedes aegypti* and has a worldwide distribution in the tropics. Dengue is the most important medical arbovirus disease of the world today, with an estimated annual 100 million cases and several hundred thousand of them severe.

Distribution

Dengue fever (DF) was first described in 1779 in Jakarta, Indonesia, and in Cairo, Egypt and 1 year later in Philadelphia, USA. From 1823 to 1905, major epidemics of dengue-like disease occurred in Zanzibar, India, the Caribbean and Hong Kong. In the 20th century, the largest outbreaks of dengue occurred in Australia (1925, 1942), the USA (1922), the Seychelles (1926), Tunisia and Greece (1927), Taiwan (1931) and Japan (1942). During the 1980s and the 1990s an increasing number of dengue epidemics have been responsible for hundreds of thousands of cases in South-East Asia and in tropical and subtropical America, where the virus has become endemic and regularly associated with disease outbreaks.

One of the severe forms of the disease, dengue haemorrhagic fever (DHF), became epidemic in Manila, Philippines, in 1953 and has since spread throughout South-East Asia. Increasing numbers of DHF cases have been reported every year in the Caribbean and other parts of the Americas since a major epidemic in Cuba in 1981.

Before the 1980s, little was known about dengue (DEN) virus distribution in Africa. Since then, outbreaks have occurred in East and West Africa, with major transmission reported in the Seychelles, Kenya, Sudan and Somalia. In addition, sporadic cases of disease, clinically compatible with DHF, have been reported from Mozambique, Djibouti and Saudi Arabia.

Virus

Virus structure

There are four antigenically different DEN virus serotypes, namely dengue-1, dengue-2, dengue-3 and dengue-4, based on plaque reduction neutralization and other tests. They belong to the genus *Flavivirus*, family Flaviviridae. Flaviviruses are enveloped nucleocapsid spherical viruses 40–50 nm in diameter. The virion has a density of about 1.23 g cm^{-3} in sucrose gradients and a sedimentation coefficient of around 210 $S_{20, w}$. The mature virion contains three structural proteins: the core protein (C), a membrane-associated protein (M) and the envelope protein (E). The viral nucleocapsid consists of the core protein and a single-stranded, positive-sense RNA approximately 11 kilobases in length. The genomic RNA has a type I 5′ cap of m^7 GpppA and lacks a 3′-end poly(A) track. The non-coding region at the 5′ end is about 110 nucleotides long and that of the 3′ end ranges from 300 to 600 nucleotides. The flavivirus genome encodes a polyprotein precursor of about 3390 amino acids, which is processed by co-translational proteolytic cleavage by cellular (signalases and convertase) and viral proteases. The gene order for the structural proteins from the 5′ terminus is C-prM(M)-E-NS1-NS2A-NS2B-NS3-NS4A-NS4B-NS5. The properties of the viral proteins are indicated in Table 1.

Virus replication and morphogenesis

Flaviviruses replicate in a wide variety of cultured cells of both vertebrate and insect

Table 1.   Biological characteristics of flavivirus proteins.

Proteins	Amino acids	Functions	Comments
C	102–126	Nucleoprotein. Forms the capsid	Cytoplasmic
PrM	166–183 (Glycoprotein)	Stabilizes E protein at acidic pH in the immature intracellular virion	Precursor of M. Forms heterodimers with E protein in the immature virion. N-glycosylation on one site
M	75	Membrane protein	Present on the mature extracellular virion
E	495 (Glycoprotein)	Binding to a cell receptor, fusion on the mature viron, induction of neutralizing antibodies	Dimeric envelope protein. N-glycosylation on one site
NS1	352 (Glycoprotein)	Functions in the viral RNA replication. Other functions (extracellular form)?	Forms intracellular dimers and extracellular hexamers. N-glycosylation on two sites
NS2A	348–354	Role in the cleavage of NS1–NS2A?	Hydrophobic protein
NS2B		Cofactor in NS3 protease activity	Hydrophobic protein
NS3	618–623	Protease, helicase, NTPase	Cytoplasmic protein
NS4A	395–405	RNA replication	Hydrophobic protein
NS4B		RNA replication	Hydrophobic protein
NS5	900–905	Polymerase, methyltransferase	Cytoplasmic protein

origins. Dengue viruses bind to susceptible cells by three known mechanisms. Gluco-aminoglycans, which are present on a multitude of cell membranes, are target molecules for DEN virions and may represent a first non-specific step of virus binding. Alternatively, non-neutralizing anti-virus envelope immunoglobulin G (IgG) antibodies form immune complexes, which may mediate virion attachment and uptake by binding to macrophages or monocytes via Fc receptors found at the cell surface. In addition, DEN viruses may bind to cells via an as yet unknown protease-sensitive receptor. Dengue viruses enter cells by endocytosis, with the formation of coated vesicles (Fig. 1). Uncoating of the nucleocapsid is accomplished by an acid-dependent fusion of viral and endosomal membranes. Viral fusion is mediated by the E protein, which undergoes an irreversible conformational change at acidic pH.

Uncoated viral genome is immediately translated into viral proteins, including NS3 helicase and NS5 polymerase, involved in RNA replication. The replication process includes transcription of the positive-strand RNA to negative-strand RNA, which then

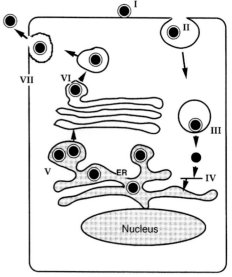

Fig. 1.   Dengue virus morphogenesis. Viruses bind to an unknown receptor (I) and enter into the cells by endocytosis (II). After fusion of the viral envelope with the endosomic membranes (III), the nucleo-capsid is processed in the cytoplasm and viral RNA replicates (IV). Immature viral particles are formed in the endoplasmic reticulum (ER) (V) and are transported through the Golgi network (VI) to the internal side of the cell surface. Viral particles are released from the cells by reverse pinocytosis (VII).

serves as template for additional positive strands. Positive-strand RNA may serve either as a template for further transcription and translation into viral proteins, or for encapsidation and virus assembling, which occur during late eclipse, approximately 15 h after virus infection. All flavivirus nucleocapsids appear to form immature enveloped virus-like particles containing E and prM protein heterodimers through a process of budding, in which virus particles assemble in the cisternae of the rough endoplasmic reticulum. Release of virus from the infected cells occurs via secretory exocytosis as virus-containing vesicles fuse with the plasma membranes (Fig. 1). The final cleavage step of prM by furin-like convertase of the Golgi apparatus leads to release of fully infectious virus particles.

Cytopathic effects of virus infection range from inapparent to severe, depending on the cell line and virus strain used. Cell fusion is sometimes observed in mosquito cells, whereas cell rounding and shrinking in mammalian cells may be associated with apoptotic cell death. Persistent infections with production of infectious DEN virus have been established in vertebrate and invertebrate cell cultures.

Clinical symptoms

The incubation period of DEN virus infection is 3–10 days. According to the World Health Organization (WHO) definition, infection by a DEN virus causes either an asymptomatic infection or a spectrum of illness, ranging from fever through relatively mild disease, known as classic dengue fever (DF), to a more severe form (DHF).

Classic DF occurs in adults as a febrile illness with abrupt onset, lasting 2–7 days and characterized by malaise, headache, retro-orbital pain, myalgia and arthralgia. A maculopapular rash develops with defervescence. Hepatomegaly occurs in 10–30% of DF cases; myocarditis has been observed. In 5–30% of DF cases, a variable degree of bleeding can occur, including petechiae, purpura, epistaxis, gingival bleeding, haematuria and hypermenorrhoea. Dengue fever can be confused with influenza, chikungunya (see entry), measles, rubella,

typhoid, malaria, leptospirosis and enterovirus infections, and differential diagnosis must be based on laboratory tests.

The clinical definition of DHF established by the WHO in 1986 is based on the presence of fever, haemorrhagic manifestations, thrombocytopenia and haemoconcentration. The WHO classification further subdivides DHF (Fig. 2) into four grades of severity. Grades III and IV are characterized by circulatory failure and may become life-threatening because of the occurrence of profound shock (dengue shock syndrome (DSS)). Plasma leakage due to an increase in vascular permeability is the main pathophysiological hallmark of DHF. However, in clinical practice the distinction between DF and DHF remains sometimes difficult.

In addition to DHF, several severe and fatal forms of DEN virus infection have been reported which do not fit the DHF description. Severe hepatic disorders have been reported and there is evidence that dengue is associated with Reye's syndrome and fulminant hepatitis. Liver involvement may also contribute directly to bleeding. Severe neurological manifestations include depressed sensorium, lethargy, confusion, seizures, paresis and coma. Encephalopathy, which may occur after infection, can include paralysis, epilepsy, tremor, amnesia, dementia and Guillain–Barré syndrome. Other severe manifestations have been reported with lungs, kidneys, gall-bladder and pancreatic involvement. Recently, co-infections of humans with two viruses have been described. These may modify the clinical presentation of dengue.

Infection with any of the four serotypes may cause severe illness. In endemic areas, DHF/DSS occurs in 0.1–2% of dengue cases, leading to a less than 1% mortality rate when patients are treated under appropriate intensive care.

Convalescence is usually brief, but may take weeks, with attendant weakness and bradycardia; there are no known sequelae associated with dengue.

Clinical laboratory findings associated with DF include neutropenia and lymphocytosis, with presence of large B lymphoblastoid cells. Liver enzymes (aspartate

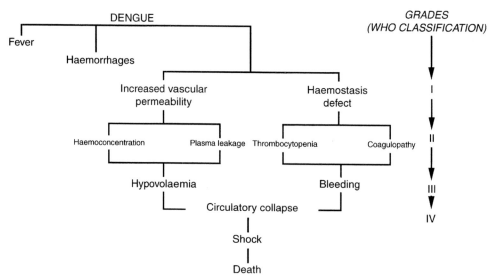

Fig. 2.   Spectrum of dengue fever, dengue haemorrhagic fever and dengue shock syndrome.

aminotransferases usually higher than alanine aminotransferases) are mildly elevated but in some cases levels of liver enzymes are very high. Hypoalbuminaemia and prolonged prothrombin times are observed. Disseminated intravascular coagulopathy is frequent. Thrombocytopenia is common and platelet counts can be very low < 20,000 mm^{-3}. Signs of plasma leakage include haemoconcentration (at least 20% increase of haematocrit), hypoproteinaemia and hypoalbuminaemia.

Pathology

Due to the risk of bleeding, it has not been possible to obtain tissues from living patients and most of what is known about the pathology of DHF is limited to observations made at autopsy. There are no significant pathognomonic lesions at the organ level. Haemorrhages appear as petechial rashes or purpura in the nose, gums and gastrointestinal tracts, underneath the capsule of the liver and in the meninges and the brain. Haemorrhages appear in patches in subcutaneous tissues. Serous effusions are present in the pericardial, pleural and abdominal cavities. The liver is enlarged in one-third of the cases and may show fatty

metamorphosis. Histological analysis of the liver shows midzonal and paracentrilobular necrosis, swelling of Kupffer cells with hyaline necrosis and formation of acidophilic cells similar to the Councilman bodies observed in yellow fever (see entry). Dengue virus replication in hepatocytes and in Kupffer cells induces apoptotic cell death *in vivo* and *in vitro*, a correlate of the presence of Councilman bodies in liver of dengue-infected patients. Microsteatosis in hepatocytes is often observed. Viral antigens are present in Kupffer cells and in hepatocytes. Oedema and haemorrhages have been observed in the brain and spinal cord without evidence of encephalitis-related pathological changes. Bone marrow examinations show in all cases a hypocellular marrow with abnormal megakaryocytopoiesis during the febrile phase of the illness. At the time of defervescence, the bone marrow appears normocellular or hypercellular with a large numbers of blast cells. Dengue virus antigens have also been localized in cells of reticuloendothelial origin and in mononuclear phagocytes in the spleen, thymus, lymph nodes and liver. Most observations, however, do not support direct cellular pathology caused by the virus.

Pathogenesis

The pathogenesis of DHF/DSS is controversial. Both viral and host factors may influence the severity of dengue. Considerable evidence supports the assumption that more severe dengue is observed with particular genotypes of virus, but the molecular basis for such an association remains elusive. The rapid onset of capillary leakage and minimal endothelial damage suggest that immunopathological events with sudden release of cytokines from activated cells might be at the origin of DHF and DSS. It has been suggested that cells of the mononuclear lineage become infected by DEN virus–antibody complexes bound to their Fc receptor. Therefore cross-reactive non-neutralizing antibodies in patients infected for the second time may enhance the infection and replication of DEN virus in these cells (antibody-dependent enhancement), which then produce and secrete vasoactive mediators, leading to an increased vascular permeability. However, this hypothesis has never been demonstrated *in vivo*. In addition cytotoxic T-cell activation may occur in patients with primary and secondary infections and may be influenced by genetic factors of the host. Several cytokines, such as tumour necrosis factor (TNF), interferon (IFN), tumour growth factor (TGF) and interleukin-8 (IL-8) have been observed to be associated with capillary leakage syndrome, and elevated titres have been noticed during the acute phase of DHF and DSS. Coagulation disorders may be linked in part to autoimmunity against clotting factors containing epitopes similar to those present on the envelope protein of DEN viruses. Thrombocytopenia might be due to bone marrow failure. An indirect effect of DEN virus infection on haematopoiesis mediated by a suppressive cytokine has been demonstrated *in vitro*.

In addition, autodestruction of endothelial cells and platelets displaying at their surface epitopes similar to that present on the non-structural NS1 protein of DEN virus may occur. The mechanism of immunopathogenesis remains hypothetical and further analyses of human specimens and the development of animal models which can reproduce DHF and DSS as observed in humans are needed urgently.

Diagnosis

Laboratory diagnosis of DEN virus infections depends on isolation of infectious virus, detection of virus-specific RNA or antigens in serum and tissues, or identification of specific antibodies in the patient's serum. Circulating virus remains readily detectable in the blood up to 5 days after onset of symptoms, with titres reaching 10^7 mosquito infectious dose (MID_{50}) per ml of serum and then is rapidly cleared by the appearance of IgM antibody (Fig. 3). Therefore, an acute-phase blood sample should be taken as soon as possible after onset of symptoms and preserved cold or frozen

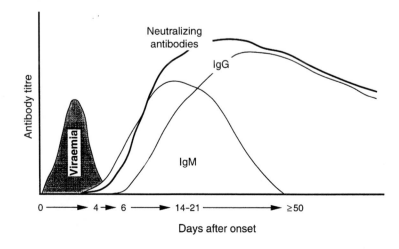

Fig. 3. Viraemia and humoral response to dengue virus infection.

at −80°C for virus isolation. Ideally, a convalescent-phase sample should be taken 10–15 days later for identification of virus antibody. Information on the patient (e.g. age, sex, date of onset of fever, travel and vaccination history) and clinical data are required to help laboratory staff in selecting and interpreting tests.

Virus isolation

Isolation of DEN virus is the most accurate method of diagnosis. Four isolation systems are used for DEN viruses. In order of decreasing sensitivity, these are: (i) intrathoracic inoculation of mosquitoes; (ii) inoculation of mosquito cell cultures; (iii) inoculation of mammalian cell cultures; and (iv) intracerebral inoculation of suckling mice. The latter two methods are not recommended for isolation of DEN viruses because their low sensitivity requires multiple passages to adapt the virus. The only advantage of these methods is the possibility of isolating other viruses that may cause dengue-like illnesses. Although 10–15% more sensitive than mosquito cell cultures, intrathoracic inoculation of mosquitoes (male *Aedes aegypti* or *Toxorhynchites amboinensis*) has the disadvantage of being tedious and requiring an insectary for mosquito rearing. Four to 7 days post-inoculation, virus is detected in neural tissues and salivary glands by indirect fluorescence assay (IFA), using polyclonal and monoclonal antibodies. Cultures of mosquito cell clones, *Aedes albopictus* C6/36 and *Aedes pseudoscutellaris* AP61, are widely used for DEN virus isolation. Cells are tested by IFA 3–7 days after inoculation.

Detection of viral RNA and antigens

Detection of DEN virus antigens in viraemic sera has not been used extensively. However, detection of DEN virus has been reported by direct capture of viral antigens using monoclonal immunoassay. Soluble NS1 antigens were detected in sera of patients who were secondarily infected with DEN virus. Such methods are potentially extremely valuable, because they require only a few hours to complete and can detect virus produced during the very early stages of the acute phase of illness, before any IgM antibodies can be detected. A commercial diagnostic kit for direct detection of virus antigens in patient sera is now available.

Reverse transcription–polymerase chain reaction (RT-PCR) has been extensively used for virus detection in human clinical samples, autopsy tissues or mosquitoes and is particularly suited for DEN virus, in providing a rapid, sensitive, simple and reproducible serotype-specific diagnosis. When properly controlled to avoid amplicon contamination, this method circumvents problems encountered with virus isolation, such as time-lags for virus isolation, loss of virus viability in serum samples maintained in poor storage conditions or the presence of neutralizing antibody. Several techniques have been developed for RT-PCR which differ in the procedure of RNA extraction from clinical specimens, in the specificity of the oligonucleotide primers and in the identification of the amplified genes. However, RT-PCR should not be used as an alternative to virus isolation, which is still required for virus characterization.

By immunohistochemistry it is possible to detect virus antigens in a variety of tissues from fatal dengue cases. Methods using polyclonal or monoclonal antibodies for immunofluorescence tests or peroxidase or phosphatase conjugate-labelled antibody on fresh tissue slices are simple methods for dengue diagnosis and can be completed in just a few hours. Alternatively, formalin-fixed and paraffin-embedded tissues can be tested for DEN viruses.

Serological diagnosis

Historically, methods for measuring antibodies, such as haemagglutination inhibition (HI), complement fixation (CF) and neutralization (N), tests have been used as reliable tests for measuring antibodies. These tests required acute- and convalescent-phase samples to measure significant increases in antibody.

The NT is the most specific serological test for DEN virus in first infections. In second infections, the specificity of the NT test is less reliable. The enzyme-linked immunosorbent assay (ELISA) has provided more rapid and simple quantitative methods to measure IgG and IgM antibody isotypes. Due to cross-reactivity between the flaviviruses the antigen battery for most of the serological tests should include all four DEN serotypes and one or several other flavivirus (e.g. yellow fever, Japanese encephalitis. West Nile – see entries). Immunoglobulin M antibody-capture ELISA (MAC-ELISA) is widely used for early IgM detection, because at day 5 of illness 80% of the patients develop IgM antibody and 99% have detectable IgM antibody between 6 and 10 days after onset. Immunoglobulin M antibody usually persists for about 60 days. Immunoglobulin M antibody-capture ELISA-positive results obtained with a single serum sample are only presumptive of DEN virus infection, because this test, like the others, is broadly reactive, in particular in secondarily infected patients or in patients with pre-existing flavivirus antibodies (vaccinated or flavivirus serially infected patients). Generally, IgG antibody can be detected about 24 h after IgM antibody in primary DEN virus infection and is broadly cross-reactive. Dengue IgM titre is usually higher than IgG titre in a primary infection, but it is lower in a secondary infection. Therefore the ratio of antibody titres in IgG-ELISA and MAC-ELISA can be used to differentiate primary and secondary infections. A number of commercial kits for dengue IgM and IgG serological diagnosis are available. The specificity of these kits may be improved in the future with the use of recombinant proteins.

Transmission

Anthropozootic cycles in rain forests involving *Aedes* mosquitoes and monkeys have been described in Malaysia, Vietnam and West Africa. Although such cycles may play a role in the maintenance of DEN viruses in nature, there is no evidence that enzootic strains are involved in epidemics. Dengue epidemics which emerge in large tropical urban centres are due to inter-human transmission of DEN virus by *A. aegypti* mosquitoes (Fig. 4). Hyperendemic situations may occur when multiple serotypes co-circulate in the same urban area. Biting rates of *A. aegypti* are highest after sunrise and before sunset. Females frequently need multiple blood meals during their gonotrophic cycle and this enhances the probability of multiple virus transmission. *Aedes aegypti* oviposits in peridomestic and usually shaded, man-made containers (e.g. water-storage pots outside or inside houses) containing more or less non-polluted water.

Ochlerotatus[1] *albopictus* is an Asian mosquito that has since the 1970s become established in parts of the USA, several Latin American countries, a few Afrotropical countries, some Pacific islands and even in European countries, such as Albania and Italy. Oviposition occurs in both natural (e.g. tree holes) and artificial containers (e.g. vehicle tyres, water pots) in peridomestic environments. *Aedes albopictus* is a known vector of DEN viruses in Asia, but, being less anthropophagic than *A. aegypti*, is usually considered a less important vector. Nevertheless, it could serve as an alternate vector of DEN viruses in its newly colonized areas.

Ochlerotatus[1] *mediovittatus*, a forest species that has encroached into peri-urban areas, may contribute to the maintenance of DEN viruses in the Caribbean region, while *Aedes polynesiensis* and *Aedes scutellaris* may act as alternate vectors of DEN viruses in the western Pacific region.

Several factors influence the transmission of DEN viruses. In some areas, such as South-East Asia, there is often a strong correlation between rainfall and the incidence of DEN virus infection, with maximum transmission occurring in months with high precipitation. However, there are exceptions and dengue epidemics may occur outside the rainy season. Ambient temperature is epidemiologically important because it influences vector distribution, blood-feeding frequency, duration of the extrinsic incubation period and adult survival rates. There is little, if any, transmission, below 17°C. Temperature may therefore play a more important role than rainfall in DEN virus transmission. Furthermore, global warming may extend the distribution of aedine vectors to more temperate regions;

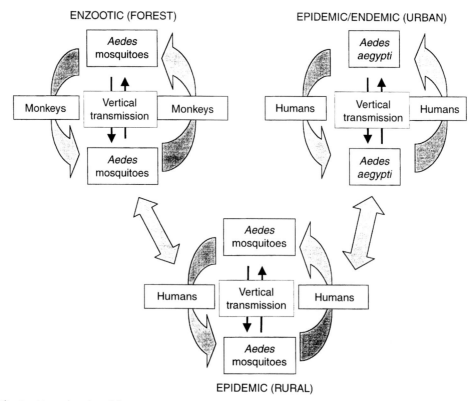

Fig. 4. Natural cycles of dengue transmission.

for example, there is concern about the possible spread of *A. albopictus* into more northern areas.

Infected mosquitoes do not disperse far after blood-feeding. Mostly *A. aegypti* and *A. albopictus* bite, and sometimes breed, in and around neighbouring houses and remain in the vicinity after blood-feeding. However, transportation of adult mosquitoes by intercontinental air travel and larvae (e.g. those of *A. albopictus*) in shipments of tyres on board ships can result in long-distance dispersal. This can involve introductions of potential vectors into countries free of them and dispersal of adult females can give rise to multiple introductions of DEN viruses in distant countries.

Human-to-human transmission in the absence of mosquito vectors is an exceedingly rare event. Congenital infection in humans is also rare. One nosocomial infection has been described in a nurse, who became infected through a needle puncture from a febrile dengue patient. Several laboratory infections have been documented; but have usually occurred after accidental needle-stick injury.

Epidemiology

Dengue viruses and *A. aegypti* mosquitoes have a worldwide distribution in tropical areas, where more than 2500 million people live. The number of DF cases is estimated to be about 100 million annually, causing several hundred thousand cases of DHF. Dengue is one of the major causes of hospitalization of children and is the most important arthropod-borne viral disease worldwide. Dengue circulation is either endemic or hyperendemic, when several serotypes co-circulate, or epidemic. Explosive outbreaks are generally first notified in cities where most of the population is non-immune. Such outbreaks affect mainly older children and adults, with an attack rate between 40 and 90%. In endemic regions of South-East Asia and more recently in South America, DEN viruses are hyperendemic and affect mainly young children.

The severity of clinical syndromes is multifactorial and depends on the virus genotype, the age, the genetic characteristics and the flavivirus/dengue immune status of the human host and of the vector (Fig. 5). Increasing incidence of DHF/DSS in most countries has been associated with the development of hyperendemicity. Factors responsible for the increasing incidence of DHF are: (i) population growth and uncontrolled urbanization; (ii) poor waste-water management systems associated with unplanned urbanization; (iii) lack of mosquito control in areas where *A. aegypti* circulates; and (iv) increasing air travel, which provides opportunities for the viruses to be transported from one endemic/epidemic area to a population-receptive area.

Because the dispersal rate of *A.aegypti* is usually low, DEN viruses are normally dispersed by movements of viraemic persons. The transmission rate is high if viraemic people enter an environment where there are both large populations of vectors and susceptible humans. Epidemics of dengue in the tropics often occur in the rainy seasons, when the vectors are usually more abundant and their survival rate is higher.

Treatment

In the absence of specific treatment for DEN virus-infected patients, management of DHF/DSS is mostly symptomatic and supportive. Antipyretics and analgesics, avoiding those which are hepatotoxic, are supportive medicaments. Salicylates, such as aspirin, should be avoided. Prognosis depends upon early diagnosis and early intervention to manage shock and coagulation disorders. The case fatality rate has decreased remarkably since fluid and electrolyte therapy has been instituted to combat impending shock.

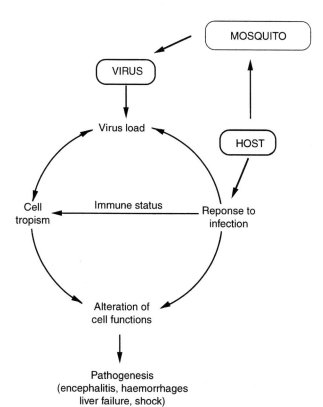

Fig. 5. Factors involved in the outcome of dengue pathogenesis.

Prevention and control

There is no fully effective method of preventing infections with DEN viruses. Candidate vaccines against DEN virus are not yet available and tools for mosquito control are somewhat limited.

Vector control

The proliferation of domestic containers (e.g. water-storage pots, discarded tin cans and tyres) in urban and rural situations and the presence of a forest DEN virus cycle reduce the likelihood of any global success in controlling the vector populations.

Space-spraying with insecticides to kill adult mosquitoes is not always very effective unless carried out in houses. However, in an epidemic urban situation, the most effective control is to use ultra-low-volume (ULV) applications of insecticides, such as malathion, fenitrothion or permethrin, to kill adult mosquitoes, especially infected ones. Best coverage is achieved by aerial spraying. This is clearly an emergency tactic and the long-term aim should be to minimize vector population size, thus circumventing an epidemic situation. The most appropriate methods are those that reduce populations of mosquito larvae. This is best achieved by eliminating mosquito breeding in peridomestic containers. The insecticide temephos (Abate) is considered safe to add to pots containing water destined for domestic purposes. Alternatively, tight-fitting lids can be placed on pots to prevent mosquito oviposition, but in practice this has generally not proved a practical, or acceptable, control measure. Larval source reduction is often advocated. Basically this consists of removing larval habitats, such as unwanted pots, tin cans and tyres and a general clean-up of house premises. This approach has sometimes been based on community participation, but people's cooperation can prove difficult to sustain.

At the individual level, personal protection can be obtained by people repeatedly space-spraying their houses. Using insect repellents on exposed skin and wearing protective clothes impregnated with repellents or insecticides, such as permethrin, may help reduce exposure to mosquito bites.

Vaccine possibilities

Several approaches have been investigated to develop protective immunity against DEN viruses. However, neutralizing antibodies raised against one DEN virus serotype are not cross-protective against other serotypes. The potential risk of DHF due to pre-existing non-neutralizing heterotypic DEN antibody would require a tetravalent vaccine for effective vaccination. Classical studies have used either inactivated DEN viruses purified from mouse brain and cell culture or attenuated DEN viruses. Dengue viruses attenuated in cell culture have, after sequential passages, been successfully tested for safety and immunogenicity in human volunteers and are promising vaccine candidates. Recombinant DEN virus vaccines using molecular technologies have raised considerable interest but their efficacy has not yet been tested in humans. In particular, synthetic peptides, purified recombinant structural and non-structural proteins as subunit vaccines, recombinant live virus vectors, infectious complementary DNA (cDNA) chimeric virus vaccines and naked DNA are future vaccine candidates.

At present, prevention of dengue outbreaks is based on laboratory-based surveillance, emergency response, education of the medical staff to ensure effective case management and community-based integrated mosquito control.

Note

[1]   *Ochlerotatus* was formerly a subgenus of *Aedes*.

Selected bibliography

Bielefeldt-Ohmann, H. (1997) Pathogenesis of dengue virus disease: missing pieces in the jigsaw. *Trends in Microbiology* 5, 409–413.

Chambers, T.J., Tsai, T.F., Pervikov, Y. and Monath, T.P. (1997) Vaccine development against dengue and Japanese encephalitis: report from a World Health Organization meeting. *Vaccine* 15, 1494–1502.

Gubler, D.J. (1998) Dengue and dengue hemorrhagic fever. *Clinical Microbiology Reviews* 11, 480–496.

Gubler, D.J. and Kuno, G. (eds) (1997) *Dengue and Dengue Hemorrhagic Fever.* CAB International, Wallingford, UK, 478 pp.

Henchal, E.A. and Putnak, J.R. (1990) The dengue virus. *Clinical Microbiology Reviews* 3, 376–396.

Innis, B.L. (1995) Dengue and dengue hemorrhagic fever. In: Porterfield, J.S. (ed.) *Exotic Viral Infections.* Chapman & Hall Medical, London, pp. 103–146.

Marianneau, P., Flamand, M., Deubel, V. and Desprès, P. (1998) Apoptotic cell death in response to dengue virus infection: the pathogenesis of dengue hemorrhagic fever revisited. *Clinical and Diagnostic Virology* 1, 113–119.

Monath, T.P. and Heinz, F.X. (1996) Flaviviruses. In: Fields, B.N., Knipe, D.M. and Howley, P. (eds) *Fields Virology,* Vol. 1, 3rd edn. Lippincott-Raven Press Publishers, Philadelphia, pp. 961–1034.

Murgue, B., Cassar, O., Deparis, X., Guigon, M. and Chungue, E. (1998) Implication of macrophage inflammatory protein-1α (MIP-1α) in the inhibition of human hematopoietic progenitor growth by dengue virus. *Journal of General Virology* 79, 1889–1893.

Rice, C.M. (1996) Flaviviridae: the viruses and their replication. In: Fields, B.N., Knipe, D.M. and Howley, P. (eds) *Fields Virology,* Vol. 1, 3rd edn. Lippincott-Raven Press Publishers, Philadelphia, pp. 931–959.

Sinniah, M. and Igarashi, A. (1995) Dengue with renal syndrome. *Reviews in Medical Virology* 5, 193–203.

World Health Organization (1997) *Dengue Haemorrhagic Fever: Diagnosis, Treatment, Prevention and Control.* World Health Organization, Geneva, 84 pp.

'Dengue' of cattle *see* **Bovine ephemeral fever.**

Dog-flies *see* **Stable-flies.**

Dog heartworm *see* **Dirofilariasis.**

Dirofilariasis

Silvio Pampiglione and Francesco Rivasi

Infection of humans and other mammals with filarial nematodes of the genus *Dirofilaria.*

Dirofilariasis, human

Of the parasitic filariae infecting domestic and wild mammals, some species of the genus *Dirofilaria* can also accidentally infect humans. Since humans are not the most suitable host, the parasites do not usually reach complete maturity in humans. Even if they do and if they mate, no microfilariae are normally found in the bloodstream. The parasite is almost always enclosed by the defensive reaction of the host and in an inflammatory nodule, or eliminated as a foreign body by a process of suppuration. Until almost 50 years ago, human dirofilariasis (HD) was considered a rare occurrence; in recent decades, however, the increase in the number of cases reported has been such that HD can now be classified as an emerging zoonosis.

There are three main species involved: *Dirofilaria repens,* a subcutaneous parasite of dogs, cats and a few other carnivores (Fig. 1); *Dirofilaria immitis,* in dogs, cats and numerous other species of mammals, parasites lodge preferably in the right ventricle of the heart (hence the name heartworm) and in the pulmonary artery and its ramifications (Fig. 2); and *Dirofilaria tenuis,* a subcutaneous parasite of the Raccoon (*Procyon lotor*). All three species are transmitted by mosquitoes. A few other *Dirofilaria* species have very occasionally been reported in humans: *D. ursi,* a parasite of the subcutaneous, perirenal and tracheal tissues of the Brown or Grizzly bear (*Ursus arctos*); *D. striata,* a subcutaneous parasite of the Puma (*Puma concolor*) and other Felidae; *D. magnilarvatum,* a subcutaneous parasite of Asiatic monkeys; *D. spectans,* a parasite of the heart of Mustelidae; *D. subdermata,* a subcutaneous parasite of the porcupine (Hystricidae);

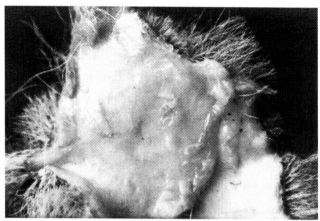

Fig. 1. *Dirofilaria repens* adults in subcutaneous tissue of a dog.

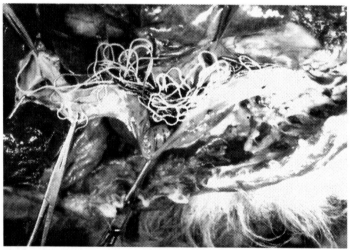

Fig. 2. *Dirofilaria immitis* adults in a dog's heart.

and perhaps also *D. linstowi*, a subcutaneous parasite of monkeys (Cercopithecidae) in Sri Lanka.

Distribution

The geographical distribution of HD coincides with the distribution of the natural reservoir hosts, which constitute the reservoir of infection for humans (i.e. dogs for *D. repens* and *D. immitis*, raccoons for *D. tenuis*) and that of the mosquito vectors.

Dirofilaria repens

This species has been found only in the Old World, being recorded from 36 countries.

The country with the highest prevalence of infection in Europe is Italy; other endemic pockets of infection exist in France, Greece and Ukraine, while sporadic cases are reported from Albania, Bulgaria, Romania, Hungary and ex-Yugoslavia. In Asia, the country most affected is Sri Lanka, followed by Turkey, Russia, Uzbekistan and other states of the ex-Soviet Union. Sporadic cases are reported in China, India, Iran, Israel, Japan, Kuwait, Malaysia and Thailand, while there are rare reports of infection from countries of the African continent, including Tunisia, Senegal, Nigeria and the Republic of South Africa. The total number of cases reported since 1885 (when the first case was published) is just over 780. However, it is likely that many other cases go unreported, either because they are not apparent and cure spontaneously, or because they are not diagnosed or reported by medical practitioners. Most infections of *D. repens* are subcutaneous or subconjunctival (hence the first designation, *Filaria conjunctivae*) but they have also been reported in the lungs, the sexual organs and in a few other visceral locations.

Dirofilaria immitis

In dogs this parasite has a virtually cosmopolitan geographical distribution, but infections in humans have been reported mainly in the USA and Japan, less frequently in Australia and Brazil and rarely in Europe. A total of about 200 cases have been reported and in almost all instances the lungs were affected. It is again possible that many asymptomatic cases go unobserved.

Dirofilaria tenuis

This species is found only in North America, particularly in the southern states of the USA and along the Atlantic seaboard. There do not appear to have been more than 70 cases of human infection (subcutaneous/conjunctival), discounting those that have gone unobserved or undiagnosed, as in the case of *D. repens*.

Of the other species of *Dirofilaria* cited as infecting wild animals, only ten or so human cases are provisionally associated with *D. ursi* in Canada and the northern states of the USA. Infection by the other species is exceptional. It is clear that in many developing countries it is almost impossible to establish whether infections due to *Dirofilaria* are rare, frequent or non-existent, because their diagnosis is largely dependent on the level of services and of public health facilities available and on the pressure of dealing with other, much more significant diseases.

Parasite

The genus *Dirofilaria* is subdivided into two subgenera, *Nochtiella* and *Dirofilaria*, in accordance with certain morphological characteristics, of which the presence or absence of longitudinal ridges running along the surface of the cuticle is a crucial distinguishing feature.

Dirofilaria (Nochtiella) repens

The male worm measures 48–70 mm × 370–450 µm, the female is 100–170 mm × 450–650 µm and microfilariae are 350–380 × 7–8 µm. In the female the vulva is about 1800 µm from the cephalic extremity, while the anus is located about 100 µm from the caudal extremity. Both sexes have inconspicuous cephalic papillae and, all over the cuticle apart from the extremities, there are prominent longitudinal ridges 4–24 µm apart. For the three species of zoonotic interest, the caudal extremity of the male features two small caudal alae, the preanal and postanal papillae and two asymmetric spicules.

Dirofilaria (Dirofilaria) immitis

The males are 120–180 mm × 700–900 µm, the females are 250–300 mm × 1000–1300 µm and microfilariae are 290–330 × 5–7 µm. The vulva of the female is about 2700 µm from the cephalic extremity, while the anus is located about 150 µm from the caudal extremity. The cuticle is smooth in both sexes apart from the cephalic extremity, where there are six papillae and the ventrocaudal region of the male, which has longitudinal ridges.

Dirofilaria (Nochtiella) tenuis

The males are 40–48 mm × 190–260 µm, the females are 80–130 mm × 260–360 µm and microfilariae are 220–250 × 4–5 µm. In the female the vulva is about 1300 µm from the cephalic extremity and the anus is 130 µm from the caudal extremity. The cuticle has longitudinal ridges about 10 µm apart.

Clinical symptoms

The nematodes can lodge in subcutaneous tissues (Fig. 3) in practically any part of the body, but usually in the upper half or under the conjunctival mucosa (Fig. 4) (*D. repens* and *D. tenuis*), more deeply in the lung (*D. immitis* and *D. repens*), in the omentum,

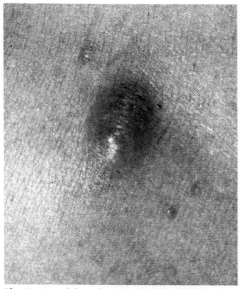

Fig. 3. A nodular subcutaneous lesion due to *Dirofilaria repens* (courtesy of *Pathologica*, 1994, 86, 396–400).

in male sexual organs or in the female breasts (*D. repens*). Wherever a nematode resides in the body, the defensive reactions of the host form a reactive nodule 1–3 cm in diameter (Fig. 3). Depending on the reactions of the host and the localization of the nodule, symptomatology can vary from infections which are completely silent to forms in which localized manifestations of an inflammatory–allergic nature (e.g. transient swellings similar to 'Calabar swellings' of Loiasis (see entry), erythema and pruritus) appear during the development of the nodule. The nodule is usually single and of an elastic or hard consistency. It may be painful spontaneously, or only when pressed. Suppuration may occur. Enlargement of satellite lymph nodes is rare, as are general manifestations. When the nematode is under the conjunctiva it causes localized reddening of the tissues, discomfort, watering, itching, oedema of the eyelids and pain. In 65% of the pulmonary cases the infection

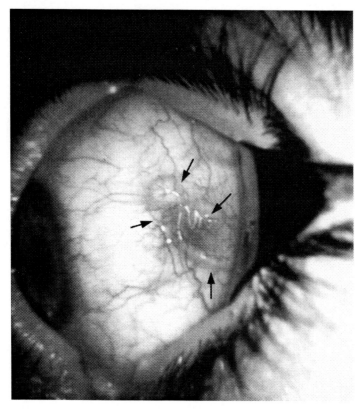

Fig. 4. *Dirofilaria repens* visible under the bulbar conjunctiva (courtesy of *Pathologica*, 1994, 86, 528–532).

is asymptomatic; a coin lesion, betraying the presence of a nodule, is discovered by chance at X-ray examination. Otherwise, the most frequent symptoms are unproductive cough, chest pain, high temperature, dyspnoea, slight haemoptysis and malaise. When the nematode lodges in the epididymis, the spermatic cord or the omentum, it can cause excruciating pain. Haematic eosinophilia is infrequent. The 40–60-year age group is most affected.

Histological examination shows a nodule to have a necrotic central area containing one or more sections of the nematode (Fig. 5) surrounded by granulomatous tissue,

ranging from acute to chronic, depending on the stage of development, rich in histiocytes, plurinucleate giant cells, plasma cells and eosinophils. In cases involving a lung, the nematode is always inside a thrombotic arterial blood-vessel, forming a small roundish infarcted area.

Diagnosis

In almost every case the initial clinical diagnosis is wrong. For example, in the subcutaneous forms the nodule is usually mistaken for a sebaceous cyst, a fibroma or some other benign tumour; when the lungs, sexual organs or breasts are affected,

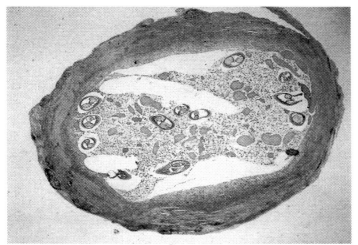

Fig. 5. Histological sections of a coiled *Dirofilaria repens* in a subcutaneous nodule (haemotoxylin and eosin original magnification × 35). Twelve sections of the nematode are visible.

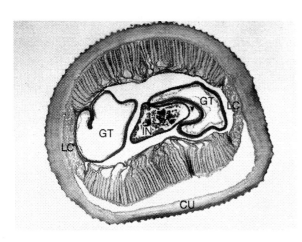

Fig. 6. Transverse section of *Dirofilaria repens* female extracted from a subcutaneous nodule (periodic acid–Schiff, original magnification × 250). Cuticula with external ridges (Cu), genital tubes (GT), intestine (IN), lateral cords (LC) and myoid fibres (MF).

it is misinterpreted as a malignant tumour. Techniques involving serological tests and molecular biology (DNA probes) are still being perfected. At the moment, the only sure way of making a correct diagnosis is by histological examination of the nodule and identification of the nematode's morphological characteristics (Fig. 6).

Transmission

The vectors are various species of mosquitoes mainly in the genera *Aedes, Ochlerotatus,*[1] *Culex, Anopheles* and *Mansonia*. Microfilariae are ingested by a vector during feeding on an infected reservoir host and pass from the insect's stomach to the Malpighian tubules, from where they enter the haemocoel and finally the labium of the proboscis (Fig. 7). When the mosquito feeds on another host, the third-stage larvae emerge from the labium and actively penetrate the skin, taking advantage of the puncture caused by the mosquito bite.

In humans larvae take about 6 months to reach maturity. There appears to be no substantial difference between the biological cycles of the various species of *Dirofilaria*, apart from the fact that *D. repens* and *D. tenuis* are almost always located in the subcutaneous tissue, while *D. immitis* enters the cardiac blood-vessels.

Treatment

The most practical treatment consists of the surgical removal of the nodule containing the nematode. Antifilarial chemotherapy is not recommended.

Control

Control of HD is based on the reduction of infection in reservoir hosts (dogs, in the case of *D. repens* and *D. immitis* and

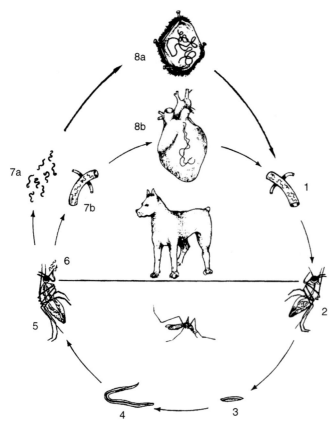

Fig. 7. Biological cycle of (a) *Dirofilaria repens* and (b) *Dirofilaria immitis* (1) Microfilariae in bloodstream (a) through lymphatic circulation and (b) directly from the heart. (2) Ingestion of microfilariae by the vector. (3) and (4) Development of the larvae in the vector. (5) Passage of larvae in the Malpighian tubules, haemocoel and labium of proboscis. (6) Active penetration of the larvae into dog during biting. (7a) Larvae in subcutaneous tissue (*D. repens*) or (7b) in bloodstream (*D. immitis*). (8a) Adults mating in the subcutaneous tissue (*D. repens*) or (8b) in the heart (*D. immitis*).

raccoons, in the case of *D. tenuis*); animals testing positive can be treated with filaricides. Where HD is endemic, it may be possible to treat all the reservoir hosts with filaricidal drugs and/or give them the chemoprophylactic drug ivermectin. Anti-mosquito campaigns, including measures to protect humans from mosquito bites, are important concomitant strategies.

Note

[1] *Ochlerotatus* was formerly a subgenus of *Aedes*.

Selected bibliography

Avdiukhina, T.I., Supryaga, V.G., Postnova, V.F., Kuimova, R.T., Mironova, N.I., Murashov, N.E. and Putinzeva, E.V. (1997) Dirofilariasis in the countries of the Commonwealth of the Independent States: an analysis of the cases over the years 1915–1996. *Meditzinskaiya Parazitologiya i Parazitarnye Bolezni* 1997(4), 3–7. (In Russian, English summary.)

Beaver, P.C. and Orihel, Th.C. (1965) Human infection with filariae of animals in the United States. *American Journal of Tropical Medicine and Hygiene* 14, 1010–1029.

Dissanaike, A.S., Abeyewickreme, W., Wijesundera, M. de S., Weerasooriya, M.V. and Ismail, M.M. (1997) Human dirofilariasis caused by *Dirofilaria (Nochtiella) repens* in Sri Lanka. *Parassitologia* 39, 375–382.

Flieder, D.B. and Moran, C.A. (1999) Pulmonary dirofilariasis: a clinicopathologic study of 41 lesions in 39 patients. *Human Pathology* 30, 251–256.

Makiya, K. (1997) Recent increase of human infections with dog heart worm *Dirofilaria immitis* in Japan. *Parassitologia* 39, 387–388.

Orihel, Th.C. and Eberhard, M.L. (1998) Zoonotic filariasis. *Clinical Microbiology Reviews* 11, 366–381.

Pampiglione, S., Canestri Trotti, G. and Rivasi, F. (1995) Human dirofilariasis due to *Dirofilaria (Nochtiella) repens*: a review of world literature. *Parassitologia* 37, 149–193.

Pampiglione, S., Rivasi, F. and Canestri Trotti, G. (1984) Human pulmonary dirofilariasis in Italy. *The Lancet* 2, 333.

Pampiglione, S. Rivasi, F. and Canestri Trotti, G. (1999) Pitfalls and difficulties in histological diagnosis in human dirofilariasis due to *Dirofilaria (Nochtiella) repens*. *Diagnostic Microbiology and Infectious Disease* 34, 57–64.

Ro, J.Y., Tsakalakis, P.J., White, V.A., Luna, M.A., Chang Tung, E.G., Green, L., Cribbett, L. and Ayala A.G. (1989) Pulmonary dirofilariasis: the great imitator of primary or metastatic lung tumor. *Human Pathology* 20, 69–76.

Dirofilariasis, animal

There are at least 27 species belonging to the genus *Dirofilaria* and they can affect 111 species of mammals. The zoonotic importance of some of them has been reported in the preceding account of human dirofilariasis. Of these, two parasites (*D. immitis* and *D. repens*) are of particular veterinary interest, since they infect dogs.

Canine dirofilariasis
Dirofilaria immitis (dog heartworm)

This is the nematode responsible for heart infections in dogs, cats and many species of wild mammals. Distribution is worldwide. The adults (length, 12–30 cm; diameter, 1–1.3 mm) live in the right ventricle and the pulmonary artery and its ramifications, releasing microfilariae into the bloodstream and exerting a mechanical and phlogistic effect that debilitates the cardiac muscle, the pulmonary circulation and, ultimately, the entire organism. The microfilariae are ingested by mosquitoes belonging to various genera (e.g. *Aedes*, *Ochlerotatus*,[1] *Culex*, *Anopheles*, *Psorophora*), which, during subsequent feeding, transmit them in turn, after an extrinsic incubation period of 13–18 days, to a new host in the form of infective larvae. In dogs, they cause mainly cardiac–respiratory and circulation disorders, ranging from mild to fatal, depending on the number and location of the filarial worms. Cats can also be affected, but more rarely, as can, by chance, humans. The prevalence of infection in dogs can vary from just a few cases to more than 40–50% of the animals examined. The dogs most at risk are those living outdoors at night during the summer when there are large populations of vector mosquitoes.

Dirofilaria repens

This nematode causes the subcutaneous form of canine dirofilariasis, but it can also affect domestic cats and other carnivores, as well as humans. It is found only in the Old World. For the veterinary surgeon it is far less important than *D. immitis*, because it causes only slight cutaneous lesions in its habitual host, or may even go unobserved owing to lack of symptoms. However, it is of greater importance in public health, because it infects humans more frequently than does *D. immitis*.

Diagnosis

Microfilariae can be identified in the blood or following filtration by a modified Knott procedure. Serological tests, such as enzyme-linked immunosorbent assay (ELISA) and immunofluorescent antibody (IFA) and polymerase chain reaction (PCR) techniques can be used to detect infections.

Treatment

Drugs of choice are triacetarsamide or melarsomine (macrofilaricide), administration of which can be followed by ivermectin (microfilaricide).

Control

Reduction in the numbers of both mosquito larvae and adults is of fundamental importance in minimizing transmission. Dogs should be given prophylactic treatment with ivermectin to protect them against infection. It is also vital to inform and educate dog-owners about canine dirofilariasis and how it is spread.

Note
[1]   *Ochlerotatus* was formerly a subgenus of *Aedes*.

Selected bibliography
Boreham, P.F.L. and Atwell, R.B. (1988) *Dirofilariasis*. CRC Press, Boca Raton, Florida, 249 pp.

Genchi, C., Venco, L. and Vezzoni, A. (eds) (1998) *La dirofilariosi cardiopolmonare del cane e del gatto*. Società Culturale Italiana Veterinari per Animali da Compagnia (SCIVAC), Cremona, 198 pp.

Rossi, L., Pollono, F., Meneguz, P.G., Gribaudo, L. and Balbo, T. (1996) An epidemiological study of canine filariose in North West Italy. What has changed in 25 years? *Veterinary Research Communications* 20, 308–315.

Webber, W.A.F. and Hawking, F. (1955) Experimental maintenance of *Dirofilaria immitis* and *Dirofilaria repens* in dogs. *Experimental Parasitology* 4, 143–164.

Dysenteries *see* **Cockroaches** *and* **Flies.**

East Coast fever *see* **Theilerioses**.

Eastern equine encephalitis

Scott C. Weaver

Eastern equine encephalitis is a serious and often fatal disease of humans, equines and other domesticated animals. Although outbreaks are sporadic, both temporally and spatially, and generally involve smaller numbers of cases than do Venezuelan equine encephalitis and western equine encephalitis (see entries), the high mortality rates and serious sequelae make eastern equine encephalitis a feared disease. Control measures are extensive in many coastal North American communities, making this an economically important disease.

Distribution and history
Outbreaks date back at least to 1831, when the first clinical descriptions consistent with eastern equine encephalitis were reported in Massachusetts. The aetiological agent, eastern equine encephalitis (EEE) virus, was first isolated in 1933 from a horse during a major equine epizootic in Maryland, Virginia, Delaware and New Jersey in the USA. Five years later, the first human isolate was made from brain tissue of a fatal case in Massachusetts. North American epidemics and epizootics involving up to tens of thousands of equines and dozens of humans continued sporadically during the 20th century, primarily along the Atlantic coast from Massachusetts to Florida and the Gulf coast to eastern Texas. From 1964 to 1995, the highest mean annual human incidence (≥ 0.011 per 10,000) occurred in Florida, Massachusetts and Georgia. During the past two decades, eastern equine encephalitis incidence and mortality have declined in North America.

The distribution of enzootic EEE virus in North America coincides with that of the principal enzootic mosquito vector, *Culiseta melanura*. Inland foci have also been documented where *C. melanura* occurs, in the Canadian provinces of Quebec and Ontario and in the states of New York, Wisconsin, Michigan, South Dakota, Minnesota, Ohio and Tennessee. Beginning in 1908, equine outbreaks were also documented in Argentina, and the distribution of EEE virus is now known also to extend through much of South and Central America (Fig. 1). Equine epizootics have also been documented on the Caribbean islands of Jamaica and Hispaniola, as well as in north-eastern Mexico. Virus strains isolated during these outbreaks are clearly of the North American variety (see below), suggesting transport beyond the presumed enzootic range by migratory birds.

Virus
Viral replication
Eastern equine encephalitis virus, like other alphaviruses in the family Togaviridae, is an enveloped RNA virus about 70 nm in diameter with a plus or messenger-sense RNA genome of about 11,700 nucleotides (Fig. 2). The genome encodes four non-structural proteins (nsP1–4), while a subgenomic 26S messenger RNA (mRNA), identical to the 3' one-third of the genome, encodes the structural proteins (capsid, E1 and E2 glycoproteins).

Alphaviruses are believed to enter the cytoplasm of vertebrate cells via receptor-mediated endocytosis, although specific EEE virus receptors have not been investigated. Genomic RNA is translated by cellular components to produce a non-structural polyprotein, and is the template for minus-strand RNA synthesis involving non-structural proteins. The 26S mRNA is also translated as a polyprotein; the capsid protein is cleaved in the cytoplasm and

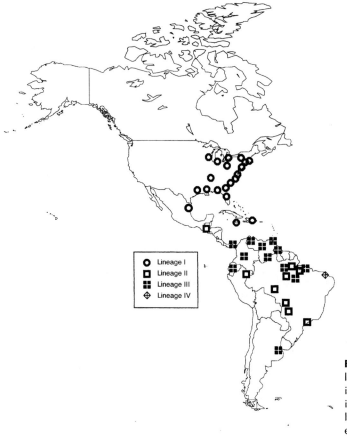

Fig. 1. Map showing the location of EEE virus isolation in the Americas. Symbols indicate distinct genetic lineages of virus circulating in each region (see Fig. 3).

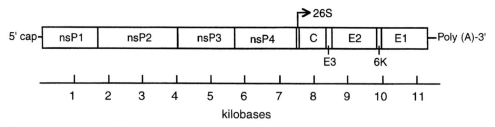

Fig. 2. Genome map of EEE virus showing the genes encoding the four non-structural proteins (nsP1–4), the capsid (C) and the E2 and E1 envelope glycoproteins.

the remaining polyprotein is processed and cleaved in the secretory pathway to yield the E1 and E2 glycoproteins, which are inserted into the plasma membrane as a heterodimer. Following encapsidation of genomic RNA in the cytoplasm, enveloped virions mature when nucleocapsids bud through the plasma membrane.

Antigenic relationships

Eastern equine encephalitis is the only virus (species) in the EEE antigenic complex of alphaviruses. North and South American antigenic varieties were first distinguished using kinetic haemagglutination inhibition (HI) studies, and later using monoclonal antibodies (Mabs). One of these

Mabs specifically recognizes an E1 glycoprotein epitope of North American isolates, regardless of year or location of isolation, demonstrating antigenic conservation within North America. In contrast, South American EEE viruses exhibit greater antigenic diversity, as demonstrated by the inability to produce a South American variety-specific Mab. Humans receiving the formalin-inactivated EEE vaccine, developed from a North American strain, develop neutralizing antibodies against North but not South American strains, further supporting their antigenic distinction.

Genetic relationships

Ribonucleic acid (RNA) fingerprinting provided the first genetic corroboration of antigenic conservation of EEE virus within North America. More recent studies using restriction fragment length polymorphism ((RFLP) of polymerase chain reaction (PCR) products from the North and South American varieties yielded different patterns,

with more variability within the South American viruses. This technique could be useful as a rapid molecular method for distinguishing the two EEE virus varieties.

Molecular phylogenetic evidence, based on sequences from several regions of the EEE genome, has demonstrated that the North and South American varieties comprise distinct lineages (Fig. 3). North American isolates are highly conserved over a 63-year time-period and over a geographical range exceeding 2000 km, comprising a single, highly conserved lineage. The South American variety exhibits greater genetic diversity, with three major lineages identified, and appears to evolve more rapidly. Based on recent evaluations of antigenic and genetic relationships, four subtypes of EEE virus have been proposed (Fig. 1).

The differences in genetic diversity between North and South American EEE viruses may reflect differences in their enzootic ecology. In North America, where passerine birds serve as reservoir hosts,

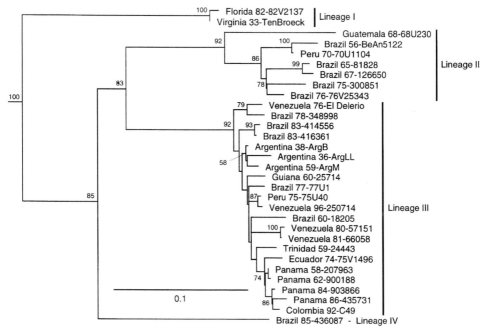

Fig. 3. Phylogenetic tree of EEE virus isolates generated from partial nsP4, E2 and 3′ untranslated sequences. The tree topology was generated using the maximum parsimony method, and the branch lengths were drawn using the neighbour-joining method, with the Kimura two-parameter distance formula to correct genetic distance for superimposed nucleotide substitutions. Bootstrap values indicate support levels for groups to the right. The scale shows a genetic distance of 0.1.

avian mobility may maintain genetic homogeneity when virus populations are occasionally mixed following dispersal of viraemic hosts. Overall, genetic relationships among North American EEE viruses are correlated with the year or decade of isolation rather than geographical location. However, detailed studies indicate geographically restricted evolution for time-periods of a few years. In contrast, South American isolates group by geographical region rather than year of isolation, indicating that multiple virus lineages circulate for periods of decades or more. Some South American strains may be transmitted among small rodents with limited dispersal, resulting in discrete genotypic foci that evolve under the influence of genetic drift or different selection due to different hosts or vectors.

Clinical symptoms

Eastern equine encephalitis causes high rates of mortality in humans, equines, turkeys, chickens, Emus (*Dromaius novaehollandiae*), Whooping cranes (*Grus americana*) and pigs. In North America, most human infection is subclinical or inapparent. The incubation period prior to apparent disease is probably 3–10 days, and a prodromal illness lasting from several days to over a week may precede acute symptoms. Early symptoms typically include fever, headache, myalgias, photophobia and dysthesias. Fifty to 90% of apparent cases proceed to encephalitis, characterized by irritability, restlessness, headache, drowsiness, anorexia, diarrhoea, convulsions and coma. Laboratory findings often include elevated leucocyte counts of 15,000–35,000 mm^{-3}, with a neutrophilic predominance and left shift. The cerebrospinal fluid (CSF) also shows an elevated white blood cell count, with a polymorphonuclear cell predominance in most cases.

The fatality rate from eastern equine encephalitis is higher in patients over 10 years of age, but surviving children generally suffer more severe sequelae. Death due to encephalitis usually occurs 2–10 days after the onset of signs and symptoms, and

survivors generally suffer progressive, disabling mental and physical sequelae. In 36 human cases reported in the USA between 1988 and 1994, the mortality rate was 36% and 35% of survivors were moderately or severely disabled. The prognosis for a good recovery is correlated with age (i.e. those over 40 years have a higher rate of complete recovery than younger people), a long prodromal course (5–7 days) and the absence of coma. The average total medical cost per transiently affected human case is US$21,000. Patients who suffer permanent neurological sequelae usually live a normal lifespan, but without gainful employment. Insecticidal interventions designed to avert eastern equine encephalitis epidemics cost between US$0.7 million and US$1.4 million, depending on the extent of the treated region, far less than the US$3 million cost of one person suffering residual sequelae.

In equines infected in North America, rates of encephalitis are also high, with up to 80–90% of infected horses developing acute and lethal disease. As with human cases, many equine survivors develop severe neurological sequelae. Typical equine signs and symptoms include fever, depression, incoordination, circling, anorexia, stupor, convulsions, prostration, ataxia and paralysis. Domestic birds suffer either from central nervous system or viscerotropic disease. Some wild birds, especially immature passerines, including both native and introduced species, also suffer natural mortality.

In South and Central America, equine outbreaks are common in some regions but there is little evidence of human disease. A single human case attributed to EEE virus based on serological grounds was reported in a Brazilian child. Eastern equine encephalitis virus-specific human antibodies have been reported in many regions of Latin America. However, no evidence of human disease has been found in Argentina, despite intensive epidemiological studies following extensive equine epizootics. It is likely that the South American variety of EEE virus is less infectious and/or less virulent for humans than is the North American variety. However, more detailed studies of human exposure and response to EEE virus infection are needed in regions of Latin America where continuous enzootic transmission is detected.

Diagnosis

Diagnosis of eastern equine encephalitis relies on virus isolation, detection of viral antigens or specific immunoglobulin M (IgM) antibodies or demonstration of sero-conversion. Immunoglobulin M capture enzyme-linked immunosorbent assay (ELISA) is highly sensitive in detecting antibodies, which generally appear in serum or CSF within 7 days of infection. Serum IgM can persist for several months, while its presence in CSF indicates recent infection. A fourfold or greater increase in antibodies detected using HI, ELISA, complement fixation (CF), plaque reduction neutralization (PRN) or indirect immunofluorescence (IF) is also considered diagnostic. High antibody titres in single serum specimens (e.g. HI ≥ 160; CF ≥ 40; IF ≥ 60; PRN ≥ 80) are suggestive but not diagnostic of recent infection. However, the sequential application of these tests can be used to arrive at a specific diagnosis, because IF, ELISA and HI antibodies are broadly reactive among alphaviruses, while CF and PRN antibodies are highly specific.

Isolation of EEE virus from human serum is unusual by the time neurological disease occurs, but virus can often be isolated from the brain in fatal cases. Virus isolation from vertebrate or mosquito samples is accomplished using intracerebral inoculation of newborn mice, or cell cultures such green monkey kidney (VERO) or baby hamster kidney (BHK-21) cells, which show cytopathic effects (CPE) 1–2 days after infection, followed by antigenic identification. Mosquito cells, such as C6/36, are also susceptible to infection but do not generally show CPE. Enzyme-linked immunosorbent assay, nucleic acid hybridization and PCR-based methods have been shown to be more rapid and nearly as sensitive as virus isolation. Immunohistochemical detection of EEE antigen in brain tissues has also been used for diagnosis. Radiological imaging of the brain, using computed tomographic scans and magnetic resonance imaging, sometimes, but not always, shows abnormal findings.

Transmission

In temperate climates, enzootic EEE virus transmission is seasonal, peaking in the late summer or early autumn. In tropical and subtropical regions, including South and Central America and the southern USA, nearly continuous transmission occurs. In North America, *Culiseta melanura*, a highly ornithophagic mosquito that rarely feeds on mammals, is the principal enzootic vector (Fig. 4). This mosquito is susceptible to infection with relatively small oral doses of virus, and biological transmission can occur as little as 48–72 h after an infectious blood meal. Pathological lesions in the mosquito mid-gut, caused by EEE virus, may facilitate rapid dissemination into the haemocoel and to the salivary glands. Horizontal transmission among passerine birds occurs primarily in forested coastal and inland hardwood swamps. Red maple (*Acer rebrum*), Hornbeam (*Carpinus caroliniana*). Cedar (*Thuja occidentalis*) and Loblolly bay (*Gordonia lasianthus*) trees provide root systems favourable for the larval development of *C. melanura*. The geographical distribution of EEE virus coincides with that of another alphavirus, Highlands J, which is also transmitted by this mosquito.

Culiseta melanura larvae develop in swamp 'crypts' (i.e. water-filled cavities under roots of trees) and emergence is bivoltine in the north-eastern USA; an overwintering generation of larvae emerges as a spring brood and a later generation emerges in the autumn. Higher water temperatures may hasten development of the later generation and increase the probability for EEE virus amplification in juvenile birds. Water temperatures in the 'crypts' may regulate the northern limit for virus amplification each year. Fledgling and nestling birds are considered the most important amplification hosts because they develop higher-titre and longer-lasting viraemia than adults, and are less defensive toward biting mosquitoes. Although the passerine fauna has not been extensively evaluated for reservoir

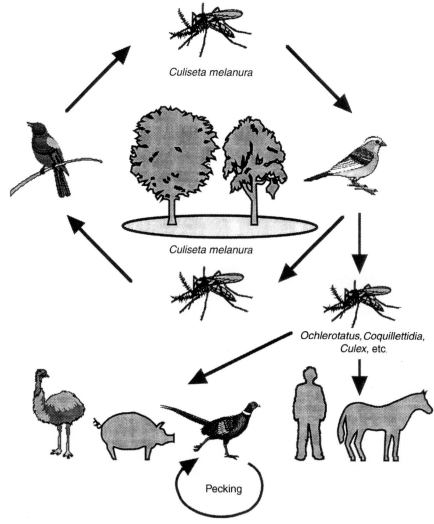

Fig. 4. Cartoon representing the enzootic and epizootic/epidemic EEE virus transmission cycles.

competence, European starlings (*Sturnus vulgaris*) exhibit more intense and longer-lasting viraemia than American robins (*Turdus migratorius*) and other birds, and can infect about three times as many mosquitoes. Infection of a wide variety of secondary hosts, including mammals, amphibians and reptiles, is also indicated by the presence of antibodies in natural populations.

Epidemics are usually preceded by detection of EEE virus in mosquitoes or birds and often by equine cases. Because equines and humans generally do not develop high-titre viraemia, they are considered dead-end hosts. Equine and human infections seldom occur more than a few kilometres from an enzootic swamp habitat, also suggesting that humans and equines do not serve as amplification hosts. Therefore, eastern equine encephalitis epidemics/epizootics do not spread geographically like Venezuelan equine encephalitis (see entry), which exploits equines as efficient amplification hosts. An association between the occurrence of human cases and excess rainfall indicates that mosquito population sizes probably regulate epidemic transmission to some extent. Passerine birds develop very high-titre viraemia of up to 10^{12} infectious units per ml of blood, so many different mosquito species are probably capable of transmitting following an infectious blood meal. Wading shore birds, including fledgling Glossy ibises (*Plegadis falcinellus*) and Snowy egrets (*Egretta thula*), also develop moderate-titre viraemia and some infections are fatal.

The mosquito vectors responsible for human and equine infection have not been identified conclusively. *Culiseta melanura* resides in hardwood swamp habitats where enzootic transmission occurs, but also disperses upland to areas where human and equine cases often occur. However, because *C. melanura* rarely feeds on hosts other than birds, other mosquito species are believed to transmit to mammals. During a recent Connecticut epizootic, *C. melanura*, *Culex pipiens*, *Culiseta morsitans*, *Ochlerotatus*[1] *sollicitans*, *Ochlerotatus cantator*, *Ochlerotatus trivittatus*, *Aedes vexans* and *Coquillettidia perturbans* were found to be infected. Other studies implicated *C. perturbans*, *Ochlerotatus canadensis*, *O. sollicitans*, *Culex salinarius* and *Anopheles quadrimaculatus* as potential epizootic/epidemic vectors, based on their catholic feeding behaviours, abundance during epizootics and laboratory transmission experiments. *Aedes albopictus* is also highly susceptible to experimental infections and has been found naturally infected in Florida. However, it has not been incriminated in natural transmission. Direct transmission via pecking among penned game-birds has been documented, and chicken mites (*Dermanyssus gallinae*) can transmit EEE virus between birds following ingestion of moderate-titre bloods meals.

Epidemiological and phylogenetic data support the hypothesis that EEE virus overwinters in temperate latitudes. However, the mechanism(s) of overwintering remains enigmatic. Although there are reports of EEE virus isolation from overwintering *C. melanura* larvae and adult males, and from *C. perturbans* eggs, most field, and all experimental, studies have failed to demonstrate transovarial transmission. Because *C. melanura* overwinters as diapausing larvae, transovarial transmission would be required for virus overwintering in this species. Migration of viraemic birds has been suggested as a possible means for EEE virus reintroduction each spring. However, phylogenetic studies indicate that genetically distinct EEE virus populations remain in the same enzootic foci from year to year, suggesting that the virus is not reintroduced into temperate regions from a common, subtropical source.

The first annual isolations of EEE virus in New Jersey are generally made from juvenile birds, prior to virus isolation from mosquito pools, indicating that persistently infected resident birds may be responsible for annual reinitiation of transmission. Experimental infections of avian hosts are needed to test this hypothesis. Meteorological data have also shown a correlation between wind patterns and the appearance of eastern equine encephalitis, suggesting the possibility that infected mosquitoes may transport the virus via low-level (surface) winds. For example, climatic data indicate that the virus may have been introduced into Quebec province, Canada, by infected mosquitoes carried on low-level winds from Connecticut in 1972. The 400-km distance could have been covered in 14–16 h at a speed of 25–30 km h^{-1} and at a temperature of 15°C or higher. However, regular, widespread transport of EEE virus via low-level winds is inconsistent with genetic studies indicating that the virus undergoes regionally independent evolution for time periods up to several years.

The transmission cycles of EEE virus have not been well characterized in most parts of Latin America, primarily because human disease has rarely been documented and enzootic sylvatic foci are often in remote locations. A preponderance of isolations in South and Central America from *Culex* mosquitoes of the subgenus *Melanoconion* have implicated them as probable enzootic vectors, with *C.* (*Melanoconion*) *taeniopus* incriminated in several locations. Antibody prevalence indicates that both small mammals and birds probably serve as reservoir hosts. Viruses isolated during Caribbean and Mexican outbreaks have been of the North American variety and were probably introduced via viraemic migratory birds. Although EEE virus has been isolated from migratory birds in the southern USA and Cuba, the genetically and antigenically distinct nature of all North vs. Central/South American viruses indicates that introductions do not often result in stable enzootic transmission.

Treatment

No antiviral treatment is available for eastern equine encephalitis. Elevated intracranial pressure, which probably contributes to morbidity and mortality, can be treated, as can convulsions. Airway protection may be needed in patients exhibiting loss of consciousness, along with hyperventilation accompanied by anaesthesia and sedation, Cerebral blood flow should be maintained via regulation of arterial partial pressure of carbon dioxide ($PaCO_2$). Brain swelling can be minimized by regulating serum sodium and osmolarity. Nosocomial infections, especially pneumonia, should be prevented and treated aggressively when they occur.

Control and prevention

Vectors

Because EEE virus is maintained in zoonotic transmission cycles in swamp habitats, little can be done in an ecologically acceptable manner to control levels of virus circulation. Control of EEE virus generally relies on early detection of enzootic amplification in birds, followed by mosquito control to reduce vector populations in inhabited regions. Sentinel Ring-necked pheasants (*Phasianus colchicus*) or chickens used for detection of seroconversion, as well as adult female mosquito collections for virus isolation, can detect high levels of virus circulation. The abundance of *C. melanura* is also an indicator of potential epizootic amplification, and high rates of infection indicate hyperenzootic transmission levels. Because equine cases

usually precede human infection by a few weeks, they are also indicators of the need for large-scale adulticide programmes.

As with many arthropod-borne diseases, personal protection against mosquito bites is often the most effective means of prevention of EEE virus infections. This is especially important for individuals who reside, work or take recreation near swamp habitats known or suspected of harbouring enzootic transmission. Diethyltoluamide (DEET) (≤35% formulations recommended; ≤10% for children) is the most effective mosquito repellent generally approved for use on the skin, and permethrin insecticide can be applied to clothing and camping gear to enhance protection. Education of persons likely to contact enzootic habitats is also an important ingredient in preventing human infection.

Mosquito control to reduce vector populations generally relies on large-scale application of adulticides in regions of enzootic transmission. Larvicides directed at breeding sites can also be useful in controlling some potential epizootic vector, such as *Culex salinarius*, *Ochlerotatus sollicitans* and *Anopheles quadrimaculatus*. The inaccessibility of enzootic swamp habitats often necessitates aerial insecticide applications. Recently, remote sensing using satellite imagery has proved valuable for identifying EEE virus foci. This approach can be used to target surveillance, as well as prevention and control measures.

Vaccines

A formalin-inactivated EEE virus vaccine is used to protect laboratory workers at high risk for infection, as well as to immunize equines, pigs and domestic birds, such as emus and pheasants. However, antibodies generated in response to the vaccine, which was derived from a North American EEE virus strain, are short-lived and do not appear to cross-react strongly with South American strains.

Note

[1]   *Ochlerotatus* was formerly a subgenus of *Aedes*.

Selected bibliography

Brault, A.C., Powers, A.M., Chavez, C.L., Lopez, R.N., Cachon, M.F., Gutierrez, L. F., Kang, W., Tesh, R.B., Shope, R.E. and Weaver, S.C. (1999) Genetic and antigenic diversity among eastern equine encephalitis viruses from North, Central and South America. *American Journal of Tropical Medicine and Hygiene* 61, 579–586.

Crans, W.J., Caccamise, D.F. and McNelly, J.R. (1994) Eastern equine encephalomyelitis virus in relation to the avian community of a coastal cedar swamp. *Journal of Medical Entomology* 31, 711–728.

Letson, G.W., Bailey, R.E., Pearson, J. and Tsai, T.F. (1993) Eastern equine encephalitis (EEE): a description of the 1989 outbreak, recent epidemiologic trends, and the association of rainfall with EEE occurrence. *American Journal of Tropical Medicine and Hygiene* 49, 677–685.

Morris, C.D. (1988) Eastern equine encephalomyelitis. In: Monath, T.P. (ed.) *The Arboviruses: Epidemiology and Ecology*, Vol. III. CRC Press, Boca Raton, Florida, pp. 1–36.

Sabattini, M.S., Daffner, J.F., Monath, T.P., Bianchi, T.I., Cropp, C.B., Mitchell, C.J. and

Aviles, G. (1991) Localized eastern equine encephalitis in Santiago del Estero Province, Argentina, without human infection. *Medicina* 51, 3–8.

Scott, T.W. and Weaver, S.C. (1989) Eastern equine encephalomyelitis virus: epidemiology and evolution of mosquito transmission. *Advances in Virus Research* 37, 277–328.

Sprance, H.E. (1981) Experimental evidence against the transovarial transmission of eastern equine encephalitis virus in *Culiseta melanura*. *Mosquito News* 41, 168–173.

Tsai, T.F. and Monath, T.P. (1997) Alphaviruses. In: Richman, D.D., Whitley, R.J. and Hayden, F.G. (eds) *Clinical Virology*. Churchill Livingstone, New York, pp. 1217–1255.

Vaidyanathan, R., Edman, J.D., Cooper, L.A. and Scott, T.W. (1997) Vector competence of mosquitoes (Diptera: Culicidae) from Massachusetts for a sympatric isolate of eastern equine encephalomyelitis virus. *Journal of Medical Entomology* 34, 346–352.

Weaver, S.C., Powers, A.M, Brault, A.C. and Barrett, A.D. (1999) Molecular epidemiological studies of veterinary arboviral encephalitides. *Veterinary Journal* 157, 123–138.

Ehrlichiosis

S.A. Ewing

Ehrlichia species are obligate, intracelluar parasites that infect granulocytes, agranulocytes or platelets of human beings, domesticated animals and certain wild animals. This genus is currently assigned to the order Rickettsiales, tribe Ehrlichieae, and comprises numerous species, many of which are tick-borne pathogens, whereas others are helminth-borne parasites. Information currently being assembled through use of modern techniques that enable study of molecular genetics is likely to result in reclassification of these bacteria, and it seems probable that tick-borne species will be found to be more closely related to one another than to the helminth-borne agents. Inasmuch as this encyclopedia deals with arthropod-borne agents, nothing more will be said about the organisms currently considered to be helminth-borne ehrlichieae.

Distribution

Ehrlichiosis was recognized to be a problem in the Old World long before its presence in the New World was discovered. Dogs in Africa were to be found infected in the 1930s, and tick-borne fever (TBF) was recognized in ruminants in Europe and the UK around 1950. The causative agent of TBF, now known as *Ehrlichia phagocytophila*, was found to be transmitted by the tick, *Ixodes ricinus*. Unlike *Ehrlichia canis* and *Ehrlichia chaffeensis*, but similar to *Ehrlichia ewingii*, *E. phagocytophila* parasitizes granulocytes.

Following the discovery of *E. chaffeensis* as a zoonotic agent, another human pathogen was recognized in North America. At the time of writing (2000) the agent has not been assigned a specific epithet and is commonly referred to as human granulocytic ehrlichia (HGE). (Unfortunately, the disease is also called HGE (human granulocytic ehrlichiosis).) Based upon molecular genetic evidence the agent is very closely related to *E. phagocytophila*, causative agent of TBF in Europe and the UK, and to *Ehrlichia equi*, a parasite of horses found mainly in western North America. *Ixodes scapularis*, a New World relative of *I. ricinus*, has been found to transmit HGE; another member of this complex of ixodids, *Ixodes pacificus*, transmits this equine parasite in western North America, especially California. These findings, along with other evidence, have led some to postulate that an array of ehrlichial species is distributed among mammals and ticks in the Nearctic region where species have circulated continuously in endemic cycles since the end of the last ice age, only to be discovered comparatively recently. New species are being found constantly; for example, an agent genetically similar to *E. chaffeensis* was recently (2000) reported from *Ixodes ovatus* in Japan.

Ehrlichiosis has an almost worldwide distribution.

Parasite

Ehrlichia canis, the type species of the genus, was discovered in Algeria in the 1930s and was itself originally assigned to the genus *Rickettsia*. In 1945 the genus *Ehrlichia* was created to accommodate those intracellular bacteria that form clusters (known as morulae) in leucocytic host cells and are transmitted by ixodid (hard) ticks. *Ehrlichia canis* is widely distributed in domestic dogs in the Old World and New World, and is transmitted by *Rhipicephalus sanguineus*, the brown dog tick. Over time, additional ehrlichial species have been discovered in a variety of mammals and various ticks found to be vectors. New species are being recognized in mammalian hosts at a more rapid pace than in the past and it has proved impossible, in some instances, to identify the vectors responsible for transmission. Information is being assembled in both the Old World and the New World that will better delineate the taxonomic status of ehrlichial species and clarify which ixodids transmit them. Rickettsial agents attach to

host cells and are believed to gain entry by inducing phagocytosis. The molecular mechanism for achieving invasion remains unknown. These organisms must have a remarkable ability to adapt to new conditions, because they are constantly shifting between invertebrate and vertebrate hosts. There appear to be complex reproductive cycles in both types of hosts, with parasite amplification resulting in remarkable levels of organisms in the blood of vertebrates and in various tissues and the saliva of ticks.

Clinical symptoms

Ehrlichial infections cause multisystemic disorders. Patients typically present with fever, depression and anorexia and sometimes with haemorrhagic tendencies. Some species cause neurological disease; meningitis is a common feature of *E. canis* infections, as is ocular disease, especially uveitis and retinal dysfunction.

Diseases that result from ehrlichial infections vary from mild or inapparent to fatal. The factors that determine severity of disease are not well known beyond the obvious susceptibility of immunocompromised hosts, a situation recognized in domestic animals as well as in human beings. The agranulocytic parasites are generally more pathogenic than the granulocytic ones. A somewhat aberrant species, *Ehrlichia platys*, parasitizes dog platelets and is thought to be transmitted by *R. sanguineus*. It causes cyclic thrombocytopenia, which is generally relatively harmless. If, however, a dog should suffer traumatic injury or be subjected to surgery during a thrombocytopenic episode, the consequences might be fatal.

Some evidence exists for an immunopathological basis for disease in ehrlichial infections. For example, interferon (IFN) gamma is thought to mediate tissue injury, at least in so-called human granulocytic ehrlichiosis (HGE); moreover, it is posited that interleukin 10 suppresses IFN-gamma-mediated damage in HGE.

In 1987 an arthropod-borne ehrlichiosis was discovered to be a zoonotic disease and *E. chaffeensis*, a parasite principally of agranulocytes, was eventually found to be the causative agent in North America.

Central nervous system disorder is commonly seen in people with *E. chaffeensis* infections, although asymptomatic infections apparently occur. Shortly after its discovery, this agent was determined to be a parasite of White-tailed deer (*Odocoileus virginianus*) and to be transmitted by the lone star tick, *Amblyomma americanum*. More recently *E. ewingii*, long recognized as parasitizing dog granulocytes, was also found to infect people; the lone star tick also transmits this species.

Diagnosis

Diagnosis of ehrlichial infections is often problematic. Finding morulae in leucocytes by light microscopy is difficult even during acute infection. A variety of serological tests have been used successfully; one difficulty with these is that patients who recover spontaneously or are cured by antibiotic therapy remain seropositive for extended periods. Moreover, cross-reactivity among ehrlichial species is common and diagnostic reagents are unavailable for those species (such as *E. ewingii*) that have not been cultivated *in vitro*. Polymerase chain reaction (PCR) techniques have been developed in recent years and are proving to be valuable diagnostic aids; these techniques are both more specific and more sensitive than earlier diagnostic methods.

Transmission and epidemiology

The developmental cycle of *Ehrlichia* species within ticks is not well documented. So far as is known, only trans-stadial transfer occurs. Attempts to demonstrate transovarial transmission have been made, in part, because *E. canis* has commonly been found in combined infections with *Babesia canis*, a protozoan parasite, which is also transmitted by the same vector, *R. sanguineus* (see Babesiosis). Ticks have been found to harbour more than one ehrlichial agent concurrently, as well as simultaneously supporting ehrlichial agents and *Borrelia burgdorferi* (see Lyme borreliosis) and/or *Babesia microti*.

Experimental evidence with HGE in larval/nymphal ticks indicates that organisms find their way to the salivary glands in the fourth week after exposure, about the time digestion of the blood meal is completed. At first, organisms are arranged around the host cell nucleus. At 6 weeks, infected salivary acinar cells become hypertrophied and large numbers of organisms are found; these findings suggest that few ehrlichial organisms reach the salivary glands until moulting of the tick vector is completed.

Considerable work must be done to determine the phylogenetic affiliation of known members of the genus *Ehrlichia*. More importantly, perhaps, epidemiological studies are needed to determine the extent to which ehrlichial agents are exchanged among vertebrate hosts as a result of the feeding habits of ixodid ticks. If the biology of the numerous three-host ticks that are available candidates to serve as vectors in various parts of the world is explored thoroughly, the potential for zoonotic disease and the possibility for exchange of these obligate intracellular parasites can be better predicted. Transmission is trans-stadial and apparently ticks must remain attached for several hours for transfer of the parasite to occur. Experimental transmission is easily effected by blood transfusion, and care must be exercised in selecting blood donors in veterinary hospitals because asymptomatic convalescent carriers are common.

Treatment

Like other rickettsial agents, the tick-borne ehrlichieae are sensitive to antibiotics of the tetracycline group. This fortunate circumstance means that, with timely diagnosis, treatment of the parasitized host is easily accomplished. Absence of pathognomonic signs or lesions renders diagnosis difficult and delayed treatment results, sometimes with fatal consequences. Doxycycline is reported to control acute *E. canis* infections effectively, but efficacy of tetracycline derivatives in clearing chronic ehrlichial infections remains controversial.

Control

Control of ehrlichial infections is largely a matter of tick control. This can involve removal of ticks from pets, such as dogs, and/or systematic use of pesticides to keep animal quarters free of acarines. Although the epidemiological features of classic canine ehrlichiosis, caused by _E. canis_, are fairly well studied, the same cannot be said for most other ehrlichial diseases. In North America _Rhipicephalus sanguineus_ lives in homes, kennels and other protected places and it feeds almost exclusively on dogs. As a consequence, classic canine ehrlichiosis is not seasonal. In contrast, those ehrlichial species that are transmitted by ticks such as _Amblyomma americanum_ (_E. chaffeensis_ and _E. ewingii_) and _Ixodes pacificus_ (_E. equi_) are far more likely to be seasonal, appearing from spring to autumn. Cognizance of the risk of tick exposure and appropriate efforts to minimize risks will automatically reduce the likelihood of ehrlichial infections in both domestic animals and human beings.

Selected bibliography

Anderson, B.E., Greene, C.E., Jones, D.C. and Dawson, J.E. (1992) _Ehrlichia ewingii sp. nov._, the etiologic agent of canine granulocytic ehrlichiosis. _International Journal of Systematic Bacteriology_ 42, 299–302.

Breitschwerdt, E.B., Hegarty, B.C. and Hancock, S.I. (1998) Sequential evaluation of dogs naturally infected with _Ehrlichia canis, Ehrlichia chaffeensis, Ehrlichia equi, Ehrlichia ewingii_ and _Bartonella vinsonii._ _Journal of Clinical Immunology_ 36, 2645–2651.

Chang, Y.-F., McDonough, S.P., Chang, C.-F., Shin, K.-S., Yen, W. and Divers, T. (2000) Human granulocytic ehrlichiosis agent infection in a pony vaccinated with a _Borrelia burgdorferi_ recombinant ospA vaccine and challenged by exposure to naturally infected ticks. _Clinical and Diagnostic Laboratory Immunology_ 7, 68–71.

Dawson, J.E. and Ewing, S.A. (1992) Susceptibility of dogs to infection with _Ehrlichia chaffeensis,_ causative agent of human ehrlichiosis. _American Journal of Veterinary Research_ 53, 1322–1327.

Dawson, J.E., Anderson, B.E., Fishbein, D.B., Sanchez, J.L., Goldsmith, C.S., Wilson, K.H. and Duntley, C.W. (1991) Isolation and characterization of an _Ehrlichia_ sp. from a patient diagnosed with human ehrlichiosis. _Journal of Clinical Miciobiology_ 29, 2741–2745.

Ewing, S.A. (1969) Canine ehrlichiosis. _Advances in Veterinary Science and Comparative Medicine_ 13, 331–353.

McBride, J.W., Corstvet, R.E., Gaunt, S.D., Chinsangaram, J., Akita, G.Y. and Osburn, B.I. (1996) Polymerase chain reaction detection of acute _Ehrlichia canis_ infection in dogs. _Journal of Veterinary Diagnostic Investigation_ 8, 441–447.

Maeda, K., Markowitz, N., Hawley, R.C., Ristic, M., Cox, D. and McDade, J.E. (1987) Human infection with _Ehrlichia canis_, a leukocytic rickettsia. _New England Journal of Medicine_ 316, 853–856.

Neer, T.M. (1999) Ehrlichiosis. In: Greene, C.E. (ed.) _Infectious Diseases of the Dog and Cat_, 2nd edn. W.B. Saunders, Philadelphia, Pensylvannia, pp. 139–147.

Rikihisa, Y. (1991) The tribe Ehrlichieae and ehrlichial diseases. _Clinical Microbiology Reviews_ 4, 286–308.

Walker, D.H. and Dumler, J.S. (1996) Emergence of the ehrlichioses as human health problems. _Emerging Infectious Diseases_ 2, 18–29.

Elaeophora species _see_ Elaeophorosis.

Elaeophorosis

Danny B. Pence

This is an infection of the blood-vessels of domesticated and wild herbivores with filarial nematodes of the genus _Elaeophora_. Infections range in clinical severity from non-pathogenic to life-threatening.

Distribution

Elaeophora schneideri occurs in the lumen of the carotid, iliac and mesenteric arteries of sheep, goats and several species of wild ruminants in the southern and western

USA. It is a normal parasite of Mule deer (*Odocoileus hemionus hemionus*) and Black-tailed deer (*Odocoileus hemionus columbianus*) in the western USA and, to a much lesser extent, White-tailed deer (*Odocoileus virginianus*) in the southern and western USA. In domestic sheep and goats, other native cervids, including Elk (*Cervus elaphus*) and Moose (*Alces alces*), native Bighorn sheep (*Ovis canadensis*) and certain introduced exotics, such as Sika deer (*Cervus nippon*), Barbary sheep (*Ammotragus lervia*) and Ibex (*Copra ibex*), *E. schneideri* is pathogenic. Prevalence of elaeophorosis in domestic sheep in New Mexico, Arizona and Colorado was about 1% in the early 1970s, but this seems to have declined dramatically in recent years. Likewise, prevalence seems to have declined in Elk in Arizona and New Mexico. *Elaeophora bohmi* occurs in the tunica media of metacarpal, metatarsal and distal extremity veins and arteries in equines in Europe (Austria), and *Elaeophora poeli* is found in the aortic intima of cattle and buffalo in Africa and Asia. *Elaeophora elaphi* infects the portal veins of Red deer (*C. elaphus*) in Europe (Spain).

Parasite
Females of *E. schneideri* are slender, loosely coiled nematodes that reach 120 mm in length; males are smaller, reaching 85 mm.

Females are ovoviviparous, producing numerous sheathless microfilariae (280 μm long) that migrate to the capillaries of the skin of the face of sheep, goats, deer, Elk and Moose; they may also localize in the capillaries of the skin on the lower extremities and in the mucous membranes of the head of sheep and goats. Adults of *E. poeli* are long and threadlike; females reach 300 mm long. *Elaeophora bohmi* and *E. elaphi* are similarly long and entwined within the vascular tissues.

Clinical symptoms
Elaeophorosis in North America is a variable disease, depending on the host involved. In the normal definitive Mule deer and Black-tailed deer hosts, there are no clinical signs of disease. Likewise, lesions are minimal in White-tailed deer. In domestic sheep and goats, Bighorn sheep, Barbary sheep, Sika deer and Ibex, a filarial dermatitis, known as 'sore head', results from an allergic response to microfilariae in the skin. An exudative dermatitis is characterized by haemorrhage, vesiculation and ulceration of the skin, with serum, erythrocyte and leucocyte extravasation on the poll and face (Figs 1 and 2), sometimes with lesions also on the abdomen and lower parts of the legs. The intensely pruritic lesions often result in severe self-induced trauma from rubbing and scratching.

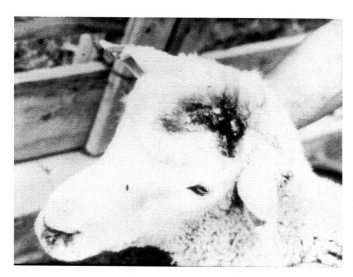

Fig. 1. Bloody lesions from rubbing on the poll of a domestic sheep with sore head caused by elaeophorosis (courtesy of C.P. Hibber, Wildlife Disease Association Study Set on Elaeophorosis).

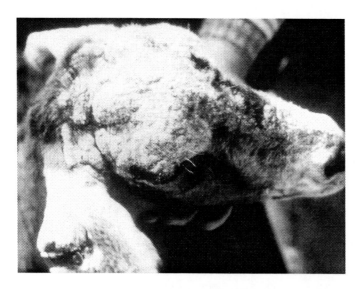

Fig. 2. Extensive proliferative encrustations on the head and muzzle of a domestic goat with sore head resulting from elaeophorosis (courtesy of C.P. Hibler, Wildlife Disease Association Study Set on Elaeophorosis).

Lesions may persist for years. The disease is more severe in Elk and Moose, and lesions result not from the microfilariae, but from adult nematodes, which evoke a severe arteritis, with hyperplasia and occlusion of cephalic and sometimes other arteries. Ischaemic necrosis and haemorrhage in the brain lead to ataxia, circling and blindness in Moose and Elk. Additionally in Elk, thrombosis, causing ischaemic damage to the eyes, optic nerves, ears, muzzle and other tissues, may lead to blindness, dry gangrene of the ear tips, muzzle and nostrils, abnormal antler growth and emaciation. Calves and yearlings, as well as adults, are affected. Death may occur within weeks to months.

Infections of *E. poeli* in cattle and *E. bohmi* in horses seem to be of little clinical significance. Although it evokes an intense arteritis and periportal multifocal granulomas, the clinical importance of *E. elaphi* remains to be determined.

Diagnosis

Unsheathed microfilariae of *E. schneideri* can be demonstrated microscopically in skin snips taken from the head or legs of sheep and goats. Microfilariae are often not abundant and the diagnosis is frequently presumptive for elaeophorosis in any sheep or goat with a facial dermatitis in the summer months from an endemic area. Diagnosis is usually presumptive or at necropsy in wild herbivores.

Transmission

Horse-flies (i.e. tabanids) are the vectors for *E. schneideri*. Vectors and the life cycles for the other species are unknown. Skin lesions in domestic sheep and goats are most pronounced during the summer months, coinciding with peak horse-fly abundance. At least 16 species, representing two genera, *Hybomitra* and *Tabanus*, of horse-flies have been implicated as vectors of *E. schneideri*. *Hybomitra laticornis* and *Hybomitra aatos* are common vectors in the south-western USA, whereas *Tabanus lineola hinellus* is important in the south-eastern USA. In any single area there appears to be one primary vector and one or more species of lesser importance in transmission of these nematodes.

Prevalence of nematode larvae in tabanids varies from as high as 20% to as low as 0.3%. Intensities of larvae in individual flies range from 1 to 181. The preferred feeding sites for these flies are the facial area or legs. Horse-flies are infected by ingestion of microfilariae in the skin of the definitive host when they take a blood meal. Ingested microfilariae migrate to the fat bodies, where they develop to first-stage larvae.

They then migrate to the haemocoel, where they grow and moult through second-stage to third-stage larvae, which, after a period of growth and maturation, migrate to the fly's head and mouthparts. The infective third-stage larvae are a replicate of the adult nematode without the reproductive system. The entire cycle in the fly takes about 2 weeks. Infective third-stage larvae are released from the horsefly's mouthparts when it takes a blood meal. Once established in a suitable vertebrate host, third-stage larvae enter the leptomeningeal arteries and moult to migrating subadults, which localize and mature to adults mostly in the common carotid arteries and their terminal branches, especially the internal maxillary arteries, but they can occur in any other arteries in the body large enough to accommodate them. The nematodes reach sexual maturity in about 6.5–7.5 months following initial infection; they live about 4 years.

Treatment

Sheep and goats can be treated with repeated administration of diethylcarbamazine, but not without risk of fatality due to dead nematodes in the arteries. Apparently, there have been no clinical trials with ivermectin.

Control

With the major decline in population levels of the Mule deer reservoir host and lower numbers of horse-flies, presumably from loss of breeding habitat due to a several-year drought in previously hyperendemic areas of Arizona and New Mexico, the risk of elaeophorosis to sheep, goats and elk has greatly decreased. Widespread use of insecticide spraying and dipping and the use of ivermectin for gastrointestinal nematode control may also have reduced the prevalence of elaeophorosis in sheep and goats in many areas.

Selected bibliography

Hibler, C.P. and Adcock, J.L. (1971) Elaeophorosis. In: Davis, J.W. and Anderson, R.C. (eds) *Parasitic and Infectious Diseases of Wild Mammals.* Iowa State University Press, Ames, Iowa, pp. 263–278.

Jensen, L. and Seghetti, L. (1955) Elaeophorosis in sheep. *Journal of the American Veterinary Medical Association* 130, 220–224.

Kemper, H.E. (1938) Filarial dermatosis of sheep. *North American Veterinarian* 19, 36–41.

Maxie, M.G. (1993) The vascular system. In : Jubb, K.V.C., Kennedy, P.C. and Palmer, N. (eds) *Pathology of Domestic Animals*, Vol. 3, 4th edn. Academic Press, Orlando, Florida, pp. 34–81.

Pence, D.B. (1991) Elaeophorosis in wild ruminants. *Bulletin of the Society for Vector Ecology* 16, 149–160.

Encephalitis *see named infections, such as* **Eastern equine encephalitis**.

Encephalomyelitis *see named encephalitis infections*.

Endemic relapsing fever *see* **Tick-borne relapsing fever**.

Endemic typhus

Karim E. Hechemy and Abdu F. Azad

Endemic typhus, murine typhus or flea-borne typhus is an important zoonosis and a widespread infectious disease of urban areas, with an apparent low prevalence. This is probably a result of the protean manifestations that this disease exhibits.

Endemic typhus is difficult to diagnose because it is a relatively less severe rickettsial disease and its clinical presentation and course resemble those of other infectious diseases. As a result, endemic typhus is probably under-diagnosed. The disease is caused by *Rickettsia typhi* (formerly known as *Rickettsia mooseri*, after Herman Mooser, who delineated the differences between the bacteria that cause endemic and epidemic typhus – see entry). More recently it has been shown that endemic typhus is also caused by another organism, identified as *Rickettsia felis*. Both rickettsiae are transmitted from the animal host/carrier, e.g. rodents, cats and opossums (*Didelphis* species), to humans by fleas.

Distribution

Endemic typhus is one of the most widely distributed arthropod-borne infections, endemic to many coastal areas, to ports throughout the world and in inland areas. It occurs in individual cases or in sporadic epidemics. For example, individual human cases are reported annually in the USA. Outbreaks have been reported in Australia and recently in China, Greece, Israel, Kuwait and Thailand. Recent serosurveys have demonstrated high prevalence of antityphus group (TG) rickettsiae in Asia and southern Europe. It is often unrecognized and significantly under-reported.

Aetiological agent

Taxonomy

Rickettsia typhi is a member of the typhus group (TG) which belong to the genus *Rickettsia* → tribe *Rickettsiae* → family *Rickettsiaceae* → order *Rickettsiales* → α group proteobacteria. Recently, another rickettsia, *R. felis*, which is maintained in opossums (*Didelphis* species) and cat fleas (*Ctenocephalides felis*) has been found to occur in typhus endemic areas, particularly in south Texas and California. It has certain characteristics that place this organism in the typhus group, but its phylogeny puts it in the spotted fever group (SFG) rickettsia. Although *R. felis* is placed within the SFG based on the sequence homologies of selected groups of genes, it is closer to TG rickettsiae in its utilization of an insect vector. Immunological characterization with monoclonal and polyclonal antibodies to rickettsial proteins and lipopolysaccharide shows reactivity with both TG and SFG rickettsiae.

Bacteria

Both *R. typhi* and *R. felis* are small, 0.2–0.5 μm by 0.3–2.0 μm, obligate intracellular bacteria. Ultrastructurally, these bacteria have a typical Gram-negative prokaryotic cytoplasm containing ribosomes and indistinct strands of DNA in an amorphous cytosol, which is surrounded by a plasma membrane. The G + C content of DNA is 28.5–29.7 mol% and the genome size is 1.1×10^9 Da. Typhus group rickettsiae grow in the cytoplasm of eukaryotic host cells. During growth, very few bacteria exit the infected cells. Instead they grow and fill the cytoplasm until the large number of cells overwhelms the host cell capabilities to support the growth of the bacterium. As a result, the host cells burst and the released bacteria initiate infections of neighbouring cells. The mechanism by which a cell is lysed is not well understood. However, it appears that haemolysins and phospholipase A stimulate the host cell to internalize the rickettsiae, and possibly help them to escape the phagosome to live in the cytoplasm.

Culture

The pure bacterium can be grown in the yolk-sac of 5–7-day-old embryonated chicken eggs or in vertebrate cell lines, e.g. VERO cells and L929 cells, and incubated at 37°C in 5% CO_2 for 4–7 days.

Isolation

Rickettsia typhi is preferably isolated from clinical or survey specimens suspected of containing the rickettsiae by animal inoculation, e.g. into mouse, rat or guinea-pig. For the production of seed inoculums of the bacterium, spleen and other organs are collected from the moribund animal and inoculated into the egg yolk-sac of embryonated chicken eggs. Rickettsiae can be maintained for decades at −70°C or in liquid nitrogen. The bacteria lose viability in a few days when they are repeatedly frozen and thawed or maintained at 4°C. Also they lose viability within hours when left at room temperature. However, they may be quite stable in desiccated arthropod faeces and in this state they have been the source of infection in humans.

Clinical symptoms

Both urban (*R. typhi*) and rural (*R. felis*) types of endemic typhus are usually mild illnesses. The incubation period ranges from 1 to 2 weeks. The major features of endemic typhus are abrupt onset of fever, headache, myalgias and, in most cases, a non-purulent maculopapular skin rash, which starts on the trunk and later spreads to the extremities. The rash may be fleeting or absent. In addition, patients have been reported to have chills, cough, arthralgias and nausea followed by vomiting. An untreated illness may last up to 2 weeks. The patient is immune from recurrent infection for life and acquires a partial resistance to epidemic typhus, i.e. *Rickettsia prowazekii* (see Epidemic typhus). Severe cases of endemic typhus infection have been associated with old age, delayed diagnosis, hepatic and renal dysfunction, central nervous system abnormalities and pulmonary compromise. Death occurs in up to 4% of hospitalized patients.

Pathology

Vascular lesions can largely account for the pathological manifestations observed in rickettsioses. The rickettsiae multiply in the endothelial cells lining the small blood-vessels, causing endothelial proliferation, thrombosis, perivascular haemorrhage and extravasations of plasma, which lead to haemoconcentration and shock in extreme cases. Vascular lesions occurring in the skin produce the rash. In extreme cases, the changes in vascularity in heart and kidney may lead to myocardial/and or renal failure.

Diagnosis

For antigen diagnosis, e.g. typhus bacterium isolation, a laboratory equipped with a biological safety level 3 facility is required and all the proper precautions must be taken by laboratory workers. As a result, rickettsial isolation is performed in very few laboratories. Blood should be collected in a heparinized vial before any antibiotic is administered to the patient. Blood should be stored for the short term at 4°C and processed as rapidly as possible. If processing is delayed for more than 24 h, the blood should be centrifuged, and the white buffy coat separated and frozen at −70°C. The classic but cumbersome methods are animal inoculation, e.g. male guinea-pigs, rats, mice or the yolk-sacs of embryonated chicken eggs. Direct cell culture isolation has been done from clinical specimens with mixed results. One of the more promising is the shell-vial technique containing several coverslips, each with a confluent layer of host cells, e.g. VERO cells. Samples containing the clinical material are mixed with tissue culture medium at a ratio if 1 : 1 and centrifuged at $700 \times g$ for 1 h at 25°C. The supernate is then decanted and fresh medium is added in the vial and the vial incubated at 34°C in 5% CO_2. A coverslip is removed at time intervals and examined by direct fluorescent antibody, using fluorescein-tagged antibodies to the TG bacteria. An alternative method is to use indirect fluorescent antibody (IFA), using group-, species- and strain-specific monoclonal antibody as the first antibody, and then to probe this immunoreaction with a fluorescein-tagged antibody to the mouse monoclonal antibody. If present, rickettsiae are usually detected within 72 h. Alternatively, or in addition, the tissue culture can be tested for the presence of the typhus bacterium by molecular methods, such as the polymerase chain reaction (PCR), using specific primers such as the gene encoding the 17-kDa protein, citrate synthase gene and 16S ribosomal RNA (rRNA).

Direct detection of the rickettsiae has also been performed, using punch biopsies from the rash area on the patient's skin. For maximum sensitivity, biopsies should be obtained before starting the patient on antibiotics. Formalin-fixed and paraffin-embedded sections of the maculopapular rash are tested as above for the shell-vial modality. Alternatively, the unfixed skin biopsy can be tested by molecular techniques.

The most common test to detect rickettsial infection is done by the detection of antibodies to the typhus organism, but these tests are not species-specific. The test cannot differentiate between the various species of the typhus group *Rickettsia*. The extent of cross-reactivity by all present modalities of serological testing are extensive, both qualitatively, i.e. the number of specimens, and quantitatively, i.e. titre levels. Because the titres are within one dilution in at least 90% of the cases, speciation cannot be undertaken.

Serological tests are based on two modalities: particle agglutination and probe-based modality. The agglutination-based assays include indirect haemagglutination and latex antigen. Both assays use the erythrocyte-sensitizing antigen (i.e. substance) (ESS). The ESS is derived from boiling a suspension of purified rickettsiae in a water-bath for 30 min. The ESS is then absorbed on sheep erythrocytes or adsorbed on latex particles. For the haemagglutination assay, equal volumes are mixed on a microtitre plate, incubated at 37°C for 2 h and left at 5°C overnight. Unsensitized erythrocytes are run with each test serum to determine the presence of anti-erythrocyte globulins that may be naturally present. Neither particle agglutination test distinguishes between the presence of immunoglobulin G (IgG) and IgM antibodies to typhus antigen. However, a titre of ≥ 128 is usually indicative of an active infection. Particle agglutination-based test titres are usually higher in the presence of IgM antibodies as determined by the IFA (see below). Both tests can be used only for the diagnosis of active infections. They are not suitable for serosurveys. The probe-based modality for the detection of antibody to TG antigen includes the IFA assay and enzyme-linked immunoassay. The IFA is at present the 'gold standard'. After incubating the slides containing the acetone-fixed antigen with the test serum, the immunoreaction is probed with a fluorescein-tagged probe to IgM or IgG antibodies. The IFA can be used to detect, in retrospect, an active infection or could be used for serosurveys using a fluorescein-tagged probe to IgG antibodies. A minimum titre of 128 for IgG and 32 for IgM is indicative of the presence of antibodies. Immunoglobulin G antibodies to the TG could last for

years at high titres; therefore, unless a second test performed 2–3 weeks later shows a change in titre levels, the IFA test cannot distinguish between an active infection and an 'old' one. In contrast, IgM titre levels usually, but not always, decrease after the first 3 months to below the minimum significant level, but sometimes a relatively low titre that is above the significant level may persists for up to 6 months. As a result, two serum specimens drawn from a patient at least 2 weeks apart are needed to determine the status of the infection. An increase in titre ≥fourfold in IgM and/or IgG antibodies indicates an active infection; a ≤fourfold decrease in IgM titre may indicate a recent infection. A static titre or changes in titre of <fourfold in IgG and IgM antibodies indicates an infection at an undetermined time.

Transmission and ecology

The major cycle of *R. typhi*, the aetiological agent of endemic typhus, involves rats (*Rattus rattus* and *Rattus norvegicus*) and the rat flea, *Xensopsylla cheopis*, which has been considered the main vector. Rickettsiae ingested by fleas while blood-feeding multiply enormously in the gut, but, unlike plague transmission (see entry), they do not cause any blockage in the proventriculus. Neither fleas nor rats appear to be harmed by their infection with either *R. typhi* or *R. felis* (see below). Rat-to-rat transmission can also involve the rat louse, *Polyplax spinulosa*, as a vector.

Once infected, fleas remain infected for life and the bacteria are transmitted transovarially. Field data, epidemiological surveys and new molecular techniques have prompted a reconsideration of the established components of the typhus vector-reservoir transmission cycle and their interaction with humans. Endemic typhus exists in some endemic disease foci where both rats and rat fleas are absent. Reported cases of murine typhus in the USA are focused largely in central and south central Texas and Los Angeles and Orange counties in California; however, infected rats and their fleas are hard to document in these areas. Cases of locally acquired endemic typhus in Los Angeles county have been associated with seropositive domestic cats and opossums (*Didelphis* species). *Ctenocephalides felis*, the cat flea, was the most prevalent flea species collected from opossums, cats and dogs (but not rats) in southern Texas. Surveys in other areas of the country have given similar results, which further minimizes the role of rat fleas in the maintenance of endemic typhus within the USA. The maintenance of *R. typhi* or an *R. typhi-* like organism in the cat flea/opossum cycle is, therefore, of potential public health importance, since *C. felis* is a widespread pest that avidly bites humans.

Recently a new typhus-like rickettsia (initially designated ELB), *R. felis*, was identified in cat fleas and opossums (*Didelphis* species) from the Californian and Texas murine typhus foci. Both *R. typhi* and *R. felis* were found in fleas and in opossum, (*Didelphis* species) tissues. Additionally, a retrospective investigation using molecular techniques demonstrated that four patients were infected with *R. typhi* and a fifth had been infected with *R. felis.* The implication of documented human infections with *R. felis* and its presence in opossums, and possibly other wildlife associated with human habitation, raises concerns about the extent of *R. felis* infection in human populations. As a result of these observations, two types of endemic typhus can be described: the urban type, which involves the classical rat/rat flea cycle, and the other is the rural type, which involves the opossum, cat/cat flea cycle.

Vertebrate reservoir hosts and humans are infected with *R. typhi* or *R. felis* when infected fleas taking a blood meal defecate on the host. In turn, the host self-inoculates by abrading the skin via scratching areas containing the rickettsia-contaminated faeces. The rickettsia then passes through the abraded skin, infecting the vertebrate host.

Alternatively, infection through the mucosal surfaces, such as the conjunctivae, can occur if contaminated faecal material is deposited on the mucosal surface. Rickettsiae in dry flea faeces can remain viable, possibly for 1–3 months.

Endemic typhus can occur throughout the year if climatic conditions are favourable for the survival of rats and their ectoparasites. The majority of cases occur during the late spring and early autumn, or whenever warm and humid climates prevail. Although it is a clinically mild disease, it can cause severe illness leading to death.

Treatment
Tetracycline is the drug of choice and is taken for 10 days. Usually the patient defervesces and recovers promptly within 24 h from the start of medication. Relapses do not occur if the full regimen of the tetracycline is taken.

Control
There are usually no specific control measures, but killing rats with rodenticides and fleas, on or off the host, with insecticides, as practised in plague control (see Plague), might be appropriate in some situations. Such control measures may help reduce the chance of contracting the disease but will not eliminate it.

Selected bibliography
Azad, A.F. (1990) Epidemiology of murine typhus. *Annual Review of Entomology* 35, 553–569.

Azad, A.F. and Beard, C.B. (1998) Interactions of rickettsial pathogens with arthropod vectors. *Emerging Infectious Diseases* 4, 179–186.

Azad, A.F., Radulovic, S., Higgins, J.A., Noden, B.H. and Troyer, M.J. (1997) Flea-borne rickettsioses: some ecological considerations. *Emerging Infectious Diseases* 3, 319–328.

Entamoeba **infections** *see* **Cockroaches** *and* **Flies.**

Eperythrozoonosis *see* **Haemotrophic mycoplasmas.**

Eperythrozoon **species** *see* **Haemotrophic mycoplasmas.**

Ephemeral fever *see* **Bovine ephemeral fever.**

Epidemic haemorrhagic fever *see* **Haemorrhagic fever with renal syndrome.**

Epidemic relapsing fever *see* **Louse-borne relapsing fever.**

Epidemic typhus

Karim E. Hechemy and Abdu F. Azad

The origin of the name typhus is from the Greek *typhos,* which means stupor arising from fever, one of the symptoms of the disease. Classical epidemic typhus, also known as louse-borne typhus, is the only rickettsial disease that can cause explosive epidemics in humans. Throughout history, epidemic typhus and plague have decided the outcome of more military campaigns than all the generals of history. In the past, epidemic typhus was associated with wars and human disasters. After the First World War (1914–1918), it is estimated that over 20 million people were infected with *Rickettsia prowazekii,* the aetiological agent of epidemic typhus, with a mortality rate of ~20% in eastern Europe. After the Second World War (1939–1945), it is estimated that 7 million people died from epidemic typhus. Today typhus still occurs in war-torn countries and remains endemic in cold areas of tropical regions, where it is maintained in the human–louse cycle.

In addition, *R. prowazekii* causes recrudescent typhus or Brill–Zinsser disease (see Transmission below).

Distribution

Classic louse-borne typhus was world-wide in the pre-antibiotic era. Even in the antibiotic era, the disease is still endemic, but restricted to the highlands and cold areas of Africa, Asia, Central and South America and parts of eastern Europe. For example, it is found during the winter in regions such as the Sahara and Arabian deserts, when heavy clothing is worn continuously; in tropical regions, among people wearing ornamental waist bands or arm and leg coverings that can harbour the body louse; and in other cold regions, such as the mountainous regions of Guatemala and Mexico, the Andean highlands and the Himalayan region. Depending on many factors, epidemic typhus can occur as a truly epidemic disease, as a prolonged endemic–epidemic infection, or as an endemic infection with sporadic outbreaks of limited geographical scope, as in a village in, for example, the Andean mountains. Large outbreaks have occurred through the years since the Second World War (1939–1945) in war-torn countries of Africa, such as Burundi, Ethiopia and Rwanda. Twenty thousand cases were reported from Burundi for the period from January to March 1997.

Bacterium

Rickettsia prowazekii has the same morphological and growth characters as *R. typhi,* the causative agent of endemic typhus (see entry). The bacterium is a small, 0.2–0.5 µm by 0.3–2.0 µm, obligate intracellular bacteria. Ultrastructurally, it has a typical Gram-negative prokaryotic cytoplasm containing ribosomes and indistinct strands of DNA in an amorphous cytosol, which is surrounded by a plasma membrane. The G + C content of DNA is 28.5–29.7 mol% and the genome size is 1.1×10^9 daltons. Typhus group (TG) rickettsiae grow in the cytoplasm of eukaryotic host cells. During growth, very few bacteria exit the infected cells. Instead they grow and fill the cytoplasm until the sheer number of cells overwhelms the host cell capabilities to support the growth of the bacterium. As a result, the host cells burst and the released bacteria initiate infections of neighbouring cells. The mechanism by which the cell is lysed is not well understood.

The complete genome of *R. prowazekii* was recently characterized. The genome contains 834 protein-coding genes. The functional profiles of these genes show similarities to those of mitochondrial genes, indicating that *R. prowazekii* is more closely related to mitochondria than to any other microorganisms studied to date. Genes for encoding anaerobic glycolysis are not found in either *R. prowazekii* or mitochondria; but both have the gene encoding components of the tricarboxylic cycle and the respiratory-chain complex for the production of adenosine triphosphate (ATP). In addition, many genes involved in the encoding and regulation of the biosynthesis of amino acids and nucleosides that are present in free-living bacteria are missing in *R. prowazekii* and in mitochondria. The proportion of non-coding DNA in the *R. prowazekii* genome is the highest (24%) of non-coding DNA in the many bacterial genomes studied so far.

Taxonomy

Rickettsia prowazekii is a member of TG, which belongs to the genus *Rickettsia* → tribe *Rickettsiae* → family *Rickettsiaceae* → order *Rickettsiales* → α group proteobacteria. While DNA analyses of *R. prowazekii* isolated from Flying squirrels (*Glaucomys volans*) differ slightly from human/lice isolates of *R. prowazekii*, biologically these isolates are very similar; nevertheless the significance of the observed differences remains to be determined.

Clinical symptoms

Classic epidemic typhus is one of the most virulent diseases known to humanity. Symptoms appear about 10 days after an infected body louse has bitten a person. Symptoms include a high fever of ~42°C, extreme pain in the muscles and joints, stiffness, headaches that have been characterized as worse than migraines, and cerebral impairment. About the third to the fifth day of illness, a maculopapular rash, consisting of elevated dark red spots, appears on the trunk and then spreads to the rest of the body. The rash may not occur in 10% of the affected persons. During the second week, the patient may become delirious with neurological symptoms and may experience stupor. In extreme untreated cases, hypotension, oliguria, azotaemia, secondary bacterial bronchopneumonia, otitis media and parotitis may occur. Thrombosis may affect the large arteries, leading to hemiplegia. Gangrene and necrosis may occur, due to thrombosis of the small vessels in the extremities. The mortality rate in untreated patients is ~20%. In a severe epidemic, the mortality rate is often as high as 40%. After 14–21 days, untreated patients may undergo a sudden remission of fever and their mental and physical states undergo quick recovery. However, full strength returns more slowly, often taking 2–3 months.

In Brill–Zinsser cases (see Transmission below), the symptoms are less pronounced than those described in classic epidemic typhus, the fever is less, the rash is usually absent or, if present, is less intense, and the mortality rate is <1%. The clinical picture of sylvatic typhus (see Transmission below) is similar but milder than that of epidemic typhus. The illness is characterized by the abrupt onset of the illness, headache, fever, myalgias and the characteristic exanthems of rickettsial infection. No deaths have been reported from patients with sylvatic typhus.

Pathology

The hallmark of epidemic typhus pathogenesis, as well as members of the genera *Rickettsia* and *Orientia*, is vasculopathy. After penetration into the body, the bacterium spreads throughout via the bloodstream, enters the endothelial cells and proliferates intracellularly until the bacteria reach a critical number. The cells then burst and release the bacteria to spread and reinfect intact cells. This seems to be the major cause of cellular injury, since it is not mediated via toxins (none has been detected to date) and it occurs in the absence of immune and inflammatory response. Cellular injury leads to extensive vasculitis, increased vascular permeability, resulting in oedema, and activation of humoral inflammatory and coagulation mechanisms. In addition, lymphocytes and macrophages accumulate around the injured small blood-vessels. Besides the vascular lesions on the skin, lesions can also be found in the heart, brain, kidney, skeletal muscle and testes. In severe infection in untreated patients, the changes in permeability in the host cells are such that plasma and plasma proteins permeate to the interstitium from the intra-vascular spaces.

Diagnosis

The modalities for the laboratory diagnosis of epidemic typhus are similar to those for endemic typhus (see entry). Antigeno-diagnosis by isolation of the organism is discouraged and should only be done in specialized laboratories that have level 3 biological safety. The isolation should be performed with specimens from patients before instituting antibiotic therapy. Simi-larly, antigenodiagnosis by direct immuno-fluorescence on skin biopsies should be done on biopsies before antibiotic therapy is administered to the patient. Serodiagno-sis is the modality of choice, even though the diagnosis is made in retrospect. Neither the particle-mediated serodiagnosis, using sheep erythrocytes or latex sensitized with the erythrocyte-sensitizing substance from *R. prowazekii*, nor the immunoprobe assays, e.g. indirect immunofluorescence or enzyme-linked immunosorbent assay (ELISA), speciate the typhus fever group agent that is causing the disease. This is because of the extensive quantitative (titre levels) cross-reactivity among the typhus fever group. It has been shown that speciation of the causative agents could be done with immunoprobe assays by an inhibition reaction.

To differentiate between an endemic typhus infection and an epidemic typhus infection, the patient serum is first incu-bated with both organisms separately. Each immune reaction is then probed with a monoclonal antibody specific to the TG rickettsia used in the first incubation. The monoclonal antibody reactivity is then probed with tagged anti-mouse immuno-globulin G (IgG) antibodies. It is expected that, if the first reaction was a homologous antigen/antibody reaction, the monoclonal antibody will not react with the specific epitope. On the other hand, if the first reac-tion was a heterologous reaction, the specific epitope will be free and available to react with the monoclonal antibody. While both standard immunoprobe and particle assays can be used for the serodiagnosis of active infection, only immunoprobe-based assays should be used for serosurveys. Titres of ≥128 in the particle agglutination assays are often indicative of active infection. In con-trast, single titres of ≥128 in the immuno-probe assays may not necessarily indicate an active infection, but an infection in the recent past. Anti-rickettsial IgG antibody titres have been known to remain at very high levels 2 years post-infection while anti-rickettsial IgM antibody titres decrease; nevertheless, they remain at diagnostic levels for up to 6 months.

Transmission and epidemiology

The main vector of classical epidemic typhus is *Pediculus humanus*, the human body louse. Although experimentally *Pedi-culus capitis*, the head louse, is capable of maintaining *R. prowazekii*, its role in the transmission of this rickettsiosis is not well established. Body lice feed only on humans and all three stages of the louse life cycle, namely eggs, nymphs and adults, occur on the same host. After adult lice, or their nymphal stages, take a blood meal from *R. prowazekii*-infected human, they become infected. Patients are infective to lice during the febrile illness and possibly for 3–4 days after the temperature returns to normal. In the louse the rickettsiae invade the gut cells, where they multiply enormously, and after about 4 days the cells burst, releasing rickettsiae into the lumen of the gut and contaminating the faeces. During a blood meal, the louse excretes faeces that contain millions of live infectious *R. prowazekii*. A minimal amount of the excreta rubbed on the skin or any exposed mucous area, such as the cornea, will cause the disease to erupt in humans. Rickettsiae can remain alive in dry faeces for about 70 days.

Body lice seek locations on the human body where the temperature is approximately 20°C. These temperatures are normally found in the folds of clothing. The body louse will abandon a patient with a temperature ≥40°C, as well as the body of a dead person. When the body louse is not feeding on the blood of its victim, it lives in seams and folds of clothing. Body louse infestation occurs through contact with discarded infested clothing and bedding, as well as by direct contact with an infected person via the migration of the louse from the patient to another person. Lice may feed several times a day and thus may transmit rickettsiae to several people in close contact, such as in crowded conditions. The body louse proliferates and spreads very rapidly in refugee camps and other crowded conditions. The risk can be expected to increase in rainy seasons, when more clothing and blankets are used and clothes are not changed. Body lice do not transmit *R. prowazekii* to their offspring. The rupturing of the gut cells in the louse often allows blood to seep through into the haemocoel, giving the louse a reddish colour; such sick lice may die after 8–12 days.

Humans are the essential reservoir host for maintaining the *R. prowazekii* infection during interepidemic periods. Young patients who survive the illness may harbour the organisms in their lymphatics and develop recrudescent typhus or Brill–Zinsser disease at a much older age. This is a full-blown infection of typhus, and body lice feeding on a Brill–Zinsser patient become infected and the cycle then repeats itself from human to louse to human. Brill–Zinsser is named for Nathan Brill, who first recognized and described the disease and Hans Zinsser, who suggested that the disease was a relapse of a past epidemic typhus infection.

Although epidemic typhus rickettsiae were considered to be maintained only in the human–louse cycle, the discovery in the late 1970s of a sylvatic cycle in the eastern USA revealed the existence of an enzootic cycle involving Flying squirrels (*Glaucomys*

volans) and their fleas (*Orchopeas howardi*) and lice (*Neohaematopinus sciuropteri*). Most of the cases have occurred in the eastern USA in rural environments, namely in the states of Georgia, Tennessee, Pennsylvania, Virginia and Massachusetts, during the colder time of the year when squirrels may seek refuge in the attics of residences. Serosurveys of flying squirrels have demonstrated the presence of antibodies to TG antigens. Seroconversion was also observed in serially trapped animals during the cold months of the year. While the organism resembling *R. prowazekii* was isolated from the flying squirrels and their ectoparasites, no organisms were isolated from humans presumed to have sylvatic typhus. Further studies will be crucial in determining the underlying mechanisms involved in the survival and persistence of this rickettsiosis.

Treatment

As with all rickettsial infections, antibiotics of the family of tetracyclines or their derivatives, such as doxycycline, are the drugs of choice. For epidemic typhus, intravenous fluids and oxygen may also be necessary as supportive therapy in addition to the antibiotics. Patients with typhus are usually expected to recover completely with prompt antibiotic therapy, although they could remain infected with *R. prowazekii* and develop Brill–Zinsser disease later in life and infect a louse if they are exposed to one.

Prevention

It is possible to reduce epidemic louse–human–louse transmission of *R. prowazekii* by using simple precautions, because the disease is not transmitted from person to person. Patients with epidemic typhus infections should be immediately deloused and provided with clean clothing. Heating clothes to 70°C will kill lice and prevent the infection from spreading. DDT powder can be applied to the body to kill lice. However, there is widespread resistance to DDT and, if this is known to occur, other insecticides, such as permethrin or temephos (Abate), can be used. In addition, impregnating clothing and bedlinen with pyrethroid insecticides, such as permethrin, may provide long-lasting protection against louse infestations. Because insecticidal dusts come into close and prolonged contact with peoples' bodies, they must have very low mammalian toxicities.

Selected bibliography
Azad, A.F. and Beard, C.B. (1998) Interactions of rickettsial pathogens with arthropod vectors. *Emerging Infectious Diseases* 4, 179–186.

McDade, J.E. (1980) Evidence of *Rickettsia prowazekii* in the United States. *American Journal of Tropical Medicine and Hygiene* 29, 277–283.

Murray, E.S., Gaon, J.A., O'Connor, J.M. and Mulahasanovič, M. (1965) Serologic studies of primary endemic typhus and recrudescent typhus (Brill Zinsser). *Journal of Immunology* 94, 723–733.

Niang, M., Brouqui, P. and Raoult, D. (1999) Epidemic typhus imported from Algeria. *Emerging Infectious Diseases* 5, 716–719.

Tarasevich, I., Rydkina E. and Raoult, D. (1998) Outbreak of epidemic typhus in Russia. *The Lancet* 352, 1151.

World Health Organization (1997) A large outbreak of epidemic louse-borne typhus in Burundi. *Weekly Epidemiological Record* 21, 152–153.

Epizootic cerebrospinal nematodiasis *see* **Setariosis.**

Epizootic haemorrhagic disease

P.S. Mellor

Epizootic haemorrhagic disease of deer is a non-contagious, infectious, insect-borne disease of ruminants, especially certain species of deer.

Distribution
Epizootic haemorrhagic disease has a very wide distribution and occurs in North, Central and South America, Africa, South-East Asia, Japan and Australia.

Aetiological agent
The virus causing epizootic haemorrhagic disease is a member of the genus *Orbivirus* in the family Reoviridae and is therefore closely related to bluetongue virus (see entry), the type species of the genus. The virion is icosahedral and unenveloped, and has a diameter of about 80 mm, with a core particle containing ten segments of double-stranded RNA (dsRNA) surrounded by a diffuse outer capsid. Eight serotypes of the virus have been identified to date.

Epizootic haemorrhagic disease (EHD) virus serotype 1 has been isolated in North America and Australia, serotype 2 in North America, the Middle East, Australia and Japan, serotypes 3 and 4 in Africa and

serotypes 5, 6, 7 and 8 in Australia. A further, untyped, EHD virus, designated '318' has also been isolated from Bahrain. In addition, specific antibodies to EHD virus have been detected in cattle across much of South-East Asia.

Clinical signs
In most ruminants, infection with EHD virus is usually inapparent but in certain species of deer and other wild ruminants, particularly in North America (e.g. White-tailed deer (*Odocoileus virginianus*), Mule deer (*Odocoileus hemionus hemionus*), Black-tailed deer (*Odocoileus hemionus columbianus*), Pronghorn antelope (*Antilocapra americana*)), the disease can be severe and is then indistinguishable from bluetongue (see entry). Cattle are usually subclinically infected but in 1959 Ibaraki virus, a variant of EHD virus serotype 2, caused a bluetongue-like disease in 39,000 Japanese cattle, killing approximately 4000 of them. More recently suspicions have been growing that EHD virus may also be a cause of disease in cattle in other parts of the world, including the USA and South Africa.

Pathology and post-mortem findings

Epizootic haemorrhagic disease virus can be very pathogenic in some ruminant species, especially in White-tailed deer, causing a syndrome referred to as haemorrhagic disease (HD). This syndrome is sometimes divided into three categories: peracute, acute and chronic. The peracute form of the disease is characterized by oedema of the head, neck and lungs and sudden death. The acute form also causes oedema but in addition produces haemorrhages in the heart, gastrointestinal tract and other organs, and erosions on the dental pad, tongue and palate. The chronic form of HD is actually a convalescent state resulting from the slow healing of lesions of the acute disease. If damage to the epithelial surfaces has been severe, the animal may succumb to starvation or to secondary bacterial infections.

Diagnosis

Most infections with EHD virus are inapparent and, when clinical disease is caused, it is indistinguishable from bluetongue. Laboratory confirmation of infection is therefore essential. Confirmation is by virus isolation from or identification in whole blood or organs (spleen, kidney, liver, lung, lymph nodes) or by the demonstration of rising antibody titres in paired serum samples. A variety of diagnostic tests are available, but the tests of choice are neutralization tests, which are serotype-specific, the competitive enzyme-linked immunosorbent assay (cELISA) (for antibody detection) and the sandwich ELISA (for antigen detection), which are both serogroup-specific.

Transmission

Epizootic haemorrhagic disease virus is transmitted between its vertebrate hosts almost entirely via the bites of certain species of *Culicoides* biting midges, which are true biological vectors. In North America the most important vector species is *C. variipennis*, but *C. lahillei* has also been implicated and other species may be involved to a lesser extent. In Africa the virus has been isolated from *C. nevelli*, *C. cornutus* and *C. schultzei* group midges,

while in Australia numerous isolations have been made from *C. brevitarsis*. The vectors in Central America, South America, Japan and South-East Asia are at present unknown.

In addition to transmission via the bites of vector species of *Culicoides*, EHD viruses have been reported to be transmitted transplacentally to the fetus from cows and ewes infected during gestation. However, the route is not considered to be of significance in epizootic haemorrhagic disease epidemiology.

Vertebrate hosts

Epizootic haemorrhagic disease virus infects and replicates in a wide range of domestic and wild ruminant species.

Treatment

Apart from supportive treatment there is no specific therapy for epizootic haemorrhagic disease.

Prevention and control

Following an outbreak of epizootic haemorrhagic disease in a country or zone previously free of the disease, attempts should be made to limit further transmission of the virus and to achieve eradication as quickly as possible through control of animal movements, housing of susceptible stock and vector abatement measures.

In enzootic situations, control of epizootic haemorrhagic disease is unlikely to be feasible since it is primarily a disease of wildlife. However, since the risk of disease is minimized in deer herds that do not exceed the carrying capacity of their habitat, it has been suggested that the size of susceptible deer populations should be regulated through properly managed hunting. There are no vaccines available for the control of epizootic haemorrhagic disease.

Selected bibliography

Gibbs, E.P.J. and Greiner, E.C. (1988) Bluetongue and epizootic hemorrhagic disease. In: Monath, T.P. (ed.) *The Arboviruses: Epidemiology and Ecology*, Vol. II. CRC Press, Boca Raton, Florida, pp. 39–70.

Omori, T., Inaba, Y., Morimoto, T., Tanaka, Y., Ishitani, R., Kurogi, H., Munakata, K., Matsuda, K. and Matumoto, M. (1969) Ibaraki virus, an agent of epizootic disease of cattle resembling bluetongue. I. Epidemiologic, clinical and pathologic observations and experimental transmission to calves. *Japanese Journal of Microbiology* 13, 139–157.

Smith, K.E., Stallknecht, D.E. and Nettles, V.F. (1996) Experimental infection of *Culicoides lahillei* (Diptera: Ceratopogonidae) with epizootic hemorrhagic disease virus serotype 2

(Orbivirus: Reoviridae). *Journal of Medical Entomology* 33, 117–122.

Sohn, R. and Yuill, T.M. (1991) Bluetongue and epizootic hemorrhagic disease in wild ruminants. *Bulletin of the Society for Vector Ecology* 16, 17–24.

Thevasagayam, J.A. (1998) The epizootic haemorrhagic disease virus serogroup. PhD Thesis submitted to the University of Hertfordshire, UK, 152 pp.

Walton, T.E. and Osburn, B.I. (1992) *Bluetongue, African Horse Sickness and Related Orbiviruses.* CRC Press, Boca Raton, Florida, 1042 pp.

Equine biliary fever *see* **Theilerioses.**

Equine infectious anaemia

C.J. Issel

Commonly referred to as EIA, or swamp fever, this persistent lentivirus infection of equid host species is mechanically transmitted between equids in close proximity by haematophagous insects and is best thought of as a blood-borne infection. Although EIA virus is not an arbovirus (the agent does not replicate in the vector), it provides an excellent model for the investigation of the dynamics of mechanical transmission of retroviruses.

Distribution

Infections with EIA virus are found worldwide where people have transported infected equids. As the majority of infections with EIA virus today are without overt clinical signs, it is reasonable to assume that, historically, the distribution of EIA virus silently followed the movement of humans accompanied by equids, and thrived where conditions were optimal (areas with high vector populations and/or where humans facilitated the transfer of blood between horses under domestication.) As a disease, EIA has been recognized since the middle of the 19th century, but it is not officially recognized in wild or domesticated equids in some areas. Where testing for the infection is common, foci may be found with infection rates exceeding 30% on ranches and individual premises or in bands of free-roaming horse populations. In the USA, over a million horses (of an estimated 6 million) are tested each year, with about 1000 new cases found every year. In recent years, the majority of infections have been found in areas or on premises where testing for EIA had not been practised routinely.

Virus

Equine infectious anaemia virus is in the genus *Lentivirus* in the family Retroviridae. It has a relatively simple genetic organization for a lentivirus: gag, pol, env genes encode structural proteins and enzymatic functions; regulatory proteins are coded by three small open-reading frames. The virus replicates predominantly in mature tissue macrophages *in vivo*. Equine infectious anaemia virus and other lentiviruses exist as quasispecies because of inherently high mutation rates. Mutations appear at highest frequency within hypervariable regions of the surface unit protein gene. These mutations can result in the emergence of novel antigenic variants that escape immunosurveillance, perhaps with higher capacity to replicate and induce disease.

Clinical signs

The majority of infections in equid host species appear to be clinically inapparent when first detected by routine surveillance testing. Research suggests that most strains have the capacity to regain the ability to cause disease through selection by rapid serial passage in equids; exposure to high doses of these strains can result in death within 20 days of exposure. The clinical signs associated with infection with EIA virus include fever, thrombocytopenia, lethargy and petechial haemorrhages on mucous membranes. Frequently, these acute signs of disease are short-lived and not observed by the owner or attending veterinarian. Most infected horses appear to recover from the initial bout, but some develop recurring febrile episodes. This chronic form of the disease is more commonly diagnosed and may be additionally characterized by anaemia, dependent oedema and profound weight loss. Classical studies of the chronic form of the disease have proved that antigenic variation of EIA virus was occurring.

Diagnosis

Equine infectious anaemia was not reliably diagnosed until practical serological tests were defined in 1970, and correlated with the presence of EIA virus. Foals of test-positive dams, however, may test positive because of active infection and/or passively acquired colostral antibodies. Since 1970, the agar gel immunodiffusion (AGID or Coggins) test has received wide international acceptance, and detects antibodies against the major core protein of EIA virus. The incubation period – that is, time from exposure to first positive test – is generally within 21–45 days in horses; once positive, the equid remains test-positive for life. The accuracy and reliability of the AGID test has encouraged the adoption of regulations for EIA control in local, national and international jurisdictions. Additional enzyme-linked immunosorbent assay (ELISA)-based tests have received approval as official tests for EIA, but confirmatory AGID tests are required. In some cases, application of more sensitive immunoblot tests has proved useful. Infections with EIA virus are more readily diagnosed by serological methods because EIA virus strains from the field are not easily cultivated in the laboratory, and because clinical signs, clinicopathological changes and pathology findings are not specific.

Transmission

The major determinants of EIA virus transmission between equids by individual insects are the amount of EIA virus in the blood and the volume of blood transferred by the vector to a second host (via interrupted feeding). The plasma viraemia with EIA is highest during acute febrile episodes and may approach 10^6 ml^{-1}. In contrast, equids without clinical disease have lower levels of virus (generally $\geq$1000-fold less), making transmission by a haematophagous insect less probable. Any blood-feeding insect has the theoretical potential to transmit EIA virus. In critical laboratory experiments, tabanids such as horse-flies (*Tabanus* species) and deer-flies (*Chrysops* species) have proved the most efficient, followed by stable-flies (*Stomoxys* species). Under experimental conditions, virus infectivity was retained and transmitted to a recipient by 25 *Tabanus fuscicostatus* held for 30 min (but not 4 h) after their partial feeding on a donor with acute disease.

In wild, free-roaming EIA virus-infected populations, an exceptionally high rate of infection in mature/dominant stallions has been observed, suggesting that their combative behaviour may increase the risk of acquiring EIA virus.

Treatment

Although the anti-retrovirus drugs, such as reverse transcriptase inhibitors, are able to interfere with EIA virus replication *in vitro*, no drugs have been found to cure EIA virus-infected equids, nor have serious attempts been made because of the expense of drugs and the uniform failure of anti-human immunodeficiency virus (HIV) (a closely related lentivirus) drug regimens to cure acquired immune deficient syndrome

(AIDS) patients. Thus, the slogan 'once infected, always infected' is appropriate. Although antipyretic drugs may reduce the severity of a febrile episode, no treatments have been shown to have long-term effects on an infection. The routine use of cortico-steroids in equids should be avoided unless accompanied by a negative serological test for EIA, because of the possible recrudes-cence of clinical signs of EIA through the use of such drugs.

Control

Serological testing for EIA provides a sense of protection and, when rigorously applied to populations, can lead to the eradication of the disease and the infection. Adoption of uniform methods for the control of EIA has facilitated the international movement of horses. The strict adherence to quaran-tine recommendations (200-metre spatial separation of test-positive individuals from other equids) has proved effective in the field. In many jurisdictions, owners are not given the option to maintain the test-positive equid; in some cases, this discour-ages testing of potential reservoir hosts and leaves the population at higher risk.

International control depends on the appli-cation and accuracy of testing in the mobile horse population. As no practical preven-tive immunization is available, more wide-spread testing is required to continue to reduce the threat of EIA.

There are no practical methods for con-trolling the arthropod mechanical vectors.

Selected bibliography

Cook, R.F., Issel, C.J. and Montelaro, R.C. (1996) Equine infectious anemia. In: Studdert, M.J. (ed.) *Virus Infections of Equines*, Vol. 6. In the series *Virus Infections of Vertebrates*, Horzinek, M.C. (series ed.), Elsevier, Amster-dam, pp. 295–323.

Foil, L.D. and Issel, C.J. (1991) Transmission of retroviruses by arthropods. *Annual Review of Entomology* 36, 355–381.

Foil, L.D., Adams, W.V. McManus, J.M. and Issel, C.J. (1987) Blood meal residues on mouthparts of *Tabanus fuscicostatus* (Diptera: Tabanidae) and the potential for mechanical transmission of pathogens. *Jour-nal of Medical Entomology* 4, 613–616.

Issel, C.J., Rushlow, K., Foil, L.D. and Montelaro, R.C. (1988) A perspective on equine infec-tious anemia with an emphasis on vector transmission and genetic analysis. *Veteri-nary Microbiology* 17, 251–286.

Equine piroplasmosis *see* **Babesiosis** *and* **Theilerioses.**

Escherichia coli *see* **Cockroaches** *and* **Flies.**

Espundia *see* **Leishmaniasis.**

Eye-flies (Chloropidae)

M.W. Service

The family Chloropidae comprises several genera, some of which contain flies of agri-cultural importance, e.g. frit-flies (*Oscinella frit*), but the genera *Hippelates* and *Siphun-culina* contain species of minor veterinary and medical importance, and are commonly known as eye-flies or eye-gnats. They are small flies about 2 mm long and shiny black. Species of *Siphunculina* occur in

Asia, while the genus *Hippelates* is found only in the Americas and probably contains the more important vector species.

Biology

Eggs of *Hippelates* are laid in light, well-drained sandy soils, especially culti-vated land: they hatch after about 2 days. The maggot-like larvae (Fig. 1) are mainly

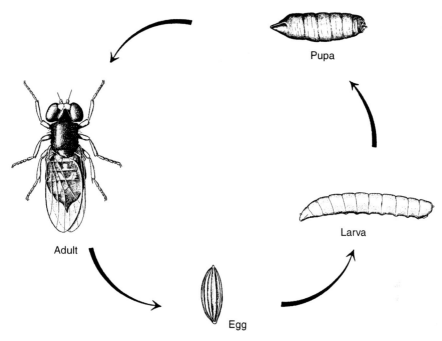

Fig. 1. Life cycle of an eye-fly (*Hippelates pusio*) (modified from D.G. Hall (1932) *American Journal of Hygiene* 16, 854–864).

saprophagous and coprophagous, feeding on decaying organic matter. In warm weather larval development is completed in 7–12 days. The puparial period lasts about a week. Larval and puparial durations are greatly lengthened by low temperatures. The life cycle is completed in about 3 weeks. Adults, which can appear in large numbers in the spring and autumn, are very persistent and tormenting pests of domesticated animals and humans. They commonly settle on or around the eyes, especially if they have discharges, and are also attracted to sores, pus, blood, sweat and other bodily secretions. The flies do not bite but spines on the proboscis scarify tissues and so facilitate transmission of infections. Adults are strong fliers, sometimes dispersing as much as 7.5 km.

The life cycle of *Siphunculina* species is similar to that of *Hippelates*, but in hot weather can be as short as about 10 days. In Asia species of *Siphunculina* are attracted to the eyes and sores of cattle and horses, to wounds and blood on animals caused by biting flies, such as stable-flies (*Stomoxys* species), and also to human and animal faeces.

Diseases

Hippelates and *Siphunculina* species are involved in the mechanical transmission of bacteria causing infection of the conjunctiva in humans, a condition often called pink-eye or red-eye. They have sometimes been considered as transmitting the causal agents of yaws (*Treponema pertenue*) and pinta (*Treponema carateum*). They have also been considered to play a minor role in the transmission of some types of tropical ulcers, but there is little evidence for this. In Trinidad a tropical skin infection caused by *Streptococcus pyogenes* can apparently be spread to humans by *Hippelates* species. Eye-flies can also spread, to a certain extent, trachoma (*Chlamydia trachomatis*) and anaplasmosis (see entry). Eye-flies have sometimes been suspected of transmitting mastitis, but there is little evidence for this. In Colorado *Hippelates* species have been associated with vesicular stomatitis (see entry), a disease of livestock.

Control

There are no easy control options. Concerns over environmental contamination largely prevent insecticidal spraying of soils to kill the larvae. Some temporary relief from the annoyance caused by adult eye-flies to both people and livestock may be obtained by ultra-low-volume (ULV) spraying of pesticides. The best measures are probably cultural control, involving discing of agricultural land and especially weed control, and traps employing attractants such as fish oil. In the USA 10,000–12,000 traps are employed in the Coachella valley, California, while there are 12,000–14,000 baited traps in Yuma county, Arizona.

Eye-worms *see* **Thelaziasis.**

Selected bibliography

Francy, D.B., Moore, C.G., Smith, G.C., Jakob, W. L., Taylor, S.A. and Calisher, C.H. (1988) Epizootic vesicular stomatitis in Colorado 1982: isolation of virus from insects collected in the northern Colorado Rocky Mountain Front Range. *Journal of Medical Entomology* 25, 343–347.

Greenberg, B. (1971) *Flies and Disease*, Vol. 1, *Ecology, Classification and Biotic Associations*. Princeton University Press, Princeton, New Jersey, 856 pp.

Greenberg, B. (1973) *Flies and Disease*, Vol. 2, *Biology and Disease Transmission.* Princeton University Press, Princeton, New Jersey, 447 pp.

Mulla, M.S., Axelrod, H. and Ikeshoji, T. (1974) Attractants for synanthropic flies: area-wide control of *Hippelates collusor* with attractive baits. *Journal of Economic Entomology* 67, 631–638.

Fièvre boutonneuse *see* **Tick-borne typhuses.**

Filaria *see* **Nematoda.**

Five-day fever *see* **Phlebotomus fevers.**

Flea-borne typhus *see* **Endemic typhus.**

Fleas (Siphonaptera)

M.W. Service

There are some 2500 species and subspecies of fleas, belonging to 239 genera, but only a few are of medical or veterinary importance. Fleas have an almost worldwide distribution, and about 94% of species feed on mammals, the others on birds. The most important vectors belong to the genus *Xenopsylla*.

Biology

Adult fleas are small insects (1–4 mm) and are flattened laterally. Wings are absent, but the hind legs are specially modified for jumping.

Both sexes of adults suck blood and are therefore equally important in the transmission of diseases. When ready to lay eggs the

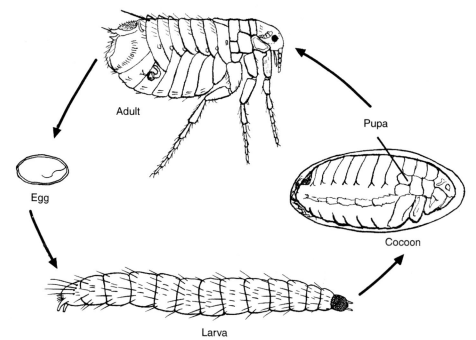

Fig. 1. Life cycle of a flea (modified from M.W. Service (2000) *Medical Entomology for Students,* Cambridge University Press, Cambridge).

female flea may leave the host (e.g. commensal and wild rodents, cats and dogs) to deposit her eggs among debris littering the host's dwelling-place, such as rodent burrows. Fleas that attack humans and domestic pests usually lay eggs in cracks and crevices of floors or among dust and debris. Occasionally eggs are laid on the host but they generally fall off. The whitish eggs are sticky and soon become covered with dirt and dust. Fleas usually live for 10–45 days, but sometimes they live for 6–12 months. During her lifetime a female flea may lay 300–1000 eggs.

Eggs hatch within 2–14 days into minute legless larvae (Fig. 1), which avoid light and are found on floors and carpets of houses, on pet's bedding and in rodent burrows. Larvae feed on almost any organic debris, including the host's faeces, as well as on partially digested blood excreted by adult fleas. There are usually three larval instars. The larval period may be as short as 10–21 days, but, in unfavourable conditions, such as lack of food or coldness, this can be extended to about 200 days. Mature larvae are about 4–10 mm long. They spin a silken cocoon around themselves and then pupate within this. Adults can emerge from the cocoons within 5–14 days, but they require stimuli to do so, such as vibrations caused by host movements in burrows or houses. Adults may remain alive in their cocoons for up to a year, and this explains why people occupying buildings that have remained empty for months may be bitten by numerous hungry fleas, which have been stimulated to emerge and are taking their first blood meal.

The life cycle from egg to adult emergence (Fig. 1) may be only 2–3 weeks, but is often considerably longer.

Adult fleas avoid sunlight and are found sheltering among the hairs of hosts or under people's clothing. Fleas may feed several times a day. Although fleas have one or two favourite host species, most are not entirely host-specific. For example, rat fleas in the genus *Xenopsylla* will feed on humans in the absence of rats, and cat (*Ctenocephalides felis*) and dog (*Ctenocephalides canis*) fleas readily attack humans. Fleas rapidly abandon dead hosts, which is of epidemiological importance in plague transmission when fleas leave dead rats and jump on humans.

Diseases

The most important infection spread by fleas is plague (*Yersinia pestis*), which is transmitted among rats and to humans by rat fleas of the genus *Xenopsylla*, in particular *X. cheopis*. Fleas also spread flea-borne endemic typhus (murine typhus), caused by *Rickettsia typhi*, and play a role in the transmission of rural epidemic typhus (*Rickettsia prowazekii*) and animal parasites, such as *Mansonella reconditum*. Other infections spread by fleas include mechanical, not biological, transmission of cat-scratch disease (*Bartonella henselae*), fowl pox virus and the virus causing myxomatosis in rabbits.

Control

Insect repellents can give some protection from flea bites when visiting flea-infested areas. Despite insecticide resistance being reported in cat and rat fleas, insecticides form the basis of flea control. Insecticides can be liberally applied to floors of houses and to rodent burrows and runways. Insecticidal fogs or aerosols have sometimes been used to fumigate buildings. When controlling fleas in urban outbreaks of plague and endemic (murine) typhus, rodenticides should be used to kill rat populations; however, if fast-acting 'one-dose' rodenticides are employed, these should only be applied several days after insecticide usage – otherwise fleas leaving dead rats will switch their attention to humans.

Cat fleas can be killed by insecticidal spraying of houses, carefully applying insecticides to cats or using insecticide-impregnated cat collars. Alternatively, insecticides formulated as 'spot-on' can be applied to the cat's skin. These are absorbed into the cat's blood and so poison blood-feeding fleas. Insect growth regulators (IGRs) can be applied topically to cats or given orally and, through the production of non-viable eggs, give flea control for 4–6 weeks.

Selected bibliography
Hinkle, N.C., Koehler, P.G. and Patterson, R.S. (1995) Residual effectiveness of insect

growth regulators applied to carpet for control of cat flea (Siphonaptera: Pulicidae) larvae. *Journal of Economic Entomology* 88, 903–906.

Holland, G.P. (1964) Evolution, classification, and host relationships of Siphonaptera. *Annual Review of Entomology* 9, 123–146.

Rothschild, M. (1975) Recent advances in our knowledge of the order Siphonaptera. *Annual Review of Entomology* 20, 241–259.

Rust, M.K. and Dryden, M.W. (1997) The biology, ecology, and management of the cat flea. *Annual Review of Entomology* 42, 451–473.

Traub, R. and Starcke, M. (eds) (1980) *Fleas. Proceedings of the International Conference on Fleas, Ashton Wold, Peterborough, UK, 21–25 June 1977.* Balkema, Rotterdam, 420 pp.

Whitely, H.E. (1987) Flea-control, tips from experts. *Veterinary Medicine* 82, 913–916.

Flies (Diptera)

M.W. Service

There are possibly 150,000 species of flies; they have an almost worldwide distribution. Except for a few wingless species, such as the sheep ked (*Melophagus ovinus* (see Hippoboscids)) flies have just one pair of membranous wings; the hind-wings are replaced by a pair of balancing knob-like structures called halteres. There are two suborders of the Diptera: the Nematocera, comprising small and slender-bodied flies, such as mosquitoes, biting midges, simuliid black-flies and phlebotomine sand-flies, and the suborder Brachycera, which includes the larger more robust flies, such as house-flies, bluebottles, greenbottles, tsetse-flies and horse-flies. Although mosquitoes are technically flies, the term fly is usually reserved for species in the suborder Brachycera. Separate entries in the encyclopedia are given to flies belonging to the Nematocera, such as mosquitoes and simuliid black-flies, which transmit medical or veterinary infections. Here the role of the stouter-built brachyceran flies belonging to the infraorder Muscomorpha, formerly called Cyclorrhapha, in mechanically transmitting infections is considered. The flies concerned with such transmission are mainly house-flies, belonging to the family Muscidae, and greenbottles and bluebottles (blow-flies) in the family Calliphoridae.

Biology
House-flies (Muscidae)

There are about 66 species of flies in the genus *Musca*, the most common of which is *Musca domestica*, the house-fly, which occurs more or less throughout the world. In some parts of Africa, Asia and the Pacific areas, another similar species, called *Musca sorbens*, is a great nuisance. The biology of the two species is almost identical and can be summarized as follows.

Female house-flies lay their eggs on a variety of materials, such as freshly prepared or waste foods from kitchens and hotels, household rubbish, decomposing organic debris found in rubbish dumps, animal and human faeces and animal feeds. Eggs can hatch within 6–12 h, but this period is extended in cool weather. The resultant larvae, called maggots, are whitish, cylindrical and without legs. They feed on liquid food resulting from decomposing and decaying organic matter. There are three distinct larval instars. In hot weather the larval period can be as short as 3–5 days, but in cooler conditions it is often 7–10 days, and sometimes can be as long as about 24 days. The third-instar larva measures about 8–14 mm, and its whitish skin turns brown and hardens to form a barrel-shaped puparium (Fig. 1). In warm weather the puparial period lasts 3–5 days, but during cooler weather can be 7–14 days.

Developmental time from egg to adult fly is about 49 days at 16°C, 25 days at 20°C, 16 days at 25°C, 10–12 days at 30°C and 8–10 days at 35°C. Very occasionally the period from egg to adult can be just a week. Adult flies avoid direct sunlight and prefer to shelter in buildings occupied by humans or animals. They frequently regurgitate their food and defecate at random, resulting in

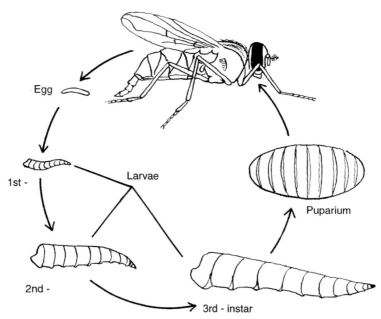

Egg

1st -

Larvae

Puparium

2nd -

3rd - instar

Fig. 1.   Life cycle of flies, such as house-flies (*Musca* species) and blow-flies (*Lucilia, Calliphora* species) (modified from M.W. Service (2000) *Medical Entomology for Students*, Cambridge University Press, Cambridge).

unsightly 'fly spots' on windows and walls, etc. Although adults can fly up to 5 km, most flies remain within about a 500 m radius of their larval habitats. Adults of *M. sorbens* frequent the face more often than do typical house-flies (*M. domestica*).

Blow-flies (Calliphoridae)

The so-called greenbottles (*Lucilia* species) and bluebottles (*Calliphora* species) are often referred to collectively as blow-flies. The adults are considerably larger than house-flies and, as to be expected, green-bottles have a metallic or coppery green body, while in bluebottles the body is dull metallic-bluish or bluish-black. Green-bottles occur in most areas of the world, the commonest species being *Lucilia* (= *Phoenicia*) *sericata*. Bluebottles have a more or less worldwide distribution, although they are more common in north-ern temperate regions than in tropical or southern temperate areas.

The biology of both greenbottles and bluebottles is very similar to that of house-flies, the developmental stages being the eggs, larvae (maggots), puparia and adults. Eggs are laid on meat, fish and carrion and also on or near festering, often foul-smelling, wounds of mammals. The life cycle usually takes 12–24 days, depend-ing mainly on temperature. Adults are common in houses and around slaughter-houses, piggeries, butcher's shops and local markets where fish and meat are uncovered.

Diseases

House-flies are involved in the cyclical transmission of a number of filarial parasites to livestock, such as *Habronema muscae* and *Draschia megastoma* to cattle and horses (see Habronemiasis), *Parafilaria bovicola* to cattle and *Parafilaria multi-papillosa* to equines (see Parafilariasis), *Stephanofilaria assamensis* to cattle (see Stephanofilariasis) and *Thelazia callipaeda* to cattle and humans (see Thelaziasis). *Phormia* species, sometimes called black blowflies and belonging to the family Calliphoridae, are vectors of rabbit haemor-rhagic disease (see entry).

In addition, because house-flies, and related flies, almost indiscriminately visit faeces, garbage, festering wounds and food, they have the potential to mechanically transmit a variety of pathogens to humans and animals. The principal routes of transmission are as follows.

1. By flies' contaminated feet, body hairs and mouthparts. However, most pathogens remain viable on flies for less than 24 h and there are usually too few organisms to cause direct transmission, except possibly with *Shigella*. The human infective dose for viral and bacterial infections is often about 10^5–10^6 organisms. However, if pathogens are first transferred to food, they may multiply and reach sufficient numbers for an infective dose (this does not apply to viruses or most rickettsiae, as they require a host cell for replication).

2. By flies' frequently regurgitating their stomach contents on food during feeding.

3. Probably the most important route of transmission is through flies' defecating on food.

Over 100 different pathogens have been recorded from house-flies, of which at least 65 have been shown to be mechanically transmitted to a greater or lesser extent, and these include the following.

- *Viruses.* Coxsackie, infectious hepatitis, myxomatosis, poliomyelitis.
- *Bacteria.* Anthrax (*Bacillus anthracis*), bovine mastitis, *Campylobacter*, cholera (*Vibrio cholerae*), bacterial conjunctivitis (pink-eye), bovine infective keratitis, dysenteries (*Shigella* species), enterotoxic *Escherichia coli* (ETEC), haemolytic streptococci, leprosy (*Mycobacterium leprae*), tropical ulcers, typhoids (*Salmonella typhi*) and paratyphoids (*Salmonella paratyphi*), *Staphylococcus aureus*, trachoma (*Chlamydia trachomatis*), yaws (*Treponema pertenue*).
- *Rickettsiae. Coxiella burnetii.*
- *Protozoans.* Amoebic dysenteries (*Entamoeba histolytica, Giardi lamblia*).

The recovery of pathogens from flies does not prove that they can transmit infections, or, if they do, how important they are in the spread of diseases. This is because there are usually more direct routes, such as faeces-contaminated hands and improperly cleaned food utensils. However, it has often been noted that seasonal increases in fly populations are accompanied by outbreaks of diarrhoeal diseases. An experiment over 50 years ago reported that, in a town in Texas which had been sprayed with DDT to control house-flies, the incidence of acute diarrhoeal infection in children caused by *Shigella* declined, although there was no significant reduction in diarrhoea due to *Salmonella*. In a similar town left unsprayed, there was no such reduction in disease. It is interesting to note that only about 100 *Shigella* bacteria can result in a human infection, but many more are required to establish a *Salmonella* infection.

More recent trials involving controlling house-flies appear to support the belief that under certain circumstances flies may be important in disease transmission. For example, when in 1988 attractant traps were used to control house-fly numbers in an Israeli army camp there was a reduction in *Shigella* infections and also apparently ETEC infections. In 1995 and 1996 when breeding sites in Pakistan villages were sprayed with insecticides, fly populations decreased by 97% and the incidence of childhood diarrhoea decreased by 23%. Similarly, ultra-low-volume (ULV) spraying with deltamethrin in The Gambia caused an 87% reduction in fly densities, and the prevalence of trachoma was four times lower in villages that had been sprayed compared with unsprayed villages. Moreover, diarrhoea in children was reduced by 25%. Other, even more recent, investigations in The Gambia have suggested that, because of the frequency of *M. sorbens* landing on the eyes of children, this fly may be a vector of trachoma.

It now seems that house-flies, and probably other common synanthropic flies, such as blow-flies, contribute to disease transmission to humans, and probably also to livestock.

Control

Larvae

Garbage and refuse heaps, manure piles, the insides of dustbins and other known or suspected larval breeding sites can be sprayed with insecticides to kill the maggots (larvae). But large volumes are often needed to penetrate the surface layers and reach the larvae.

Adults

Flies, together with other obnoxious insects, can be prevented from entering buildings by placing plastic-mesh screens over doors, windows and other openings, but screening becomes ineffective unless it is well maintained and any damage is repaired. The well-known practice of placing curtains made of numerous, often coloured, vertical strips of plastic or beads in doorways is a simple but effective way of excluding flies. Ultraviolet light traps are often used to kill flies entering restaurants, food stores and dairies. Flies attracted to the traps are electrocuted on entering them by contact with an electric grid.

Environmental sanitation can be adopted to reduce flies, such as placing household and farm refuse in plastic bags or in bins with tight-fitting lids, ensuring that dustbins are emptied once or twice a week and preventing the accumulation of decaying vegetable or animal matter and other rubbish. Refuse should be placed in pits and covered daily with a 15 cm layer of earth and, when full, covered with 60 cm of compacted earth to prevent rats from digging up buried garbage.

Residual insecticides can be sprayed on the interior walls, doors and ceilings of animal shelters and houses; such treatments should remain effective in killing adult flies for 1–2 months. Exterior walls of dairies and piggeries can also be sprayed, but the duration of effectiveness will depend on whether deposits are washed off by rain. Outdoor applications of insecticidal aerosols from ground-based spraying machines or aerial ULV spraying can give relief from flies

around dairies, cattle markets and recreational areas – but the effects are short-lived.

Cords or rope strips soaked in insecticides, and preferably dyed red to alert people of their toxic nature, can be hung up in dairies and cowsheds to kill flies landing on them. Dichlorvos (DDVP)-impregnated resin strips, often sold as Vapona strips (in some countries, however, they are no longer available), are commonly used in houses, hotel kitchens, restaurants and hospitals. Their fumigant effect can last for 2–3 months. Commercially available sticky tapes (flypapers) incorporating sugar as an attractant can be relatively effective, although unsightly, in attracting and catching flies.

Liquid or solid baits incorporating an attractant, such as sugar, and insecticides are sometimes used to control house-flies. Sometimes the house-fly sex pheromone called muscalure is added to baits to enhance their attractiveness.

Selected bibliography

Chavasse, D.C., Shier, R.P., Murphy, O.A., Huttly, S.R.A., Cousens, S.N. and Akhtar, T. (1999) Impact of fly control on childhood diarrhoea in Pakistan: community-randomised trial. *The Lancet* 353, 22–25.

Cohen, D., Green, M., Block, C., Slepon, R., Ambar, R., Wasserman, S.S. and Levine, M.M. (1991) Reduction of transmission of shigellosis by control of houseflies (*Musca domestica*). *The Lancet* 337, 993–997.

Echeverra, P., Harrison, B.A., Tirapat, C. and McFarland, A. (1983) Flies as a source of enteric pathogens in a rural village in Thailand. *Applied and Environmental Biology* 46, 32–36.

Emerson, P.M., Lindsay, S.W., Walraven, G.E.L., Faal, H., Bøgh, C., Lowe, K. and Bailey, R.L. (1999) Effect of fly control on trachoma and diarrhoea. *The Lancet* 353, 1401–1403.

Emerson, P.M., Bailey, R.L., Olaimatu, O.S., Walraven, G.E.L. and Lindsay, S.W. (2000) Transmission ecology of the fly *Musca sorbens*, a putative vector of trachoma. *Transaction of the Royal Society of Tropical Medicine and Hygiene* 94, 28–32.

Fischer, O. (1999) The importance of Diptera for transmission, spreading and survival of agents of some bacterial and fungal diseases in humans and animals. *Veterinarni Medica* 144, 133–160.

Foil, L.D. and Gorham, J.R. (2000) Mechanical transmission of disease agents by arthropods. In: Eldridge, B.F. and Edman, J.D. (eds) *Medical Entomology. A Textbook on Public Health and Veterinary Problems Caused by Arthropods.* Kluwer Academic Publishers, Dordrecht, pp. 461–514.

Greenberg, B. (1971) *Flies and Disease*, Vol. 1, *Ecology, Classification and Biotic Associations.* Princeton University Press, Princeton, New Jersey, 856 pp.

Greenberg, B. (1973) *Flies and Disease*, Vol. 2, *Biology and Disease Transmission.* Princeton University Press, Princeton, New Jersey, 447 pp.

Keiding, J. (1986) The house-fly: biology and control. WHO/VBC/86.937, World Health Organization mimeographed document, Geneva, 63 pp.

Levine, O.S. and Levine, M.M. (1991) Houseflies (*Musca domestica*) as mechanical vectors of shigellosis. *Review of Infectious Diseases* 13, 688–696.

Olsen, R.A. (1998) Regulatory action criteria for filth and other extraneous materials: III. Review of flies and foodborne entereic diseases. *Regulatory Toxicology and Pharmacology* 28, 199–211.

Skidmore, P. (1985) *The Biology of the Muscidae of the World.* W. Junk, Dordrecht, 550 pp.

Flinders Island spotted fever *see* **Tick-borne typhuses**.

Fortuna disease *see* **Theilerioses**.

Fowl pox

Antony J. Della-Porta

Fowl pox is an infection of poultry and wild birds caused by avipoxviruses of the family Poxviridae.

Avian pox is a common viral disease of poultry and of wild birds. These viruses have infected over 60 species of birds in 20 families. Of the domestic bird species, those that are infected with poxviruses include chickens, turkeys, Pigeons (*Columba livia*) and Canaries (*Serinus canaria*). The disease has a worldwide distribution. Fowl pox was originally used to describe poxvirus infections of all avian species but more recently has been used to refer to poxvirus infections of chickens. There are two forms of the disease: a cutaneous form, characterized by proliferative skin lesions, and the diphtheritic form, characterized by lesions in the respiratory tract.

Distribution

Fowl pox has a worldwide distribution. The incidence of the disease is variable because of differences in management and hygiene or the use of vaccination to limit infection. It is a relative slow-spreading disease.

Virus

Fowlpox virus is the type species of the *Avipoxvirus* genus in the family Poxviridae (subfamily Chondropoxvirinae). The virion is enveloped and contains one molecule of double-stranded DNA of a total genome length of between 130,000 and 150,000 nucleotides (EMBL/GenBank accession number X17202/D00295). The virus multiplies in the cytoplasm of epithelial cells, with the formation of large intracytoplasmic inclusion bodies (Bollinger bodies), which contain smaller elementary bodies (Borrel bodies).

Clinical symptoms

The cutaneous form of the disease is characterized by the appearance of nodular lesions on various parts of the bare skin of the bird. The disease can be seen as a mild form with only small focal lesions, usually on the wattles and comb. It can also be seen as a severe form, where lesions can occur on any part of the body; they may be small and discrete or they may coalesce to cover large areas. The surface of these lesions is moist only for a short period of time before it dries and forms rough yellow-brown scabs. Removal of such lesions before the scab is completely dry can leave behind a haemorrhagic moist surface. When the scab dries, it will fall off to leave a scar.

In the diphtheritic form, the lesions occur mainly around the mucous membranes in the mouth, nostrils, pharynx, oesophagus, larynx and trachea. The bird has difficulty feeding if the lesions are in the mouth. Breathing becomes difficult if the lesions are in the trachea, and the clinical signs may appear similar to those of infectious laryngotracheitis (ILT). In commercial poultry, fowl pox and turkey pox can cause serious economic loss. Egg production is reduced in layers and the growth of young chickens is retarded. In birds with the diphtheritic form involving the respiratory tract, mortality can be as high as 50%.

Diagnosis

There are two forms of fowl pox seen in birds, and these relate to the route of infection. The cutaneous form is transmitted by contact with infected lesion material or by virus-contaminated insect mouthparts. The lesions are typical of poxviruses and must be confirmed by histology (the presence of cytoplasmic inclusions) or by virus isolation. The respiratory or diphtheritic form of the disease must be differentiated from ILT, an infection caused by a herpesvirus.

Virus identification

Smear technique for fowl pox
Elemental bodies (Borrel bodies) can be detected in smears prepared from lesions and stained with Wright's stain or by the Gimenez method.

Histology
Tissue sections from lesions, stained with haematoxylin and eosin, show cytoplasmic inclusions. The main lesion is hyperplasia of the epithelium and enlargement of cells, with associated inflammatory changes. Characteristic eosinophilic A-type cytoplasmic inclusion bodies (Bollinger bodies) are observable by light microscopy. These bodies can also be seen using acridine orange or Giemsa's stains. The specific nature of these

bodies can be demonstrated using fluorescent antibodies or by immunoperoxidase, using a specific anti-fowlpox virus serum.

Electron microscopy
Electron microscopy can be used to demonstrate the typical morphology of the virus by negative staining or by thin section. Fowlpox virus, the type species of the _Avipoxvirus_ genus, is a brick-shaped or rectangular virus, with dimensions of around 250 nm × 354 nm, with what appears to be a random distribution of surface tubules. In thin section, the virion consists of an electron-dense, centrally located, biconcave core or nucleoid, with two lateral bodies in each cavity and surrounded by an envelope.

Virus isolation
BIRD INOCULATIONS Inoculations of susceptible birds by applying a suspension of lesion material to the scarified comb or the denuded feather follicles of the thigh, or by the wing-stick method. The lesions usually develop within 5–7 days, giving cutaneous lesions typical of poxviruses.

IN CHICKEN EMBRYOS Nine to 12-day-old embryonated chicken eggs are inoculated on to the chorioallantoic membrane (CAM), using standard CAM inoculation techniques. Pocks of a diffuse or focal nature develop on the membrane after incubation of the embryos for 4–7 days at 37°C.

IN CELL CULTURE A range of primary chicken cells (chicken embryo fibroblasts, kidney or dermis) or the continuous Japanese quail cell line, QT35, can be used to grow fowlpox virus. Some isolates may require adaptation to be grown in these cells. Isolation in cell lines is not, however, used in primary identification of fowlpox virus.

Restriction endonuclease mapping
Restriction endonuclease mapping has been applied to distinguish _Avipoxvirus_ genus members in a range of species of birds. The genomes of fowl- and pigeon poxvirus isolates, analysed using _Bam_HI and _Hind_III endonucleases, were found to be very similar, with only one or two bands different.

Polymerase chain reaction (PCR) identification

Using specific DNA primers, PCR has been useful for the detection and identification of fowlpox virus. This technique can detect small qualities of virus and distinguish fowlpox from other avian poxviruses.

Serological tests

Virus neutralization

Virus neutralization in chick embryos or cell culture may be used for antibody determination. It is rarely used in diagnostic testing because of the time it takes and the cost. Avian poxviruses are immunogenically distinct, although varying levels of cross-reactivity exists. Virus neutralization may be used to identify virus isolates.

Agar gel immunodiffusion

Immunodiffusion may be used for differential identification of poxviruses or their antisera. It is of no value for quantifying antibody responses.

Passive haemagglutination

A passive haemagglutination assay has been developed for fowl pox and is of use for the quantification of antibody levels in serum.

Enzyme-linked immunosorbent assay (ELISA)

An ELISA can be used for the quantification of antibody levels in serum. It is probably the assay of preference in most laboratories that have adopted ELISAs as the standard serological technique for antibody quantification.

Transmission

Individuals handling birds at the time of vaccination may carry virus on their hands or clothes and may inadvertently infect birds by transferring it to lesions on the skin or depositing it in the eyes. If the bird-holding facility is contaminated, virus in feathers or dried scabs can generate an aerosol that can infect the birds via the respiratory tract and/or through cutaneous lesions.

Mosquitoes have been shown to be able to transmit the virus to birds following feeding on infected animals. The species that have been associated with this transmission include *Aedes aegypti*, *Aedes vexans*, *Ochlerotatus*[1] *stimulans*, *Anopheles maculipennis*, *Culex nigripalpus*, *Culex pipiens*, *Culex quinquefasciatus*, *Culex tarsalis*, *Culiseta annulata* and *Wyeomyia vanduzeei*. The stable-fly, *Stomoxys calcitrans*, has also been incriminated as a vector. Virus has also been shown to be transmitted by the mite *Dermanyssus gallinae*. The sticktight flea, *Echidnophaga gallinacea*, has also been associated with possible transmission of fowl pox virus. Arthropod transmission is also undoubtedly associated with transmission of reticuloendotheliosis (RE) virus, because of its integration in the fowlpox genome. In all instances transmission involving arthropods is mechanical, by contamination with the vector's mouthparts; there is no replication of the virus in the vector.

Treatment

It is difficult to eliminate fowlpox virus from the environment because of its high resistance to chemical and physical treatments. When desiccated, the virus shows remarkable resistance. It can survive in dried scabs for periods from months to years. For this reason, vaccination is recommended where fowl pox is endemic or on premises where infection has been diagnosed.

There is no treatment for birds infected with avian poxviruses. Care should be taken to exercise good husbandry of the birds and to reduce environmental stress.

Control

Modified live fowl- or pigeon pox virus vaccines are available commercially. These should be used where fowlpox is endemic or where it occurred the previous year.

The immune status of the birds needs to be taken into consideration when administering the vaccine. If the birds have recently come from a vaccinated flock or one in which there was a recent fowl pox infection, the vaccination should be delayed until the immunity has waned. The vaccination is applied using the wing-stab method of vaccination.

It has recently been reported that there is an association between vaccination of flocks with fowl pox vaccine and the occurrence of reticuleoendotheliosis in the flock. Originally it was suggested that the vaccine might have been contaminated with RE virus, but recent studies show that the RE virus genome has been integrated into the fowl pox genome. Fowlpox virus carrying RE provirus has a global distribution and RE virus seems to be restricted to fowlpox virus and is not present in other avipox viruses of non-domestic poultry (D. Boyle, personal communication).

Note

[1]   *Ochlerotatus* was formerly a subgenus of *Aedes.*

Selected bibliography

Akey, B.L., Nayar, J.K. and Forrester, D.J. (1981) Avian pox in Florida wild turkeys: *Culex nigripalpus* and *Wyeomyia vanduzeei* as experimental vectors. *Journal of Wildlife Diseases* 17, 597–599.

Fadly, A.M., Witter, R.L., Smith, E.J., Silva, R.F., Reed, W.M., Hoerr, F.J. and Putnam, M.R. (1996) An outbreak of lymphomas in commercial broiler breeder chickens vaccinated with a fowlpox vaccine contaminated with reticuloendotheliosis virus. *Avian Diseases* 25, 35–47.

OIE (1996) Fowl pox. In: *Manual of Standards for Diagnostic Tests and Vaccines*, 3rd edn. Office International des Epizootics, Paris, pp. 701–705.

Tripathy, D.N. and Hanson, L.E. (1976) A smear technique for staining elementary bodies of fowl pox. *Avian Diseases* 20, 609–610.

Tripathy, D.N. and Reed, W.N. (1998) Pox. In: Calnek, B.W., Barnes, H.J., Beard, C.W., McDougald, L.R and Saif, Y.M. (eds) *Diseases of Poultry*, 10th edn. Iowa State University Press, Ames, Iowa, pp. 643–659.

Francisella tularensis see **Tularaemia.**

Gad-flies *see* **Horse-flies.**

Gall-sickness *see* **Anaplasmosis.**

Gan Gan virus

John S. Mackenzie

Infections of humans with Gan Gan virus

Gan Gan (GG) virus is a mosquito-borne, unassigned member of the family Bunyaviridae. It was first isolated in 1969 from *Ochlerotatus*[1] *vigilax* mosquitoes trapped at the Gan Gan Army camp at Nelson Bay in the sand-dunes and swamp country of the Port Stephens Peninsula of New South Wales.

Distribution

Gan Gan virus has been obtained from mosquitoes collected in New South Wales and Queensland.

Virus

Gan Gan virus has been grouped with three other antigenically related viruses in the Mapputta antigenic group. This group comprises two other Australian viruses, Trubanaman virus (see entry) and Mapputta virus, and a virus from Papua New Guinea, Maprik virus.

Clinical symptoms and pathogenesis

Only three cases of acute polyarthalgia or polyarthritis disease due to infection with GG virus have been recognized. All three cases were observed during a widespread outbreak of epidemic polyarthritis due to Ross River virus in 1983–1984, but they were negative serologically to Ross River virus (see entry). The three patients lived at Griffith in the Murrambidgee irrigation area of New South Wales, and suffered acute febrile illnesses, with malaise, myalgia, polyarthralgia or polyarthritis with or without sore eyes or rash. These were self-limiting illnesses of several days' duration, with complete recovery. Antibodies to GG virus were found in paired sera.

Diagnosis

Diagnosis is made serologically by standard serological techniques, such as immunoglobulin M (IgM) capture enzyme-linked immunosorbent assay (ELISA), with confirmation by neutralization tests.

Transmission

Gan Gan virus has been isolated from *Ochlerotatus vigilax* in New South Wales, and from *Ochlerotatus theobaldi theobaldi*, *Ochlerotatus theobaldi eidsvoldensis* and *Culex annulirostris* in Queensland. The role of these species in transmission cycles is not known.

Ecology

Little is known about the ecology of GG virus. It is believed that the vertebrate hosts of the virus are probably terrestrial animals. Human infections appear to be widespread in New South Wales, with an overall prevalence of 4.7%, but with some pockets of higher prevalence rates.

Note

[1]   *Ochlerotatus* was formerly a subgenus of *Aedes*.

Selected bibliography

Boughton, C.R., Hawkes, R.A. and Naim, H.M. (1990) Arbovirus infection in humans in NSW: seroprevalence and pathogenicity of certain Australian bunyaviruses. *Australia and New Zealand Journal of Medicine* 20, 51–55.

Newton, S.E., Short, N.J., Irving, A.M. and Dalgarno, L. (1983) The Mapputta group of arboviruses: ultrastructural and molecular studies which place the group in the *Bunyavirus* genus of the family Bunyaviridae. *Australian Journal of*

Experimental Biology and Medical Science 61, 201–217.

Vale, T.G., Carter, I.W., McPhie, K.A., James, G.S. and Cloonan, M.J. (1986) Human arbovirus infections along the South Coast of New South Wales. *Australian Journal of Experimental Biology and Medical Science* 64, 307–309.

Ganjam virus *see* **Nairobi sheep disease.**

Germiston virus

Michèle Bouloy

Germiston (GER) virus, a member of the Bunyaviridae family and the genus *Bunyavirus,* was isolated for the first time by R.H. Kokernot and colleagues from mosquitoes collected in South Africa near the town of Germiston. This virus infects humans but, like many viruses of this family, it causes only mild febrile illness. It also infects wild and domestic animals, as revealed by virus isolations or by the presence of specific antibodies. However, the circulation of GER virus has not been reported to be responsible for any large epidemics or epizootics and as a consequence it has no great social and economic impact. Whereas very little information on the epidemiology of the virus has been reported during the last 20 years, the molecular organization of the particle and its genome has been deciphered.

Human infections
Distribution

The virus is endemic in southern Africa, particularly in South Africa, Angola, Botswana, Zimbabwe and Mozambique. Strains of GER virus have also been isolated in Kenya and Uganda.

Virus

As are all members of the Bunyaviridae, GER virus is a spherical particle approximately 100 nm in diameter, composed of an envelope with protruding spikes and three internal circular and helical nucleocapsid structures. These ribonucleoproteins consist of three single-stranded RNA molecules (L, M, S, for large, medium and small, respectively) forming the tripartite genome, associated with many copies of the N nucleoprotein and a few molecules of L protein, the RNA-dependent RNA polymerase. A characteristic feature of the viruses of the genus *Bunyavirus* is the fact that the genome segments possess the 3′ terminal consensus nucleotides UCAUCACA . . ., which are complementary to the 5′ terminal sequences and form panhandle structures. These sequences are identified at the termini of the GER virus genome.

The genome is of negative polarity. The L segment (approximately 7000 nucleotides) codes for the L protein, the M segment (4534 nucleotides) for the precursor to the envelope glycoproteins and the S segment (980 nucleotides) for the N protein (26 kDa) and for a non-structural protein NSs (11 kDa) from two overlapping open-reading frames. The M segment messenger (mRNA) synthesizes a polypeptide precursor (162 kDa), which is cleaved co-translationally and generates, in this order, the envelope glycoprotein G1 (98 kDa), the NSm (16 kDa) protein and the glycoprotein G2 (37 kDa). The role of the non-structural proteins NSm and NSs is still unknown. The whole replication cycle occurs in the cytoplasm of infected cells. During transcription, three subgenomic mRNAs are synthesized: they are slightly shorter than their corresponding templates because transcriptase terminates synthesis some 60–100 nucleotides before the end of the template is reached. Messenger RNAs lack poly-A at their 3′ ends and possess a 5′ methylated cap and 10–18 additional non-viral nucleotides derived from cellular RNAs, which are used to initiate the mRNA synthesis with a cap-snatching mechanism, like that of influenza virus. Morphogenesis occurs by budding through the membranes of the Golgi complex.

In an attempt to gain a picture of bunyavirus evolution, sequences of several viruses of the Bunyamwera, California and Simbu serogroups have been analysed. The resulting dendrogram (Fig. 1) shows that the viruses are classified into three groups, confirming earlier classification using data of complement fixation and other tests.

However, whereas GER virus (as well as Guaroa and Kairi viruses) was distinct from the viruses of the Bunyamwera complex by complement fixation, it was shown to belong to the complex when analysed by the neutralization test. This suggests that the segmented genome of GER virus may result

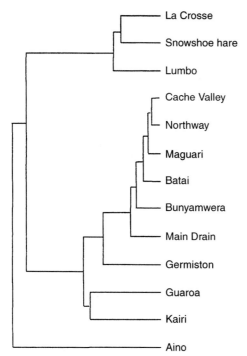

Fig. 1. Relationships between the N protein sequences of bunyaviruses. The dendrogram was generated by the PILEUP program in the UWGCG package. The distance along the axis is proportional to the similarity between sequences. (Adapted from Dunn, E.F., Pritlove, D.C. and Elliott, R.M. (1994) *Journal of General Virology* 75, 597–608.)

from reassortment with ancestral viruses of different origins.

Clinical symptoms
As with other viruses of the genus, the most frequent symptoms of GER virus infection are fever, rash and headache. Two human cases occurred from laboratory contamination: the disease was mild and of brief duration (37 h to 3 days).

Diagnosis
When an infection with GER virus, or any other virus, is suspected, the method of choice for diagnosis is virus isolation. Germiston infects mice and most of the strains were isolated after intracerebral inoculation of the biological specimens to suckling mice, which develop encephalitis and die within a few days. At present, there is a tendency to use cell cultures, such as VERO, LLC-MK2 or BHK-21, which are susceptible to the virus and exhibit cyto-pathic effect. Mosquito cells (C6/36 or AP61 derived from *Aedes albopictus* and *Aedes pseudoscutellaris*, respectively) may also be used for isolation but, in contrast to mammalian cells, virus infection does not produce any cytopathic effect.

Although there are serological cross-reactions between viruses of the Bunyamwera group, identification of viruses by complement fixation and neutralization tests have been classically used as sero-logical methods. Nowadays, enzyme-linked immunosorbent assays (ELISA) have been established for the detection of immuno-globulin G (IgG) and IgM antibodies against many arboviruses.

As molecular diagnosis has been developed for many viruses, reverse transcription–polymerase chain reactions (RT-PCR) with appropriate primers can be used to detect the presence of the viral genome.

Transmission
Germiston virus has been repeatedly iso-lated from the culicine mosquito *Culex rubinotus* in South Africa, Zimbabwe, Mozambique, Kenya and Uganda. It seems likely that transovarial transmission occurs in this species.

Animal infections

As suggested by the presence of neutralizing antibodies, livestock such as goats, sheep and cattle, as well as horses, can be infected by GER virus. A high seroprevalence to GER virus was also reported in wild rodents (e.g. Nile rat (*Arvicanthis niloticus*), Black rat (*Rattus rattus*), Brush-furred rats (*Lophuromys sikapusi*, *Lophuromys flavopunctatus*), Water or Marsh rat (*Dasymys incomtus*)) and the Large grey mongoose (*Herpestes ichneumon*). A transmission cycle involving rodents and *C. rubinotus* is likely to be responsible for the maintenance of virus in nature.

Laboratory rodents (mice and hamsters) are sensitive to the virus: Germiston virus causes death of weaned mice inoculated by the peripheral route and sentinel hamsters have been used successfully to isolate strains of GER virus in Mozambique and South Africa.

Monkeys experimentally infected develop viraemia but exhibit mild disease or inapparent infections.

Treatment and control

No treatment or vaccine for human or veterinary use is available. Because of the absence of epidemics, the low pathogenicity and the low economic impact, no control measures against the virus have been considered.

Selected bibliography

Gonzalez, J.P. and Georges, A.-J. (1986) Bunyaviral fevers: Bunyamwera, Ilesha, Germiston, Bwamba and Tataguine. In: Monath, T.P. (ed.) *The Arboviruses: Epidemiology and Ecology*, Vol. II. CRC Press, Boca Raton, Florida, pp. 87–98.

Kokernot, R.H., Smithburn, K.C., Paterson, H.E. and McIntosh, B.M. (1960) Isolation of Germiston virus, a hitherto unknown agent, from culicine mosquitoes, and a report of infection in two laboratory workers. *American Journal of Tropical Medicine and Hygiene* 9, 62–69.

Okuno, T. (1961) Immunological studies relating two recently isolated viruses, Germiston virus from South Africa and Ilesha virus from West Africa, to the Bunyamwera group. *American Journal of Tropical Medicine and Hygiene* 10, 223–226.

Getah virus

T. Kumanomido

Distribution

The virus was initially isolated from *Culex gelidus* mosquitoes in Malaysia in 1955 but has since been isolated from mosquitoes in other Asian countries, Australia and north-eastern Russia. The first outbreaks of disease caused by Getah (GET) virus occurred among racehorses in Japan in 1978. Since then, further research has shown that GET virus is an equine pathogen.

Aetiological agent

Getah virus is a member of the Semliki Forest (SF) (see entry) antigenic complex, family Togaviridae, genus *Alphavirus*. It is a typical alphavirus and is readily propagated in cell culture from a wide variety of species lines, including mosquito cells.

Antigenicity of the virus is best revealed by virus neutralization (VN) tests, but haemagglutination inhibition (HI) and complement fixation (CF) tests are also useful for preliminary group and complex assignment. Cross-reactivity has been demonstrated among the four SF complex viruses: Getah, Sagiyama, Bebaru and Ross River viruses (see Ross River virus). Getah viruses from different geographical areas differ slightly but cluster by area, although there is no identity even among strains in the same locality in the same year. Plaque variants and mutants of GET virus are isolated in many cell cultures.

The genome of GET virus is single-stranded RNA (ssRNA) of positive polarity, containing approximately 12,000 nucleotides. In the 3′ untranslated region, GET and Ross River viruses share considerable sequence homology. Serological surveys have detected antibodies to GET virus in humans, horses, pigs and a variety of other species in Malaysia, Japan and several Australasian countries. Antibodies in humans vary regionally, from 1.2–9% in Japan, to 10.3% on Hainan island, China, and 7% (HI) in eastern Siberia, to 41–54% among older people in north-eastern Australia (not implicated in human disease). In animals, high antibody prevalences (20–80%) have been found in pigs and in horses, although these differ by regions, years and ages. These findings suggest that GET virus is widespread, in particular, infecting pigs and horses, which are highly susceptible to GET virus.

Pathogenicity of GET virus is relatively mild and limited to horses and pigs. Getah virus prevalence may occur throughout the year in the tropical climates, but seasonally, between summer and autumn in temperate climates.

Incidence of disease

The first outbreaks of Getah disease occurred among race horses during the autumn at different habitats in training centres and farms in the suburbs of Tokyo. A total of 884 of 2661 (33.2%) racehorses suffered from pyrexia, limb oedema and rash. The morbidity in one epizootic site was 722/1903 (37.9%) during a 43-day period. Getah virus strains MI-110 and Sakai were isolated from plasma and nasal swabs from ill horses. Recurrence of the disease in horses occurred sporadically in western Japan in 1979 and 1983. A similar outbreak of disease, characterized by depression, anorexia, fever, limb oedema and lymphocytopenia, occurred on a thoroughbred farm in India in 1990; serological studies indicated that the outbreak was caused by GET virus.

Clinical symptoms

Getah virus infection in horses is characterized by a complex of pyrexia, rash (Fig. 1), and oedema of the limbs, affecting approximately 80%, 50% and 43% of the horses, respectively. Complete recovery follows

7–10 days after onset. Major histological changes observed in infected horses suggest immunoreactive responses and imply that the rash, which appears closely related in time with development of neutralizing antibody, may be caused by anaphylactic or immune complex-mediated hypersensitivity. Occasionally, slight perivascular cuffing with mononuclear cells in the cerebrum and small haemorrhagic foci in the spinal cord are detectable in horses infected experimentally, suggesting that the central nervous system may be involved to a certain extent, although not implicated clinically. Getah virus has been recovered from blood plasma, nasal mucous membrane, lung, spleen, spinal cord, bone marrow and various lymph nodes of diseased horses. Highest virus titres were demonstrated in axillary ($10^{3.5}$ tissue culture infective dose ($TCID_{50}$) g^{-1}) and inguinal lymph nodes ($10^{6.5}$ $TCID_{50}$ g^{-1}) in the acute stage.

Pigs are also highly susceptible to the virus. However, adult pigs are not apparently infected but produce a relatively high titre of prolonged viraemia and antibody. Getah virus may occasionally cause deaths in newborn piglets or in fetuses by transplacental infection. Dead fetuses are frequently observed in pregnant sows infected with Japanese encephalitis (JE) virus (see entry), which is widely distributed in Asia, and this may lead to non-recognition of damage for which GET virus is responsible.

Diagnosis

Serological diagnosis of GET virus infection is routinely performed by VN, HI and CF tests with paired acute- and convalescent-phase serum samples. The VN test is more specific for defining the infecting virus than is HI or CF, which are more cross-reactive.

Virus neutralization and HI antibodies are detectable in horses 4–6 days after infection and persist for a relatively long period, and CF antibody is detectable a few days later than VN and the HI antibodies. Enzyme-linked immunosorbent assay (ELISA), particularly immunoglobulin M (IgM) capture ELISA, is of great use for rapid and relatively specific laboratory diagnosis.

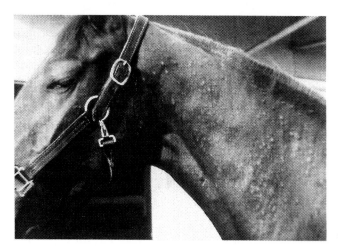

Fig. 1. Pyrexia rash on the neck of a horse.

Virus isolations are routinely performed using cell cultures. Intracranial inoculation of suckling mice with plasma, platelets or lymphocytes is also useful for virus isolation at the febrile stage of illness, but not by the time a rash has appeared.

Transmission

The viraemia titres in pigs and horses suggest that pigs play an important role as major amplifying hosts or may serve as natural hosts for maintenance of the virus, and that horses are also involved as natural hosts, or occasionally act as an ancillary amplifying host during epizootics. Getah virus has been isolated from various species of mosquitoes, such as *Culex tritaeniorhynchus*, *C. gelidus*, *Culex pseudovishnui*, *Culex fuscocephala*, *Culex vishnui*, *Culex bitaeniorhynchus*, *Aedes euedes*, *Ochlerotatus*[1] *communis*, *Anopheles amictus*, *Armigeres subalbatus*, *Mansonia bonneae* and *Mansonia dives*. In particular, GET virus has been isolated from *Culex* species in tropical and temperate regions of South-East Asia and in north-eastern Australia, whereas it has been isolated predominantly from *Aedes* species in eastern and western Siberian tundra zones.

Studies of GET virus from mosquitoes at an epizootic site revealed that 15/18 were from synchronously emerging (autumn) *Aedes vexans*; the rest were from *C. trit-*

aeniorhynchus. A survey in western Japan revealed that only a few strains were from *C. tritaeniorhynchus*, the predominant species at these sites. Laboratory experiments suggest that *A. vexans* is a better vector than are *Culex* species, and may be the major vector in Japanese epizootics. However, many species are probably involved in transmission and the principal vectors may differ according to local ecology and environmental factors. It may be that *Aedes* and *Ochlerotatus* mosquitoes are more important in cold temperate climates and in tundra zones, whereas *Culex* mosquitoes may be better vectors in warmer temperate and tropical zone regions. The maintenance mechanism of GET virus remains unknown. Terrestrial vertebrates or migrant birds may be involved in the cycle, and overwintering by transovarial transmission in mosquitoes has not been ruled out.

Prevention

A formalin-inactivated vaccine of whole virus of the MI-110 strain, propagated in porcine kidney cell culture, has been developed and used to protect horses in Japan. There are no vector control strategies aimed at the prevention of transmission.

Note

[1]   *Ocherotatus* was formerly a subgenus of *Aedes*.

Selected bibliography

Calisher, C.H. and Walton, T.E. (1966) Getah virus infections. In: Studdert, M.J. (ed.) *Virus Infections of Equines,* Vol. 6. In the series *Virus Infections of Vertebrates,* Horzinek, M.C. (series ed.). Elsevier, New York, pp. 157–165.

Calisher, C.H., Shope, R.E., Brandt, W., Casals, J., Karabatsos, N., Murphy, F.A., Tesh, R.B. and Wiebe, M.E. (1980) Proposed antigenic classification of registered arboviruses: I. *Togaviridae, Alphavirus. Intervirology* 14, 229–232.

Kamada, M., Ando, Y., Fukunaga, Y., Kumanomido, T., Imagawa, H., Wada, R. and Akiyama, Y. (1980) Equine Getah virus infection: isolation of the virus from racehorses during an enzootic in Japan. *American Journal of Tropical Medicine and Hygiene* 29, 984–988.

Kono, Y. (1988) Getah virus disease. In: Monath, T.P. (ed.) *The Arboviruses: Epidemiology and Ecology,* Vol. III. CRC Press, Boca Raton, Florida, pp. 21–36.

Kumanomido, T., Fukunaga, Y., Ando, Y., Kamada, M., Imagawa, H., Wada, R., Akiyama, Y., Tanaka, Y., Kobayashi, M., Ogura, N. and Yamamoto, H. (1986) Getah virus isolation from mosquitoes in an enzootic area in Japan. *Japanese Journal of Veterinary Science* 48, 1135–1140.

Peters C.J. and Dalrymple, J.M. (1990) Alphaviruses. In: Fields, B.N. and Knipe, D.M. (eds) *Virology,* 2nd edn. Raven Press, New York, pp. 713–753.

Sentsui, H. and Kono, Y. (1980) An epidemic of Getah virus infection among racehorses: isolation of the virus. *Research in Veterinary Science* 29, 157–161.

Shibata, I., Hatano, Y., Nishimura, M., Suzuki, G. and Inaba, Y. (1991) Isolation of Getah virus from dead fetuses extracted from a naturally infected sow in Japan. *Veterinary Microbiology* 27, 385–391.

Takashima, I., Hashimoto, N., Arikawa, J. and Matsumoto, K. (1983) Getah virus in *Aedes vexans nipponi* and *Culex tritaeniorhynchus*: vector susceptibility and ability to transmit. *Archives of Virology* 76, 299–305.

Wada, R., Kamada, M., Fukunaga, Y., Ando, Y., Kumanomido, T., Imagawa H., Akiyama, Y. and Oikawa, M. (1982) Equine Getah virus infecion: pathological study of a horse experimentally infected with the MI-110 strain. *Japanese Journal of Veterinary Science* 44, 411–418.

Yago, K., Hagiwara, S., Kawamura, H. and Narita, M.A. (1987) A fatal case in newborn piglets with Getah virus infection: isolation of the virus. *Japanese Journal of Veterinary Science* 49, 989–994.

Giardia infections *see* **Cockroaches** *and* **Flies.**

Greenbottles *see* **Flies.**

Greenheads *see* **Horse-flies.**

Habronemiasis of horses

E.T. Lyons

Habronemiasis is usually a benign infection of nematodes in the stomach of equids. Aberrant infective larvae produce 'summer sores' and other cutaneous lesions and may be more of a problem than adult worms.

Distribution

Habronemiasis is ubiquitous. Countries where this disease is commonly reported include China, England, Japan, Russia and the USA.

Parasite

Three species of parasites cause habronemiasis in horses: *Habronema muscae*, *Habronema majus* (synonym *Habronema microstoma*) and *Draschia megastoma* (formerly *Habronema megastoma*). These nematodes are in the order called Spirurida. The adults of the three species have varying total lengths: *H. muscae* males are 8–14 mm and females 13–22 mm in length; *H. majus* males are 16–22 mm and females 15–25 mm long; and *D megastoma* males are 7–10 mm and females 10–13 mm long. Maturation occurs in the glandular portion of the stomach. Both species of *Habronema* reside on the mucous exudate of the glandular stomach, but their heads may attach to the gastric mucosa. *Draschia megastoma* live in tumour-like lesions, usually along the margo plicatus, which separates the white oesophageal region from the glandular portion of the stomach. Most of these lesions are less than 50 mm in diameter, have one or two central openings and contain numerous worms embedded in necrotic and caseous exudate. Some lesions as large as a 'child's head' have been described.

Clinical symptoms

Usually, infections of spirurids in the stomach are asymptomatic and not diagnosed in live animals. Presence of these parasites and the subclinical problems they cause are typically detected only at necropsy of the infected horses. *Habronema muscae* and *H. majus* have been associated with chronic gastritis, resulting in emaciation and debilitation.

Draschia megastoma is the most pathogenic of the three species. Clinical signs of this parasite and the gastric abscesses it causes are usually not apparent. However, deaths may result when there is suppurative gastritis that leads to perforation of the stomach wall and peritonitis. Perforating abscesses may involve the spleen with a fistulous tract-like formation. Nodules located near the pylorus may interfere with closure of the pyloric sphincter.

The third-stage larvae (L$_3$) of all three species are quite detrimental when located outside the gastrointestinal tract, especially in cutaneous infections. Damaged areas of the skin, mainly on the lower limbs, abdomen and shoulders, attract infected flies, resulting in deposition of L$_3$. In these areas L$_3$ produce pruritus, which is pronounced in severe cases. Infected wounds do not heal and chronic, proliferative, granulomatous masses that bleed freely can result. These lesions tend to be seasonal in temperate climates and are commonly called 'summer sores'. They subside in the cold winter months when fly breeding is inhibited.

Eye infections result in photophobia and conjunctivitis, with excessive lachrymation and eventual formation of granulomatous growths on the eyelids and nictitating membranes. Lesions of the conjunctival sac are typically in the medial canthus and are wart-like in appearance. Here, they are red at first and then turn yellowish as a result of caseation and calcification.

In male equids, spirurid L$_3$-infected lesions on the glans penis, on the prepuce and around the urethral orifice are irritating. This results in difficult and increased frequency of urination. Occurrence of aberrant spirurid larvae in the lungs is associated with abscesses and pneumonia. Both *Streptococcus equi* and *D. megastoma* larvae have been found in the same lung abscesses.

Diagnosis

Laboratory examination by faecal flotation is not a satisfactory method of detecting spirurid eggs because they are thin-walled and collapse in the flotation fluids used. Xenodiagnosis is impractical since it involves application of eggs from uninfected flies to the faecal sample and examination of resultant adult flies for *Habronema* and *Draschia* L_3. Indirect diagnosis has been used and involves examination of flies from stable areas for spirurid L_3.

Clinical diagnosis by gastric lavage has been used for recovery of spirurid adults, larvae and eggs. Also, endoscopic examination of the stomach has been advocated, especially in detecting tumours caused by *D. megastoma*.

Habronema and *Draschia* L_3 in cutaneous and ocular lesions are specifically diagnosed by biopsy and by saline flush techniques. Detection of gritty conjunctival plaques is pathognomonic for conjunctival habronemiasis.

Transmission

The parasites require dipteran intermediate hosts, such as the non-biting house-fly, *Musca domestica*, and the blood-feeding stable-fly, *Stomoxys calcitrans*. Adult female worms lay embryonated eggs that are voided in the faeces of the horse. The first-stage larvae (L_1) are quite active in the loose-fitting eggshell. They have a stylet at the anterior end and are sometimes called 'aciculate larvae'. Fly maggots (larvae) ingest the L_1, which use the stylet to penetrate the alimentary canal of the insect larvae and locate in the body cavity. Larvae of *D. megastoma* develop in the Malpighian tubules and *Habronema* species in the fat bodies. Synchronization occurs for concurrent development of both the nematode L_1 to the infective L_3 and the fly larva to adult. Interestingly, if environmental factors delay development of the insect larvae, similar retardation occurs in the nematode larvae.

Infection of horses results from L_3 crawling from the proboscis of the flies as they feed on the mouth, lips, nostrils, eyes and other external areas, especially in wounds. The flies are attracted to horses by warmth and moisture. Adult worms in the stomach result from L_3 deposited by the flies on the lips, and possibly nostrils, of the horses or when infected flies are swallowed by horses. The pre-patent period is about 2 months. When L_3 invade horses, other than orally or possibly intranasally, they do not mature.

Treatment

Two currently marketed macrocyclic lactones, ivermectin and moxidectin, are efficacious on stomach worms and aberrant larvae. These compounds are not usually administered for specific removal of the gastric species of spirurids, but efficacy is achieved whenever the drugs are used primarily for control of other internal parasites. Dramatic clinical response of cutaneous lesions is effected by these drugs.

Control

Modern chemical fly control methods are indirectly effective in decreasing transmission of spirurids. Composting manure in tight enclosures prevents, or at least curtails, the breeding of flies and also kills spirurid larvae. Treatment of horses with macrocyclic lactones and removing the stomach parasites reduces their transmission.

Usage of macrocyclic lactones for primary control of strongyles and other endoparasites has the added benefit of stomach worm control. Marked reductions in prevalence of stomach worms has been documented in central Kentucky in thoroughbred horses after several years of ivermectin usage in parasite control programmes.

Selected bibliography

Campbell, W.C., Leaning, W.H.D. and Seward, R.L. (1979) Use of ivermectin in horses. In: Campbell, W.C. (ed.) *Ivermectin and Abamectin.* Springer-Verlag, New York, pp. 234–244.

Drudge, J.H. and Lyons, E.T. (1989) *Internal Parasites of Equids with Emphasis on Treatment and Control*, revised. Monograph, Hoechst-Roussel Agri-Vet, Somerville, New Jersey, 26 pp.

Roubaud, E. and Descarzeaux, J. (1992) Evolution of *Habronema muscae* in the housefly and of *H. microstomum* in *Stomoxys*. *Bulletin de la Société Pathologie Exotique* 15, 572–574.

Schwartz, B., Imes, M. and Foster, A.O. (1948) *Parasites and Parasitic Disease of Horses*, revised. Circular No. 148, USDA, Washington, DC, 56 pp.

Soulsby, E.J.L. (1965) *Textbook of Veterinary Clinical Parasitology*, Vol. 1, Helminths. F.A. Davis, Philadelphia, 1120 pp.

Haematobia see **Horn-flies.**

Haemobartonella canis see **Haemotrophic mycoplasmas.**

Haemoproteosis

Carter T. Atkinson

Species of *Haemoproteus* are common vector-transmitted intraerythrocytic parasites of domestic and wild birds. They share many morphological and developmental features with closely related haemosporidian parasites in the genera *Plasmodium* and *Leucocytozoon*, but are distinguished by the presence of highly refractive granules of golden-brown or black pigment in mature gametocytes and by the absence of schizogony in circulating blood cells. More than 100 valid species of *Haemoproteus* are currently recognized. They are separated by gametocyte morphology and limited experimental evidence suggesting that they are specific to host family or subfamily. Vectors and detailed life cycles for most of these species are unknown and it is likely that many will be synonymized with further work. Species of *Haemoproteus* are traditionally believed to be non-pathogenic, but evidence is accumulating that pre-erythrocytic tissue stages of these parasites are capable of causing severe myopathy and fatal infections in both domestic and wild birds.

Haemoproteus meleagridis

Distribution

Found in the USA south of New York and east of Texas with some reports from domestic turkeys in Venezuela. *Haemoproteus meleagridis* is primarily a parasite of Wild turkeys (*Meleagris gallopavo*) that infects domestic turkeys when suitable reservoir hosts and vectors are present.

Parasite

The life cycle begins when infective sporozoites are inoculated into a susceptible turkey by a ceratopogonid fly in the genus *Culicoides*. Two generations of pre-erythrocytic schizogony occur in skeletal and cardiac muscle (Fig. 1). The first begins when infective sporozoites invade capillary endothelial cells and myofibroblasts and develop into thin-walled schizonts measuring 12–20 µm in diameter. Between 5 and 8 days post-infection, these produce long, slender merozoites, which subsequently invade new capillary endothelial cells in skeletal and cardiac muscle and develop as second-generation schizonts. Early second-generation schizonts are 5–8 µm in diameter and 28 µm in length. These grow rapidly to form large, fusiform, thick-walled megaloschizonts measuring up to 500 µm in length. Megaloschizonts reach maturity at 17 days post-infection and rupture to release small spherical merozoites, which invade erythrocytes and develop into gametocytes. Mature gametocytes, which completely encircle the host erythrocyte nucleus, develop within 7–10 days after red blood cells are invaded. Parasitaemias reach their peak intensity in the peripheral circulation at approximately 21 days post-infection and fall rapidly within 7 days to

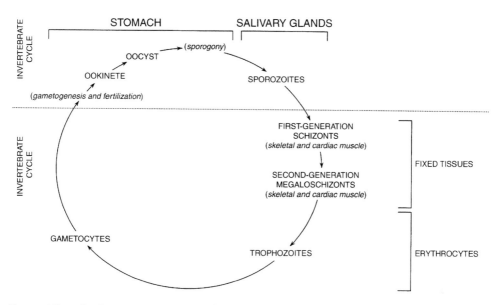

Fig. 1. Life cycle of *Haemoproteus meleagridis.*

low intensities. A second, smaller peak in parasitaemia may occur at approximately 35 days post-infection. Birds probably remain chronically infected for life.

Closely related species

Closely related *Haemoproteus* species that occur in other galliform hosts include *H. pratasi* in Guinea fowl (*Numida meleagris*), *H. lophortyx* in California quail (*Callipepla californica*), *H. rileyi* in Peafowl (*Pavo cristatus*) and *H. stableri* and *H. mansoni* in Red grouse (*Lagopus lagopus*) and Ruffed grouse (*Bonasa umbellus*), respectively. With the exception of *H. lophortyx*, virtually nothing is known about the vectors or pathogenicity of these other species. Proved vectors for *H. lophortyx* are the hippoboscid flies, *Stilbometopa impressa* and *Lynchia hirsuta*. This species may be pathogenic, but evidence is limited.

Clinical symptoms

Clinical signs are not evident in light infections, but severe pathology is associated with the development of megaloschizonts in cardiac and skeletal muscle in heavy infections. Domestic turkey poults with experimental infections exhibit lameness

in one or both legs and have lower weights and growth rates than uninfected controls (Fig. 2). Gross and microscopic lesions in infected birds include extensive deposition of parasite pigment in tissue macrophages of the liver and spleen, enlargement of these organs, and necrosis and calcification of muscle fibres adjacent to developing megaloschizonts (Fig. 3).

Diagnosis

Parasites are identified from Giemsa-stained thin blood smears (Fig. 4). *Haemoproteus meleagridis* is the only haemoproteid that has been described from turkeys. Presence of circumnuclear erythrocytic gametocytes with prominent golden-brown or black pigment granules and absence of erythrocytic schizonts are diagnostic for this species.

Transmission

Proved vectors are ceratopogonid flies in the genus *Culicoides*. *Culicoides edeni*, *C. hinmani* and *C. arboricola* support complete sporogonic development of *H. meleagridis* in the south-eastern USA and it is likely that other ornithophagic ceratopogonids are capable of transmitting the

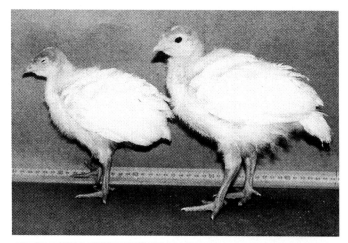

Fig. 2. Three-week-old domestic turkey poults at 12 days post-inoculation with approximately 58,000 sporozoites of *Haemoproteus meleagridis* (left) or with physiological saline (right). The infected bird (left) subsequently died from severe myopathy associated with developing megaloschizonts.

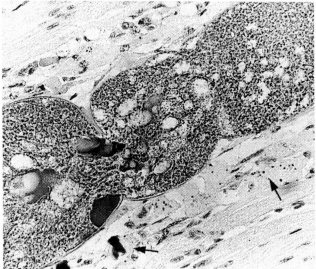

Fig. 3. Megaloschizont of *Haemoproteus meleagridis* in skeletal muscle of an experimentally infected domestic turkey poult. Areas of necrosis and calcification (arrows) surround the megaloschizont.

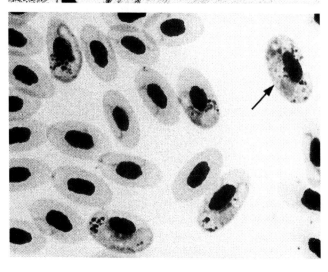

Fig. 4. Giemsa-stained blood smear with mature (arrow) and immature gametocytes of *Haemoproteus meleagridis.*

parasite in other parts of its range. The sporogonic cycle begins when a blood meal containing mature macrogametocytes and microgametocytes is taken from an infected host. These undergo gametogenesis, fertilization and ookinete formation in the mid-gut of the vector. Ookinetes subsequently penetrate the mid-gut wall and develop under the mid-gut basal lamina as spherical oocysts, which measure approximately 10 μm in diameter. Sporogony typically takes 4–6 days, eventually producing fewer than 100 sporozoites, which bud from a single sporoblast (Fig. 5). Oocysts subsequently rupture, releasing sporozoites into the haemocoel of the insect. These invade the salivary glands and pass through the salivary ducts during the next blood meal.

Transmission of *H. meleagridis* is seasonal and limited to the spring and summer months in more temperate parts of its range, but can occur throughout the year in subtropical habitats in Florida, where suitable vectors are present year-round.

Treatment

With the exception of rare fatal infections involving large numbers of megaloschizonts, infections are self-limiting and treatment is not necessary. Effective

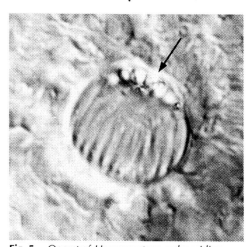

Fig. 5. Oocyst of *Haemoproteus meleagridis* on the mid-gut wall of *Culicoides edeni*. The oocyst contains densely packed, slender sporozoites and a small residual body (arrow).

chemotherapeutic treatments for the pathogenic tissue stages of *H. meleagridis* have not been developed.

Control

Reduction of populations of ceratopogonid fly vectors can, in theory, reduce transmission of *H. meleagridis*, but this method has not been tested. When possible, isolation of domestic birds from sylvatic cycles involving wild reservoir hosts may be the most effective way to prevent infections.

Haemoproteus columbae
Distribution

Worldwide in columbiform hosts. Prevalence in both domestic and feral populations of Common pigeons (*Columba livia*) is dependent on vector distribution and numbers, and ranges from 0% in some regions to up to 100% in others.

Parasite

The life cycle begins when infective sporozoites are inoculated by ectoparasitic hippoboscid vectors into a susceptible host. Sporozoites invade capillary endothelial cells of the lungs, where they undergo pre-erythrocytic development to form thin-walled, branching schizonts, which radiate along pulmonary capillaries. The pre-patent period ranges from 17 to 37 days, after which merozoites bud from the periphery of schizonts, enter the circulation and invade erthryocytes. Development of large, thick-walled megaloschizonts has also been reported in heart, gizzard and skeletal muscle of Bleeding-heart doves (*Gallicolumba luzonica*) and may occur in other host species as well. Merozoites in circulating erythrocytes develop to mature halteridial microgametocytes and macrogametocytes, which partially encircle the erythrocyte nucleus within approximately 5–10 days. Gametocyte numbers peak in the peripheral circulation approximately 10–20 days after first appearing and then decline in numbers. Infected birds may undergo relapses at later dates, but remain immune to reinfection as long as the initial chronic infection persists.

Closely related species

Haemoproteus sacharovi is a closely related species that occurs in columbiform hosts, including *C. livia*. Gametocytes of *H. sacharovi* cause gross hypertrophy of host erythrocytes, while those of *H. columbae* have little effect on host cell size. Natural vectors of *H. sacharovi* are not known, although the hippoboscid fly, *Pseudolynchia maura*, can transmit the parasite in the laboratory.

Clinical symptoms

Haemoproteus columbae is believed to be relatively non-pathogenic, with few effects on hosts. Birds with intense erythrocytic infections may be lethargic and anorexic. In rare reports of fatal infections, birds were anaemic and suffered from interstitial pneumonia. Gross and microscopic lesions included congested, hypertrophic and darkly pigmented livers and spleens and cellular infiltrates in the alveolar septae. In one report of a fatal *H. columbae* infection, extensive tissue damage was associated with numerous developing megaloschizonts in skeletal, cardiac and gizzard muscle.

Diagnosis

Parasites are identified in Giemsa-stained thin blood smears. In *C. livia*, the presence of erythrocytic gametocytes with prominent golden-brown or black pigment granules that partially encircle the host cell nucleus and the absence of erythrocytic schizonts are diagnostic for this species.

Transmission

Proved vectors are ectoparasitic hippoboscid flies and include *Ornithomyia avicularia*, *Pseudolynchia canariensis*, *Pseudolynchia brunnea*, *Pseudolynchia capensis* and *Microlynchia pusilla*. Suspected vectors are ceratopogonid flies in the genus *Culicoides*, but their ability to transmit columbiform haemoproteids has never been conclusively demonstrated. The sporogonic cycle begins when a hippoboscid fly takes a blood meal from an infected host and ingests mature macrogametocytes and microgametocytes. These undergo gametogenesis, fertilization and ookinete formation in the mid-gut of the vector. Ookinetes subsequently penetrate the midgut wall and develop under the mid-gut basal lamina as spherical oocysts, which measure approximately 40 µm in diameter. Sporogony in developing oocysts typically takes up to 10 days, eventually producing thousands of sporozoites, which bud from multiple sporoblasts. Oocysts subsequently rupture, releasing sporozoites into the haemocoel of the insect. These invade the salivary glands and pass through the salivary ducts during the next blood meal and are injected into a new pigeon.

In temperate North America, transmission of *H. columbae* is seasonal and closely correlated with changes in vector populations, generally increasing in the autumn and winter months and then declining as vector density decreases. More limited data from tropical and subtropical parts of the world, where populations of hippoboscid flies remain more constant, indicate that high rates of transmission and high prevalences of infection can be maintained throughout the year.

Treatment

Infections are self-limiting and birds subsequently develop chronic, low-intensity infections and concomitant immunity to reinfection. Treatment is usually not necessary, but Butalex (Buparvaquone, Mallinckrodt Veterinary Ltd, UK) at a single dose of 2.5 mg kg^{-1} has been found to be effective in eliminating gametocytes from the peripheral circulation. Infections that produce megaloschizonts may be rapidly fatal at about the time when gametocytes appear in the peripheral circulation, making treatment difficult. Efficacy of chemotherapy against megaloschizonts and pre-erythrocytic stages of the parasite is unknown.

Control

Reduction of hippoboscid fly vectors is the most efficient approach to control. This should include dusting infested birds and nesting boxes with a suitable insecticide to kill adult flies, and treatment of premises to eliminate habitats for puparial development.

Haemoproteus nettionis
Distribution
Worldwide in domestic ducks and geese. *Haemoproteus nettionis* is primarily a parasite of wild waterfowl that infects domestic birds when suitable vectors and wild reservoir hosts are present.

Parasite
The life cycle begins when infective sporozoites are inoculated into a susceptible host by a ceratopogonid fly in the genus *Culicoides*. Details about the pre-erythrocytic development of the parasite are poorly known. Oval, thin-walled schizonts have been described in capillary endothelial cells of the lungs and occasionally the heart and spleen. Large megaloschizonts have not been observed, but critical studies to document their development have not been done. The pre-patent period ranges from 14 to 17 days.

Once circulating erythrocytes have been invaded by pre-erythrocytic merozoites, mature gametocytes, which partially encircle the host erythrocyte nucleus, develop in approximately 6 days. Parasitaemias reach their peak intensity in the peripheral circulation at approximately 22 days after infection and fall rapidly. Birds probably remain chronically infected for life and experience periodic relapses, particularly during the breeding season.

Closely related species
Haemoproteus greineri has been reported from a variety of anatid hosts in North America, while *Haemoproteus gabaldoni* is known only from Muscovy ducks (*Cairina moschata*) in Venezuela. Both species can be distinguished from *H. nettionis* by gametocyte morphology. Gametocytes of *H. greineri* completely encircle the host cell nucleus, while gametocytes of *H. gabaldoni* partially encircle the host cell nucleus and have highly amoeboid outlines. Nothing is known about their vectors or pathogenicity.

Clinical symptoms
Haemoproteus nettionis is believed to be non-pathogenic, with no clinical signs in infected hosts. Minor gross and microscopic lesions have been described in tissues of experimentally infected Pekin (= Mallard) (*Anas platyrhynchos*) and Muscovy ducks, but infected birds showed no signs of clinical illness. These lesions included accumulation of parasite pigment in tissue macrophages and moderate infiltrates of lymphocytes and granulocytes in various organs.

Diagnosis
Giemsa-stained thin blood smears will identify the parasites. In ducks and geese, the presence of erythrocytic gametocytes with prominent golden-brown or black pigment granules that partially encircle the host cell nucleus and the absence of erythrocytic schizonts are diagnostic for this species.

Transmission
Proved vectors are ceratopogonid flies in the genus *Culicoides*. *Culicoides downesi* supports complete sporogonic development of *H. nettionis* in North America, while other ornithophagic ceratopogonids are presumed vectors in other parts of the world. The sporogonic cycle begins when a blood meal containing mature macrogametocytes and microgametocytes is taken from an infected host. These undergo gametogenesis, fertilization and ookinete formation in the mid-gut of the vector. Ookinetes subsequently penetrate the mid-gut wall and develop under the mid-gut basal lamina as spherical oocysts, which measure approximately 10 μm in diameter. Sporogony typically takes 4–6 days, eventually producing fewer than 100 sporozoites, which bud from a single sporoblast. Oocysts subsequently rupture, releasing sporozoites into the haemocoel of the insect. These invade the salivary glands and pass through the salivary ducts during the next blood meal.

Transmission of *H. nettionis* occurs during the spring and summer months, when ceratopogonid populations reach their peak. Detailed epidemiological studies have not been done.

Treatment
Infections are self-limiting and birds subsequently develop chronic, low-intensity

parasitaemias, which do not require treatment. Effective chemotherapeutic treatments
for *H. nettionis* have not been developed.

Control

Reduction of populations of ceratopogonid
fly vectors can, in theory, reduce transmission of *H. nettionis*, but this method has
not been tested and may not be feasible,
since the vectors are unknown outside of
North America. When possible, isolation of
domestic birds from sylvatic cycles involving wild reservoir hosts may be the most
effective way to prevent infections. Given
the apparent low pathogenicity of the parasite, costs associated with control probably
outweigh any potential benefits.

Selected bibliography

Atkinson, C.T. (1991) Vectors, epizootiology, and
    pathogenicity of avian species of *Haemo-*
    proteus (Haemosporina: Haemoproteidae).
    Bulletin of the Society for Vector Ecology 16,
    109–126.
Atkinson, C.T., Forrester, D.J. and Greiner, E.C.
    (1988) Pathogenicity of *Haemoproteus mele-*
    agridis (Haemosporina: Haemoproteidae) in
    experimentally infected domestic turkeys.
    Journal of Parasitology 74, 228–239.
Bennett, G.F. and Peirce, M.A. (1988) Morpho-
    logical form in the avian Haemoproteidae
    and an annotated checklist of the genus
Haemoproteus Kruse, 1890. *Journal of*
    Natural History 22, 1683–1696.
Bennett, G.F., Pierce, M.A. and Earle, R.A. (1994)
    An annotated checklist of the valid avian
    species of *Haemoproteus, Leucocytozoon*
    (Apicomplexa: Haemosprida) and *Hepato-*
    zoon (Apicomplexa: Haemogregarinidae).
    Systematic Parasitology 29, 61–73.
Earle, R.A., Bastianello, S.S., Bennett, G.F. and
    Krecek, R.C. (1993) Histopathology and mor-
    phology of the tissue stages of *Haemoproteus*
    columbae causing mortality in Columbi-
    formes. *Avian Pathology* 22, 67–80.
el-Metenawy, T.M. (1999) Therapeutic effects of
    some antihaematozoal drugs against *Haemo-*
    proteus columbae in domestic pigeons. *Deut-*
    sche Tierärztliche Wochenschrifte 106, 72.
Fallis, A.M. and Wood, D.M. (1957) Biting midges
    (Diptera: Ceratopogonidae) as intermediate
    hosts for *Haemoproteus* of ducks. *Canadian*
    Journal of Zoology 35, 425–435.
Garnham, P.C.C. (1966) Avian haemoproteid:
    Haemoproteus columbiae. In: *Malaria Para-*
    sites and Other Haemosporidia. Blackwell
    Scientific Publications, Oxford, pp. 941–947.
Greiner, E.C. and Forrester, D.J. (1980) *Haemo-*
    proteus meleagridis Levine 1961: redescrip-
    tion and developmental morphology of the
    gametocytes in turkeys. *Journal of Parasitol-*
    ogy 68, 652–658.
Sibley, L.D. and Werner, J.W. (1984) Suscepti-
    bility of pekin and muscovy ducks to
    Haemoproteus nettionis. *Journal of Wildlife*
    Diseases 20, 108–113.

Haemoproteus species *see* **Haemoproteosis.**

Haemorrhagic fever with renal syndrome

Rongman Xu

Haemorrhagic fever with renal syndrome
(HFRS), known also as epidemic haemorrhagic fever and Korean haemorrhagic
fever, is endemic in China, Korea and parts
of Eurasia. The aetiological agent of HFRS is
Hantaan (HTN) virus (family Bunyaviridae,
genus *Hantavirus*). Viruses of this genus
cause chronic, inapparent infections of
rodents. Hantaan virus was first isolated
from the Striped field mouse, *Apodemus*
agrarius, by H.W. Lee, Korea University,
Republic of Korea, in 1976.

Distribution

Seroepidemiological surveys and documented case reports show that hantaviruses
are widely distributed throughout much of
the world, but most cases of HFRS (>90%)
are from China. There were 1,289,746
reported cases up to 1995, 92.7% of which

were in Asia and 7.3% in Europe, with just a few cases reported from the Americas. There are three epidemiological patterns of HFRS, depending on the location of the outbreak and the reservoir host of the disease: rural, urban and from animal houses (vivaria). Each hantavirus has a principal rodent host and it appears that there has been coevolution or parallel evolution of these viruses and their hosts. The reservoir hosts in rural areas are mainly rodents, such as *Apodemus* species in Asia and Europe, *Clethrionomys* species in eastern Europe and the Far East and *Microtus* and *Peromyscus* species in the Americas. The reservoir hosts for the urban type are domestic rats (*Rattus* species). The reservoir hosts for animal house infections are colonized experimental rats.

Aetiological agent

Four viruses have been associated with HFRS: HTN virus, which is the type species for the genus *Hantavirus*, and which was isolated from the Hantaan River area of Korea; Dobrava (DOB) virus, which causes HFRS in the Balkans; Seoul (SEO) virus, which produces many urban cases of HFRS in China, Korea, Japan and South-East Asia, and laboratory infections in many parts of the world; and Puumala (PUU) virus, which causes nephropathia epidemica in Scandinavia and other parts of Europe.

Clinical symptoms

All known diseases caused by these hantaviruses are characterized by proteinuria and azotaemia. Typical HFRS infections are characterized by fever, haemorrhagic diathesis and renal disorders. There are five phases: febrile, hypotensive, oliguric, diuretic and convalescent. The febrile phase usually lasts 3–8 days, with sudden onset of fever up to 40°C, chills, general malaise, weakness and generalized myalgias. This may be followed by severe anorexia, dizziness, headache and pain in the eyeballs. The hypotensive phase can last from several hours to 3 days, with shock, including tachycardia, low pulse pressure, hypotension, cold and clammy skin and dulled sensorium. The oliguric

phase usually lasts 3–7 days. During this phase blood pressure begins to return to normal, but many patients become hypertensive and may have severe nausea and vomiting associated with persistent oliguria. About 50% of fatalities occur during the oliguric phase. Clinical recovery begins with the onset of the diuretic phase, which lasts from days to weeks. The convalescent phase takes 2–3 months and is characterized by a progressive recovery of the glomerular filtration rate. The above description applies to the more severe cases of HTN virus infection in Asia or DOB virus infection in the Balkans, both of which have a case fatality of 5–15%. Milder cases caused by these viruses, or the generally less severe HFRS from SEO virus or PUU virus infection, do not usually display the full spectrum of clinical manifestations and have a case fatality rate of less than 1%.

Diagnosis

There is no specific clinical test to confirm HFRS. The appearance of fever, abdominal pain and severe retching, marked proteinuria, flush, shock, haemorrhagic diathesis, pulmonary oedema, leucocytosis, thrombocytopenia, haemoconcentration and azotaemia are virtually diagnostic. Haemorrhagic fever with renal syndrome is confirmed by serological tests that demonstrate increasing or decreasing antibody titres to a hantavirus in paired acute- and convalescent-phase samples.

Transmission

Hantaviruses are usually transmitted by contamination of wounds by the saliva, urine or faeces of rodents, by aerosols of these products or by rodent bites. Human-to-human spread has not been reported for HTN virus but has been reported for Andes virus, an aetiological agent of hantavirus pulmonary syndrome.

Some evidence has been obtained for transmission of HTN virus by mites. *Ornithonyssus bacoti* (tropical rat mite) and *Leptotrombidium* species (trombiculid mites) are the principal suspected mite vectors among domestic and wild rodents, respectively. In China, *Leptotrombidium scutellaris* has been confirmed as a vector both in nature and in the laboratory, and *Leptotrombidum subpalpale* has been shown to be a vector, at least in the laboratory. These are also the prevalent mite species in HFRS foci in China. Virus replication in mites has not been proved, so transmission by mites might be mechanical, rather than replicative. Transovarial transmission and virus multiplication have been reported from China, but this requires further research to determine whether this route of transmission really occurs. The epidemiological significance of mite transmission remains unclear.

Treatment

There is no specific treatment of HFRS, so the management of the patient must be supportive and based on an understanding of the pathophysiological characteristics of the disease. Early diagnosis and hospitalization before the onset of the hypotensive and haemorrhagic phenomena are very important. The febrile phase requires bedrest, mild sedation, analgesics and strict maintenance of fluid balance, especially avoiding overhydration. Treatment in the hypotensive phase requires administration of an intravascular volume expander. Treatment in the oliguric phase is the same as for acute renal failure. In the diuretic phase, attention must be paid to adequate replacement of fluids and electrolytes. Intravenous ribavirin given within the first 4 days of onset has been shown to lessen renal failure, decrease bleeding manifestations and decrease case fatality in a Chinese setting,

in which results of dialysis and other supportive measures were less than optimum.

Control

Rodent control, such as improving people's living conditions to reduce contacts with rodents, should be considered in the control of HFRS. Insecticide spraying, to kill mites, has been recommended in endemic outbreaks of HFRS in China, but vaccination is also very important in endemic regions of HFRS and for those undertaking research on HFRS.

Selected bibliography

Fisher-Hoch, S.P. and McCormick, J.B. (1985) Haemorrhagic fever with renal syndrome: a review. *Abstracts on Hygiene and Communicable Diseases* 60(4), R1–R20.

Lee, H.W., Calisher, C.H. and Schmaljohn, C. (1998) *Manual of Hemorrhagic Fever with Renal Syndrome and Hantavirus Pulmonary Syndrome.* WHO Collaborating Centre for Virus Reference and Research (hantaviruses), Asian Institute for Life Sciences, Seoul, Korea, 250 pp.

Peters, C.J., Simpson, G.L. and Levy, H. (1999) Spectrum of hantavirus infection: hemorrhagic fever with renal syndrome and hantavirus pulmonary syndrome. *Annual Review of Medicine* 50, 531–545.

She, J.J., Zhang, Y., Huang, C.A., Yu, M.M., Jiang, K.J. and Wu, G.H. (1998) Preliminary study on *Leptotrombidium* (*L.*) *subpalpale* as spreading medium of HFRS. *Chinese Journal of Vector Biology and Control* 9, 47–50. (In Chinese with English abstract.)

Song, G. (1999) Epidemiological progressses of hemorrhagic fever with renal syndrome in China. *Chinese Medical Journal* 112, 472–477.

Haemotrophic mycoplasmas

(Containing species from the former genera *Haemobartonella* and *Eperythrozoon*)

Harold Neimark

Haemobartonella and *Eperythrozoon* were the names given to uncultivated bacteria that parasitize the surface of erythrocytes of a wide range of vertebrate animals hosts. Formerly *Haemobartonella* and *Eperythrozoon* species were classified as rickettsiae

(order *Rickettsiales*), which they appeared to resemble because of their small size and staining properties, their uncultivated status, their transmission by arthropod vectors and their haemotrophic character. The latter property seemed to relate these bacteria to *Anaplasma* (family *Anaplasmataceae*), which grow as inclusion bodies within erythrocytes. However, *Haemobartonella* and *Eperythrozoon* differed from *Anaplasma* (see Anaplasmosis) in that they attach to the surface of red cells, do not invade erythrocytes and, notably, lack cell walls.

Distribution
The agents in domesticated animals probably occur on most continents but extensive studies have not been done; organisms in wild animals may be more localized.

Aetiological agents and phylogeny
Recently, the 16S ribosomal RNA (rRNA) genes of several *Haemobartonella* and *Eperythrozoon* species were sequenced and their phylogenetic position determined. These studies demonstrated unequivocally that these uncultivated wall-less bacteria are not rickettsia but rather that they are mycoplasmas. Thus, presumably all the members of the genera *Haemobartonella* and *Eperythrozoon* are actually members of a single genus, *Mycoplasma*. The formal transfer of *Haemobartonella felis* and *Haemobartonella muris* and *Eperythrozoon ovis*, *Eperythrozoon suis* and *Eperythrozoon wenyonii* from the rickettsiae to the genus *Mycoplasma* has been proposed in order to recognize their actual phylogenetic affiliation. The demonstration that these haemotrophic bacteria are mycoplasmas has provided an entirely new perspective for studying these bacteria. The remaining officially named species of *Haemobartonella* and *Eperythrozoon* are also wall-less and all share identical properties with the haemotrophic mycoplasma species described here, and it seems likely that they too will be found to be mycoplasmas (Table 1).

Mycoplasmas (class Mollicutes, order Mycoplasmatales) are prokaryotes with the general characteristics of lactic acid bacteria (particularly streptococci) but they lack cell walls and are notable for their small cell size and for containing the smallest chromosomes of any cells capable of independent replication. Mollicutes occur as pathogens or commensals in a broad range of hosts including vertebrate animals, arthropods and plants. Until recently, mycoplasmas infecting vertebrates appeared to colonize only the mucous membranes of their hosts; at these sites pathogenic mycoplasmas cause respiratory or urogenital disease, often with an arthritic component. The former *Haemobartonella* and *Eperythrozoon* represent a novel group of parasitic mycoplasmas that possess a pathogenic capacity previously unrecognized among the mollicutes. The haemotrophic mycoplasmas form a new phylogenetic cluster within the so-called pneumoniae group of *Mycoplasma* and share properties with other members of the pneumoniae group.

Cell structural features
All the species parasitize the erythrocytes of their hosts and adhere to the erythrocyte surface; all have been shown by electron microscopy to lack a cell wall and to be coccoidal in shape. Many produce an indentation on the red cell membrane at the site of attachment and also, in some, fine fibrils can be seen connecting the bacteria and the erythrocytes. Some members of the pneumoniae group possess tip or bleb structures, which are involved in host cell attachment; similar bleb structures have been observed in a haemotrophic mycoplasma from the South American monkey, *Saimiri sciureus*, and in an agent from the Owl monkey, *Aotus trivirgatus*.

Surface components of haemotrophic mycoplasmas involved in erythrocyte adherence have not been identified. Experiments with lectins in *Mycoplasma wenyonii* infection suggest that the erythrocyte membrane is altered, as shown by increased recognition of both soybean agglutinin and peanut agglutinin receptor carbohydrates.

Nomenclature
To avoid confusion in nomenclature, rickettsial species names have been retained where there was no conflict with existing *Mycoplasma* species names; where rickettsia and mycoplasmas contained identical names (e.g. *felis*, *muris* and *suis*) rather than proposing completely new names, the prefix *haemo* was used to form new species

Haemotrophic mycoplasmas

Table 1. Haemotrophic mycoplasmas of domesticated and laboratory animals.

Host	Bacterium	Disease	Other features	Vector(s)
Dog	*Haemobartonella canis**	Mild to severe anaemia can be fatal	Can induce cold agglutinins	Ixodid ticks suspected
Cat	*Candidatus* species Mycoplasma haemofelis	Agent of feline infectious anaemia, severe illness can be fatal	Acute-stage cold agglutinins	Cat flea suspected (oral, vertical transmission reported)
	Candidatus species Mycoplasma haemominutum	Clinical signs mild or absent	Cell size smaller than M. haemofelis	
Wild, laboratory mice, rat, hamster, rabbit	*Eperythrozoon coccoides**	Anaemia, infection often inapparent	Infection also by ingesting blood	*Polypax serrata* (mouse louse), other biting arthropods
Wild, laboratory mice, rat	*Candidatus* species Mycoplasma haemomuris	General illness, splenomegaly can be fatal		*Polypax spinulosa* (rat louse)
Pig	*Candidatus* species Mycoplasma haemosuis	Icteroanaemia more severe in young animals	Can induce cold agglutinins	*Stomoxys calcitrans*[†] (stable-fly)
	*Eperythrozoon parvum**	Non-pathogen	Cell size smaller than M. haemosuis	*Aedes aegypti*[†] (mosquito)
Sheep, goat	*Candidatus* species Mycoplasma ovis	Haemolytic anaemia poor weight gain, young animals unthrifty		Ticks suspected, other arthropods[†]
Cattle	*Candidatus* species Mycoplasma wenyonii	Mild anaemia, occasionally acute, infection often inapparent		*Dermacentor andersoni* (tick)

*These cell wall-less haemotrophic bacteria share characters with the haemotrophic mycoplasmas and will probably prove to be mycoplasmas, but their phylogenetic relationship remains to be established.
[†]Mechanical transmission.

names (*Mycoplasma haemofelis*, *Mycoplasma haemomuris*, *Mycoplasma haemosuis*, *Mycoplasma ovis* and *M. wenyonii*). The haemotrophic mycoplasmas have been given the vernacular name 'hemoplasmas'.

Related bacteria

Numerous reports have described erythrocytic bodies resembling these bacteria in a wide variety of vertebrate animals. Often these bodies were given bacterial species names merely on the basis of observing structures in stained blood smears. Careful evaluation of blood smears is required to distinguish these bacteria from erythrocytic structures, such as Pappenheimer bodies, Heinz bodies, Howell–Jolly bodies or other structures, and it may be difficult to differentiate haemotrophic mycoplasmas from basophilic structures without the aid of molecular diagnostic methods or electron microscopy. In a few cases the erythrocytic bodies were examined critically and shown by electron microscopy to be wall-less bacteria. Erythrocytic bodies identified by electron microscopy as wall-less *Eperythrozoon* or *Haemobartonella* have been described in a Raccoon (*Procyon lotor*), Llamas (*Lama glama*) and various monkey species used in laboratory studies. One of these, an agent in the South American Squirrel monkey (*Saimiri sciureus*) has been shown to be a new haemotrophic *Mycoplasma* species, and others probably represent new haemotrophic *Mycoplasma* species or new hosts for known haemotrophic *Mycoplasma* species.

Host range

As a group, these haemotrophic bacteria infect the erythrocytes of a wide range of animal hosts. Individual species appear to have a narrow host range, but in fact the host range of most species has not been fully examined.

Possible human infections

Transmission by blood-feeding vectors may result in cross-infection between domestic and wild animal populations, and possibly humans, and the host ranges of these bacteria need to be investigated. Reports of rare occurrences of haemotrophic bacteria from human cases, some of which were demonstrated to be wall-less by electron microscopy, will be discussed in a separate publication.

Clinical symptoms

Infections caused by haemotrophic mycoplasmas are frequently clinically inapparent but some species are pathogenic and cause visible disease in healthy, immunocompetent hosts. Clinical disease usually includes haemolytic anaemia, which may vary from mild to severe. Poor weight gain is characteristic in young animals. These bacteria can persist for years in latently infected animals without causing clinical disease; apparently they are cleared from the circulation by sequestration in the spleen. Splenectomy, stress or other predisposing factors often result in the appearance of large numbers of infected erythrocytes in the circulation, which may or may not be accompanied by clinical disease.

Diagnosis

These bacteria have not been cultivated and are maintained by serial passage in animal hosts. Microscopic examination of blood smears stained with Romanowsky-type stains (Wright–Giemsa's stain is particularly suitable) shows small (diameter less than 0.9 μm) blue- to purple-stained coccoid, ring- or rod-shaped structures on the surface of red cells (the rod-shaped structures are probably composed of coccoidal bodies). Fluorescent staining provides greater sensitivity. The number of infected red cells can range from just detectable to more than 80% of erythrocytes infected and individual erythrocytes can be infected by many organisms. Detection of inapparent infection by haematological methods can be difficult and may require daily sampling for prolonged periods, but molecular diagnostic methods should improve detection. Serological tests have been described. For most purposes, blood is best collected with citrate as the anticoagulant, since these bacteria lose infectivity when collected with ethylenediamine tetra-acetic acid (EDTA) and heparin interferes with the polymerase chain reaction (PCR). Deoxyribonucleic acid (DNA) from organisms in blood is well preserved on FTA blood-cards (Fitzco). Haemotrophic mycoplasmas can readily be dissociated from erythrocytes by gently shaking erythrocytes in phosphate-buffered saline, pH 7.2. Infected blood has been cryopreserved by freezing in liquid nitrogen, but 10% glycerol–10% horse serum commonly used for preserving mycoplasmas at −70°C may be adequate.

Transmission

Vectors are thought to be involved in the transmission of all species; all have been demonstrated to be, or are suspected of being, transmitted by blood-feeding arthropods, although sometimes only mechanically. Vectors include ixodid (hard) ticks, lice (*Polyplax* species), fleas (e.g. *Ctenocephalides felis*), flies (e.g. *Stomoyxs calcitrans*) and mosquitoes (e.g. *Aedes aegypti*) (see Table 1).

Treatment

All species that have been examined are sensitive to tetracycline but are resistant to penicillin and other antimicrobial agents that target the bacterial cell wall.

Control

Lack of detailed knowledge on the vectors precludes any vector control measures.

Selected bibliography

Clark, K.G.A. (1975) A basophilic micro-organism infecting human red cells. *British Journal of Haematology* 29, 301–304.

Contamin, H. and Michel, J.C. (1999) Haemobartonellosis in squirrel monkeys (*Saimiri sciureus*): antagonism between *Haemobartonella* sp. and experimental *Plasmodium falciparum* malaria. *Experimental Parasitology* 91, 297–305.

Duarte, M.I., Oliveira, M.S., Shikanai-Yasuda, M.A., Mariano, O.N., Takakura, C.F., Pagliari, C. and Corbett, C.E. (1992) *Haemobartonella*-like microorganism infection in AIDS patients: ultrastructural pathology. *Journal of Infectious Diseases* 165, 976–977.

Foley, J.E., Harrus, S., Poland, A., Chomel, B. and Pedersen, N.C. (1998) Molecular, clinical, and pathologic comparison of two distinct strains of *Haemobartonella felis* in domestic cats. *American Journal of Veterinary Research* 59, 1581–1588.

Gwaltney, S.M. and Oberst, R.D. (1994) Comparison of an improved polymerase chain reaction protocol and the indirect hemagglutination assay in the detection of *Eperythrozoon suis* infection. *Journal of Veterinary Diagnostic Investigation* 6, 321–325.

Kreier, J.P. and Ristic, M. (1984) Genus III *Haemobartonella*; Genus IV *Eperythrozoon*. In: Kreig, N.R. and Holt, J.G. (eds) *Bergey's Manual of Systematic Bacteriology*, Vol. 1, 8th edn. Williams & Wilkins, Baltimore, pp. 724–729.

Kreier, J.P., Gothe, R., Ihler, G.M., Krampitz, H.E., Mernaugh, G. and Palmer, G.H. (1992) The haemotrophic bacteria: the families Bartonellaceae and Anaplasmataceae. In: Balows, A., Trüper, H.G., Dworkin, M., Harder, W. and Schleifer, K.-H. (eds) *The Prokaryotes: a Handbook on the Biology of Bacteria: Ecophysiology, Isolation, Identification, Applications*, Vol. 4. Springer-Verlag, Berlin, pp. 3994–4022.

Maede, Y. (1979) Sequestration and phagocytosis of *Hemobartonella felis* in the spleen. *American Journal of Veterinary Research* 40, 691–695.

Messick, J.B., Cooper, S.K. and Huntley, M. (1999) Development and evaluation of a polymerase chain reaction assay using the 16S rRNA gene for detection of *Eperythrozoon suis* infection. *Journal of Veterinary Diagnostic Investigations* 11, 229–336.

Neimark, H. and Kocan, K.M. (1997) The cell wall-less rickettsia *Eperythrozoon wenyonii* is a mycoplasma. *FEMS Microbiological Letters* 156, 287–291.

Neimark, H., Johansson, K.-E., Rikihisa, Y. and Tully, J. (2001) Proposal to transfer some members of the genera *Haemobartonella* and *Eperythrozoon* to the genus *Mycoplasma* with descriptions of *Mycoplasma hemofelis*, comb. nov., *Mycoplasma hemomuris*, comb. nov., *Mycoplasma hemosuis* comb. nov. and *Mycoplasma wenyonii* comb. nov. *International Journal of Systematic and Evolutionary Microbiology* 51, 891–899.

Prullage, J.B., Williams, R.E. and Gaafar, S.M. (1993) On the transmissibility of *Eperythrozoon suis* by *Stomoxys calcitrans* and *Aedes aegypti*. *Veterinary Parasitology* 50, 125–135.

Rikihisa, Y., Kawahara, M., Wen, B., Kociba, G., Fuerst, P., Kawamori, F., Suto, C., Shibata, S.

and Futohashi, M. (1997) Western immuno-blot analysis of *Haemobartonella muris* and comparison of 16S rRNA gene sequences of *H. muris*, *H. felis*, and *Eperythrozoon suis. Journal of Clinical Microbiology* 35, 823–829.

Heartwater (cowdriosis)

Keith J. Sumption

Heartwater is a disease caused by infection of ruminants with the rickettsia *Cowdria ruminantium*.

The infection is frequently fatal in cattle, sheep and goats in sub-Saharan Africa, and also on a few islands in the Indian and Caribbean regions. It is transmitted predominantly by ixodid (hard) ticks of the genus *Amblyomma*, which feed preferentially on domestic and wild ruminants. The name refers to the frequent post-mortem finding of excessive fluid around the heart. Cowdriosis is a synonym, reflecting the classification of the causal organism and the contribution of E.V. Cowdry to the identification of the aetiology.

Distribution

The disease is found in most of sub-Saharan Africa, except in very arid areas, which are unsuitable for maintenance of the vector ticks, but has also been maintained on a few islands in the Caribbean and Indian oceans (Madagascar, Mauritius) where vector populations have become established. An efficient vector species is also present in the Yemen, but the existence of heartwater has not been reported. Potential extension of the disease range to mainland America is possible because some of the *Amblyomma* species present could act as vectors. In Africa the majority of cases occur in areas with farming systems involving non-indigenous animal breeds and cross-breeds, where some or most animals lack genetic resistance to the occurrence of disease. In areas where the majority of animals have a high genetic resistance, disease is seldom reported.

Aetiological agent

Cowdria ruminantium (Eubacteria, Proteobacteria, alpha subdivision; classification in *Bergey's Manual*; order *Rickettsiales*, family *Rickettsiaceae*, tribe *Ehrlichiae*) is known to replicate only within mammalian or tick cells. In mammalian infections, the detection of infection in endothelial cells lining the major and minor blood-vessels is used in diagnosis and it is likely that the excessive fluid accumulation in body cavities relates to the altered function of the endothelium. Electron-dense extracellular forms (elementary bodies) are produced in endothelial cell cultures and are infective to other animals and cell cultures, and are probably in the same life-cycle phase as the forms seen free in the plasma of infected animals during acute infection.

Clinical signs

Under natural tick exposure the incubation period is usually between 2 and 3 weeks, with nymphal transmission occurring slightly earlier than adult tick transmission. The severity of clinical signs and the frequency of occurrence differ between individuals and breeds, but the signs are generally more severe in exotic breeds, non-indigenous to heartwater-endemic areas, and also in animals over 1 month of age. Disease usually starts with a sudden rise in body temperature, rising in large and small ruminants over 2–3 days to often exceed 41°C. Listlessness and nervous signs may be observed; the animal can appear anxious, with hypersensitive responses to light and hand/air movements about the eye, and may develop muscular tremors, trembling, altered gait and locomotor control, leaning or circling. Mild diarrhoea may be seen in cattle. The occurrence of these signs, usually accompanied by increased respiratory rate and effort in breathing, can occur in other diseases, but usually proceed quickly in heartwater to recumbency, coma and death. Fits may occur, and animals that develop increased respiratory effort or distress usually die within 3–12 h. Under natural conditions where stock-persons have the care of many animals, animals are commonly found dead without clinical signs having been observed. In more resistant animals, fever and increased respiratory rate may be the extent of the signs observed. Animals often continue to eat until very shortly before death and may be found dead with grass in their mouths. Mortality rates can reach 50% in exotic cattle and 90% in small ruminants, although under conditions of routine tick control sporadic deaths over a prolonged period are more frequent than outbreaks.

Diagnosis

Gross pathology signs are frequently the first indicator of a case of heartwater. Presence of feeding ticks on the body can indicate that tick control is not effective in preventing tick feeding, but absence of ticks does not indicate that tick control was effective 2–3 weeks previously. Heartwater should be suspected when excessive fluid is found in the thorax (0.5 l in small ruminants, 1–2 l in cattle) and around the heart, and/or when there is a full gall-bladder with bile staining on the omentum. The disease is best confirmed by making a smear of the brain (cerebral cortex or brain stem) and staining with Giemsa for detection of intracellular morulae in capillary endothelial cells, which is indicative of infection. Alternative tests where facilities permit include culture of neutrophils and use of polymerase chain reaction (PCR) techniques. Serological tests, including enzyme-linked immunosorbent assay (ELISA), are difficult to interpret, because the specificity of many tests is poor as result of cross-reactions with ehrlichial infections and/or poor sensitivity for the detection of recovered cattle, which leads to underestimates of infection prevalence.

In many cases, if *Amblyomma* ticks are frequently observed to feed on domestic stock, it is likely that heartwater is present and that most adult animals will have encountered the infection.

Transmission

The tick–mammal cycle is predominantly via feeding of nymphs or adult *Amblyomma* ticks. Only *Amblyomma* species have been proved to be field vectors. Both African and non-African species of *Amblyomma* have been shown to be possible vectors, but in the natural situation *A. variegatum* and *A. hebreum* are the most widespread and significant vectors, in West–Central–East Africa and southern Africa, respectively. The former tick species is also present in the Caribbean and Madagascar, and in semi-arid areas of East Africa *Amblyomma gemma* and *Amblyomma lepidum* are also important vectors. Transmission is considered almost entirely trans-stadial, with larvae acquiring infections and subsequently transmitting when the larvae become nymphs and then adults. The pre-transmission period – that is, the interval from when ticks are placed on a host to the transmission of infection – is in the region of 1–3 days for nymphs and 3–4 days for adults. During this time maturation of infection occurs, with increased infectivity for the ruminant host; this appears to coincide with increase in infection in tick salivary glands.

Ticks become infected while feeding on animals with acute infections and also for some time after recovery (carrier state), with animals such as the Cape buffalo (*Syncerus caffer*) being proven to be carriers for 8 months. A wide range of ruminant and non-ruminant species may be involved as sources of infection for ticks. The most significant sources are probably those favoured by feeding larvae and nymphs, since infection of domestic stock is by nymphs and adult ticks. Vertical transmission between dam and calf has been reported and might have some importance in the frequency of early exposure/resistance in endemic areas, but horizontal transmission is not known except through needle transmission involving contaminated blood products.

Treatment

Cowdria is susceptible to tetracyclines and these are the drugs of choice. Treatment must be commenced early, since recovery after respiratory effort has developed is often ineffectual. In commercial sheep flocks, treatment of febrile animals with long-acting tetracycline antibiotics is prudent; in outbreak situations a flock treatment should be considered. Animals should be rested, and a subsequent treatment, 2–3 days after the first administered dose, is often justified, as relapses are common.

Control

In most African countries control of the disease in susceptible stock has been by application of acaricides to livestock, which should be at short intervals, because transmission can occur with nymphs feeding on the host for as little as 2 days. With resistant indigenous stocks, vector control is rarely considered necessary, although sporadic losses can occur, especially in sheep, but are frequently not recognized. In eastern Africa control by acaricides of the more feared disease East Coast fever (see Theilerioses) also has the benefit of simultaneously controlling heartwater. However, relaxation of tick control in such situations could result in outbreaks of disease, since the level of herd immunity will be low.

A live, virulent vaccine (for infection and treatment) is currently available only in southern Africa and is impractical for widespread use. The prophylactic use of long-acting antibiotics is feasible in susceptible bought-in animals with no immunity, providing that conditions of high tick attack rates prevail, with the aim of immunity developing under controlled challenge.

Selected bibliography

Bezuidenhout, J.D., Prozesky, J.L., Du Plessis, J.L. and Van Amstel, S.R. (1994) Heartwater. In: Coetzer, J.A.W., Thomson, G.R. and Tustin, R.C. (eds) *Infectious Diseases of Livestock with Special Reference to Southern Africa*, Vol. 1. Oxford University Press, Cape Town, pp. 351–370.

Camus, E., Barre, N., Martinez, D. and Uilenberg, G. (1996) *Heartwater (Cowdriosis). A Review.* Office International des Epizooties, Paris, France, 177 pp.

Uilenberg, G. and Camus, E. (1993) Heartwater (Cowdriosis). In: Woldehewit, Z. and Ristic, M. (eds) *Rickettsial and Chlamydial Diseases of Domestic Animals*. Pergamon Press, Oxford, pp. 293–332.

Heartworm *see* **Dirofilariasis.**

Haemoplasmas *see* **Haemotrophic mycoplasmas.**

Hepatozoonosis, canine

Gad Baneth

Two distinct *Hepatozoon* species infect canids: *Hepatozoon canis*, which is primarily found in haemolymphatic tissues and causes anaemia and lethargy, and *Hepatozoon americanum*, which infects muscular tissues and induces severe myositis and lameness.

Distribution

Canine hepatozoonosis has been reported from tropical, subtropical and temperate regions of all continents except Australia.

Hepatozoon canis infection in dogs was first described from India in 1905 and has since been recorded in southern Europe, the Middle East, Africa and the Far East. *Hepatozoon canis* infection is often referred to as Old World canine hepatozoonosis. American canine hepatozoonosis was described from Texas in 1978 and following that report also from several southern states in the USA, including Louisiana, Alabama, Georgia, Tennessee, Oklahoma and Florida.

Parasite

Hepatozoon canis and *H. americanum* are tick-borne protozoal parasites from the family Haemogregarinidae.

The life cycles of *H. canis* (Fig. 1) and *H. americanum* are complex and involve tick hosts that become infected when they are feeding on the blood of a dog with hepatozoonosis. *Hepatozoon* gamonts from the dog's blood are released from neutrophils within the tick and sexual reproduction of the parasite takes place, followed by the formation of oocysts, which are found in the haemocoel. Infection of a dog occurs when it ingests a tick containing mature oocysts. Sporozoites released in the gut of the dog penetrate the intestinal wall and disseminate to the spleen, lymph nodes and bone marrow in *H. canis* infections and to skeletal and myocardial muscles in *H. americanum* infections. Merogony takes place in these organs, and merozoites that are released from mature meronts penetrate neutrophils and form gamonts, which circulate in the peripheral blood.

Hepatozoon americanum was initially considered a strain of *H. canis*, until it was described in 1997 as a separate species based on differences in clinical signs, tissue tropism, pathological findings, parasite morphology and tick vectors (Table 1). Subsequent genetic and antigenic comparisons have supported the separation of these parasites.

Clinical signs

Hepatozoon canis infection

Old World canine hepatozoonosis varies from being asymptomatic in apparently healthy dogs to a severe and life-threatening disease in animals, with extreme lethargy, cachexia and anaemia. An asymptomatic to mild disease is the most common presentation of the infection and it is usually

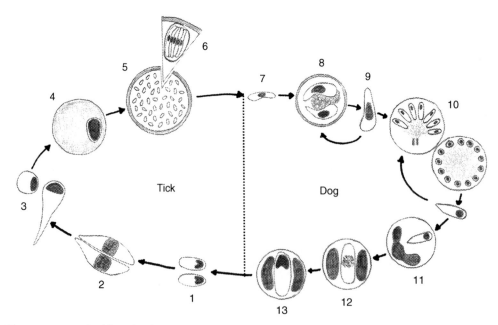

Fig. 1. Stages in the life cycle of *Hepatozoon canis*: (1) free gamonts in the tick following a blood meal; (2) gamonts associate in syzygy; (3) male and female gametes develop while in syzygy prior to fertilization; (4) fertilization results in the formation of a zygote; (5) mature oocyst containing sporozoites; (6) a section through an oocyst showing a sporocyst containing sporozoites; (7) free sporozoites in a dog's gut; (8) merogony–meronts containing macromerozoites; (9) free macromerozoite; (10) merogony – longitudinal and cross-sectional views of meronts containing micromerozoites; (11) penetration of a myeloid cell by a micromerozoite; (12) developing gamont with 'scattered' chromatin; and (13) mature gamont within a neutrophil in the blood.

associated with a low level of *H. canis* parasitaemia (1–5%), while a severe illness is found in dogs with a high parasitaemia, often approaching 100% of the peripheral blood neutrophils. High parasitaemia rates are frequently accompanied by extreme neutrophilia reaching as high as 150,000 leucocytes μl^{-1}.

Most dogs infected with *H. canis* appear to undergo a subclinical infection. A survey of dogs from Israel showed that 33% had been exposed to the parasite, as indicated by the presence of anti-*H. canis* antibodies. Only 3% of the seropositive dogs had detectable blood gamonts and only 1% had severe clinical signs associated with the infection. A case–control study of dogs with *H. canis* parasitaemia admitted to a veterinary hospital in Israel indicated that 15% had a high number of circulating parasites (>800 gamonts μl^{-1}) accompanied by elevated body temperature, lethargy, weight loss, anaemia, hyperglobulinaemia and hypoalbuminaemia. Post-mortem examination of

dogs with a high parasitaemia revealed hepatitis, pneumonia and glomerulonephritis associated with *H. canis* meronts. Meronts and developing gamonts were also found in the spleen, bone marrow and lymph nodes, often with no apparent host inflammatory response.

Concurrent infections of dogs with *H. canis* and other canine pathogens that have been reported include: parvovirus, canine distempter, *Babesia canis*, *Ehrlichia canis*, *Toxoplasma gondii* and *Leishmania infantum* (see entries on Babesiosis, Ehrlichiosis and Leishmaniasis). Immune suppression induced by an infectious agent, an immature immune system in young animals or immunodeficient conditions are hypothesized to influence the pathogenesis of new *H. canis* infections or the reactivation of pre-existing ones.

Hepatozoon americanum infection

American canine hepatozoonosis is a chronic disease that is almost always severe

Table 1. Comparison of findings from dogs with *H. canis* and *H. americanum* infections.

	H. canis	H. americanum
Common clinical signs	Fever, lethargy, emaciation	Gait abnormalities, muscular hyperaesthesia, fluctuating fever, lethargy, mucopurulent ocular discharge
Severity of clinical signs	Often mild. A severe disease is seen in dogs with a high parasitaemia	Severe
Haematological findings		
Peripheral blood gamonts	Common	Infrequent
% parasitaemia of neutrophils	1–100%	Usually <0.1%
Extreme leucocytosis	Rare. Found in dogs with a high parasitaemia	Common
Anaemia	Common	Common
Radiographical findings	Non-specific	Periosteal proliferation of long bones
Main method of diagnosis	Demonstration of gamonts in blood smears	Demonstration of cysts and pyogranuloma by muscle biospy
Main target tissues	Spleen, bone marrow, lymph nodes	Skeletal muscle
Histopathological findings	Hepatitis, splenitis, pneumonia	Pyogranulomatous myositis
Distinct morphological features	'Wheel spoke' meront	'Onion skin' cyst
Vector tick	*Rhipicephalus sanguineus*	*Amblyomma maculatum*
Treatment	Imidocarb dipropionate, doxycyline	Trimethoprim/sulfa, pyrimethamine, clindamycin, decoquinate
Prognosis	Good	Poor

and leads to debilitation and death. Most dogs diagnosed with H. americanum infection are presented with gait abnormalities and muscular pain induced by myositis. In a study of dogs with canine hepatozoonosis from Alabama and Georgia, 86% were febrile, 82% suffered weight loss, 77% had mucopurulent ocular discharge, induced in some cases by parasitic myositis of the extraocular muscles, 64% had generalized muscle atrophy and hyperaesthesia was recorded in a similar percentage of animals. Signs of pain were generalized or localized in the lumbar and cervical spine or in joints. Gait abnormalities included stiffness, hind-limb paresis, ataxia and inability to rise. The mean survival time was 1 year, despite anti-protozoal therapy and supportive treatment. A marked neutrophilia is one of the consistent haematological findings in American canine hepatozoonosis, with white blood cell counts ranging from 30,000 to 200,000 μl^{-1}. Serum biochemical abnormalities include increased alkaline phosphatase activity, hypoalbuminaemia and a false hypoglycaemia, induced by the glucose metabolism of white blood cells in blood taken with anticoagulants other than sodium fluoride.

Post-mortem examination of dogs with American canine hepatozoonosis reveals cachexia and muscular atrophy. Histopathology of specimens from muscular and cardiac tissues shows pyogranulomatous myositis and typical round to oval cysts (250–500 μm diameter) containing a central nucleus surrounded by concentric rings of membranes. These cysts are sometimes referred to as having an 'onion peel' appearance, due to the structure of the membranes surrounding a core mass. The cystic forms of H. americanum are more numerous than the pyogranulomas in muscular tissues and, while the cysts are frequently not associated with a host inflammatory response; pyogranulomas contain parasites that have ruptured from meronts and induced a cell response characterized by the presence of neutrophils and macrophages. Hepatozoon americanum meronts and multifocal pyogranulomas are found less frequently in non-muscular tissues, including lymph nodes, spleen and pancreas. Amyloid deposition may be evident in lymphoid organs and kidneys. Periosteal bone proliferation of the long bones, pelvis and vertebrae, and the formation of bone exostosis are common findings in American canine hepatozoonosis and contribute to the painful sensation and stiffness of infected dogs.

Diagnosis

The main method used to diagnose Old World canine hepatozoonosis is by microscopic detection of intracellular H. canis gamonts in blood smears stained by Giemsa's or Wright's stain. The parasitaemia level is usually 0.5–5% of the neutrophils and may reach as high as 100% in heavy infections. The gamonts are ellipsoidal corpuscles, about 11 μm × 4 μm, found in the cytoplasm of neutrophils and rarely in monocytes (Fig. 2). Hepatozoon canis meronts in infected tissues are usually round to oval, about 30 μm in diameter, and include numerous elongated micromerozoites with defined nuclei. A cross-sectional cut of the meront through the midshaft of the micromerozoites reveals a form with a clear core surrounded by a circle of micromerozoite nuclei, which is often referred to as a 'wheel spoke' (Fig. 3). This form is typical for H. canis meronts and not found in H. americanum infection.

Gamonts of H. americanum are morphologically similar by light microscopy to H. canis gamonts, but they are relatively rare in the blood and the level of parasitaemia does not usually exceed 0.1%. The common way of confirming H. americanum infection is by muscle biopsy and demonstration of parasites in cysts or granulomas. The parasites appear to be widely dispersed in the muscular tissues and it is recommended to sample the biceps femoris, semitendinosus or epaxial muscles. Radiography of the limb bones or pelvis demonstrating periosteal proliferation can be used for screening a suspected animal, although the appearance of lesions on X-rays may vary from being subtle to marked.

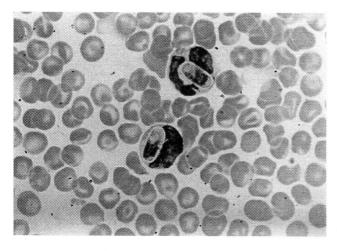

Fig. 2. *Hepatozoon canis* gamonts in a Giemsa-stained blood smear from a naturally infected dog.

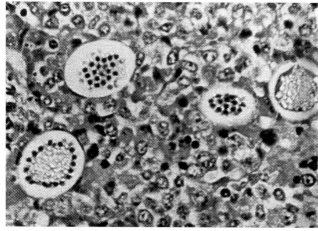

Fig. 3. *Hepatozoon canis* meronts in a histopathological section of lymph node tissue from a dog with naturally occuring Old World canine hepatozoonosis.

An indirect fluorescent antibody test for anti-*H. canis* antibodies using gamont antigens has been developed and used for epidemiologcial studies in Israel and Japan. Sera from dogs infected with *H. americanum* showed only a low degree of cross-reactivity with *H. canis* antigens and there is currently no assay available for the reliable detection of anti-*H. americanum* antibodies.

Transmission

The brown dog tick, *Rhipicephalus sanguineus*, is the main vector for Old World canine hepatozoonosis caused by *H. canis*, while American canine hepatozoonosis is transmitted by the Gulf Coast tick, *Amblyomma maculatum*. Trans-stadial transmission of *H. canis* and of *H. americanum* has been shown to occur in both *R. sanguineus* and *A. maculatum*.

Transmission to dogs occurs by oral ingestion of ticks having mature oocysts and has been demonstrated by experimental infections of dogs with *H. canis* or with *H. americanum*. Vertical transmission of *H. canis* was reported in puppies born to an infected dam and raised in a tick-free environment, but it is not currently clear how important this mode of transmission is to the epidemiology of the disease.

Naturally occurring American canine hepatozoonosis has been reported in Coyotes (*Canis latrans*) in Oklahoma and it is suggested that Coyotes are important wildlife reservoir hosts for the disease in the USA.

Treatment

Old World canine hepatozoonosis is treated with imidocarb dipropionate injected subcutaneously or intramuscularly at 5–6 mg kg^{-1} every 14 days until gamonts are no longer present in blood smears. Elimination of *H. canis* gamonts from the peripheral blood may require as much as 8 weeks. Oral doxycyline at 10 mg kg^{-1} day^{-1} for 21 days has also been used in combination with imidocarb dipropionate for treatment of *H. canis* infection.

American canine hepatozoonosis currently remains a disease with no treatment that can effectively eliminate *H. americanum* from its host. Research from Auburn University in Alabama has indicated that temporary remission of clinical signs can be achieved with a combination oral therapy of trimethoprim/sulfa (15 mg kg^{-1} every 12 h), pyrimethamine (0.25 mg kg^{-1} every 24 h) and clindamycin (10 mg kg^{-1} every 8 h) for 14 days. Most dogs, however, treated only with this combination relapse and die within 12–24 months. Remission can be prolonged with the oral administration of the coccidiostat decoquinate at 10–20 mg kg^{-1} mixed in the food every 12 h. Addition of decoquinate achieved an apparent cure of about 80% of treated dogs, but, because therapy discontinuation resulted in the recurrence of clinical signs in several dogs, it is recommended that treatment be continued for 1–2 years. Supportive therapy with non-steroidal anti-inflammatory drugs is effective in relieving pain and fever in dogs with American canine hepatozoonosis.

Control

Prevention of exposure of dogs to ticks by the use of acaricides is warranted to control the spread of both forms of canine hepatozoonosis.

Selected bibliography

Baneth, G. and Weigler, B. (1997) Retrospective case–control study of hepatozoonosis in dogs in Israel. *Journal of Veterinary Internal Medicine* 11, 365–370.

Baneth, G., Shkap, V., Presentey, B.-Z. and Pipano, E. (1996) *Hepatozoon canis*: the prevalence of antibodies and gamonts in dogs in Israel. *Veterinary Research Communications* 20, 41–46.

Baneth, G., Shkap, V., Samish, M., Pipano, E. and Savitsky, I. (1998) Antibody response to *Hepatozoon canis* in experimentally infected dogs. *Veterinary Parasitology* 74, 299–305.

Craig, T.M. (1998) Hepatozoonosis. In: Greene, C.E. (ed.) *Infectious Diseases of the Dog and Cat*, 2nd edn. W.B. Saunders, Philadelphia, pp. 458–465.

Craig, T.M., Smallwood, J.E., Knauer, K.W. and McGrath, J.P. (1978) *Hepatozoon canis* infection in dogs: clinical, radiographic and hematological findings. *Journal of American Veterinary Medical Association* 173, 967–972.

Macintire, D.K., Vincent-Johnson, N., Dillon, A.R., Blagburn, B.L., Lindsay, D.S., Whitley, E.M. and Banfield, C. (1997) Hepatozoonosis in dogs: 22 cases (1989–1994). *Journal of the American Veterinary Medical Association* 210, 916–922.

Mathew, J.S., Ewing, S.A., Panciera, R.J. and Woods, J.P. (1998) Experimental transmission of *Hepatozoon americanum* Vincent-Johnson et al., 1997 to dogs by the Gulf Coast tick, *Amblyomma maculatum* Koch. *Veterinary Parasitology* 80, 1–14.

Panceira, R.J., Ewing, S.A. Mathew, J.S., Cummings, C.A., Kocan, A.A. and Fox, J.C. (1998) Observations on tissue stages of *Hepatozoon americanum* in 19 naturally infected dogs. *Veterinary Parasitology* 78, 265–276.

Vincent-Johnson, N.A., Baneth, G. and Macintire, D.K. (1997) Canine hepatozoonosis: pathophysiology, diagnosis and treatment. *The Compendium on Continuing Education* 19, 51–65.

Vincent-Johnson, N.A., Macintire, D.K., Lindsay, D.S., Lenz, S.D., Baneth, G., Shkap, V. and Blagburn, B.L. (1997) A new *Hepatozoon* species from dogs: description of the causative agent of canine hepatozoonosis in North America. *Journal of Parasitology* 83, 1165–1172.

Hepatazoon **species** *see* **Hepatozoonosis, canine.**

Hippoboscids (Hippoboscidae)

M.W. Service

Adult hippoboscids (louse-flies, flat-flies, tick-flies, keds) are peculiar flies that are greatly flattened dorsoventrally and have large toothed and recurved claws and a leathery integument. The degree of development of the wings differs greatly in different genera; in the genus *Hippobosca* they are fully formed, whereas in *Melophagus* both wings and halteres are absent (Fig. 1). There are three subfamilies. The largest is the Ornithomyinae, most species of which are

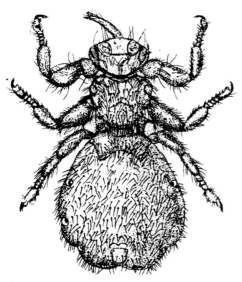

Fig. 1. Example of a wingless adult hippoboscid fly, the sheep-ked (*Melophagus ovinus*).

parasites of birds, *Pseudolynchia canariensis* (Fig. 2) being a parasite of pigeons. The Melophaginae contain flies parasitic on bovids and cervids, the best known being the sheep-ked (*Melophagus ovinus*), which is wingless. The Hippoboscinae contain species that parasitize mostly equines and bovids. Hippoboscids only rarely bite humans.

Biology

Female flies suck the blood of their hosts and, like the females of tsetse-flies, are viviparous – that is, larvae develop one at a time in the uterus of the female fly and, when a larva is mature, it is deposited by the fly and shortly afterwards becomes a puparium.

The sheep-ked (*Melophagus ovinus*) (Fig. 1) is found throughout most of the temperate areas and in cooler parts of the tropics where there are sheep. A mature, fully grown larva is deposited on the fleece of sheep when the fly is about 2 weeks old; thereafter additional larvae are deposited every 7–8 days. Within a few hours the deposited larva pupates to form a brown puparium. Puparia are firmly glued to sheep's wool, especially around the neck and on the forelegs and flanks. An adult fly emerges from a puparium after about 3–4 weeks, but in cool weather after 5–7 weeks. Adults of both sexes blood-feed on sheep. The entire life

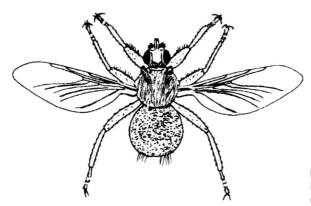

Fig. 2. Example of a winged adult hippoboscid adult, the pigeon-fly (*Pseudolynchia canariensis*).

cycle is spent on the host and the time from newly emerged adult to the next generation adult is about 5 weeks.

Pseudolynchia canariensis (the pigeon-fly) (Fig. 2) is an important parasite of domestic pigeons and seems more or less restricted to these birds in the Americas. In the Old World *P. canariensis* is also found parasitizing several species of wild birds, especially raptors. The fly is found throughout the tropics and in warmer areas of temperate regions. Adults have long thin wings and fly from host to host and, on alighting, suck blood, mainly from the less feathered areas. Larvae are deposited at 3–4-day intervals when the adults are either on or off the host. The puparial stage is found at the bottom of cages or nests and, at 23°C, lasts about 30 days. In the USA adults not infrequently bite humans.

Diseases
In Africa sheep-keds transmit the trypanosome *Trypanosoma melophagium* (see Animal trypanosomiasis). *Pseudolynchia canariensis* and other *Pseudolynchia* species together with *Microlynchia pusillus* and *Ornithomyia avivularia* are vectors of *Haemoproteus columbae*, while *Stilbometopa impressa* and *Lynchia hirsuta* transmit *Haemoproteus meleagridis* (see Haemoproteosis).

Control
Shearing sheep clearly rids them of most keds. Applications of organophosphate or pyrethroid insecticides to the fleece or oral administration of the drug ivermectin can greatly reduce fly infestations.

Probably the best control of pigeon-flies involves cleaning out pigeons' nests and houses at 3-weekly intervals to get rid of the puparia. Alternatively, nesting-boxes can be dusted with insecticides.

Selected bibliography
Bequaert, J.C. (1953) The Hippoboscidae or louse-flies (Diptera) of mammals and birds. Part II. Structure, physiology and natural history. *Entomologia Americana* (new series) 32, 1–209 and 33, 211–442.

Pfadt, R.E. (1976) Sheep ked populations on a small farm. *Journal of Economic Entomology* 63, 313–316.

Radostis, O.M., Gay, C.C., Blood, D.C. and Hinchcliff, K.W. (1999) *Veterinary Medicine. A Textbook of the Diseases of Cattle, Sheep, Pigs and Horses*, 9th edn. Baillière-Tindall, London, 1881 pp.

Horn-flies (Muscidae)

M.W. Service

Horn-flies (e.g. *Haematobia* species) are in the subfamily Stomoxyinae. Adults are greyish and somewhat similar in appearance to stable-flies (see entry) but are smaller (about 4 mm long) and more slender. Previously these flies were placed in the genera *Lyperosia* or *Siphona*. The species *Haematobia exigua*, which attacks buffaloes, is often called the buffalo-fly. (Unfortunately simuliid black-flies (see Black-flies) are sometimes called buffalo-flies.) Horn-flies have an almost worldwide distribution.

Biology
When cattle defecate, female horn-flies that are flying around and biting the animals lay their eggs in the freshly dropped faeces. The eggs hatch to produce slender cylindrical (maggot-shaped) larvae, which feed on semi-fluid dung; the third and final larval instar pupates to form a brown puparium. Development time depends on temperature. In hot weather (24–26°C), eggs can hatch within 24 h, larvae pupate within 7 days and the puparial period lasts about 5–7 days. In cooler weather, however, the life

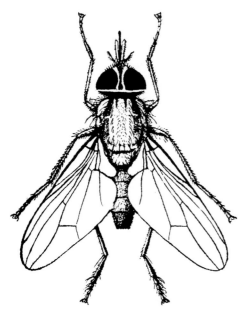

Fig. 1. An adult of a horn-fly (*Haematobia irritans*).

Diseases

Horn-flies rarely bite humans but can be serious pests of cattle. There are often several hundred flies on and around a single cow or buffalo, and sometimes up to about 5000 flies. Such high numbers are considered to reduce weight gains in beef cattle and lower milk production in dairy herds. It has been estimated that *Haematobia irritans* causes more than US$160 million annual loss to the cattle industry in the USA.

Horn-flies transmit *Stephanofilaria stilesi* to cattle (see Stephanofilariasis) and *Parafilaria multipapillosa* to equines (see Parafilariasis).

Control

Spraying cattle with residual insecticides can give some control, but there may be objections to or restrictions on this practice because it could result in pesticide residues in meat and milk. Insecticide-impregnated ear tags have sometimes proved effective in protecting cattle. Another approach is the introduction of insect growth regulators (IGRs) to animal feeds, or administering the drug ivermectin, either orally or by subcutaneous injection. These treatments prevent the life cycle from being completed in the animal's faeces.

cycle from egg to puparium may last up to 6 weeks and, in very cold weather, it may extend to several months, with the puparium entering a state of diapause (overwintering). After emergence, adult flies (Fig. 1) of both sexes soon blood-feed on cattle, and females can lay eggs in as little as 3 days after emergence. Flies congregate mainly on the shoulders and flanks, where the animal's switching tail causes them little disturbance; they frequently cluster around the bases of the horns – hence their name, horn-flies. Horn-flies spend nearly all their time settling on or flying around cattle. They probably live for 1–2 months and take two to three blood meals a day; in so doing they cause considerable distress to the animals.

Horses and sheep are attacked much less than cattle because their drier and harder faecal droppings are not so suited to larval development as are the moist and softer buffalo- and cow-pats.

Selected bibliography

Bruce, W.G. (1964) The history and biology of the horn fly, *Haematobia irritans* (Linnaeus); with comments on control. *North Carolina Agricultural Experimental Station Technical Bulletin* 157, 1–32.

Hillerton, J.E. (1985) Sexing of *Haematobia irritans* (L.) (Dipt., Muscidae). *Entomologist's Monthly Magazine* 121, 211–212.

McLintock, J. and Depner, K.R. (1954) A review of the life history and habits of the horn fly, *Siphona irritans* (L.) (Diptera, Muscidae). *Canadian Entomologist* 86, 20–33.

Roberts, F.H.S. (1952) *Insects Affecting Livestock with Special Reference to the Important Species Occurring in Australia*. Angus & Robertson, Sydney, 267 pp.

Horse-flies (Tabanidae)

M.W. Service

The horse-flies (clegs, deer-flies, gad-flies, greenheads, stouts, tabanids) are the largest (6–30 mm long) biting flies that attack animals and humans. They comprise about 4000 species, belonging to 30 genera, of which the most important from the veterinary and medical points of view are *Chrysops*, *Tabanus* and *Haematopota*. Tabanids have a worldwide distribution, although the genus *Haematopota* is uncommon in North America and absent from South America and Australia.

Biology

Only adult females take blood meals from humans and a wide spectrum of animals, including livestock; males feed on naturally occurring sugary secretions. Eggs are laid on the underside of leaves, twigs and small branches and on grasses, plant stems, rocks and stones that are near or overhanging larval habitats, which are mainly muddy, semi-aquatic or aquatic sites. Eggs hatch within 4–14 days and the resultant larvae drop down on to the underlying mud or water. Larvae are cylindrical and rather maggot-shaped (Fig. 1), but have distinct, raised, tyre-like rings encircling most body segments; in addition, the first seven segments have laterally and ventrally six roundish protuberances called pseudopods. Larvae are found in mud, damp soil, humus, rotting vegetation and muddy waters and on the edges of pools and ponds and may

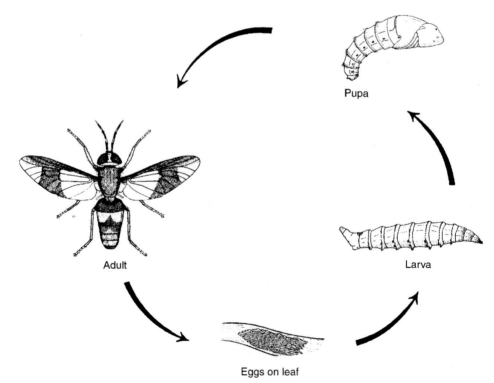

Pupa

Adult

Larva

Eggs on leaf

Fig. 1. Life cycle of a horse-fly (tabanid). The adult shown is a *Chrysops* species. (Modified from M.W. Service (2000) *Medical Entomology for Students,* Cambridge University Press, Cambridge.)

adhere to floating vegetation, such as leaves, twigs and logs. They breathe in air through the very short and conical siphon positioned on the last body segment.

Larvae of some tabanids, especially *Chrysops* species, feed on detritus and decaying vegetable and animal matter, whereas larvae of *Tabanus* and *Haematopota* are mainly predacious. Larval development takes a long time, often extending over 1–2 years, while in temperate regions larvae may live for 3 years before pupating. Larvae grow to 1–6 cm in length, depending on the species. The pupal period lasts about 5–20 days.

Adult females bite during the daytime and are especially active in sunshine, but a few species feed at dusk and during the night. Tabanids are strong fliers and may travel several kilometres. They locate their hosts mainly by colour and movement. Many species inhabit woods and forests, but others bite in more open areas and feed on cattle and deer in pastures. Bites can be painful and because of the fly's coarse mouthparts wounds often continue to bleed after the female has departed. Because of the pain inflicted by biting, feeding is often interrupted, which results in several blood meals being taken from the same or different hosts before the fly is satisfied, behaviour which can enhance mechanical transmission of infections.

In both temperate and tropical countries, the occurrence of adults is seasonal. In the tropics, populations often reach a peak towards the beginning of the rainy seasons, decreasing in size in the dry seasons, but often not completely disappearing. In temperate countries, adults usually die off at the end of the summer, with a new population emerging the subsequent spring.

Diseases

In Africa, species of *Chrysops*, such as *C. silaceus*, are of medical importance because they are involved in the cyclical transmission of the filarial worm *Loa loa* (see Loiasis). Tabanids of several genera, but in particular *Tabanus*, are known or suspected mechanical vectors of the pathogens causing anaplasmosis, anthrax, *Elaeophora schneideri*, surra (*Trypanosoma evansi*), *Trypanosoma vixax*, tularaemia, Issyk-Kul virus disease and possibly vesicular stomatitis (see entries for all these infections).

Control

There are very few practical control measures that are effective in reducing tabanid populations. Insecticidal spraying of cattle and other livestock and the application of insect repellents to humans and animals may reduce numbers trying to bite. Attractant traps, consisting of coloured screens coated with adhesive, have sometimes been employed to trap horse-flies, but there are no real solutions for combating tabanids.

Selected bibliography

Anderson, J.F. (1985) The control of horse flies and deer flies (Diptera: Tabanidae). *Myia* 3, 547–598.

Anthony, D.W. (1962) Tabanids as disease vectors. In: Maramorosch, K. (ed.) *Biological Transmission of Disease Agents. Symposium Held under the Auspices of the Entomological Society of America, Atlantic City, 1960.* Academic Press, New York, pp. 93–107.

Foil, L.D. (1989) Tabanids as vectors of disease agents. *Parasitology Today* 5, 88–95.

Krinsky, W.L. (1976) Animal disease agents transmitted by horse flies and deer flies (Diptera: Tabanidae). *Journal of Medical Entomology* 13, 225–275.

Human granulocytic ehrlichia *see* **Ehrlichiosis.**

Hydrotaea irritans (Muscidae)

M.W. Service

Species of *Hydrotaea*, known as sweat-flies, are muscid flies, as are house-flies, which they somewhat resemble. *Hydrotaea irritans* is particularly annoying and is often called the sheep head-fly. It has a wide geographical distribution but is most abundant in the Holarctic regions (i.e. North America and Europe).

Biology

Female adult flies can be troublesome and very persistent pests of humans and animals, being attracted in large numbers by sweat and secretions from the nose, mouth, ears, eyes and sores, upon which they feed. They also suck up blood oozing from wounds, but they do not actively bite and penetrate the skin, although their rasping mouthparts can aggravate the flow of blood. Adults also feed on carrion, decaying matter and faeces, as well as on sugary secretions.

Eggs are usually laid in the soil of pastures and on leaf litter in woodlands, although they may sometimes occur in animal faeces. The second-instar larva is saprophagous, but the third-instar larva is predatory on larvae of other insects. The puparium occurs in the soil.

Diseases

Apart from being troublesome pests, they are mechanical vectors of pathogens and have been involved in the transmission of mastitis (see entry).

Control

There are no practical control measures, apart from judicious use of insect repellents on the face, use of insecticide-impregnated ear tags in livestock and application of pour-on pyrethroid insecticides.

Icteroanaemia *see* **Anaplasmosis.**

Ilesha virus

Jack Woodall

A mosquito-borne infection of humans and possibly domestic animals, restricted to equatorial Africa and Madagascar and causing fever with rash, rarely fatal haemorrhagic symptoms and (possibly) meningoencephalitis.

Distribution

In a belt from Senegal and Nigeria through Cameroon, the Central African Republic, Burundi, Uganda and Kenya to Madagascar. Neutralizing antibody rates in human populations have been found as high as 38% in children and 44% in adults in Nigeria, rising to 54% overall in savannah areas (less in plateau and rain-forest areas).

Domestic animals

Neutralizing antibodies were also found in cows and goats in Nigeria (inadequate numbers of sheep and pigs were tested). However, in the absence of virus isolation from animals, this finding could be due to cross-reactions with one or more other bunyaviruses.

Virus

A bunyavirus, most closely related to Cache Valley virus (see entry), which is a virus transmitted by anopheline and culicine mosquitoes in North America, and to Bunyamwera virus (see entry), from Africa. Ilesha (ILE) virus was first isolated from the serum of a 9-year-old girl presenting with a few days of fever and weight loss at Ilesha Hospital, western Nigeria, in April 1957. Two further isolations, also from children, were made there a month later. Isolation was by intracerebral inoculation of newborn mice. There have been 24 subsequent isolations from cases of acute febrile illness, 21 of them with rash, in the Central African Republic, Uganda and Cameroon, and from fatal cases of haemorrhagic fever in Madagascar and meningoencephalitis in the Central African Republic.

Clinical symptoms

Like many other mosquito-borne viral infections, the predominant symptom is fever, sometimes accompanied by a rash on one or more areas of the body. The haemorrhagic fever case was a 44-year-old female resident of urban Tananarive, the capital of Madagascar, who presented in May 1990 with a history of fever without rash, myalgia of 7 days' duration, haematemesis and melaena; her platelet count was 200,000 mm^{-3}, prothrombin time 90% and cephalin–kaolin time 32 s. Two days later, despite a blood transfusion, her fever rose to 41°C, she had anaemia, leucopenia, a prothrombin time of only 50%, a cephalin–kaolin time of 50 s, cardiovascular collapse and another digestive tract haemorrhage. She died within 24 h. The virus isolated from her acute-phase blood reacted reciprocally with ILE virus in a plaque reduction neutralization test.

The fatal case of meningoencephalitis was an approximately 15-year-old African boy from the rural savannah region in the north of the Central African Republic, with a 1-week history of an illness in August 1964 which resembled rabies, but with no history of any animal bite. He was evacuated to the hospital in the capital, Bangui, and died on the night of his arrival. His family refused an autopsy. Ilesha virus was isolated from his cerebrospinal fluid (CSF) but not from his blood. Ilesha virus had also been isolated during the previous month from a 24-year-old European who had camped in the forest at the edge of Bangui and fallen ill with transient influenza-like symptoms and a rash, followed by complete recovery. A clinical spectrum ranging from cases of mild fever to more severe arthralgia and myalgia to rare cases of neurological manifestations is characteristic of many arbovirus infections. However, the virus from the mild case was being worked on in the same laboratory at the time of the isolation from the fatal case. This fact, plus the rarity of isolating arboviruses from CSF, the lack of a confirmatory isolation from the blood, the absence of autopsy material and the impossibility of obtaining a convalescent serum for antibody tests, means that laboratory contamination cannot be ruled out. This was before the time that sequencing became available to show whether one strain is identical to or different from another.

Diagnosis

Because of serological cross-reactions with other bunyaviruses in the haemagglutination inhibition (HI) and complement fixation (CF) tests, the definitive diagnosis must be made by virus isolation from whole blood or serum taken in the febrile phase (inoculated into newborn mice intracerebrally, or into primary chick embryo cells, VERO, LLC-MK2 or other susceptible cell lines), followed by neutralization testing in weanling mice or tissue culture.

Transmission

The vector is probably the malarial mosquito *Anopheles gambiae*, in contrast to the majority of other mosquito-borne viruses, which are transmitted by culicines. In fact, ILE virus has been isolated from that species in the Central African Republic and Kenya. In the laboratory, after 12 days' extrinsic incubation in parenterally inoculated *Aedes aegypti*, the virus was transmitted by bite to infant mice, but ILE virus has not been recovered from *A. aegypti* in nature. The virus replicates in *Aedes albopictus* cell culture. This is a South-East Asian mosquito that was not found in Africa prior to 1990, but has been introduced, most probably as dry but viable eggs in exported vehicle tyres originating from Asia, into several African countries, including Nigeria, Burkina Faso, South

Africa and Madagascar. This mosquito is an efficient vector of dengue viruses and may therefore be a potential vector of ILE virus. Attempts to infect embryonated birds' eggs and African and Asian monkeys in the laboratory have failed, suggesting that the virus may not have birds or monkeys as its natural host; its wild reservoir host is unknown, but, since it does infect infant mice in the laboratory, a rodent host could be suspected.

Treatment

As for most viral infections, antibiotics are ineffective and treatment is supportive, involving medication to reduce fever and pain, and fluid replacement. Treatment of haemorrhagic disease would involve whole-blood and platelet transfusions where available.

Control

Mosquito repellents, window screens, mosquito bed nets, especially insecticide-impregnated ones, and clothing that covers the arms and legs, plus avoidance of going outdoors after dark, reduce exposure to mosquito bites.

Selected bibliography

Digoutte, J.P., Salaun, J.J., Robin, Y., Brès, P. and Cagnard, V.J.M. (1980) Minor arboviral diseases in Central and West Africa. *Médecine Tropicale* 40, 523–533.

Fagbami, A.H. and Fabiyi, A. (1975) A survey for Ilesha Bunyamwera group virus antibodies in sera from domestic animals and humans in three ecological zones of Nigeria. *Virologie* 26, 27.

Johnson, B.K., Shockley, P., Chanas, A.C., Squires, E.J., Gardner, P., Wallace, C., Simpson, D.I., Bowen, E.T., Platt, G.S., Way, H., Chandler, J.A., Highton, R.B. and Hill, M.N. (1977) Arbovirus isolations from mosquitoes: Kano Plain, Kenya. *Transactions of the Royal Society of Tropical Medicine and Hygiene* 71, 518–521.

Morvan, J.M., Digoutte, J.P., Marsan, P. and Roux, J.F. (1994) Ilesha virus: a new aetiological agent of haemorrhagic fever in Madagascar. *Transactions of the Royal Society of Tropical Medicine and Hygiene* 88, 205.

Okuno, T. (1961) Immunological studies relating two recently isolated viruses, Germiston virus from South Africa and Ilesha virus from West Africa, to the Bunyamwera group. *American Journal of Tropical Medicine and Hygiene* 10, 223–226.

Ilheus virus

Alan D.T. Barrett

Infection of humans and other animals with Ilheus (ILH) virus, a member of the genus *Flavivirus* of the family Flaviviridae.

Ilheus, human

Ilheus virus causes a febrile illness followed by complete recovery. It is not considered to be a public health problem as few cases of Ilheus virus disease have been reported since the discovery of the virus in 1944.

Distribution

Ilheus virus has been isolated in Brazil, Colombia, French Guyana, Guatemala, Honduras, Panama and Trinidad. There is also serological evidence that the virus may be found in Argentina. To date, there have been no successful attempts to detect serological evidence of ILH virus infection in Peru.

Virus

The first isolate of ILH virus was made in Ilhéus city, Bahia State, Brazil, in 1944 from a pool of *Ochlerotatus*[1] and *Psorophora* mosquitoes. The first human isolate was made in 1957 from a febrile patient.

Ilheus virus is a member of the *Flavivirus* genus of the family Flaviviridae. The genus contains approximately 70 viruses. Virus particles are approximately 50 nm in diameter and icosahedral in shape, with a lipid envelope that is derived from the host cell. Virions contain three structural proteins. The small capsid (C) protein surrounds the genome of the virus and the envelope contains two proteins, known as the envelope (E) and membrane (M) proteins. The E protein is the viral haemagglutinin (i.e. the protein that binds to red blood cells) and contains most of the epitopes recognized by neutralizing antibodies. The E protein is the major virion protein. Two types of virions are recognized; mature extracellular virions contain M protein, while immature intracellular virions contain precursor M (prM), which is proteolytically cleaved during maturation to yield M protein. The genome is one positive-sense, single-stranded RNA of approximately 11,000 nucleotides which is infectious. The 5' terminus of the genome posesses a type I cap (m-^{7}GpppAmp), followed by the conserved dinucleotide AG. There is no terminal poly-(A) tract at the 3' terminus. The gene order is C-prM-E-NS1-NS2A-NS2B-NS3-NS4A-NS4B-NS5.

Serological tests involving haemagglutination inhibition, neutralization and complement fixation tests have all shown that ILH virus is a member of the *Flavivirus* genus of the family Flaviviridae, but have been inconclusive about the serological classification within the genus. The virus was initially classified as a member of the Japanese encephalitis serogroup. Subsequently, ILH virus was described as being a serologically distinct ungrouped flavivirus, on the basis of neutralization tests. However, recent nucleotide sequencing studies based on the NS5 gene indicated that ILH virus is a member of the Ntaya subgroup of the *Flavivirus* genus. This subgroup includes Bagaza, Rocio (see entry), Israel Turkey meningoencephalomyelitis, Ntaya and Tembusu viruses. Ilheus virus was most closely related to the South American Rocio virus at the nucleotide level. At one time, it was suggested that Rocio virus was a virulent variant of ILH virus. Limited nucleotide sequencing studies, however, suggest that Rocio and ILH are distinct viruses.

The virus grows in a number of cell cultures including primary rhesus kidney cells, VERO and LLC-MK2 monkey kidney cell lines, BHK-21 baby hamster cell lines and PS pig kidney cell lines. The virus is virulent in newborn and weanling mice and causes encephalitis after intracerebral or intraperitoneal inoculation.

Clinical symptoms

Human infections are reported as the sudden onset of an acute illness, characterized by a high fever, severe headache, chills and myalgia. Some patients have respiratory problems, photophobia and/or pleocytosis. Clinical symptoms continue for 3–5 days and are followed by complete recovery, although one patient had a viraemia for 73 days. However, two cases of encephalitic disease have been reported, but with no sequelae. There have been few reports (less than 15) of isolation of virus from human infections. The majority of human isolates came from cases of febrile illness with headache and myalgias. Two isolates were from encephalitic patients, while two were from asymptomatic patients.

Epidemiology

Other than antibodies against yellow fever and the dengue viruses (see entries), the highest rate of haemagglutination inhibition antibodies against flaviviruses in the Amazon basin (St Louis encephalitis, yellow fever, dengue 1–4, Bussuquara, Cacipacore, Ilheus and Rocio) is against ILH virus. Seroprevalence varies from 3.4 to 26% of the human population, with higher values in areas where virus isolates have been made. Although antibody levels are high, it has proved difficult to isolate ILH virus from humans, with fewer than 15 isolates being made. This may be due to brief or low viraemias, or most human infections may be asymptomatic. Alternatively, the serological cross-reaction between ILH and Rocio viruses (see entry) may complicate interpretation of the haemagglutination inhibition antibody titres.

Diagnosis

There is serological cross-reaction between ILH and Rocio viruses in haemagglutination inhibition tests; thus diagnosis of infection requires neutralization tests. There is no enzyme-linked immunosorbent assay (ELISA). Virus isolation from humans has proved difficult.

Transmission

Ilheus virus is transmitted by mosquitoes, infects mammals (including monkeys, bats and horses) and causes human infections. The sylvatic transmission cycle is thought to involve mosquitoes and birds. The virus has been isolated from febrile patients (eight isolates), sentinel monkeys (two isolates), once from a bat and several times from mosquitoes, including *Psorophora albipes*, *Psorophora lutzii*, *Ochlerotatus*[1] *serratus*, *Ochlerotatus fulvus*, *Ochlerotatus scapularis*, *Anopheles cruzii* and *Haemagogus leucocelaenus*. However, most isolates have been made from *Psorophora ferox*, suggesting that this may be the principal vector of the virus. A number of animals have antibodies to ILH virus, including bats, monkeys, rodents, marsupials and birds.

Treatment

There is no treatment for ILH virus infections.

Control

No control measures have been used since Ilheus disease is not considered to be a public health problem.

Note

[1]   *Ochlerotatus* was formerly a subgenus of *Aedes*

Selected bibliography

Calisher, C.H., Karabatsos, N., Dalrymple, J.M., Shope, R.E., Porterfield, J.S., Westaway, E.G. and Brandt, W.E. (1989) Antigenic relationships among flaviviruses as determined by cross-neutralizations tests with polyclonal antisera. *Journal of General Virology* 70, 37–43.

Karabatsos, N. (1985) *International Catalogue of Arboviruses Including Certain Other Viruses of Vertebrates*, 3rd edn. American Society for Tropical Medicine and Hygiene, San Antonio, Texas, 1146 pp.

Kuno, G., Chang, G.-J.J., Tsuchiya, K.R., Kara-batsos, N. and Cropp, C.B. (1998) Phylogeny of the genus *Flavivirus. Journal of Virology* 72, 73–83.

Laemmert, H.W. and Hughes, T.P. (1947) The virus of Ilheus encephalitis. Isolation, serological specificity and transmission. *Journal of Immunology* 55, 61–67.

Indian tick-borne typhus *see* **Tick-borne typhuses.**

Israeli spotted fever *see* **Tick-borne typhuses.**

Issyk-Kul virus disease

Irina N. Gavrilovskaya

Commonly referred to as Issyk-Kul fever because it is caused by Issyk-Kul (IK) virus, which is transmitted to people through bites of *Argas* ticks or mosquitoes that have fed on infected bats. Sporadic cases of this disease have been recorded in south Tadzhikistan (the former Tadzhik Republic, USSR), in 1975 and 1978. Outbreaks of Issyk-Kul fever were described in the same region in 1982 and 1985. The disease is manifested by non-specific symptoms, such as high fever, headache and muscle pain. Lethal cases have not been recorded. The disease is endemic to the central Asian countries (of the former USSR) and western Malaysia.

Distribution

Clinically manifest cases of Issyk-Kul fever have been described only in Tadzhikistan, but immunoprevalence to IK virus among healthy human populations of neighbouring countries has been found in Kyrgyzstan (or Kyrgyz Republic) (up to 3.2%) and in Turkmenistan (up to 9%). The natural habitat of the virus is wider and includes south Kazakhstan, western Malaysia and probably some parts of Iran, Afghanistan, India and Pakistan. There is a possibility that Issyk-Kul fever cases occur in these territories. Antibodies to IK virus have also been found in the House mouse (*Mus musculus*), Libyan jird (*Meriones libycus*), sheep and cattle.

Virus

The IK virus was first isolated in 1970 from bats and *Argas vespertilionis* ticks collected from bats. Specimens were collected in the north of Kyrgyzstan in a settlement situated in the coastal region along the Issyk-Kul lake, longitude 77° 40′ East and latitude 42° 15′ North. The IK virus belongs to the family Bunyaviridae, as shown by electron microscopy, and has no serological relationship with 39 arboviruses belonging to 14 groups or to 23 ungrouped bunyaviruses. Issyk-Kul virus is serologically identical to Ketarah virus isolated from bats (*Scotophilus kuhlii*[1]) and ticks (*Argas pusillus*) in western Malaysia (1966). Issyk-Kul virus is an ungrouped RNA virus. Its particle size (estimated by filtration through filters of 220, 110 and 50 nm pore size) is about 50 nm. Issyk-Kul virus is sensitive to lipid solvents. The virus is pathogenic for suckling white mice, 2-week-old white mice and adult white mice when inoculated intracerebrally or subcutaneously. In mice the virus causes death on days 6–7 post-infection, with histological findings of meningoencephalitis, interstitial pneumonia, hepatitis, nephritis and inflammation of the spleen. Intracerebral and subcutaneous infection of hamsters and African green monkeys (*Chlorocebus aethiops*[2]) were not lethal; histological findings were less prominent but similar to those described in mice. Issyk-Kul virus is a pantrophic agent that causes generalized infection in experimentally infected animals.

Clinical symptoms

Descriptions of clinical symptoms are based on the observation of a sporadic case of Issyk-Kul fever in a staff member infected during fieldwork with bats and of 34 cases of Issyk-Kul fever during outbreaks of the disease in 1982 and 1985 in Tadzhikistan. The incubation period is 5–7 days, followed by an abrupt onset of high fever (39–41°C) for 3–8 days, headache (80%), dizziness (50%), pharyngitis, a cough and muscle pain (30%), nausea and vomiting (25%), rash, abdominal pain, chills, pain in the eyes, tear-shedding (epiphora) and photophobia (6%). The acute period of the disease lasts about 8 days. The convalescent period is rather long (1–1.5 months) and is always followed by weakness. No deaths have been recorded.

Diagnosis

The diagnosis is performed by isolation of virus strains from the blood of patients in the acute phase of the disease. Isolations have been made by intracerebral injection of patient blood in 2-day-old laboratory mice, which develop the symptoms of paralysis in their extremities, clonic spasms and death. Serological diagnosis was done by a study of paired sera of patients by complement fixation tests and diffuse precipitation in agar reactions. All tests were undertaken with sucrose–acetone antigens prepared from the brains of laboratory mice infected with arboviruses isolated in the territory of the former USSR. The increase of the antibody titre to IK virus antigen from 8–16 in the first serum to 32–256 in the second serum to IK virus antigen confirmed the diagnosis of Issyk-Kul fever.

Transmission

The first isolation of IK virus was from Noctule bats (*Nyctalus noctula*). Numerous strains were isolated later from six species of bats (Table 1). These findings confirmed that bats are the main host of IK virus in nature. The habitats of these species coincide with endemic areas in the countries of central and southern Asia. There are many possible means of viral transmission to humans: transmissive, respiratory and alimentary (Table 2). Issyk-Kul virus has been simultaneously isolated from bats and *Argas vespertilionis* ticks. Thirty-two per cent of *Argas* ticks collected from bats were infected. Penetration of these ticks into houses and their attaching themselves to humans have been recorded. Female *Argas* ticks feed in June and lay eggs 4 months later. Most cases of Issyk-Kul disease occur in June–August, which coincides with the peak of tick activity. *Ixodes vespertilionis* ticks (Tadzhikistan, Kyrgyzstan) and gadflies (*Tabanus agrestis*) (Kazakhstan) are also involved in virus transmission.

The other vectors for viral transmission are two species of mosquitoes: *Ochlerotatus*[3] *caspius* and *Anopheles hyrcanus*. These mosquitoes are the most abundant species in endemic areas and the peak of their activity coincides with the peak number of Issyk-kul cases. A study of food preferences of these species was made by the detection of antibodies to IK virus in the sera of humans, bats, cattle, dogs and horses. It was shown that these two species, and also *Culex pipiens*, attack humans and bats equally. The role of mosquitoes in viral transmission has been verified by isolation of the virus from naturally infected *O. caspius* and *A. hyrcanus* (Table 1) and by successful experimental infection of *O. caspius*. The mosquitoes were fed on experimentally infected laboratory mice and Common pipistrelle bats (*Pipistrellus* (= *Vespertilio*) *pipistrellus*). About 63% of female mosquitoes became infected and 80% of infected females transmitted the virus to laboratory suckling mice by bite.

It is most likely that mosquitoes transmit the virus to birds (Table 1), from which six strains of IK virus have been isolated. These observations have led to the conclusion that ticks (*A. vespertilionis*, *A. pusillus*, *I. vespertilionis*) and mosquitoes (*O. caspius* and *A. hyrcanus*) are the principal vectors of IK virus in Tadzhikistan, Kyrgyzstan and Malaysia.

Respiratory and alimentary routes of infection can occur when people visit bats

Table 1. Isolation of Issyk-Kul virus from humans and natural reservoirs.

Source of isolation	Geographical location	Dates of isolation	No. of strains
Humans	Tadzhikistan:		
	Kumsangir, Dushanbe, Parhar	1975–1982	19
Bats			
Nyctalus noctula	Kyrgyztan:		
	Dzhety-Oguz	1970	1
Myotis oxygenathus	Kyrgyzstan:		
	Sokuluk	1971, 1973	2
Eptesicum serotinus	Kyrgyzstan:		
	Sokoluk	1971	2
Pipistrellus pipistrellus	Tadzhikistan:		
	Leninsk	1974	2
	Kumsangir	1973	1
Rhinolophus ferrumequinuum	Kumsangir	1982	1
Scotophilus kuhlii	Malaysia:		
	Kelantan	1966	1
Birds			
Passer hispaniolensis	Kyrgystan:		
	Moskovsk	1973	1
Alcedo atthis			1
Motacilla alba			1
Hirundo rustica			1
Jynx torquilla	Tadzhikistan:		
	Dzhirgtal	1976	1
Phoenicurus phoenicurus	Komsomolobad	1976	1
Motacilla cinerea	Komsomolobad	1976	1
Ticks (from bats):			
Argas vespertilionis	Kyrgyztan:		
	Sokoluk	1970, 1971	2
	Osh	1972	1
	Frunze	1971	1
	Leninsk	1973	6
	Kalininsk	1972, 1974	3
Argas pusillus	Malaysia:		
	Kelantan	1966	2
Ixodes vespertilionis	Kyrgyzstan:		
	Frunze	1972	1
Mosquitoes			
Ochlerotatus caspius	Kyrgyzstan:		
	Moskovsk	1973	1
Anopheles hyrcanus	Moskovsk	1974	1
Tabanid	Kazakhstan		
Tabanus agrestis	Aktyubinsk	1981	1

in their habitats and also by eating food contaminated with bat excreta.

Treatment

The treatment of Issyk-Kul fever is mainly supportive. Bedrest is important. The clini-cal manifestation of the first phase of illness can be treated at the primary health care level; this includes administration of antipyretics (e.g. paracetamol). The use of antibiotics is often necessary to combat secondary bacterial infections. The use of

Table 2.   Transmission of Issyk-Kul virus.

Virus type	Geograhical location	Natural vertebrate hosts	Vectors	Mechanisms of transmission to humans
Bunyavirus Ungrouped	Kyrgyzstan Turkmenistan Tadzhikistan Kazakhstan Uzbekistan W. Malaysia (Keterah)	Bats	*Argas* species *Ochlerotatus caspius* *Culex pipiens* *Anopheles hyrcanus*	Insect bite Respiratory (direct contact with bats) Alimentary (contact with food) contaminated with bat's excreta)

antiviral drugs, such as ribavirim, should be evaluated through careful clinical trials.

Control

The number of ticks attached to bats in their natural habitats can be controlled, possibly by spraying with acaricides. This and the application of effective chemical repellents for personal protection of people living in endemic areas, may be implemented.

Notes

[1]   This bat was formerly known as *Scotophilus temmincki.*
[2]   This species was formerly in the genus *Cercopithecus.*
[3]   *Ochlerotatus* was formerly a subgenus of *Aedes.*

Selected bibliography

Anon. (1992) Classification and nomenclature of viruses. *Archives of Virology* 2 (suppl.), 223–227.

Bulychev, V.P., Alekseev, A.N, Kostyukov, M.A., Gordeeva, Z.E. and Lvov, D.K. (1979) Transmission of Issyk-Kul virus by mosquitoes *Aedes caspius caspius* Pall. by bite in the experiment. *Medical Parasitology and Parasitological Diseases* 6, 53–56. (In Russian, English summary.)

Lvov, D.K. (1988) Issyk-kul fever. In: Monath, T.P. (ed.) *The Arboviruses: Epidemiology and Ecology,* Vol. III. CRC Press, Boca Raton, Florida, pp. 53–62.

Lvov, D.K., Karas, F.R., Timofeev, E.M., Tsyrkin, Yu., M., Vargina, S.G., Veselovskaya, O.V., Osipova, N.Z., Grebenyuk, Yu., I., Gromashevski, V.L., Steblyanko, O.N. and Fomina, K.B. (1973) Issyk-Kul virus, a new arbovirus isolated from bats and *Argas* (*Carios*) *vespertilionis* (Latr., 1802) in the Kirghiz S.S.R. *Archive für die Gesampte Virusforschurg* 42, 207–209.

Lvov, D.K., Kostyukov, M.A., Pak, T.P. and Gromashevski, V.L. (1980) Isolation of an arbovirus antigenically related to Issyk-Kul virus from the blood of a sick person. *Voprosy Virusologii* 1, 61–62. (In Russian, English summary).

Lvov, D.K., Kostyukov, M.A., Danijaroiv, O.A., Tukhtaev, T.M., Sherikov, B.K., Bunietbekov, A.A., Bulychev, V.P. and Gordeeva, Z.E. (1984) An outbreak of arbovirus infection in the Tadzhik S.S.R. caused by Issyk-Kul virus (Issyk-Kul Fever). *Voprosy Virusologii* 1, 89–92. (In Russian, English summary.)

Jamestown Canyon virus

Paul R. Grimstad

Jamestown Canyon (JC) virus (family Bunyaviridae, genus *Bunyavirus*, California serogroup) has been recognized as a potentially serious human pathogen for the past two decades in North America. A number of cases of severe central nervous system (CNS) disease, including encephalitis and probably one or more deaths, have been reported from several midwestern USA regions, upper New York State and southern Canada. Routine medical surveillance and diagnostic targeting of JC virus do not exist. Wherever efforts have been made to study this pathogen, serosurveys have demonstrated widespread human and large vertebrate infections throughout North America. Minimal evidence of overt disease in wild or domesticated animals exists; JC virus infection was associated with one documented occurrence of high mortality in newborn White-tailed deer fawns (*Odocoileus virginianus*) in north-central Michigan (USA). Concern has been expressed about its potential as a human teratogen following laboratory animal studies. Jamestown Canyon virus is known to be transmitted by several *Aedes* and *Ochlerotatus*[1] mosquito species and to overwinter vertically (transovarially) in their eggs. Involvement of *Anopheles* species in a secondary amplification and overwintering cycle is likely.

The disease

From a clinical standpoint, JC virus and other California (CAL) serogroup viral CNS infections differ only in severity. However, from a public health standpoint, the precise identification of the agent and attachment of the correct name are critical to our understanding of the medical ecology of each virus, as each is quite distinct in many respects. Unfortunately, there is considerable confusion in the literature as to the names of clinical diseases associated with CAL serogroup viral infections in North America. The first virus in this serogroup to be isolated was California encephalitis virus in 1943. Following the isolation of La Crosse (LAC) virus from a fatal human case in 1964, references to both 'La Crosse encephalitis' (see entry) and 'California encephalitis' cases appeared in scientific literature and other types of reports. With the identification in 1980 of JC virus and snowshoe hare (SSH) virus as additional North American CAL serogroup viruses causing severe encephalitis, as well as the association of trivittatus virus and other North American CAL serogroup members with milder CNS illness, the confusion was magnified. Thus, referring to any single untyped or every CAL serogroup CNS case as 'California encephalitis' is incorrect. Reference to a case of encephalitis as 'California serogroup encephalitis' is provisionally acceptable because it describes milder illness as a 'California group viral infection'. However, when the agent is typed, it is most appropriate to link the disease and correct name of the aetiological agent, e.g. Jamestown Canyon virus encephalitis (or Jamestown Canyon encephalitis), La Crosse virus encephalitis (or La Crosse encephalitis). Also erroneous is the use of the names 'Jamestown Canyon encephalitis virus', 'La Crosse encephalitis virus' (also LaCrosse or Lacrosse), etc., appearing in the literature. Given the problems of obtaining a correct identification of any California group viral infection in the USA, other than probably LAC virus, the reader should not attribute disease reports to any one agent in this serogroup unless neutralization tests (NT) or another definitive assay utilizing multiple CAL serogroup viruses or antigens were employed. As an example (see Grimstad, 1994) of how reports can change, a retrospective review of serological results by one US public laboratory found that 62% of what had previously been termed CAL encephalitis (presumably La Crosse) were in fact caused by JC virus infection. Failure to accurately type the viral aetiological agent in this age of sophisticated diagnostics is a disservice to the patient and to public health.

Distribution

Jamestown Canyon virus has one of the widest geographical ranges of any CAL serogroup virus, as well as viruses in other genera and families in North America, even surpassing St Louis encephalitis virus (see entry). Jamestown Canyon virus was first isolated in 1961 from *Culiseta inornata* mosquitoes collected in Jamestown Canyon west of Denver, Colorado, USA. Subsequently, many isolates were obtained from a wide range of mosquito species, including species of the genera *Aedes*, *Ochlerotatus*, *Anopheles*, *Coquillettidia* and *Psorophora*, and from three tabanid (*Chrysops* and *Tabanus*) species collected in Wisconsin, USA. Vertebrate isolations have been quite uncommon in comparison. The largest number of isolates have come from White-tailed deer (*O. virginianus*) populations; a recent report noted that JC virus was isolated from vesicular lesions of a horse in the USA. There are apparently no confirmed human virus isolations on record. In total, virus isolations and serological evidence of past infection in vertebrates indicate that JC virus may be found from Alaska east across virtually all Canadian provinces, including the Maritime provinces, south through New York and other Atlantic seaboard states to Florida, then west through Texas, into north-eastern Mexico, on to California and northward along the Pacific coast, thus encircling North America. Evidence of JC virus transmission has also been found in virtually every one of the encircled states where any effort has been made to document arboviral presence. Jamestown Canyon virus has been isolated from northern boreal forests in Canada to marshy areas in the southern USA; in California it has been isolated from mosquitoes in the hot Central Valley, as well as from partially snow-covered mountainous regions of that state. Monoclonal antibody characterization of multiple Canadian JC virus isolates with the prototype Colorado isolate and the closely related South River virus (New Jersey, USA) suggests the possible existence of multiple antigenically distinct forms, not unlike Cache Valley virus (see entry).

Virus

As is common to all bunyaviruses, JC virus is an enveloped virus whose genome is composed of three single-stranded negative-sense RNA segments. The large (L) segment of bunyaviruses encodes a probable viral polymerase. The middle (M) segment encodes two glycoproteins, G1 and G2, plus a non-structural protein; G1 functions in vertebrate cell infection while G2 appears critical for mosquito infection. The third and shortest (S) segment encodes for the nucleocapsid and a second non-structural protein. Nucleotide sequences are conserved within the genus. Recent work has demonstrated that LAC virus and JC virus could co-infect *Aedes albopictus* mosquitoes in the laboratory and result in the formation of all six possible reassortant genotypes.

Clinical symptoms and record of infection

In Canada, the majority of CAL serogroup viral infections appear to be SSH virus; however, in one study, 6.5% of Newfoundland residents were positive for antibodies against JC virus. In the USA, inapparent human infection is well documented from retrospective serosurveys where anti-JC virus antibody prevalence has ranged from 3.5 to 12.9% of New York State residents, 2.5 to 10.0% of Wisconsin residents and 3.0 to 15.0% of northern Indiana residents, with a statewide average of 27.7% in Michigan premarital blood samples and 17.6% overall in a survey of 18 native Alaskan populations and even higher in select groups having extensive exposure in enzootic foci. A 1988 review suggested four generalized syndromes associated with CAL serogroup infections; JC virus typified the fourth syndrome, with cases presenting as febrile illnesses, often with acute CNS and respiratory system involvement. That review also suggested that presentation of Jamestown Canyon clinical symptoms in humans is 'perhaps the [most variable] of any of the CAL group members'. The role of JC virus in domesticated animal disease is unknown. Serosurveys have shown antibody prevalence rates exceeding 25–50% in large animals (cattle, horses) with no clear disease association. One association with foetal loss is noted below in discussing transmission.

Diagnosis

Traditional diagnoses of CAL serogroup viral infections, including JC virus, have been made using established serological procedures: complement fixation (CF), haemagglutination inhibition (HI) and/or NT and measurement of a fourfold or greater rise or fall in antibody. Virus isolation has been extremely rare and almost exclusively in fatal LAC virus infections. Surveys made in the 1980s of diagnostic practices among Canadian provincial and US state health departments demonstrated that two-thirds, at most, included an assay for CAL group infection and, of these, none routinely used the NT. Among laboratories that conducted tests, all used LAC virus antigen and most used it as the exclusive viral test antigen. This is critical, as studies in Indiana showed that use of LAC virus antigen in CF and HI tests failed to detect infections caused by JC virus, while use of LAC virus in NT would only identify approximately 5% of true JC virus infections (when compared with NT results using JC virus in parallel NTs with LAC virus). Indeed, comparison of case reports of 'California encephalitis' from one midwestern state with results of a large serosurvey performed there suggested that less than 1% of actual Jamestown Canyon CNS cases were being detected; however, these were all reported with the assumption they were LAC virus infections, as only HI with LAC virus antigen was used. The serological study results suggested >1000 cases of Jamestown Canyon encephalitis alone should have been detected had that virus been included in assays. At present, the use of enzyme-linked immunosorbent assay (ELISA) and indirect immunofluorescence with only LAC virus antigen constitutes the primary detection system in private laboratories under contract to many hospitals and health management organizations in the USA. Thus, JC virus and other CAL serogroup virus clinical infections, other than perhaps LAC virus, are thought to be extremely under-reported in the USA.

Transmission

The primary model of transmission of JC virus by various *Aedes* and *Ochlerotatus* species suggests a single seasonal peak of virus amplification in large vertebrate hosts, primarily the White-tailed deer (*Odocoileus virginianus*), with viral overwintering in the mosquito egg as a result of vertical (transovarial) transmission. This cycle has been clearly demonstrated with *Ochlerotatus*[1] *provocans* in Michigan and New York and with *Ochlerotatus stimulans* in Indiana. That other aedine species may be involved in localized transmission has been shown with the isolation of vertically transmitted JC virus from *Ochlerotatus triseriatus* (the primary vector of LAC virus) in Ohio and several *Ochlerotatus communis* group species in California. Field studies have not strongly implicated *Culiseta inornata* as the primary vector.

In an elegant 1993 study, workers in California showed that coastal populations of *C. inornata* were incompetent vectors when fed an alpine (Sierra Nevada) JC virus isolate; however, a Central Valley (California) *C. inornata* population fed the alpine isolate demonstrated excellent competence as a vector, transmitting it both horizontally and vertically. 'The differences were clearly related to both mosquito species and viral strain,' the authors noted. In a north-central Michigan study site where a captive breeding White-tailed deer herd was inadvertently maintained for several decades in a JC virus focus, a 100% seroconversion rate among all yearling deer occurred in a 2–6-week period every late spring, coincident with the emergence of vertically infected *O. provocans*. Previously infected adult does often showed serological evidence of reinfection; fawns were protected from a primary infection during their first summer of life by maternal antibodies against JC virus. Evidence demonstrated that seronegative does infected in late pregnancy with JC virus experienced a high rate of fawn loss (fawns born paralysed, dead or aborted), suggesting that JC virus may be a naturally teratogenic virus. Of importance were the observations at the Michigan study site of early autumn anamnestic responses in several does. At that site and time (mid-1980s), the only mosquitoes feeding on deer and humans were *Anopheles punctipennis* and *Anopheles quadrimaculatus*. In addition, there was seroconversion of two 9–10-month-old does in late February to early March in one year, and serological detection of anamnestic responses two years in a row in older does. There, JC virus transmission apparently occurred in the late winter and when the ground was still snow-covered; workers at the site complained of biting mosquitoes, and collected host-seeking *A. punctipennis*. Unfortunately, carefully frozen specimens were not available for virus isolation and polymerase chain reaction (PCR) techniques had not been developed at that time. Thus, it appears that JC virus may be transmitted in a dual cycle involving: (i) spring-emerging, vertically infected aedine vectors with subsequent horizontal amplification, primarily in deer; and (ii) a late-summer, early-autumn anopheline amplification, of interest primarily as an alternate means of JC virus overwintering. Interestingly, records of onset of human cases to date in the north-eastern areas of the USA and southern Canada suggest that the greater majority of human cases have onset in late summer into early autumn, coincident with late-season anopheline feeding. During this time, none of the probable spring aedine vector species is present to transmit JC virus.

Treatment

The clinical treatment of a CNS case caused by JC virus infection would be similar to that for any other arboviral neuropathogen; severe symptoms (high fever, seizures, coma) would be treated until recovery occurs. There have been no studies utilizing antiviral drugs to treat JC virus infection, as have been tried with other human arboviral infections, nor is there likely to be a vaccine produced, given the current lack of support for associating JC virus and other bunyaviruses, other than perhaps LAC virus, with clinical disease in domesticated animals and humans.

Control

Efforts to control the probable primary vectors of JC virus in North America would be likely to be ineffective, given their basic biology, the variety of their breeding sites and the environmental impact that would probably result from trying to control the geographically vast *O. communis* group and other aedine vectors, *A. quadrimaculatus*, *A. punctipennis* and perhaps even the *C. inornata* populations. Timely public education remains the key to any control or case reduction.

Note

[1] *Ochlerotatus* was formerly a subgenus of *Aedes*.

Selected bibliography

(see also selected bibliography under Cache Valley virus)

Artsob, H., Spence, L., Brodeur, B.R. and Th'ng, C. (1992) Monoclonal antibody characterization of Jamestown Canyon (California serogroup) virus topotypes isolated in Canada. *Viral Immunology* 5, 233–242.

Boromisa, R.D. and Grimstad, P.R. (1986) Virus–vector–host relationships of *Aedes stimulans* and Jamestown Canyon virus in a northern Indiana enzootic focus. *American Journal of Tropical Medicine and Hygiene* 35, 1285–1295.

Cheng, L.L., Rodas, J.D., Schultz, K.T., Christensen, B.M., Yuill, T.M. and Israel, B.A. (1999) Potential for evolution of California serogroup bunyaviruses by genome reassortment in *Aedes albopictus. American Journal of Tropical Medicine and Hygiene* 60, 430–438.

Grimstad, P.R. (1988) California group virus disease. In: Monath, T.P. (ed.) *The Arboviruses: Epidemiology and Ecology*, Vol. II. CRC Press, Boca Raton, Florida, pp. 99–136.

Grimstad, P.R. (1994) California group viral infections. In: Beran, G.W. (ed.) *Handbook of Zoonoses*, Section B: *Viral*, 2nd edn. CRC Press, Boca Raton, Florida, pp. 71–79.

Grimstad, P.R., Calisher, C.H., Harroff, R.N. and Wentworth, B.B. (1986) Jamestown Canyon virus (California serogroup) is the etiologic agent of widespread infection in Michigan humans. *American Journal of Tropical Medicine and Hygiene* 35, 376–386.

Grimstad, P.R., Williams, D.G. and Schmitt, S.M. (1987) Infection of white-tailed deer (*Odocoileus virginianus*) in Michigan with Jamestown Canyon virus (California serogroup) and the importance of maternal antibody in viral maintenance. *Journal of Wildlife Disease* 23, 12–22.

Heard, P.B. (1997) The epidemiology of California and Bunyamwera serogroup viruses in Indiana. PhD dissertation, University of Notre Dame, Notre Dame, 224 pp.

Kramer, L.D., Bowen, M.D., Hardy, J.L., Reeves, W.C., Presser, S.B. and Eldridge, B.F. (1993) Vector competence of alpine, Central Valley, and coastal mosquitoes (Diptera: Culicidae) from California for Jamestown Canyon virus. *Journal of Medical Entomology* 30, 398–406.

Zhang, M. (1993) Jamestown Canyon virus: characterization of geographic strains by molecular, cellular, and animal assays. PhD dissertation, University of Notre Dame, Notre Dame, 221 pp.

January disease *see* **Theilerioses.**

Japanese encephalitis

Alan D.T. Barrett

Infection of the central nervous system of humans and other animals with Japanese encephalitis (JE) virus, a member of the *Flavivirus* genus of the family Flaviviridae.

Japanese encephalitis, human

Japanese encephalitis virus causes a rural, zoonotic viral disease that is a major public health problem in many Asian countries. It is the most important arthropod-borne virus encephalitis and has replaced poliovirus as the major cause of human epidemic encephalitis in the world. Although a disease resembling Japanese encephalitis was described in the late 19th century, the virus was not isolated in Japan until 1935; this prototype strain is known as Nakayama. The virus is transmitted between vertebrate hosts by mosquitoes. Humans are a dead-end host, due to a low viraemia. The disease caused by JE virus is characterized by infection of the central nervous system. There are at least 50,000 clinical cases reported each year, but it is thought that the true figure is much higher. The majority of cases occur in children below the age of 10 years. The mortality rate is 15–25% and up to 70% of those who survive infection develop neurological sequelae.

Distribution

Japanese encephalitis virus is found throughout much of Asia (Fig. 1). It is epidemic in temperate regions of Asia (e.g. Japan, Taiwan, People's Republic of China, Korea, maritime areas of the former USSR, northern Vietnam, northern Thailand, Myanmar, Nepal, Sri Lanka and India) and endemic in tropical regions (e.g. Malaysia, Indonesia, southern Vietnam, southern

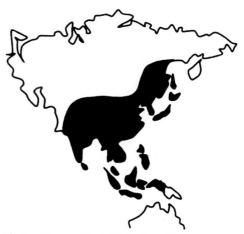

Fig. 1. Geographical distribution of Japanese encephalitis.

Thailand and the Philippines). Japanese encephalitis had not been described in Australia until 1995, when cases of Japanese encephalitis were reported on the island of Badu in the Torres Strait, and subsequently the first human case of Japanese encephalitis was reported on mainland Australia in 1998.

Virus

Japanese encephalitis virus is a member of the *Flavivirus* genus of the family Flaviviridae. The genus contains approximately 70 viruses. Japanese encephalitis virus is a member of the JE complex viruses, which are related on the basis of cross-reactivity in neutralization tests and close relatedness at the nucleotide level. The JE virus complex includes Alfuy (see entry), JE, Koutango, Kunjin (see entry), Murray Valley encephalitis (see entry), St Louis encephalitis (see entry), Usutu, West Nile (see entry) and Yaounde viruses. Japanese encephalitis virus multiplies in a large range of cell cultures derived from different animal and mosquito species. Monkey kidney cell lines – VERO and LLC-MK-2 – are usually used for infectivity titrations. A number of animal species are susceptible to JE virus. The virus is lethal for newborn mice and rats by all routes of inoculation. As the animals get older, age-related resistance to disease is observed following inoculation by peripheral routes, while adult mice are still susceptible following direct inoculation of virus into the brain (i.e. neuroinvasiveness decreases with age, while virus is still neurovirulent for all ages of mice). Japanese encephalitis virus causes a lethal disease in primates following intracerebral inoculation, while some strains are also lethal following intranasal inoculation; asymptomatic infection takes place following peripheral inoculation of virus.

Virus particles are icosahedral in shape, with a lipid envelope; the particles are approximately 50 nm in diameter. The lipid envelope is derived from the host cell. Virions contain three structural proteins. The small capsid (C) protein surrounds the genome of the virus and the envelope contains two proteins, known as envelope (E)

and membrane (M). The E protein is the viral haemagglutinin (i.e. the protein that binds to red blood cells) and contains most of the epitopes recognized by neutralizing antibodies. Thus, the E protein is the major virion protein. Two types of virions are recognized; mature extracellular virions contain M protein, while immature intracellular virions contain precursor M (prM), which is proteolytically cleaved during maturation to yield M protein. The genome is one positive-sense, single-stranded RNA of approximately 11,000 nucleotides which is infectious. The 5′ terminus of the genome possesses a type I cap (m-^{7}GpppAmp), followed by the conserved dinucleotide AG. There is no terminal poly-(A) tract at the 3′ terminus. The gene order is C-prM-E-NS1-NS2A-NS2B-NS3-NS4A-NS4B-NS5. All viral proteins are produced as one polyprotein, which is post-translationally processed by viral and cellular proteases.

The replication cycle involves the binding to cell receptors(s), which is mediated by the viral E protein. Uptake of the virus particle into cells is via receptor-mediated endocytosis, followed by pH-dependent membrane fusion activity to release the virus nucleocapsid into the cytoplasm. The input virus does not contain viral RNA-dependent RNA polymerase. Thus, the positive-sense genomic RNA is translated to generate the non-structural (NS) proteins required for replication of the virus, including the RNA-dependent RNA polymerase. RNA replication is associated with membranes and begins with transcription of the input genomic RNA to synthesize complementary negative-sense strands, which are then used as templates to transcribe positive-sense genomic RNA. The genomic RNA is synthesized by a semi-conservative mechanism involving replicative intermediates (i.e. containing double-stranded regions as well as nascent single-stranded molecules) and replicative forms (i.e. duplex RNA molecules). Synthesis of negative-sense RNA continues throughout the replication cycle. Once the polyprotein has been translated, it is processed by cellular proteases and the viral NS2B-NS3 serine protease to generate the individual structural and non-structural proteins. In addition to the three structural proteins C, prM and E, seven non-structural proteins are found in virus-infected cells: NS1, NS2A, NS2B, NS3, NS4A, NS4B and NS5. Few of the non-structural proteins have been studied in detail. NS3 is a multi-functional protein whose N-terminal one-third forms the viral serine proteinase complex together with NS2B. The C-terminal portion of NS3 contains an RNA helicase domain involved in RNA replication, as well as RNA triphosphatase activity involved in the formation of the 5'-terminal cap structure of the viral RNA. Two enzymic activities have been assigned to NS5: the RNA-dependent RNA polymerase and the methyltransferase activity necessary for methylation of the 5' cap structure. NS1 is an unusual non-structural protein, as it is glycosylated. The functions of NS2A, NS4A and NS4B are poorly understood, but current evidence suggests that NS2A, NS2B, NS4A and NS5 are all part of the replication complex and that NS1 is involved in RNA synthesis and virus assembly.

Virus particles can first be observed in the rough endoplasmic reticulum, which is believed to be the site of virus assembly (i.e. interaction of genomic positive-sense RNA molecules with structural proteins C, prM and E). Progeny virions assemble by budding through intracellular membranes into cytoplasmic vesicles. These immature virions (i.e. containing prM rather than M protein) are then transported through the membrane systems of the host secretory pathway to the cell surface, where exocytosis occurs. Shortly before virion release, the prM protein is cleaved by furin or a furin-like cellular protease to generate mature virions that contain M protein. Immature virions have low infectivity compared with mature virions. Host-cell macromolecular synthesis is not shut off during virus replication and is not decreased until cytopathic effect is evident, late in the infection process.

Epidemiology

Japanese encephalitis is endemic in tropical areas of Asia and epidemic in temperate regions of Asia. Endemicity in tropical areas is thought to be due to the availability of mosquito vectors throughout the year, while there is seasonal incidence in temperate climates. Specifically, the disease is reported annually with seasonal (peaking in June and July during the rainy season) and age (mainly children between the ages of 1 and 15 years but peaking in those 3–5 years of age) distributions. Human infections are related to increased vector densities associated with rainfall or irrigation practices. The disease is found in rural areas of Asia where the estimated population is 2000 million. Of this population approximately 700 million are children under the age of 15 years and an annual birth cohort of 70 million per year. The disease incidence is estimated to be between 1.8 and 2.5 per 10,000 children. Therefore, it is estimated that there are approximately 175,000 cases of Japanese encephalitis per year. It is estimated that the case fatality rate is 25% (rates ranging from 5 to 40% have been reported) and that approximately 45% (plus reports of up to 70%) of surviving patients have neurological sequelae. These include neurological and psychomotor retardation, motor deficits, convulsions, memory impairment, optic atrophy, limb paralysis, Parkinsonism and also psychological and behavioural disorders. Much of the information on neurological sequelae comes from case reports rather than detailed studies incorporating controls. None the less, it appears that a proportion of the patients with neurological sequelae do recover over time.

Japanese encephalitis appears to be age-related, with the majority of patients being children while the elderly also tend to succumb to encephalitis. It is thought that this is due to the high level of immunity in the adult population. All evidence indicates that there is one serotype of JE virus and that infection gives lifelong protection from re-infection.

Molecular epidemiology

Strain variation has been recognized for many years. Initially antigenic variation was detected with polyclonal antisera in neutralization, complement fixation, agar gel diffusion and haemagglutination inhibition tests, and subsequently with monoclonal antibodies. Overall, two major immunotypes of JE virus have been differentiated: Nakayama and Beijing-1/JaGAr-01. Other antigenically distinct groups of strains have been identified, including northern Thailand and Malaysia, while studies with monoclonal antibodies suggested that at least five antigenic groups could be identified. Oligonucleotide mapping was used to demonstrate the first evidence for genetic variation among strains of JE virus. Subsequent studies used direct nucleotide sequencing of portions of the genome to identify four genotypes of JE virus. Genotype I included isolates from Cambodia and northern Thailand, genotype II included isolates from Sarawak, Indonesia, southern Thailand and Malaysia, and genotype III included isolates from temperate regions of Asia: Japan, China, Taiwan, India, Nepal, Sri Lanka and the Philippines. Subsequent studies showed that isolates from Japan, Korea and India were distinct clusters within genotype III. Genotype IV included isolates from Indonesia.

Overall, the molecular epidemiological studies of JE virus have identified at least five antigenic groups and four genetic groups/genotypes. The relationship of the antigenic groups to the genotypes is not clear at the present time. The practical significance of these differences has been the subject of much debate. In particular, should strains from one or more antigenic groups/genotypes be included in vaccines to give effective protection against all JE virus strains found in nature (see below)? Also, there is very little information on the molecular basis of neurovirulence of JE virus or biological differences between genotypes of JE virus. However, it is noteworthy that JE virus isolates from Thailand can be distinguished genetically: isolates from northern Thailand are from genotype I while isolates from southern Thailand are from genotype II. The incidence of encephalitis in humans in northern Thailand is 12.2 per 100,000, while it is only 0.3 per 100,000 in southern Thailand. There are many potential explanations for this observation, but genetic differences in the viruses may contribute to the observed differences in disease incidence.

Finally, the entire genome of a number of strains of JE virus has been sequenced. However, none of these strains is from genotype IV. Therefore, the molecular epidemiology of JE virus still requires further studies.

Clinical symptoms

Following the bite of a mosquito, there is an incubation period of 6–16 days before clinical symptoms (i.e. neuroinvasion) are described. These take the form of a febrile illness/headache, aseptic meningitis or encephalitis. The most important form of the disease is acute meningomyeloencephalitis. Onset is rapid, with 1–4 days of fever, headache, chills, drowsiness, stupor, anorexia, nausea and vomiting. Generalized motor seizures are seen in children. Subsequently, patients show symptoms of nuchal rigidity, photophobia, tremors, involuntary movements, focal motor nerve impairment, involving the central and peripheral nervous systems, or coma. The cerebrospinal fluid of patients is a good indicator of infection with markers of disease including one or more of increased pressure, increased concentration of protein, increased lymphocyte counts, anti-JE virus immunoglobulin M (IgM) and virus isolation. Fatal cases usually involve respiratory complications, seizures, virus in cerebrospinal fluid and low levels of anti-JE virus IgM. Examination of brains from fatal cases shows that infection of neurons is widespread in the central nervous system, although the thalamus and basal ganglia appear to be particularly involved. Microscopic lesions include neuronal degeneration and necrosis, rather than apoptosis, plus perivascular inflammation. Non-fatal cases recover in 1–2 weeks. However, neurological and/or psychiatric sequelae are seen in a large proportion of patients who survive the acute disease (see Epidemiology above).

Diagnosis

Japanese encephalitis virus is rarely isolated from peripheral blood during the acute stage of disease in humans. This is thought to be due to a combination of a low viraemia and clinical symptoms of disease being seen after the virus has invaded the central nervous system, when the viraemia has finished. Virus can be isolated from cerebrospinal fluid early in the course of acute encephalitis, but this is consistent with a poor prognosis. Most virus isolates have been obtained from brains of patients at autopsy. Viral antigen can also be detected in the neurons of patients at autopsy by immunohistochemical techniques.

A number of procedures have been used to detect serum antibodies against JE virus: haemagglutination inhibition, complement fixation, immunofluoresence and enzyme-linked immunosorbent assay (ELISA). It is necessary to show a fourfold increase in antibody titres to JE virus between paired serum samples for all these tests to have a presumptive diagnosis of Japanese encephalitis. The presumptive diagnosis is due to serological cross-reactions with antibodies against other flaviviruses. Many other flaviviruses overlap geographically with JE virus, including the dengue and West Nile viruses (see entries), and this can result in misinterpretation of test results. In contrast, detection of IgM antibodies is considered a specific test for JE virus and is the method of choice. An ELISA is usually used to detect JE virus-specific IgM antibodies. Detection of IgM antibodies in cerebrospinal fluid is usually associated with clinical Japanese encephalitis.

Transmission

The virus is transmitted by mosquitoes between vertebrate hosts (Fig. 2). The natural cycle involves rice-field-breeding mosquitoes and domestic pigs or water birds (e.g. egrets (*Egretta* species) and herons (Ardeidae)). The most important vector, *Culex tritaeniorhynchus*, is found in most parts of Asia, where it breeds prolifically in rice fields. JE virus has also been demonstrated to infect several other mosquito species, including *Culex fuscocephala*, *Culex gelidus*, *Culex pipiens*, *Culex quinquefaciatus*, *Culex bitaeniorhynchus*, *Culex epidesmus*, *Culex vishnui*, *Culex pseudovishnui*, *Mansonia uniformis*, *Mansonia bonneae/dives*, *Aedes curtipes*, *Aedes albopictus*, *Armigeres obturbans*, *Anopheles hyrcanus* and *Anopheles barbirostris*. In

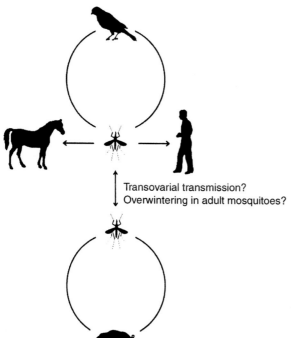

Transovarial transmission?
Overwintering in adult mosquitoes?

Fig. 2. Transmission cycle of Japanese encephalitis involving birds, horses, pigs, humans and mosquitoes.

temperate regions, the 'Japanese encephalitis season' is considered to start in June, with detection of virus in mosquitoes, and this peaks in July. This is followed by the detection of virus in pig and bird amplifying hosts with increasing frequency during July and August. Human infections are concurrent with the increased frequency in amplifying hosts. The exact timing of the 'Japanese encephalitis season' will vary depending on a number of factors, including geographical location in Asia, rainfall and migration of birds. It is not clear how JE virus survives between 'Japanese encephalitis seasons' in temperate areas. There is evidence to support vertical (transovarial) transmission by *Culex* and *Aedes* species, sexual (venereal) transmission between male and female mosquitoes and a potential role for migratory birds as a means of virus survival. Seroepidemiological studies indicate that JE virus infects a wide range of animals, including dogs, ducks, chickens, cattle, bats, snakes and frogs. The role, if any, these animals play in the ecology of JE virus is not known. However, birds and pigs are considered to be the major viraemic-amplifying hosts of the virus.

Treatment

There are no antiviral treatments to control flavivirus infections; rather, supportive therapy is the norm.

Control

Vectors

In theory, transmission of JE virus can be blocked by mosquito control measures, and in epidemic situations aerial insecticidal spraying (e.g. ultra-low-volume applications) can be the best method of curtailing transmission. However, an increasing problem is the spread of resistance in the principal vector, *C. tritaeniornynchus*, to a range of insecticides. Spraying rice-fields with insecticides is not usually practical, because of their large size, but in some areas, such as China, intermittent irrigation, whereby standing water is drawn from fields periodically, has apparently reduced both numbers of vectors and cases of Japanese encephalitis.

Vaccines

However, given that Japanese encephalitis is usually found in rural areas, human immunization is the method of choice. Although vaccination is used to control Japanese encephalitis, economic development of Asian countries is also contributing to control. Smaller areas of rice-fields, use of agricultural pesticides and reduction of the rural population at the expense of increased urbanization have all contributed to a decrease in cases of Japanese encephalitis.

There are licensed vaccines available to control Japanese encephalitis. Inactivated vaccines are based on strains Nakayama, Beijing-1 or P3. The former two are based on formalin-inactivated mouse-brain preparations, which are semi-purified to remove brain materials, while strain P3 is also formalin-inactivated, but grown in primary hamster kidney cell cultures in the People's Republic of China. Only the inactivated mouse-brain-derived vaccines are approved by the World Health Organization for international use. The above vaccines require two doses given on days 0 and 7–28 to induce protective immunity, with a booster dose at 1 year and subsequently every 3–4 years to maintain immunity. Initially, formalin-inactivated mouse-brain vaccines were based on strain Nakayama; however, in 1989 this strain was replaced with strain Beijing-1, due to a combination of being antigenically closer to recent Japanese isolates of JE virus, a high potency being retained following purification and being a better immunogen than strain Nakayama. This resulted in a vaccine that required a dose equivalent to half that needed for strain Nakayama. Inactivated vaccines are manufactured in India, Japan, Republic of Korea, People's Republic of China, Thailand and Vietnam. There is also a live Japanese encephalitis vaccine based on strain SA14-14-2 grown in primary hamster kidney cell culture. This vaccine is only licensed for use in the People's Republic of China. This vaccine appears to be very efficacious and over 100 million doses of it have been administered since 1989, with no known reports of adverse events.

The success of human vaccination has been demonstrated by the decrease in the number of cases in Japan. Prior to 1966, there were 1000–5000 cases per year, with mortality up to 50%. Following the introduction of vaccination, the number of cases has steadily decreased to the point where fewer than ten cases were reported each year during the 1990s. A similar situation has taken place in the Republic of Korea and Taiwan, and all three countries have reported a shift from cases in children to cases in adults and the elderly. Since the vast majority of Japanese encephalitis cases are in children, vaccination has focused on children.

The mouse-brain inactivated vaccine has been reported to cause occasional adverse events, including late allergic mucocutaneous and asthmatic reactions. The majority of the reactions take place after the second or subsequent dose of vaccine. There were a number of adverse events reported during the period 1989–1992, during which 15% of recipients were hospitalized and two-thirds required medical treatment. In addition, there have been, since 1983, occasional reported cases of acute disseminated encephalomyelitis.

The mechanism of protective immunity is poorly understood for most flaviviruses, although production of neutralizing antibodies appears to correlate with immunity. Most neutralizing antibodies recognize epitopes of the E protein. Cell-mediated immunity correlates with non-structural proteins, in particular NS3.

Japanese encephalitis, animal

Japanese encephalitis is the most important veterinary flavivirus disease. Two animal hosts are considered to be important: horses and pigs. Horses infected with encephalitis are considered to be dead-end hosts, due to low viraemias, while JE virus induces abortion in pigs, and these animals are considered to be a major amplifying host.

Epidemiology

Culex tritaeniorhynchus, the principal vector of JE virus, prefers to feed on animals other than humans. Consequently, high seroprevalence rates are seen in pigs, horses and birds. Significant seroconversion is seen in cattle, Water buffaloes (*Bubalus bubalis*), dogs, donkeys and monkeys. Among birds, ducks and chickens, waterhens (*Amaurornis* species), egrets (*Egretta* species) and herons (Ardeidae) seroconvert.

Pigs are important amplifying hosts in the epidemiology of the virus. Infected pigs develop sufficiently high viraemias to infect mosquitoes. Importantly, adult pigs do not show clinical signs of Japanese encephalitis. In terms of veterinary disease, infection of pregnant sows results in abortion and stillbirth, due to transplacental infection.

Infected equines can succumb to Japanese encephalitis; however, equines are considered a dead-end host, as viraemias are too low to infect mosquitoes. Cattle seroconvert and, due to low viraemias, cannot transmit the virus to mosquitoes.

Treatment of animal Japanese encephalitis

There is no treatment.

Control of animal Japanese encephalitis

Vaccination of pigs is used to reduce the incidence of abortions, as adult pigs do not show clinical signs of disease. A live vaccine has been used in the People's Republic of China to protect horses.

Selected bibliography

Burke, D.S. and Leake, C.J. (1988) Japanese encephalitis. In: Monath, T.P. (ed.) *The Arboviruses: Epidemiology and Ecology*, Vol. III. CRC Press, Boca Raton, Florida, pp. 63–92.

Burke, D.S., Tingpalapong, M., Ward, G.S., Andre, R. and Leake, C.J. (1986) Intense transmission of Japanese encephalitis to pigs in a region free of epidemic encephalitis. *Japanese Encephalitis and Haemorrhagic Renal Syndrome Bulletin* 1, 17–26.

Chen, W.-R., Tesh, R.B. and Rico-Hesse, R. (1990) Genetic variation of Japanese encephalitis in nature. *Journal of General Virology* 71, 2915–2922.

Huang, C. (1982) Studies of Japanese encephalitis in China. *Advances in Virus Research* 27, 72–100.

Lacey, L.A. and Lacey, C.M. (1990) The medical importance of riceland mosquitoes and their control using alternatives to chemical insecticides. *Journal of the American Mosquito Control Association* 6 (suppl. 2), 1–93.

Monath, T.P. and Heinz, F.X. (1996) Flaviviruses. In: Fields, B.N., Knipe, B.M. and Howley, P.M. (eds) *Fields Virology* Vol. 1, 3rd edn. Lippincott-Raven, Philadelphia, pp. 961–1034.

Rice, C.M. (1996) *Flaviviridae*: the viruses and their replication. In: Fields, B.N., Knipe, B.M. and Howley, P.M. (eds) *Fields Virology*, Vol. 1, 3rd edn. Lippincott-Raven, Philadelphia, pp. 931–960.

Tsai, T.F., Chang, G.-J.J. and Yu, Y.X. (1988) Japanese encephalitis vaccines. In: Plotkin, S.A. and Orenstein, W.A. (eds) *Vaccines*, 3rd edn. W.B. Saunders, Philadelphia, pp. 672–710.

Japanese river fever *see* **Scrub typhus.**

Japanese spotted fever *see* **Tick-borne typhuses.**

Kala azar *see* **Leishmaniasis.**

Karelian fevers *see* **Sindbis virus.**

Keds *see* **Hippoboscids.**

Kenya tick-borne typhus *see* **Tick-borne typhuses.**

Keystone virus

Bruce F. Eldridge

Keystone (KEY) virus is a mosquito-borne arbovirus transmitted to small mammals in the eastern USA. It is of no known public health importance, although neutralizing antibodies have been detected in humans.

Distribution
Mid-Atlantic to south-eastern coastal states of the USA. Usually associated with coastal pine forests and freshwater swamps (Fig. 1).

Virus
Keystone virus is a member of the genus *Bunyavirus* and the California serogroup. In common with other members of this genus, viral genomes have three single-stranded RNA segments, designated large (L), medium (M) and small (S).

Clinical symptoms
No symptomatic infections have been reported in humans. Neutralizing antibodies have been detected in human sera collected in Florida. Antibodies detected by haemagglutination inhibition tests in Louisiana were probably to KEY virus.

Diagnosis
Confirmation of arboviral disease requires isolation of virus from an infected patient or a fourfold or greater increase in antibody titre between acute and convalescent

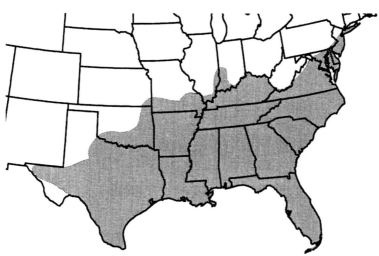

Fig. 1. Distribution of Keystone virus in the south-eastern USA.

human serum samples. Isolation of fully typed virus from mosquitoes or detection of antibodies in sentinel mammals may demonstrate enzootic viral activity.

Transmission

Keystone virus is transmitted to mammals primarily by mosquitoes classified in the *Ochlerotatus*[1] *scapularis* division. Keystone virus infects a variety of mammals, including Cotton rats (*Sigmodon hispidus*), Eastern grey squirrels (*Sciurus carolinensis*), Cottontail rabbits (*Sylvilagus floridanus*), White-tailed deer (*Odocoileus virginianus*), horses, cattle, dogs and humans, but not all of these are important maintenance hosts for the virus. Cotton rats and Cottontail rabbits play key roles in KEY virus ecology in the southern portion of the geographical range of KEY virus; Grey squirrels and Cottontail rabbits are involved in the northern portion.

Keystone virus has been isolated from many species of mosquitoes, including *Aedes* species, but the overwhelming majority of isolations have been from the genus *Ochlerotatus*, such as *O. atlanticus*, *O. tormentor* and *O. infirmatus*, all members of the *O. scapularis* division (Table 1). Isolations of virus from *O. tormentor* are equivocal, because adults of this species are virtually indistinguishable from those of *O. atlanticus*. On the other hand, there are many isolations of KEY virus from *O. atlanticus* in

areas where *O. tormentor* does not occur. There have been a few isolations from other mosquito species, including *Aedes vexans*, *Ochlerotatus triseriatus*, *Ochlerotatus canadensis*, *Culex nigripalpus*, *Anopheles crucians* and *Anopheles punctipennis*. There has been a single isolation of KEY virus from *Chrysops obsoletus*, a deer-fly.

Based on the isolation of KEY virus from *O. atlanticus* larvae collected in nature, transovarial transmission of KEY virus in *O. atlanticus* appears to be a common means of viral maintenance. Transovarial transmission of KEY virus in *O. atlanticus* has also been demonstrated in laboratory experiments. Keystone virus was the second mosquito-borne arbovirus shown conclusively to be transmitted transovarially in its mosquito host; La Crosse virus was the first. Since then, many other California serogroup viruses have been shown to be transmitted in this way, and currently it is believed that this method of transmission is common to all viruses in this serogroup. However, transovarial transmission of KEY virus has been demonstrated only for *O. atlanticus*.

The relative importance of horizontal transmission between mosquitoes and mammals in KEY virus ecology is unknown. Grey squirrels and Cottontail rabbits can be infected experimentally, and develop viraemias high enough to infect *O. atlanticus* females. Deer have a high prevalence of neutralizing antibody to KEY virus and are sources of blood meals for *O. atlanticus*. However, when infected artificially, deer do not develop high viraemias, and they are probably dead-end hosts. Prevalence of KEY virus antibodies in humans in enzootic areas is low, suggesting that humans are probably not involved in KEY virus transmission dynamics other than as occasional dead-end hosts.

The relatively high degree of host specificity of KEY virus for mosquitoes of the *O. scapularis* division and the occurrence of efficient transovarial transmission of the virus in these species suggests the possibility of coevolution of KEY virus and *O. scapularis* division mosquitoes, with both virus and mosquito vectors having evolved from tropical ancestors.

Table 1. Minimum infection rates (MIR) for KEY virus reported in the literature (two or more isolations).

Species	No. tested	No. positive	MIR*
Ochlerotatus[†] *atlanticus*	67,485	244	277
Ochlerotatus atlanticus/ tormentor	143,864	485	297
Aedes infirmatus	175,406	108	1,624
Culex (Melanoconion) species	74,221	4	18,555
Ochlerotatus taeniorhynchus	661,518	24	27,563
Ochlerotatus canadensis	126,835	4	31,709
Aedes vexans	396,845	3	132,282
Culex nigripalpus	687,508	2	343,754

*Number tested/number positive.

[†]*Ochlerotatus* was formerly a subgenus of *Aedes*.

Keystone virus occurs most frequently in lowland pine forests in coastal areas of the Atlantic Ocean and the Gulf of Mexico. *Ochlerotatus atlanticus*, *O. tormentor* and *O. infirmatus* larvae are found in woodlands and open grassy depressions flooded by spring and summer rains. Because these depressions have sandy substrata, larvae complete development only after sustained rains, after which they develop in large numbers. These species aggressively bite humans during daylight hours.

Keystone virus may occur in the same geographical and ecological setting as Jamestown Canyon (JC) virus (see entry), another California serogroup virus. Evidence of KEY enzootic viral activity usually appears earlier in the year than does that of JC virus. In the north KEY virus activity occurs during late summer and autumn and in the south after the first heavy spring rains. Jamestown Canyon virues activity occurs in early to late spring in the eastern USA, depending upon latitude. This temporal difference is probably due to differences in the ecology of the mosquito vectors of the two viruses and the differing roles of their vertebrate hosts. Appearance of larvae of KEY virus mosquito vectors is associated with spring or summer rains and those of JC virus vectors with melted snow or early spring flooding. Deer are important in the ecology of JC virus, but not KEY virus. A prior artificial infection of deer with JC virus prevents artificial infection of KEY virus for at least 30 days, suggesting an additional reason for the relative unimportance of deer as important hosts of KEY virus.

Control

Usually none. High densities of mosquito vectors tend to be limited geographically and temporally. Mosquito abatement may be indicated in specific situations, such as the close proximity of high-density housing to freshwater swamps and adjacent pine forests. In such cases, control would probably be limited to destruction of adult female mosquitoes by ground application of insecticidal fogs.

Note

[1] *Ochlerotatus* was formerly a subgenus of *Aedes*.

Selected bibliography

King, W.V., Bradley, G.H., Smith, C.N. and McDuffie, W.C. (1960) *A Handbook of the Mosquitoes of the Southeastern States*. Handbook no. 173, United States Department Agriculture, Washington, DC, 188 pp.

LeDuc, J.W., Suyemoto, W., Eldridge, B.F. and Barr, A.R. (1975) Ecology of California encephalitis viruses on the Del Mar Va Peninsula. II. Demonstration of transovarial transmission. *American Journal of Tropical Medicine and Hygiene* 24, 124–126.

Lewis, A.L., Hammon, W.McD., Sather, G.D., Taylor, D.J. and Bond, J.O. (1965) Isolations of California group arboviruses from Florida mosquitoes. *American Journal of Tropical Medicine and Hygiene* 14, 451–455.

Parkin, W.E., Hammon, W.McD. and Sather, G.D. (1972) Review of current epidemiological literature on viruses of the California arbovirus group. *American Journal of Tropical Medicine and Hygiene* 21, 964–978.

Watts, D.M., Tammariello, R.F., Dalrymple, J.M. and Eldridge, B.F. (1979) Experimental infection of vertebrates of the Pocomoke Cypress Swamp, Maryland, with Keystone and Jamestown Canyon viruses. *American Journal of Tropical Medicine and Hygiene* 28, 344–350.

Kissing bugs *see* **Triatomine bugs.**

Kokobera virus

John S. Mackenzie

Infections of humans with Kokobera virus

Kokobera (KOK) virus is a mosquito-borne flavivirus enzootic to Australia and Papua New Guinea. The virus was first isolated from *Culex annulirostris* mosquitoes collected at Kowanyama (Mitchell River Mission) in northern Queensland in 1960. Seroepidemiological studies in New South Wales, Queensland and Papua New Guinea have indicated that occasional human infections occur with KOK virus, and indeed it was subsequently shown to be the cause of rare cases of acute polyarticular disease in Queensland, Victoria and New South Wales.

Distribution

Kokobera virus has been isolated from mosquitoes collected in widely separated areas of Australia, including New South Wales, Queensland, northern and south-western Western Australia and the Northern Territory, as well as in Papua New Guinea.

Virus

Kokobera virus is a flavivirus closely related to Stratford virus (see entry), which is also enzootic to Australia. It was initially classified as a member of the Japanese encephalitis (see entry) serological complex on antigenic grounds, albeit more distant than other members, but it has recently been reclassified by the 7th International Committee for Taxonomy of Viruses (in Sydney, 1999) into a separate serological group with Stratford virus.

Clinical symptoms and pathogenesis

Only a few cases of acute polyarticular disease due to KOK virus infection have been recognized. Patients present with extreme lethargy, joint pains and a severe headache, with pain on rotation of the head rather than on flexion. A mild fever may occur, and a reddish, itchy rash with slightly raised lesions 2–3 mm in diameter was reported in one case, lasting about 4 days. Symptoms generally resolve in about 2 weeks, but full recovery may take several months.

Diagnosis

Diagnosis is usually carried out by serological tests, such as enzyme-linked immunosorbent assay (ELISA) (competitive or immunoglobulin M (IgM) capture), with confirmation by plaque reduction neutralization. Virus isolates are identified by neutralization, using monospecific sera or specific monoclonal antibodies, or by polymerase chain reaction of complementary DNA (cDNA), followed by nucleotide sequencing.

Transmission

Kokobera virus has been isolated from several mosquito species, including *C. annulirostris*, *Ochlerotatus*[1] *vigilax* and *Ochlerotatus camptorhynchus*. However, the role of each of these in transmission is unknown. In Papua New Guinea, KOK virus was isolated from a mixed pool of *Aedes* species.

Ecology

From seroepidemiological studies, the vertebrate hosts of KOK virus are thought to be marsupials, with an indication that horses may play a minor role. Although specific antibodies have occasionally been described in sentinel chicken flocks, birds are not believed to play a role in transmission cycles. Molecular epidemiological studies have shown that different topotypes of KOK virus occur in distinct geographical regions, which supports the concept that the virus has sedentary vertebrate hosts. This is in contrast to Murray Valley encephalitis (see entry) and Kunjin (see entry) viruses, which exist throughout Australia as single genotypes but which use birds as their major vertebrate hosts.

Treatment

There is no specific treatment for KOK virus.

Prevention and control

Apart from trying to avoid mosquito bites, such as by applying insect repellents, no specific measures have been invoked to present infections.

Note

[1] *Ochlerotatus* was formerly a subgenus of *Aedes*.

Selected bibliography

Boughton, C.R., Hawkes, R.A. and Naim, H. M. (1986) Illness caused by a Kokobera-like virus in south-eastern Australia. *Medical Journal of Australia* 145, 90–92.

Hawkes, R.A., Boughton, C.R., Naim, H.M., Wild, J. and Chapman, B. (1985) Arbovirus infections in humans in New South Wales: seroepidemiology of the flavivirus group of togaviruses. *Medical Journal of Australia* 143, 555–561.

Poidinger, M., Hall, R.A., Lindsay, M.D., Broom, A.K. and Mackenzie, J.S. (2000) Antigenic and genetic analysis of Kokobera virus strains. *Virus Research* 68, 7–13.

Korean haemorrhagic fever *see* **Haemorrhagic fever with renal syndrome.**

Kumlinge disease *see* **Tick-borne encephalitis.**

Kumri *see* **Setariosis.**

Kunjin virus and Kunjin encephalitis

John S. Mackenzie

Kunjin (KUN) virus is the aetiological agent of Kunjin encephalitis. Cases of Kunjin encephalitis have previously been erroneously included with cases of Murray Valley encephalitis (see entry) collectively as Australian encephalitis. Kunjin virus was first isolated from *Culex annulirostris* mosquitoes trapped at Kowanyama (Mitchell River Mission) in northern Queensland in 1960.

Distribution

Kunjin virus has been isolated from all mainland states of Australia. It has also been isolated from *Culex pseudovishnui* mosquitoes collected in Sarawak and Borneo, in the Oriental zoogeographical region. Seroepidemiological studies have indicated that KUN virus occurs in Papua New Guinea, and possibly elsewhere in the Indonesian archipelago.

Virus

Kunjin virus is a mosquito-borne flavivirus in the Japanese encephalitis serological complex, most closely related to West Nile virus (see entry) on antigenic and genetic grounds. Indeed, in a recent compilation of viral taxonomy by the 7th International Committee for the Taxonomy of Viruses (in Sydney, 1999), it has been reclassified as a subtype of West Nile virus. The complete sequence has been described and the full length genome has 10,664 nucleotides. An infectious clone has been constructed, which has provided a valuable tool for investigations of the identity and intracellular locations of flavivirus non-structural protein and of flavivirus replication strategies, and has considerable potential as a viral vector in future vaccine strategies.

Clinical symptoms and pathogenesis

Kunjin virus is a minor cause of arboviral encephalitis in Australia, compared with the principal cause of arboviral encephalitis, the closely related Murray Valley encephalitis (MVE) virus. The signs and symptoms of Kunjin encephalitis include an abrupt onset of a prodromal stage, with fever, headache, anorexia, malaise, photophobia, stiff neck, dizziness, nausea and vomiting. This may progress to obvious neurological disease, usually within 5 days of onset, manifesting in alterations in mental state, ataxia, speech disturbances or convulsions, leading to coma, pharyngeal paralysis and respiratory failure. No cases of death have been attributed to KUN virus. The first recognized case of Kunjin encephalitis was reported from Broome in Western Australia in 1978, although some of the cases during the last major outbreak of Murray Valley encephalitis in south-eastern Australia were retrospectively associated with KUN virus. Only a small number of cases of encephalitis have been recorded in recent years. Cerebrospinal fluid (CSF) findings of the Western Australian encephalitis cases showed elevated protein levels. An electroencephalogram (EEG) was taken in one case and showed nonspecific, diffuse, slow wave activity. Kunjin virus has also been associated with a mild febrile disease, with malaise, headache, myalgia and sometimes joint involvement.

There have not been sufficient numbers of cases and case follow-ups to give detailed information on sequelae. However, one severe case from Western Australia had residual facial nerve palsy and an unsteady gait.

There has been a single report of encephalomyelitis in a horse. It is not known whether KUN virus can cause disease in horses in northern Australia.

Diagnosis
Diagnosis is usually by serological tests, most commonly by immunoglobulin M (IgM) capture enzyme-linked immunosorbent assay (ELISA). As IgM antibody can last several months, diagnosis on a single specimen can only be regarded as presumptive, and may represent recent past exposure. Therefore serological diagnosis requires paired serum samples and evidence of a fourfold or greater rise in IgG antibodies using ELISA or haemagglutination inhibition (HI) tests. Immunoglobulin M antibodies are not usually found in CSF, except during a severe case of encephalitis or central nervous system (CNS) infection, when it is present, but usually transiently. Thus, finding specific IgM in the CSF in a

single specimen is often considered sufficient to diagnose infection, without the need for paired serum samples. Virus isolation is difficult and seldom achieved from serum, because patients generally present well after the viraemic phase. However, virus might be detectable in CSF or serum by reverse transcription–polymerase chain reaction (RT-PCR).

Transmission
From both field oberservations and experimental studies, the major vertebrate hosts of KUN virus are believed to be waterbirds in the order Ciconiiformes, particularly the Nankeen night heron (*Nycticorax caledonicus*). Seroepidemiological studies have also suggested a number of wild and domestic animal could be possible vertebrate hosts, including cattle, horses and some macropods, although experimental evidence is lacking. The major mosquito vector species is *Culex annulirostris*, but the virus has been isolated from a range of other mosquito vectors, including *Culex australicus*, *Culex squamosus*, *Culex quinquefasciatus* and *Ochlerotatus*[1] *tremulus*, but it is uncertain whether all these other species contribute to the transmission cycles.

Ecology and epidemiology
Although KUN virus shares a number of biological properties with the closely related MVE virus, including major vertebrate hosts and vector species, there are significant differences in their epidemiological and ecological patterns. Kunjin virus is found throughout northern Australia, and results from sentinel chicken surveillance data and mosquito isolations suggest that it is active every year in Western Australia and probably every year in the Northern Territory. Interestingly, however, the majority of sentinel chicken seroconversions in the north of Western Australia are to MVE virus rather than KUN virus, whereas evidence from cattle seroconversions, sentinel chicken seroconversions and virus isolations suggest that KUN virus is more active than MVE virus in the Northern Territory. Further south, in the arid Pilbara area of Western Australia, KUN virus

activity is more frequent than MVE virus activity except in years of exceptionally heavy rainfall. However, variations in the levels of activity of KUN or MVE viruses in the north of Western Australia are not consistent. Data from northern Queensland are not available over an extended period, but, from human seroconversions and mild febrile illness caused by KUN virus, it would appear that KUN virus is more active than MVE virus in Queensland.

Kunjin virus activity occurs more frequently than MVE virus activity in temperate areas, particularly in south-eastern Australia. This strongly suggests that KUN virus can disperse more readily than MVE virus from enzootic areas in northern Australia to epidemic areas in the south-east. Indeed, KUN virus activity has been evident from human and/or sentinel chicken seroconversions in parts of Victoria and/or New South Wales in a number of years over the past two decades, whereas MVE virus activity has not been detected since the last major epidemic in 1974. The reasons for this apparent ability of KUN virus to disperse from northern enzootic areas are unknown. Although KUN and MVE viruses share major vector species and vertebrate hosts, there is some evidence to suggest that KUN virus may be able to use additional members of the order Ciconiiformes, some of which may exhibit a greater range or may move further in different environmental conditions.

All Australian KUN virus isolates are antigenically indistinguishable by standard serological techniques using polyclonal sera. However, antigenic differences can be detected using monoclonal antibodies. All Australian isolates are also closely related genetically and comprise a single topotype, with less than 2% nucleotide divergence between any two isolates. This close antigenic relationship and high level of genomic homology observed for the Australian strains of KUN virus is consistent with the involvement of avian vertebrate hosts, allowing virus to circulate around the continent.

Treatment
No specific treatment is available for KUN virus infection.

Prevention and control
Prevention of infection has been largely directed at behavioural changes, with local warnings disseminated when epidemic activity is predicted. These warnings suggest the use of insect repellents and, in northern Australia, the use of mosquito nets. The latter has been particularly directed at Aboriginal communities, where most cases occur in young children and infants. Wearing long sleeves and long trousers at dusk and dawn are suggested. Mosquito control measures have not been invoked to prevent KUN virus infections.

Note
[1] *Ochlerotatus* was formerly a subgenus of *Aedes*.

Selected bibliography

Coia, G., Parker, M.D., Speight, G., Byrne, M.E. and Westaway, E.G. (1988) Nucleotide and complete amino acid sequences of Kunjin virus: definitive gene order and characteristics of the virus-specified proteins. *Journal of General Virology* 69, 1–21.

Dalgarno, L, Short, N.J., Hardy, C.M., Bell, J.R., Strauss, J.H. and Marshall, I.D. (1984) Characterization of Barmah Forest virus: an alphavirus with some unusual properties. *Virology* 133, 416–426.

Doherty, R.L., Carley, J.G., Filippich, C., White, J. and Gust, I.D. (1976) Murray Valley encephalitis in Australia, 1974: antibody responses in cases and community. *Australia and New Zealand Journal of Medicine* 6, 446–453.

Mackenzie, J.S., Smith, D.W., Broom, A.K. and Bucens, M.R. (1993) Australian encephalitis in Western Australia, 1978–1991. *Medical Journal of Australia* 158, 591–595.

Mackenzie, J.S., Lindsay, M.D., Coelen, R.J., Broom, A.K., Hall, R.A. and Smith, D.W. (1994) Arboviruses causing human disease in the Australasian region. *Archives of Virology* 136, 447–467.

Marshall, I.D. (1988) Murray Valley and Kunjin encephalitis. In: Monath, T.P. (ed.) *The Arboviruses: Epidemiology and Ecology*, Vol. III. CRC Press, Boca Raton, Florida, pp. 151–190.

Russell, R.C. (1995) Arboviruses and their vectors in Australia: an update on the ecology and epidemiology of some mosquito-borne arboviruses. *Reviews of Medical and Veterinary Entomology* 83, 141–158.

Russell, R.C. (1998) Vectors vs. humans in Australia – who is on top down under? An update on
vector-borne disease and research on vectors
in Australia. *Journal of Vector Ecology* 23,
1–46.

Varnavski, A.N. and Khromykh, A.A. (1999)
Noncytopathic flavivirus replicon RNA-
based system for expression and delivery
of heterologous genes. *Virology* 255,
366–375.

Kyasanur Forest disease

M.G.R. Varma

An infection of humans and monkeys caused by an arthropod-borne virus (arbovirus) and named after the locality, Kyasanur Forest in southern India, where it was first discovered. The disease is restricted to southern India, where it is locally known as 'monkey disease', because of its association with monkey deaths.

Distribution

The disease is restricted to forested areas of five districts (Uttar Kannada, Shimoga, Chikmagalur, Udupi and Dakshina Kannada) of Karnataka State in South India (Fig. 1), although antibodies to the virus have been found in humans and animals in other parts of India far removed from the endemic/enzootic zone. It was first discovered in March 1957 in Kyasanur Forest in the Shimoga District of Karnataka State, a mosaic of tropical wet evergreen forests, semi-evergreen forests, moist deciduous forests and dry deciduous forests, with bamboo and shrub jungle at the edges.

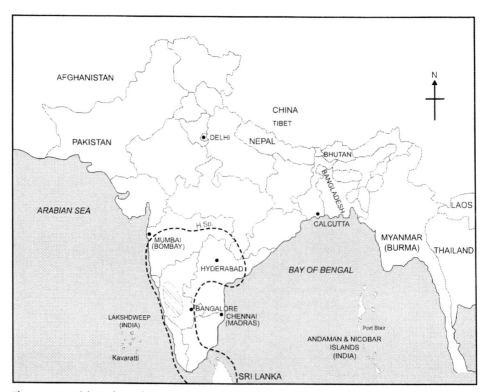

Fig. 1. Map of the Indian subcontinent showing distribution of Kyasanur Forest disease (hatched area) and of the tick vector *Haemaphysalis spinigera* (dashed line).

Kyasanur Forest forms part of the Western Ghats, a mountain range some 1300 km long running along the western edge of India from south of Bombay to the southern tip of the subcontinent through the states of Maharashtra, Karnataka, Kerala and Tamil Nadu and covering an estimated area of 159,000 km². The unprecedented and mass deaths of two species of forest monkeys, the Bonnet macaque (*Macaca radiata*) and the Common or Black-faced langur, also known as the Hanuman monkey (*Semnopithecus entellus*[1]), gave the disease its local name 'monkey disease'. Epizootics in monkeys precede epidemics of the disease in humans, and a systematic surveillance of monkey deaths is an integral part of epidemiological studies of the disease.

The initial epizootic/epidemic in 1957 covered only a few hundred square kilometres and it was thought that Kyasanur Forest disease would be restricted to this original focus, but in 1972, 1973 and 1975 there were four outbreaks of the disease to the north, west, south and south-east of the original focus. Eight years later, in 1983, there was a large epizootic/epidemic 80 km south of the previous 1975 outbreak, with several monkey deaths and 1555 human cases, of whom 150 died; this was in a part of undisturbed forest, where some 400 ha were clear-felled for the establishment of a Cashew tree (*Anarcardium occidentale*) plantation, and most of the human cases were in the immigrant labourers employed for forest clearance. The next sizeable outbreak occurred in 1988–1989 when several hundred human cases, with deaths, were reported in areas to the west, south-west, south and south-east of the Kyasanur Forest focus. In further outbreaks in 1990–1992, during which a successful vaccine trial involving 88,152 persons in 72 villages in the Kyasanur Forest disease (KFD) virus area was carried out, there were 349 cases of the diseases, 24 in vaccinees and 325 in unvaccinated individuals. As recently as April–May 2000, 21 confirmed cases of Kyasanur Forest disease and two deaths were reported in the Uttar (north) Kannada district of Karnataka State (source of information ProMED mail <www.promedmail.org>). By the late 1990s,

the known distribution of the disease covered some 5000 km².

One of the interesting features of the spread of Kyasanur Forest disease in Karnataka State has been the appearance of the disease in areas often separated by several kilometres from the original focus in Kyasanur Forest and from each other.

Virus

Kyasanur Forest disease virus is a distinct member of the tick-borne encephalitis virus complex (genus *Flavivirus*, family Flaviviridae), which includes the eastern (also known as Russian spring–summer encephalitis (RSSE) virus) and the western subtypes of tick-borne encephalitis virus and louping ill virus (see entries). It can be distinguished from other members of the complex by analysis of envelope protein epitopes using monoclonal antibodies and on the basis of the structural protein gene sequences. In 1995 a new virus, closely related to KFD virus was isolated from the blood of human patients in Jeddah, Saudi Arabia. Clinically Kyasanur Forest disease closely resembles Omsk haemorrhagic fever (see entry).

Epidemiology

There are several aspects of the epidemiology of Kyasanur Forest disease that deserve examination and explanation. When the disease first appeared suddenly in southern India in early 1957, it caused considerable alarm. The introduction of yellow fever into the subcontinent, with its fauna of susceptible monkeys and mosquito vectors, has been, and remains, a perpetual threat, and it was thought that, in spite of strict quarantine measures, yellow fever had at last been introduced into India. Prompt reporting of monkey deaths and accompanying human illness and deaths by the health authorities, together with the swift response of the National Institute of Virology (formerly the Virus Research Centre) at Pune, several hundred kilometres to the north, allayed these fears and led to what is now regarded as a classic and in-depth study of a 'new/ emerging' disease.

The outbreak was during the dry part of the year, when mosquitoes are very scarce in the forest, but the insect collectors noticed large numbers of immature ticks and were actually bitten by them. An agent, subsequently named KFD virus, was isolated from the ticks collected in the forest, and also from monkeys and humans. All these isolates were shown to be identical and antigenically similar to the virus causing Russian spring–summer encephalitis (RSSE), a disease unknown in India. The questions which were uppermost in the minds of the investigators were as follows. Was KFD virus introduced into the area or was it already there in a cryptic form, becoming overtly manifest due to ecological or behavioural factors? A foreign source of infection was a possibility, but this was complicated by the finding of antibodies to RSSE virus (closely related to KFD virus) in humans in an area several hundred kilometres to the north as early as 1952, as well as KFD-positive human sera well outside the enzootic/epidemic area. If in fact it was introduced, was it through the agency of ticks on birds migrating from the north to the enzootic area? Thousands of migrant birds were screened for ticks, but only one was infested with an exotic tick species of the genus *Hyalomma*, which is not involved in the transmission of KFD virus in nature. If KFD virus was not introduced, was it always present in an occult phase in Kyasanur Forest or indeed in the adjoining forest areas, as part of the biocenosis, appearing 'suddenly' due to ecological changes, human behaviour or other amplifying mechanisms? It is quite possible that occasional monkey deaths and sporadic cases of Kyasanur Forest disease in the area in the past were unrecognized and therefore not reported or were misdiagnosed. It was the monkey deaths on an unprecedented scale, a sight unlikely to be forgotten, and several human cases in villages adjoining the forest that alerted health authorities. During the period 1964–1973, 1046 monkey deaths were reported, of which 860 were Black-faced langur monkeys (*S. entellus*) and 186 Bonnet macaque monkeys (*M. radiata*): 50% of *S. entellus* and 18.1% of *M. radiata* necropsied were positive for KFD virus.

There are several causes for the first outbreak. The most important are environmental factors – more precisely, ecological changes. The main feature of the Kyasanur Forest ecosystem was the recent encroachment of humans into undisturbed forest due to a considerable increase in the population; the population of the Kyansanur Forest disease area had more than doubled in the 10 years since 1951. This had several consequences. The clearing or thinning of the forest for agricultural purposes, particularly rice cultivation, led to an increased contact of humans with the forest. The patches of grazing land in and adjacent to these cleared areas were suitable for cattle grazing. Cattle are important hosts for adults of the tick *Haemaphysalis spinigera*, the chief vector of the disease, and the presence of cattle in the forest increased the numbers of this vector and converted a latent zoonosis into an epizootic. Apart from the steady expansion of the paddy-fields at the expense of the forest, commercial felling of trees for timber and firewood and pruning of large areas of the forest canopy for green manure gave rise to miles of interface, which fundamentally modified the ecology of the region. One of the features of this interface was the establishment of the Lantana bush (*Lantana camara*) and more recently of the weed *Chromolaena odorata*. The Lantana bush, originally imported into Sri Lanka from tropical America for ornamental purposes, has invaded almost all regions of India. It is an aggressive weed, prospering when original forests are destroyed or disfigured. The dense impenetrable thickets of Lantana may grow to a height of 3 m above ground and are often used as shelter by ground birds, small mammals, cattle and deer.

Since the original outbreak, Kyasanur Forest disease has subsequently appeared in areas where the forests have been cleared for monocultures, such as for Teak (*Tectona grandis*) or Eucalyptus (*Eucalyptus* species), or as in the case of the Nidle forest outbreak in 1982–1983, for the commercial growing of Cashew trees (*A. occidentale*). Apart from commercial and agricultural activities, daily activities, such as gathering firewood or young girls picking forest blossoms, and herding cattle in the forest are aspects of human behaviour relevant in the natural history of the disease.

Monkeys in the forest infected with the virus either die or become immune and therefore play no further part in virus maintenance. It has been observed that, because of larval tick infestation of monkeys and squirrels, the timing of such infestations and synchronization with virus circulation in monkeys, each outbreak appears to exhaust itself by the end of the year. Such 'spent' foci may remain silent, with low-grade virus activity persisting for several years before becoming active again. It is particularly difficult to detect a cryptic focus, because the occasional monkey deaths that occur may not be reported.

Although the outbreaks of Kyasanur Forest disease appear to be isolated in time and space, they have always followed destruction of forests and intrusion of humans. The whole forested areas of the Western Ghats may be regarded as a vast enzootic area and, although timber extraction on a commercial scale has been halted from the forests of Karnataka and Kerala states, further outbreaks will occur when the stable ecosystem is disturbed or destroyed and the populations of monkeys, small mammals and ticks are amplified to reach levels required for a flare-up of virus activity.

Clinical symptoms
After an incubation period of 3–8 days following the bite of an infected tick, there is a sudden onset, with malaise and high fever, which may reach 40°C by the third or fourth day. Myalgia, particularly of the back and calf muscles, headache, cough, sore throat, diarrhoea and vomiting are common and there is marked dehydration. Severe conjunctivitis and photophobia are present. A consistent finding is papulovesicular lesions on the soft palate. Rash or discolorations of the skin are absent. In some cases there is generalized lymphadenopathy. There may be neurological signs suggestive of brain involvement, dyspnoea and cyanosis, and

occasional patients may have renal failure or signs of hepatocellular failure. In earlier studies involving poor villagers, haemorrhagic symptoms, such as bleeding from the nose, gums and intestines, were often reported, sometimes as early as the third day, but the majority of cases, including infections in laboratory personnel, have been devoid of haemorrhagic manifestations. Atypical lymphocytes are present in the peripheral blood of all patients during some stage of the disease.

After about 10 days, the fever subsides and the patient recovers but is weak. In a minority of cases (about 20%), this first phase is followed by a second phase with neurological complications. Fever returns, with severe headache, neck stiffness, mental disturbance, coarse tremors, giddiness, abnormal reflexes and cerebrospinal fluid (CSF) pleocytosis. These persist until the fever subsides, after about 7 days. The patient usually recovers, but remains weak, with a long period of convalescence. Mortality is 5–10% and complications leading to death are haemorrhage, encephalitis, bronchopneumonia, shock and renal or hepatic failure. Main post-mortem findings are haemorrhagic pneumonia, the presence of reticuloendothelial elements in the spleen and liver and degenerative changes in the larger parenchymal organs.

Diagnosis
Clinical signs useful in diagnosis are facial flushing, congestion of the conjunctiva, gingival hyperplasia, cervical lymphadenopathy, neck stiffness and hypotension, with significant gastrointestinal haemorrhage. Apart from these signs, diagnosis of Kyasanur Forest disease is by isolation of the virus from the blood, up until the 12th day, in suckling mice or vertebrate cell culture systems, such as primary monkey kidney cells or pig stable (PS) kidney cells. Rising antibody titres in serological tests, such as neutralization (NT), haemagglutination inhibition (HI) and complement fixation (CF), between acute and convalescent sera will confirm the diagnosis. A history of forest exposure is also helpful.

Transmission

The virus is transmitted by the bite of infected ticks, and young adult humans of both sexes are infected, although there are more male than female cases, reflecting the extent of occupational exposure in the forest. The two major vectors are *H. spinigera* and *Haemaphysalis turturis*. Transmission to humans is almost exclusively by the bite of nymphs of *H. spinigera*, which have acquired the infection by feeding as larvae on infected monkeys or infected rodents in the forest. Adult ticks can remain infected with the virus for up to 14 months. Nymphs of *H. spinigera* are most prevalent in the drier part of the year (December to May); their numbers start to rise in December and peak in January to March, after which they decline; they are rare in the rainy season (June to October). Peak adult populations of the tick are seen at the height of the rainy season in July and August, when there are few human cases. Monkey deaths and human cases of the disease start appearing in November or December, reaching a peak in January to February, when nymphs of *H. spinigera* are most abundant, and gradually decline by the end of May with the approach of the rainy season. A positive correlation has been shown between intensity of infection in ticks and total number of human cases. Human infections occur when villagers at the edge of the forest enter the forest for herding cattle, gathering firewood and forest blossoms, or when they walk through the forest from village to village.

The tick fauna of Kyasanur Forest and the species from which the virus has been isolated are listed in Table 1. The most frequently infected are *H. spinigera* and *H. turturis* and these are the ones involved in the maintenance cycle of the virus in nature. Old World monkeys spend more time on the ground than is generally acknowledged, the Common langur (*S. entellus*) spending as much as 80% of its active time on the ground. It is during this time that both Bonnet macaques (*M. radiata*) and the langurs pick up ticks, and 12% of Bonnet macaques and 43% of the Common langurs are commonly infested with large numbers

Table 1.   The ticks of Kyasanur Forest.

*Haemaphysalis spinigera**	Amblyomma species
*Haemaphysalis turturis**	Dermacentor auratus*
Haemaphysalis papuana kinneari *	Rhipicephalus species
Haemaphysalis wellingtoni *	Boophilus microplus
*Haemaphysalis cuspidata**	Ixodes petauristae*
*Haemaphysalis kyasanurensis**	Ixodes ceylonensis
*Haemaphysalis minuta**	
Haemaphysalis aculeata	
*Haemaphysalis bispinosa**	
Haemaphysalis cornigera	
Haemaphysalis leachi	
*Haemaphysalis intermedia**	

*KFD virus isolated from naturally infected ticks.

of immature stages of *H. spinigera* and *H. turturis*. Infected monkeys also have high viraemic levels and their activity pattern of rest and movement favours the formation of foci of infection and the dissemination of infection. Nymphs developing from fed larvae detaching from dead monkeys are often found in relatively small areas of the forest floor, so called 'hot spots', which serve as a source of infection to humans and other animals. Kyasanur Forest disease virus has also been isolated from a soft tick, *Ornithodoros chiropterphila*, collected from the insectivorous bat *Rhinolophus rouxi*, but the significance of this in the natural history of KFD virus is unknown.

In laboratory experiments, *H. spinigera*, *H. turturis*, *Haemaphysalis papuana kinneari*, *Haemaphysalis minuta*, *Haemaphysalis kyasanurensis*, *Haemaphysalis wellingtoni*, *Haemaphysalis cuspidata*, *Ixodes petauristae*, *Ixodes ceylonensis*, *Rhipicephalus haemaphysaloides* and *Dermacentor auratus* transmitted the virus. Experimental transovarial transmission of the virus was shown only in *I. petauristae*, and the role of transovarial transmission as a maintenance mechanism of KFD virus is negligible.

Small mammals, such as the White-bellied rat (*Rattus rattus wroughtoni*), the White-tailed rat (*Rattus blanfordi*), the Jungle-striped or Western Ghats squirrel (*Funambulus tristriatus tristriatus*) and the House shrew (*Suncus murinus*), are parasitized by immature stages *I. ceylonensis*, *H. p. kinneari*, *H. spinigera* and *H. turturis*.

Larvae of *H. spinigera* prefer squirrels to the other small mammals. Virus has been isolated from *R. r. wroughtoni*, *R. blanfordi*, *S. murinus* and the bat *R. rouxi* (not infested with vector ticks) and, in experimental infections, from the shrew and the squirrel, as well as the Porcupine (*Hystrix indica*) (which was infested with vector ticks), all of which have high levels of viraemia. However, because of their distribution — the squirrel is found at the extreme edge of the forest, low population levels of the hosts and low tick loads, small mammals may not play a major role in the maintenance of the virus. Nevertheless, since optimal vector–host conditions would enhance virus transmission and multiplication and lead to the exhaustion of virus activity, low tick infestation levels of rodents and shrews and the population levels of these animals would suggest that they may have a role in low-grade virus maintenance and the formation of cryptic foci.

Forest-dwelling ground birds, such as the Pea fowl (*Pavo cristatus*) and the Grey jungle fowl (*Gallus sonneratii*), carry heavy tick loads, particularly of *H. wellingtoni* and *H. minuta*, both of which have been found harbouring the virus in nature. Fledgling domestic chicks are highly susceptible to KFD virus infection and, while this finding does not allow extrapolation to wild species, it is possible that the Pea fowl and the Jungle fowl may also be highly susceptible to the virus and thus have a subsidiary role in the maintenance of the virus.

Domestic cattle are the most important hosts for adults of *H. spinigera*. Although not forest residents, village cattle are taken into the forest for grazing where they are heavily parasitized by ticks. Experimentally infected cattle have a very low viraemia and it is unlikely that they serve as donors for infecting ticks, but they have a vital role in amplifying the tick population. When one considers that the degree of infestation of humans with the vector ticks (i.e. number of ticks collected divided by number of individuals) is only 0.12, only a high population of vector ticks and a correspondingly high rate of vector infection can offset the low infestation rate of humans.

Treatment and prevention

There is no known treatment for Kyasanur Forest disease. Patients should be cared for in a tick-free environment. Medical and nursing staff should avoid contamination with the blood of the patients. Kyasanur Forest disease virus is highly infectious and well over 100 laboratory infections have been recorded, some of them probably following inhalation of infective aerosols.

A formalin-inactivated vaccine was field-evaluated in the 1990–1992 epidemic seasons in 72 villages in Karnataka State. In total 88,152 persons were vaccinated and the vaccine was shown to have a significant protective effect.

Control

The most effective way of controlling Kyasanur Forest disease is by vaccination of the population most at risk. But this requires effective surveillance, prompt reporting and expeditious delivery of the vaccine, with all the necessary infrastructure this entails.

Personal protection against ticks involves daily examination of the whole body and clothing for attached ticks, followed by their prompt removal. Repellents, such as diethyltoluamide (DEET), applied directly to the skin can provide short-term protection against ticks, while clothing impregnated with pyrethroid insecticides, such as permethrin, may give protection for longer periods. Lindane emulsion and benzene hexachloride (HCH) suspension applied at the rate of 1.12 kg ha^{-1} of forest floor has effectively controlled nymphs of *H. spinigera* and *H. turturis* for up to 6 weeks. Sprays or dusts containing 0.5% malathion, 0.25–0.5% carbaryl or 0.01–0.03% HCH have been effective against adult ticks on cattle, but the protection lasts for only 1–2 days. 'Pour-on' formulations of pyrethroids can also be applied to cattle to provide protection against ticks.

Note

[1]   This monkey was formerly in the genus *Presbytis.*

Selected bibliography

Adhikari Prabha, M.R., Prabhu, M.G., Raghuveer, C.V., Bai, M. and Mala, M.A. (1993) Clinical study of 100 cases of Kyasanur Forest disease with clinicopathological correlation. *Indian Journal of Medical Sciences* 47, 124–130.

Bannerjee, K. (1988) Kyasanur Forest disease. In: Monath, T.P. (ed.) *The Arboviruses: Epidemiology and Ecology*, Vol. III. CRC Press, Boca Raton, Florida, pp. 93–116.

Banerjee, K. (1996) Emerging viral infections with special reference to India. *Indian Journal of Medical Research* 103, 177–200.

Bhat, H.R. (1990) Analysis of various socio-economic elements affecting the Western Ghat ecosystem. *Bulletin of the National Institute of Virology, Pune* 8, 3–12.

Boshell, M.J. (1969) Kyasanur Forest disease: ecologic considerations. *American Journal of Tropical Medicine and Hygiene* 18, 67–80.

Dandawate, C.N., Desai, G.B., Achar, T.R. and Banerjee, K. (1994) Field evaluation of formalin inactivated Kyasanur forest disease virus tissue culture vaccine in three districts of Karnataka state. *Indian Journal of Medical Research* 99, 152–158.

Drummond, R.O., Rajagopalan, P.K., Sreenivasan, M.A. and Menon, P.K. (1969) Tests with ixodicides for the control of the tick vectors of Kyasanur Forest disease. *Journal of Medical Entomology* 6, 245–251.

Pavri, K. (1989) Clinical, clinicopathologic and haematologic features of Kyasanur Forest disease. *Review of Infectious Diseases* 11 (suppl. 4) S854–S859.

Simpson, D.I.H. (1996) Arbovirus infections. In: Cook, G.C. (ed.) *Manson's Tropical Diseases*, 20th edn. W.B. Saunders, London, pp. 615–665.

Venugopal, K., Gritsun, T., Lashkevich, V.A. and Gould, E.A. (1994) Analysis of the structural protein gene sequence shows Kyasanur Forest disease virus as a distinct member of the tick-borne encephalitis virus serocomplex. *Journal of General Virology* 75, 227–232.

Zaki, A.M. (1997) Isolation of a flavivirus related to the tick-borne encephalitis complex from human cases in Saudi Arabia. *Transactions of the Royal Society of Tropical Medicine and Hygiene* 91, 179–181.

La Crosse virus

Barry J. Beaty

La Crosse (LAC) virus is a member of the California (CAL) serogroup of viruses in the family Bunyaviridae, which is the largest family of vertebrate viruses. La Crosse and the other CAL serogroup viruses are maintained in nature in distinct cycles, involving preferred vector species and vertebrate hosts, respectively. A notable feature of the CAL group viruses is their ability to be trans-seasonally maintained and amplified by transovarial transmission (TOT) in their respective vector species.

Distribution

Californian serogroup viruses (14 named viruses) have been isolated in North and South America, Africa, Europe and Asia. La Crosse virus has been isolated from, and is known to cause encephalitis in, children in most states east of, or contiguous to, the Mississippi River in the USA. In the upper Midwest, LAC virus is vectored by *Ochlerotatus*[1] *triseriatus*, with Eastern chipmunks (*Tamias striatus*) and Eastern grey squirrels (*Sciurus carolinensis*) serving as the principal vertebrate hosts. *Ochlerotatus triseriatus* is known as the tree-hole mosquito, and it is widely distributed in the forested areas of the midwestern, eastern and southern USA. The vertebrate hosts are also abundant in these areas. Snowshoe hare (SSH) virus, which is an antigenic subtype of LAC virus, is sympatric with LAC virus in the northern USA; however, SSH virus has a distinct natural cycle, involving *Ochlerotatus communis* (and other *Ochlerotatus* and *Aedes* species) or *Culiseta inornata* mosquitoes and Snowshoe hares (*Lepus americanus*). Other CAL group viruses are found in Europe, Asia and Africa and have their own arbovirus cycles, comprised of preferred vertebrate hosts and arthropod vectors. For example, in Europe Tahyna (TAH) virus (see entry) is vectored by *Aedes vexans* and other *Aedes* species.

Virus

La Crosse virus is a member of the *Bunyavirus* genus of the family Bunyaviridae. Bunyavirus virions are 80–100 nm in diameter and enveloped. The negative-sense genome of bunyaviruses is tripartite, and consists of large (L), medium (M) and small (S) RNA segments. The viral nucleocapsids are circular in configuration, because of hydrogen bonding of conserved RNA sequences, with inverted complementarity at the 3′ and 5′ termini. The L, M and S RNA segments of LAC (and certain other bunyaviruses) have been sequenced and coding assignments determined. The S RNA segment codes for the nucleocapsid (N) protein and a non-structural protein NSs, which are translated from overlapping reading frames in the viral complementary sequence. The M RNA codes for a polyprotein that is post-translationally processed, yielding the G1 and G2 glycoproteins and a non-structural protein NSm. The L RNA codes for the RNA polymerase.

There is not a lot of information concerning LAC virus replication. Subsequent to virus adsorption, penetration and uncoating, nucleocapsids are released into the cytoplasm. The virion-associated RNA-dependent RNA polymerase initiates primary transcription. The three messenger RNA (mRNA) species possess short, non-viral-coded, primer sequences at their 5′ ends, which are acquired from host mRNA in both vertebrate and invertebrate cells. The LAC virion contains a primer-stimulated RNA polymerase and a methylated cap-dependent endonuclease, and LAC virus primes its own mRNA transcription using scavenged host primers. Transcription of both S and M mRNA species terminates approximately 100 nucleotides before the end of the template RNA. Little information is available concerning transcription of the L mRNA species. La Crosse mRNAs are not polyadenylated. After translation of the mRNA species, genome replication begins, and genome complementary RNA accumulates. Large quantities of viral mRNA (secondary transcription) and viral structural proteins are then synthesized. Virus morphogenesis involves budding into the cisternae of the Golgi and virus-containing vesicles fuse with the plasma membrane and release of virions.

Clinical symptoms

In most years, LAC virus is the primary cause of arboviral encephalitis in the USA. Humans are tangential hosts. La Crosse virus is a major cause of encephalitis and aseptic meningitis in children. Most cases (75%) occur in children under 10 years of age, and most cases are in boys (2–3 : 1 male : female ratio). The incubation period is from 7 to 14 days. Infection can yield clinical symptoms ranging from mild febrile illness to aseptic meningitis and fatal encephalitis. Common symptoms include fever, headache and vomiting, which can progress to seizures and disorientation. Approximately 50% of patients hospitalized with La Crosse encephalitis have seizures, and the case fatality rate in these patients is 1.0%. Recurrent seizures occur in about 25% of patients who originally presented with seizures, which is a greater frequency than that following St Louis encephalitis or western equine encephalitis infections (see entries) and is a frequency equivalent to that resulting from infection with eastern equine encephalitis (see entry). Antibody to LAC virus is three times more prevalent in people institutionalized for permanent mental disorders than in the general population. Acute care costs for patients are significant, and long-term care costs for individuals with sequelae to La Crosse encephalitis (e.g. recurrent seizures, institutionalization) can be enormous. Interestingly, specific genotypes of LAC virus seem to be associated with human central nervous system (CNS) infections. The incidence of La Crosse encephalitis in endemic areas has been estimated at 5–10 per 100,000 population (nearly equal to the rate for bacterial meningitis of all causes). It is important to note that LAC virus infections are grossly under-reported.

As noted previously, other members of the CAL serogroup are also associated with human infections and illness (including encephalitis) in the USA, including SSH, California encephalitis, Jamestown Canyon, Keystone (see entries) and trivittatus (TVT) viruses. There are an estimated 15,000 California serogroup virus infections annually in Indiana and 300,000 annually in the midwestern USA. Tahyna virus (see entry) is more associated with an influenza-like illness.

Many other viruses of the family Bunyaviridae (e.g. Akabane, Crimean–Congo haemorrhagic fever, Oropouche, Rift Valley fever (RVF), phlebotomus fevers (see entries)) are of considerable medical and veterinary importance. Rift Valley fever and Akabane viruses are major causes of abortion and teratology in domestic animals. Cache Valley virus (see entry) is emerging in the USA as a cause of abortion and teratology in animals and perhaps humans.

Diagnosis

La Crosse virus infections have classically been diagnosed serologically by demonstration of a greater than fourfold increase in serum neutralization, haemagglutination inhibition or complement fixation titres. Immunofluorescent antibody and enzyme immunoassay techniques can also provide diagnostic information using acute and convalescent sera, but can also give rapid, clinically relevant diagnosis by detection of specific immunoglobulin M (IgM) antibodies. Isolation of LAC virus from patients is rare, and most isolates have been obtained post-mortem. La Crosse virus can also be detected in specimens by reverse-transcription–polymerase chain reaction. The gold standard for serological diagnosis of LAC virus infections is demonstration of a more than fourfold increase in serum neutralization titres. Upon presentation, differential diagnosis includes herpes encephalitis and CNS tumours. Thus, provision of clinically relevant diagnostic capability for LAC virus infections is a significant advance and prevents administration of DNA antagonists or surgery, respectively, due to misdiagnosis.

Transmission

Ochlerotatus triseriatus mosquitoes transmit LAC virus orally, transovarially and venereally (Fig. 1). The anatomical bases of LAC virus productive infection (i.e. virus infection and replication in mid-gut cells, dissemination to and infection of epidemiologically significant target organs and subsequent oral transmission or TOT) in *O. triseriatus* have been described. Detection of viral antigen in salivary glands, ovarian follicles and accessory sex glands provided anatomical explanations for oral, transovarial and venereal transmission of LAC virus. Multiple barriers to productive viral infect-

ion of vectors have been demonstrated: a mid-gut infection and dissemination barrier, and salivary gland infection and dissemination barriers. The G1 and G2 glycoproteins are the determinants of mid-gut infection.

California serogroup bunyaviruses and their vectors share an unprecedented host–parasite relationship. The viruses are very efficiently transovarially transmitted by their respective vectors. The discovery of LAC virus overwintering in diapaused eggs of *O. triseriatus* was a major advance in arbovirology. In laboratory studies, the viruses seem to exert no significant observable deleterious effect on the developing oocytes and embryos, even during critical periods of embryogenesis, follicular resting stages (ovarian diapause) and diapause.

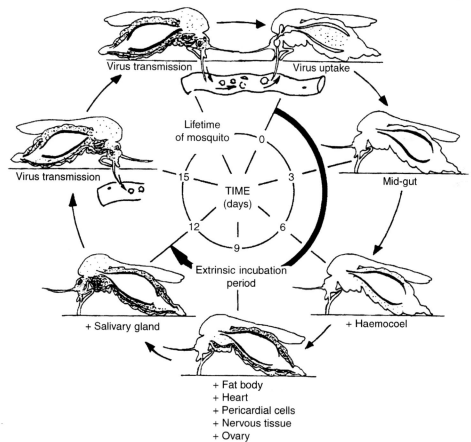

Fig. 1. The dissemination of La Crosse virus in *Ochlerotatus triseriatus* (modified from Beaty, B.J. and Marquardt, W.C. *The Biology of Disease Vectors.* University Press of Colorado, Niwot, 1996).

However, when transovarially infected embryos were compared with non-infected mosquitoes in their ability to successfully overwinter in a natural site, there was increased mortality in the infected mosquitoes. None the less, >50% of infected mosquitoes successfully overwintered.

Indeed, the virus may persist for several years in the eggs. Detection of LAC viral antigen in ovarian follicles has demonstrated that transmission is transovarial. Antigen detection and *in situ* hybridization in sections of ovaries from LAC virus transovarially infected *O. triseriatus* revealed LAC virus antigen and RNA in most ovarian tissues, including follicular epithelium, germaria, oocytes, nurse cells and calyx. The molecular basis of TOT has been elucidated; LAC and host transcription are coregulated. Thus, during diapause, LAC transcription is reduced, thereby enhancing successful overwintering of transovarially infected larvae.

Transovarial transmission of LAC virus is especially important, because this mode of transmission functions to maintain, amplify and overwinter CAL group viruses. Further, differential TOT rates could have major epidemiological consequences. Ovarian infection and transmission barriers could dramatically influence arbovirus cycle integrity, maintenance and transmission potential of bunyaviruses. These factors could also condition the vector host range and distribution of bunyaviruses. For example, geographical strains of *O. triseriatus* differ in their ability to transmit LAC virus transovarially; *O. triseriatus* from Connecticut transovarially transmits LAC virus less efficiently than that from Wisconsin, directly reflecting the distribution and endemicity of the virus.

Treatment

Treatment is typically symptomatic and follows general paediatric and critical-care measures. Recognition and appropriate treatment and management of seizures and intracranial pressure associated with cerebral oedema can be critical. Brain herniation can result from increased cranial pressure, which typically occurs soon after hospitalization. Ribavirin has been used to treat LAC virus infections. Administration of anticonvulsants for up to a year can decrease post-encephalitic epilepsy dramatically.

Control

There is no vaccine for LAC virus, which is unfortunate. A killed virus vaccine could easily be prepared and administered to children in areas of La Crosse endemicity. A killed virus vaccine could provide protection through puberty, thereby protecting children during the years when they are most susceptible to severe disease. Control is limited to prevention of mosquito bites, by encouraging children in endemic areas to wear long-sleeved shirts and long trousers, by the application of insect repellents and by discouraging playing in wooded areas, etc.

However, one of the unheralded successful control efforts of a vector-borne disease was the inititation of a vigorous source reduction campaign in La Crosse County, Wisconsin, after the natural cycle of the virus had been revealed. Removal of old tyres and other man-made breeding sites, implementation of laws mandating cleaning up of breeding sites, closure of tree holes and other breeding sites with cement, surveillance for *O. triseriatus* near premises experiencing infections and removal of the breeding sites, coupled with a vigorous public health education programme, virtually eliminated La Crosse encephalitis cases in the county. This occurred even in the face of increased population growth and movement of people into the forested area breeding sites of the vector.

Note

[1]   *Ochlerotatus* was formerly a subgenus of *Aedes*.

Selected bibliography

Beaty, B.J., Borucki, M., Farfan, J. and White, D. (1997) Arbovirus–vector interactions: determinants of arbovirus evolution In: Saluzzo, J.F. and Dodet, B. (eds) *Factors in the Emergence of Arbovirus Diseases*. Elsevier, London, pp. 23–35.

Borucki, M.K., Chandler, L.J., Parker, B., Blair, C.D. and Beaty, B.J. (1999) California group virus superinfection and segment reassortment in transovarially infected mosquitoes. *Journal of General Virology* 80, 3173–3179.

Chandler, L.J., Wasieloski, L.P., Blair, C.D. and Beaty, B.J. (1996) Analysis of La Crosse virus S segment RNA and its positive sense transcripts in persistently infected mosquito tissues. *Journal of Virology* 70, 8972–8976.

Dobie, D., Blair, C.D., Chandler, L., Rayms-Keller, A., Wasieloski, L.P. and Beaty, B.J. (1997) Analysis of La Crosse virus S mRNA 5' termini in infected *Aedes triseriatus* mosquitoes and mosquito cells. *Journal of Virology* 71, 4395–4399.

Gonzalez-Scarano, F. and Nathanson, N. (1996). *Bunyaviridae.* In: Fields, B.N., Knipe, D.M. and Howley, P.M. (eds) *Virology*, Vol. 1. Lippincott-Raven, Philadelphia, pp. 1473–1504.

Grimstad, P.R. (1988) California group viruses. In: Monath, T.P. (ed.) *The Arboviruses:*

Epidemiology and Control, Vol. II. CRC Press, Boca Raton, Florida, pp. 99–136.

McGaw, M., Chandler, L., Wasieloski, L., Blair, C. and Beaty, B. (1998) Effect of La Crosse Virus infection on overwintering of *Aedes triseriatus. American Journal of Tropical Medicine and Hygiene* 58, 168–175.

McJunkin, J.E., Khan, R.R. and Tsai, T.F. (1998) California–La Crosse encephalitis. *Infectious Disease Clinics of North America* 12, 83–93.

Rust, R.S., Thompson, W.H., Matthews, C.G., Beaty, B.J. and Chun, R.W. (1999) La Crosse and other forms of California encephalitis. *Journal of Child Neurololgy* 14, 1–14.

Woodring, J., Chandler, L., Oray, C., McGaw, M., Blair, C. and Beaty, B. (1998) Diapause and transovarial transmission rates in geographic strains of La Crosse virus infected mosquitoes. *American Journal of Tropical Medicine and Hygiene* 58, 587–588.

Langat virus

E.A. Gould

Langat (LGT) virus infects rodents, particularly ground rats (Müller's rat (*Rattus muelleri validus*) and the Noisy rat or Long-tailed rat (*Rattus sabanus vociferans*)). It is not known to cause overt disease in rodents in their natural environment, but young laboratory mice inoculated intracerebrally with the virus develop encephalitis and paralysis. Most of these infections result in death. The virus does not appear to infect mammalian species other than rodents in the wild; however, it is found in *Ixodes* and *Haemaphysalis* ticks in Malaysia. Under laboratory conditions, some other animal species are susceptible to infection and a proportion of human volunteers also developed encephalitis following experimental inoculation.

Distribution

The word Langat refers to the name of the forest in Malaysia where the prototype virus, TP21, was isolated from a pool of *Ixodes granulatus* collected from two species of Malaysian forest rats, *R. muelleri validus* (Müller's rat) and *R. sabanus vociferans* (Long-tailed or Noisy rat). As far

as is known, LGT virus occurs only in Malaysia and further north in neighbouring Thailand, where it was isolated from a pool of *Haemaphysalis papuana* collected from the underside of leaves on the edge of the forest in the Khao Yai National Park, approximately 150 km north-east of Bangkok. An unpublished report of its isolation in Siberia in 1974 has never been confirmed or repeated, and current scientific opinion, based on studies of the evolution and dispersal of the flaviviruses, does not support the view that LGT virus occurs naturally in Siberia. *Ixodes* species of ticks that feed on and thus transmit the virus to indigenous rodents survive in the moist undergrowth and rotting vegetation of the Malaysian forests. The ticks have a life cycle lasting 3–5 years. If during the first stage, i.e. the larval stage, they become infected by feeding on infected rodents, they may remain infected and capable of transmitting LGT virus to uninfected rodents throughout the nymphal and adult stages (trans-stadial transmission). A very low proportion of eggs may also become infected and pass the virus transovarially to the larval stage in the following cycle. It is now known that tick-borne flaviviruses, including LGT virus, may also be transmitted from infected to non-infected ticks when they co-feed on either susceptible or insusceptible animals. Thus LGT virus has evolved strategies for survival that ensure its perpetuation in the natural environment, even though the conditions may at times not favour efficient transmission.

Virus

The genus *Flavivirus* comprises approximately 70 recognized viruses, many of which are transmitted by mosquitoes rather than ticks, and some have no known arthropod vector. Langat is a tick-borne flavivirus, in the family Flaviviridae. It is both antigenically and genetically most closely related to a group of viruses collectively known as the tick-borne encephalitis (TBE) virus complex (see Tick-borne encephalitis). The virions have a diameter of approximately 50 nm and a spherical appearance under the electron microscope. The virions contain a positive-sense, single-stranded RNA genome, about 10.5 kb in length, which is inside a capsid (C) protein. This is enclosed by an outer lipid membrane, which supports dimers of envelope (E) glycoprotein, which are intimately associated with membrane protein (M). The viral RNA also encodes seven non-structural proteins, NS1, NS2a, NS2b, NS3, NS4a, NS4b, NS5, which encode the replicative functions of the virus, such as RNA translation, proteolytic processing of the translated polyprotein and RNA replication (for a representation of the genome strategy, see Fig. 2 of louping ill virus). Virus assembly and maturation take place in the cytoplasm of infected cells. There have been reports of virus-specific nuclear antigen in cells infected with several different flaviviruses, but these have not yet been satisfactorily explained.

Virus replication

Cells become infected when virions attach, via the envelope glycoprotein, to as yet unidentified cellular receptors. The attached virions are engulfed in endosomal vesicles, the relatively low pH of which causes a conformational change in the envelope protein, leading to its fusion with the endosomal membrane and releasing the viral RNA into the cytoplasm to initiate the translational and transcriptional processes. The positive-sense virion RNA acts as the messenger RNA (mRNA) and is translated as a polyprotein, which is either concurrently or subsequently proteolytically cleaved by virus-encoded and/or host cell proteases. The helicase (NS3) and the RNA-dependent RNA polymerase (NS5) form a replication complex with transcribed RNA and the cycle is repeated to accumulate structural proteins and progeny RNA, which are assembled into virions prior to release from the cell. Maturation of the virions occurs in association with the membranes of the endoplasmic reticulum. The pre-membrane (PrM) protein becomes intimately associated with envelope protein, which, in this form, remains inert to the relatively low pH at the endosomal membranes. As the maturing virus particles are released from the cell, the PrM protein is cleaved to M protein, resulting in development of the mature conformational form of the E protein on the surface of the virion.

Clinical symptoms

There is no evidence that LGT virus has infected humans in the natural environment. This is probably because either: (i) humans are rarely exposed to the virus via the bite of an infected tick, or (ii) infected humans develop only mild or subclinical infections and therefore do not report to hospital for examination. Several published papers state that LGT virus, prototype strain TP21, is naturally attenuated for humans; however, it can cause disease in experimentally inoculated humans. Several infected volunteers with leukaemia developed fever, leucopenia and encephalitis, but reports in Russia of trials with LGT virus as a vaccine showed that the virus induced protection against an encephalitic tick-borne virus in

88% of the volunteers, with no untoward reactions. Virulence comparisons, in monkeys or mice, of LGT virus with European and Far East Asian strains of TBE complex viruses have shown LGT virus to be the least neurovirulent and the least neuroinvasive virus.

Pathogenesis

Histopathological lesions in mice experimentally inoculated with LGT virus included perivascular cuffing and neuronal damage in the cerebrum and anterior horns of the thoracic and cervical cord.

Diagnosis

In theory it is difficult to differentiate serologically between antibodies produced in response to infection with LGT virus and those raised against other TBE complex viruses, because they are all genetically closely related. However, the presence of antibody to LGT virus in humans or rodents would be a reliable indicator of infection by this virus, since the other TBE complex viruses are not found in Malaysia or Thailand. Infection by LGT virus can be confirmed by virus isolation, either following intracerebral infection of newborn mice or infection of susceptible tissue culture cells. Since there are no unique monoclonal antibodies for identification of LGT virus by immunofluorescence microscopy, absolute identification requires nucleotide sequencing. Presumptive confirmation of infection can be obtained in a seroconversion assay either by neutralization of infectivity, complement fixation, haemagglutination inhibition or an enzyme-linked immunosorbent assay (ELISA), using acute and convalescent sera.

Transmission

Langat virus was isolated from the hard tick *Ixodes granulatus* in Ulu Langat Forest Reserve, Malaysia, and from *Haemaphysalis papuana* in central Thailand. Analysis of *I. granulatus* obtained from other areas of Malaysia failed to reveal LGT virus, suggesting that the virus is not particularly widespread throughout the entire region of Malaysia. However, this could simply reflect the limited number of ticks analysed, because various species of ground rats throughout Malaysia have been found to have antibody against LGT virus, albeit at a low frequency. The virus has also been shown experimentally to be transmissible by *Ixodes ricinus*, *Dermacentor marginatus* and *Haemaphysalis spinigera*.

Langat virus transmission to ticks is believed to occur when a viraemic rodent is fed upon by an appropriate non-infected tick. If, for example, the infected tick is a larva, it then drops off the rodent, retires to the moist undergrowth and, after a suitable interval, depending on temperature, humidity and time of season, moults to the next stage in its life cycle, i.e. the nymphal stage. The virus survives this trans-stadial process and may subsequently be transmitted to a non-infected rodent when the nymphal tick takes a blood meal. The moulting process is repeated to produce an infected adult, which subsequently takes a blood meal and lays its eggs. The entire life cycle can take between 2 and 5 years, depending upon the environmental conditions. While it is not known how long LGT virus can survive in infected rodents, there is good evidence that other TBE complex viruses can produce persistent infections in the Bank vole (*Clethrionomys glareolus*), the Wood mouse (*Apodemus sylvaticus*) and the Yellow-necked mouse (*Apodemus flavicollis*). However, as yet, there is no evidence that such persistently infected animals can transmit the virus to ticks during feeding.

Transmission of LGT virus in rodents between infected and non-infected co-feeding ticks has been shown to take place experimentally in the laboratory at a low frequency. In fact, this mode of transmission may be the main mechanism by which the virus survives and perpetuates, because Malaysian ground rats do not appear to develop high-titre viraemias when infected by LGT virus. Because most flaviviruses seem to be capable of causing infection in mammalian hosts by the oral route, transmission by oral infection – for example, when rodents eat infected ticks – is a third possible mechanism, although it is likely to be a very infrequent event.

Epidemiology

Langat virus has never been reported as a natural infection of humans, probably because: (i) the virus does not produce severe clinical symptoms in naturally infected humans; and (ii) very few humans are exposed to LGT virus because only a low proportion (probably less than 1%) of ticks are infected. There have been few studies on LGT virus in the forests of Malaysia but the evidence suggests that rodents do not develop significant clinical signs when exposed to the virus. It is therefore presumed that LGT virus persists in a relatively silent form in its natural environment.

Susceptibility of other animal species

Most flaviviruses will infect a wide variety of laboratory animals, such as monkeys, mice, rats, hamsters and some bird species, often causing encephalitis. In addition, humans inoculated with LGT virus show clinical evidence of infection. *Ixodes* species have quite catholic preferences and are therefore likely to feed on a wide range of animal species in the Malaysian jungles. Nevertheless, there is no serological evidence that wild animals other than rodents are exposed to or are susceptible to infection by LGT virus.

Treatment

Because LGT virus does not appear to be a problem for humans in Malaysian forests, no specific treatment has been developed. However, in laboratory mouse experiments, passive antibody administration increased LGT virus prevalence. It was suggested that this enhancement of virus titre resulted from immunosuppression of the host following exposure to high-titre antibody. Moreover, in some parts of Europe, people known to have been bitten by ticks in regions where TBE is prevalent were offered immune human immunoglobulin as a prophylactic measure against the disease. However, suggestive evidence that these measures might cause disease enhancement rather than amelioration led to the recommendation by the World Health Organization (WHO) that this practice should no longer be continued. It is thought that the injected immunoglobulin may cause virus–antibody complexes, resulting in pathology when such complexes occur on the surface of infected central nervous system cells.

Control

Humans are only likely to be at risk from infection by LGT virus if they become exposed to infected ticks by walking through or resting in areas of the forests where the undergrowth provides ideal conditions for tick survival. For hikers or forest workers, the use of protective clothing, such as boots and thick socks, and the application of tick repellents or acaricides to exposed areas or clothing should reduce the risk of infection.

Selected bibliography

Bancroft, W.H., Scott, R.M., Snitbhan, R., Weaver, R.E. and Gould, D.J. (1976) Isolation of Langat virus from *Haemaphysalis papuana* Thorell in Thailand. *American Journal of Tropical Medicine and Hygiene* 25, 500–504.

Begum, F. (1969) Differentiation of strains of reduced pathogenicity suitable for vaccines. *American Journal of Tropical Medicine and Hygiene* 18, 1034–1041.

Webb, H.E., Wetherley-Mein, G., Smith, C.E. and McMahon, D. (1966) Leukaemia and neoplastic processes treated with Langat and Kyasanur Forest disease viruses: a clinical and laboratory study of 28 patients. *British Medical Journal* 1, 258–266.

Latrine-fly *see* **Flies.**

Leishmaniasis

R.W. Ashford

Definition

Disease in humans or other animals caused by infection with protozoan parasites of the genus *Leishmania*. The 20 or so species of *Leishmania* which infect humans and domesticated animals cause numerous distinct diseases, collectively known as the leishmaniases.

Leishmaniasis, human

The main clinical varieties of leishmaniasis caused by *Leishmania* in humans are as follows:

- Cutaneous leishmaniasis (CL) or oriental sore, which may be anthroponotic, caused by *L. tropica* (in Asia) or *L. peruviana*, or zoonotic, caused by *L. tropica* (in Africa), *L. major*, *L. aethiopica*, *L. mexicana*, *L. amazonensis*, *L. panamensis*, *L. guyanensis* or *L. braziliensis*.
- Visceral leishmaniasis or kala azar, which may be infantile, caused by *L. donovani infantum*, or have little age specificity, caused by *L. donovani donovani*. *Leishmania d. infantum* affects people of all ages who are suffering from immunosuppressive disease.
- Mucocutaneous leishmaniasis or espundia, usually caused by *L. braziliensis*, following cure of the initial oriental sore.
- Post-kala azar dermal leishmaniasis (PKDL), caused by *L. d. donovani* following cure of the initial visceral leishmaniasis.
- Diffuse cutaneous leishmaniasis (DCL), caused by *L. aethiopica* or *L. amazonensis*.

Numerous other species of *Leishmania* have been described, mostly from Central or South America, rarely infecting humans or domesticated animals and usually responsible for simple cases of cutaneous leishmaniasis.

Distribution

The leishmaniases occur in more than 100 countries, from warm temperate through subtropical to tropical climates. South-East Asia and Australasia are the only large areas with suitable climates where the diseases are absent. Visceral leishmaniasis is concentrated in eastern Africa, particularly Sudan and Kenya, and, on the Indian subcontinent, in Bangladesh, north-east India and Nepal. Post-kala azar dermal leishmaniasis has a similar distribution, though the proportion of treated kala azar cases that develop this condition varies. Infantile visceral leishmaniasis is characteristically circum-Mediterranean in its distribution, extending east through south-west Asia to China, and west to Central and South America, where most cases occur in north-east Brazil. This last form is increasingly rare in its classical infantile form, but has expanded to infect adults who are infected with the human immunodeficiency virus (HIV) or who are otherwise immunocompromised.

Both anthroponotic and zoonotic CL, in the Old World, are mostly found in arid or semi-arid areas. The former occurs, usually as epidemics, in the densely populated cities of central and west Asia, from Aleppo in Syria to Kabul in Afghanistan, while the zoonotic form is characteristic of semi-desert rural areas, in both Asia and North Africa, where colonies of the reservoir hosts are found.

Cutaneous leishmaniasis due to *L. mexicana*, *L. amazonensis* or *L. braziliensis* is widely distributed in South and Central America. The precise distribution is focal and depends mainly on the presence of suitable vectors and reservoir hosts. *Leishmania braziliensis* has recently expanded to peri-urban foci, where it appears to be dependent on domesticated dogs and possibly equines.

Each of the other forms of leishmaniasis, such as CL due to *L. aethiopica* in the highlands of Ethiopia or due to *L. peruviana* in the western Andes, has a focal distribution, depending on the presence of reservoir hosts and/or vectors in sufficient number and proximity to humans.

The dependence of all forms of leishmaniasis on a limited choice of sand-fly vectors and of most forms on wild or domesticated reservoir hosts leads to a strong correlation between leishmaniasis and environmental features, notably climatic and vegetation zones. Only where populations of vectors and reservoir hosts coincide can the parasite survive.

Parasite

Parasites of all species of *Leishmania* are morphologically similar and, while presumptive identification may be made on circumstantial grounds, biochemical analysis is required for formal identification at species level. All species inhabit the reticuloendothelial cells of a vertebrate host and the gut of a phlebotomine sand-fly. There are two main stages in the life history: the amastigote and promastigote. Amastigotes are intracellular, rounded, some 5 μm in diameter, containing a single nucleus, a kinetoplast and a flagellar pocket with the rudiments of a flagellum. Amastigotes are the form found in the monocytes and macrophages of the vertebrate host. They divide repeatedly and spread to new cells when the initial host cell bursts.

In the sand-fly host the amastigotes in the blood meal transform to promastigotes. These are longer, with a central nucleus and anterior kinetoplast and with a well-developed flagellum, which is used either for propulsion or for attachment. Both amastigotes and promastigotes divide repeatedly by longitudinal binary fission.

Promastigotes may be cultured in various media, mostly containing defibrinated blood and inactivated serum. Amastigotes can be cultured in appropriate cell cultures. Identification requires analysis of electrophoretic migration patterns of isoenzymes, though confirmation of presumptive identification can sometimes rely on monoclonal antibody or DNA probes, the latter with or without polymerase chain reaction (PCR) amplification. Neither DNA nor monoclonal probes have yet attained sufficient reliability to replace isoenzyme analysis.

Clinical symptoms and signs

Oriental sore or cutaneous leishmaniasis first appears as a persistent insect bite. Gradually the lesion enlarges, remaining red, but without noticeable heat or pain (Fig. 1). Resolution of the lesion involves immigration of leucocytes, which isolate the infected area, leading to necrosis of the infected tissues and the formation of a healing granuloma in the floor of the lesion. The necrotic process may be rapid, causing a

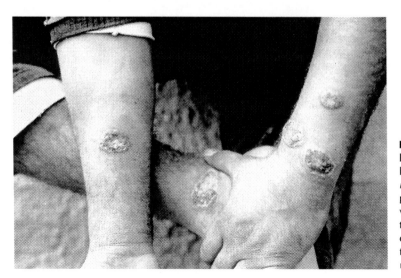

Fig. 1. Cutaneous leishmaniasis: the lesions of *Leishmania major* infection are painless, but are very unsightly for the 3 months of their duration. Infection is followed by immunity to reinfection.

large open wet ulcer (especially *L. major* and *L. braziliensis*), or may be more indolent, without frank ulceration (*L. tropica, L. aethiopica, L. peruviana*). Natural cure without treatment is the rule, but the time taken varies greatly according to the identity of the parasite and the site of the lesion. Similarly, the size of the lesion may vary between millimetres and centimetres in diameter. It is not unusual, especially with *L. major* infection, for numerous lesions to occur simultaneously, causing great disfigurement and distress. Oriental sore is not usually associated with systemic signs or symptoms, but draining lymph nodes may become enlarged and lesions may spread along lymphatic ducts (*L. guyanensis*).

Oriental sore caused by *L. tropica* or *L. major* is not usually associated with detectable serological response. A skin-test response develops prior to final cure and remains for many years. Cured patients remain immune to the homologous infection for many years.

Kala azar or visceral leishmaniasis is sometimes preceded by a dry or ulcerating lesion at the site of the infective bite. Systemic signs of intermittent medium-grade pyrexia, anaemia, splenomegaly, hepatomegaly and progressive cachexia develop at variable rates, between weeks and years following infection (Fig. 2). Less constant signs include lymphadenopathy and persistent diarrhoea. The outcome of fully developed visceral leishmaniasis is death, usually due to concomitant infection resulting from the weakened state of the subject. There is, however, increasing evidence that many people who become infected never develop full-blown disease and they recover spontaneously. The proportion of these subclinical cases varies from almost 100% with *L. d. infantum* infection in otherwise healthy adults to less than 25% during epidemics of kala azar in Africa. However, this resistance to infection is eliminated by the HIV virus, and *L. d. infantum* infection in acquired immune deficiency syndrome (AIDS) victims may present in many and bizarre ways.

Although full-blown kala azar is usually fatal, it is associated with a very strong

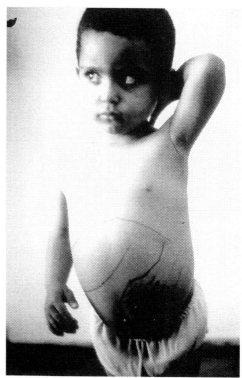

Fig. 2. Infantile visceral leishmaniasis. The outlines of the enlarged liver and spleen are marked on this Libyan child's abdomen. Although the child does not feel very sick, the outcome of *Leishmania donovani infantum* infection is almost invariably fatal without long and expensive treatment.

serological response, to the extent that the albumin/globulin ratio is reversed. The raised serum proteins are used diagnostically in a non-specific formol-gel test. Cured cases develop a positive skin-test reaction, which is frequently used for retrospective epidemiological study, though there is evidence that this may be lost in a few years. In endemic areas or during epidemics, many apparently healthy people may develop positive serology and, subsequently, skin-test reactions. This is the best evidence for the subclinical cases mentioned above.

Mucocutaneous leishmaniasis is occasionally reported from Sudan and other Old World foci. Here, it seems that the lesion commences at the site of a bite on or close to a mucosal surface. Occasional infections with *L. d. infantum* are reported from the tonsils or buccal mucosa. It is tempting to suppose that these originate from accidentally inhaled sand-flies.

Classical mucocutaneous leishmaniasis, or espundia, is, however, restricted to *L. braziliensis* infections, in which, following the apparently complete resolution of the initial oriental sore, sometimes many years later, metastatic lesions appear on the buccal or nasal mucosa. The mucosa and associated cartilage are gradually eroded until much of the face may be destroyed (Fig. 3). The initial symptom is mild irritation of the tip of the nose or other affected surface. Parasites are difficult to find in these lesions, but a history of cutaneous leishmaniasis, supported by positive serology or skin test, is an important sign.

Post-kala azar dermal leishmaniasis is normally a sequel to kala azar that has been

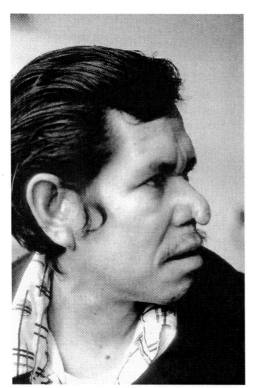

Fig. 3. Mucocutaneous leishmaniasis is caused by a relapse of infection with *Leishmania braziliensis*. The mucosa and associated cartilage are gradually destroyed, giving rise, in this Peruvian case, to the characteristic appearance of 'tapir nose'.

cured by treatment. Occasional cases of PKDL are reported with no history of kala azar. It usually appears within 2 years of the complete cure of the visceral infection, and commences with the appearance of mottling of the skin, like freckles.

Diffuse cutaneous leishmaniasis is restricted to Venezuela and the Dominican Republic and to Ethiopia and Kenya. It is usually a manifestation of infection with parasites that normally cause simple cutaneous leishmaniasis, associated with a specific anergy or immunological lack of response. The lesions may be restricted, perhaps to the border of an ear, or may be widespread all over the body. They are raised macules or patches of thin skin, which, although painless, are grossly disfiguring. The initial Ethiopian cases described were at first misdiagnosed as suffering from lepromatous leprosy. Characteristically, parasites are very numerous in the lesions.

Diagnosis

In places where they are well known and endemic, or during epidemics, all three main forms of leishmaniasis – cutaneous, mucocutaneous and visceral – can be diagnosed with some reliability by clinical examination, backed, in visceral leishmaniasis, by a blood count showing anaemia and leucocytopenia. Confirmation of the diagnosis of any of the leishmaniases generally depends on the demonstration of the amastigote parasites in infected tissue. Specimens examined are usually skin biopsies or aspirates from bone marrow or spleen. The collection of specimens requires careful preparation and training. The parasites may be demonstrated in stained microscopical preparations or in culture.

Transmission

All forms of leishmaniasis are transmitted by phlebotomine sand-flies (see entry). The amastigote parasites are ingested with a blood meal, and proceed to divide in the sand-fly gut. Very soon they transform to promastigotes, which continue to multiply rapidly. Some 3 days following a feed, the sand-fly defecates the remnants of the blood meal. At this stage, any unattached parasites are voided. The parasites which are to survive attach themselves by their flagellae either to the microvilli of the mid-gut or to the cuticular surface of the anterior part of the hind-gut, the hind-gut triangle or the pyloric valve. In either case, following defecation, the parasites detach themselves from the gut wall and again divide repeatedly, eventually attaching themselves to the chitinous piece of fore-gut that extends into the mid-gut, the cardiac valve. At this stage, some parasites become differentiated as 'metacyclic' forms, which are unattached and fast-swimming, with a small body and long flagellum. Transmission depends on the injection of these metacyclic forms when the sand-fly next takes a blood meal.

In addition to blood, sand-flies feed on honeydew, which they lap from leaf surfaces, and on sap, for which they probe leaves or petioles. The precise nature of this sugar meal may determine whether or not parasites survive in the fly.

It is generally thought that sand-flies remain infected for life, but there is evidence that infected flies have difficulty feeding, and their lifespan is reduced. A subsequent feed on bird blood may 'cure' an infected fly.

Transmission can readily be achieved by inoculation of infected material from one person to another. It was common practice in south-west Asia to deliberately infect young girls with material from an oriental sore, so that their lesion would be in an inconspicuous place, and they would subsequently be immune. More recently there is evidence that much of the visceral leishmaniasis associated with HIV infection in southern Europe is transmitted by sharing of contaminated needles and syringes for the misuse of drugs.

The reported transmission both by venereal contact and by blood transfusion is of little, if any, general significance.

The various combinations of vector and reservoir host which maintain the various *Leishmania* species in different habitats and geographical areas allow the stratification of the leishmaniases into 'nosodemiological units', a simplified version of which is given in Table 1.

Treatment

Treatment of any of the leishmaniases is slow and expensive. The first-line drugs are compounds containing pentavalent antimony, such as sodium antimony gluconate. These are delivered over a period of 20 days or more, either by intravenous injection (for visceral leishmaniasis or severe CL) or by injection into the periphery of single lesions. Second-line treatment, when antimony is ineffective or contraindicated, uses amphotericin B, allopurinol, pentamidine or paromomycin (monomycin) in diverse combinations and formulations. Recommended dosages are not given here, as they are subject to frequent change and to local variation.

Cheap, effective, short, preferably oral treatment for visceral leishmaniasis and topical treatment for CL are urgent requirements.

Control

There has rarely been any systematic attempt to control transmission of leishmaniasis and even more rarely any effective evaluation. The minimal control measures recommended by the World Health Organization (WHO) for all forms of leishmaniasis are the establishment of efficient passive case detection and treatment, where indicated, accompanied by an efficient reporting and recording system. Active case detection is indicated in areas with poor health services or during spreading epidemics.

As far as is known, all vector species are susceptible to commonly used insecticides, including DDT. Residual insecticides sprayed on internal surfaces of houses and outhouses are highly effective for controlling synanthropic sand-flies, such as *Phlebotomus argentipes*, *Phlebotomus sergenti* and certain populations of *Phlebotomus papatasi* and *Lutzomyia longipalpis*. Control of sylvatic species is much more difficult, and usually impractical. Occasionally reduction of reservoir host populations is effective in reducing human infection but, more frequently, the best recommendation is to site barracks or camps appropriately and to use personal

Table 1. Stratification of the leishmaniases of humans and domesticated animals into 'nosodemiological units'. Mammal names according to Corbet and Hill (1980).

Leishmania species	Disease spectrum in humans	Geographical distribution	Vector	Reservoir host	Other mammal hosts	Habitat
L. tropica	Oriental sore ('dry form'), leishmaniasis recidivans	Central to south-west Asia	Phlebotomus sergenti	Humans only	Dog (cutaneous leishmaniasis)	Densely populated cities
		Equatorial and southern Africa, Kenya and Namibia	Phlebotomus guggisbergi and others	Probably rock hyrax (Procavia capensis)		Rocky areas in arid to semi-arid places
L. major	Oriental sore ('wet form')	North Africa and south-west Asia, from Algeria to Saudi Arabia	Phlebotomus papatasi	Fat sand-rat (Psammomys obesus)	Gerbils (Meriones shawi, Meriones libycus, Meriones crassus), Bandicoot rat (Nesokia indica)	Saline depressions with Chenopodiaceae
		Central Asia from Iran to Uzbekistan	Phlebotomus papatasi	Great gerbil (Rhombomys opimus)	Numerous desert mammals	Alluvial fans with loess deposits
		West Africa to Kenya, Sahel belt	Phlebotomus duboscqi	Relative importance of different hosts to be determined	Rodents (Arvicanthis spp., Praomys spp., Tatera robusta, Aethomys kaiseri, Taterillus emini), Squirrel (Xerus rutilus), Vervet monkey (Cercopithecus aethiops)	Sahel savannah
L. aethiopica	Chronic oriental sore; diffuse cutaneous leishmaniasis	Highlands of Ethiopia and Kenya	Phlebotomus longipes and Phlebotomus pedifer	Rock hyraxes, Procavia capensis and Heterohyrax brucei	Giant rat (Cricetomys gambianus)	Cliffs and rocky areas, between 1500 and 2600 m altitude
		Highlands of south-west Ethiopia	Phlebotomus pedifer	Heterohyrax brucei		Relict forest with giant fig (Ficus vasta) trees, around 2000 m altitude
L. donovani donovani	Kala azar (visceral leishmaniasis); post-kala azar dermal leishmaniasis	Eastern and southern Sudan, western Ethiopia	Phlebotomus orientalis	Presumably zoonotic but reservoir host uncertain	Rodents (Acomys cahirinus, Rattus rattus, Arvicanthis niloticus, Praomys natalensis), Serval cat (Felis serval), Genet (Genetta genetta)	Alluvial flat lands with woodland of Acacia seyal and Balanites aegyptiaca
		Northern Kenya, south-western Ethiopia	Phlebotomus martini			Semi-arid bush with termitaria
		North-east India, Bangladesh, Terai region of Nepal	Phlebotomus argentipes	Humans only		Villages on alluvial plains

Species	Disease	Distribution	Vector	Reservoir host	Other hosts	Habitat
L. donovani infantum (syn. *L. chagasi*)	Infantile visceral leishmaniasis; cutaneous leishmaniasis; AIDS-associated leishmaniasis	Southern France, Cevennes hills	*Phlebotomus ariasi*	Dog (viscerocutaneous leishmaniasis)	Fox (*Vulpes vulpes*)	Forested areas at middle altitude
		Central and western Mediterranean basin, both Europe and North Africa	*Phlebotomus perniciosus*		Fox, Black rat (*Rattus rattus*)	Villages and suburbs, with calcareous outcrops, in subhumid bioclimatic zone
		Through Mediterranean basin to Iran	Various		Racoon dog (*Nyctereutes procyonides*) (China), foxes (*Vulpes* spp.), jackals, *Canis* spp.	Various
		Central and South America	*Lutzomyia longipalpis*, *Lutzomyia evansi*		Fox (*Dusicyon thous*) (records from *Dusicyon vetulus* probably represent misidentification of the fox)	Villages and homesteads in semi-arid areas
L. mexicana	Cutaneous leishmaniasis; chiclero ulcer	Central America	*Lutzomyia olmeca*	Climbing rat (*Ototylomys phyllotis*)	Rodents (*Heteromys desmarestianus*, *Nyctomys sumichrasti*, *Sigmodon hispidus*)	Lowland secondary forest
	Cutaneous leishmaniasis	Texas	*Lutzomyia anthophora*	Wood rat (*Neotoma micropus*)		Semi-arid open brush with *Opuntia*
L. amazonensis (syn. *L. garnhami*, *L. pifanoi*)	Cutaneous leishmaniasis; diffuse cutaneous leishmaniasis	South America	*Lutzomyia flaviscutellata*	Spiny rats (*Proechimys guyanesis*, *Proechimys cuvieri*)	Opossums (*Didelphis marsupialis*, *Metachirops opossum*, *Metachirus nudicaudatus*, *Marmosa cinerea*), Anteater (*Tamandua tetradactyla*), Rice rat (*Oryzomys capito*), Squirrel (*Sciurus vulgaris*), Kinkajou (*Potos flavus*), Fox (*Dusicyon thous*)	Dry forest
L. venezuelensis	Cutaneous leishmaniasis	Towns in Lara State, Venezuela	Uncertain	Uncertain	Domestic cat and equines	Peri-urban forest
Leishmania sp.	Diffuse cutaneous leishmaniasis	Dominican Republic	Uncertain	Presumably zoonotic, but reservoir host unknown		Not specified
L. braziliensis	Cutaneous leishmaniasis; mucocutaneous leishmaniasis	Central and South America from 19°N to 29°S	*Lutzomyia wellcomei*, etc.	Presumably zoonotic, but reservoir host unknown	Numerous forest animals	Primary forest
		South America	*Lutzomyia whitmani*	Dog?	Horse (*Equus caballus*), Donkey (*Equus asinus*)	Expanding in heavily populated suburbs

Continued

Table 1. *Continued.*

Leishmania species	Disease spectrum in humans	Geographical distribution	Vector	Reservoir host	Other mammal hosts	Habitat
L. peruviana	Cutaneous leishmaniasis	Peruvian Andes	*Lutzomyia verrucarum, Lutzomyia peruensis, Lutzomyia ayacuchensis*	Man and dog are thought to play an equal role		Western Andean valleys at 800 to 3000 m altitude
L. guyanensis	Cutaneous leishmaniasis with lymphatic spread: 'pian bois'	Guyanas, Brazil N. of the Amazon	*Lutzomyia umbratilis, Lutzomyia anduzei*	Sloth (*Choloepus didactylus*), Opossum (*Didelphis marsupialis*) in suburbs	Opossum (*Didelphis marsupialis*), Anteater (*Tamandua tetradactyla*), Spiny rat (*Proechimys* sp.)	Primary forest
L. panamensis	Cutaneous leishmaniasis	Central America	*Lutzomyia trapidoi, Lutzomyia ylephiletor, Lutzomyia gomezi, Lutzomyia panamensis*	Sloth (*Choloepus hoffmanni*)	Opossums (*Didelphis marsupialis, Metachirus nudicaudatus*), Sloth (*Bradypus variegatus*), rodents (*Akodon* sp., *Rattus rattus, Proechimys semispinosus, Heteromys desmarestianus*), Tree porcupine (*Coendou* sp.), dog	Primary forest
L. shawi	Cutaneous leishmaniasis	Para and Acre States, Brazil	*Lutzomyia whitmani*		Sloths (*Choloepus didactylus, Bradypus griseus*), monkeys (*Cebus apella, Chiropotes satanus*), Coati (*Nasua nasua*)	To be specified
L. lainsoni	Cutaneous leishmaniasis	Northern Para State, Brazil	*Lutzomyia ubiquitalis*		Paca (*Cuniculus paca*)	Forest, near water
L. naiffi	Cutaneous leishmaniasis	Para and Amazonas States, Brazil	*Lutzomyia ayrozai, Lutzomyia paraensis*	Armadillo (*Dasypus novemcinctus*)		To be specified

protection against sand-fly bites whenever necessary.

Although cutaneous leishmaniasis is usually self-curing and not life-threatening, individual cases may be psychologically and socially damaging, and epidemics may be seen as a major, if localized, public health priority. Attempts to control urban, anthroponotic CL have used house-spraying with residual insecticides. While this should be effective and was effective in Soviet Azerbaijan in the 1950s, more recent efforts have been inadequately thorough and have failed.

Zoonotic CL was controlled in Soviet Central Asia by aerial survey, followed by ground survey, to identify rodent colonies, which were then eliminated by deep ploughing or by poisoning. Attempts to do the same in Arabia and North Africa, where there is a different reservoir host, have given ambivalent results. In South American foci, control is even more difficult. Clearance of forest surrounding new settlements has been effective but, contrary to earlier expectations, forest clearance has sometimes led to peri-domestic transmission rather than to the elimination of the infections.

In the Indian region, visceral leishmaniasis should be controllable by house-spraying, as the vector is strictly synanthropic. Indeed, it is claimed that the disease almost disappeared during the 1960s as an incidental result of malaria control measures. Visceral leishmaniasis in Africa, on the other hand, is much more difficult to control as the vectors are sylvatic and the disease occurs in irregular epidemics in impoverished peripheral communities. The best that can be done in these circumstances is to ensure the availability of diagnosis and cure with, perhaps, the provision of fine-mesh bed-nets for individual protection, preferably impregnated with a pyrethroid insecticide.

What was probably *L. d. infantum* infection was effectively eliminated in China in the 1950s by the almost complete elimination of dogs. This has not been attempted elsewhere, and the detection and elimination of infected dogs has failed to reduce transmission in Brazil.

There are no effective vaccines for leishmaniasis, despite considerable effort. Trials have been conducted on vaccines against *L. major* infection in Iran with equivocal results, and a product has been tested for protection against *L. braziliensis* infection in Brazil. Deliberate infection, or leishmanization, is mentioned above. This procedure was carried out on millions of Iranian military recruits, but was abandoned by certain other armies when a small proportion of subjects developed unsightly, spreading, intractable lesions.

Leishmaniasis, animal

The dog is the domesticated animal most affected by leishmaniasis. In some parts of southern Europe, it is difficult to maintain dogs due to the intensity of transmission and the expense of treatment. Equines are affected in localized areas of South and Central America, and there are various reports from cats. Isolated reports of leishmaniasis in sheep and goats (Kenya), cattle (Zimbabwe) and buffaloes (India) are unconfirmed by replication and are of unknown significance.

Dogs may be infected with several *Leishmania* species causing cutaneous disease, but the most important canine leishmaniasis is that caused by *L. d. infantum*, canine viscerocutaneous leishmaniasis (CanL).

Canine viscerocutaneous leishmaniasis (CanL)
Distribution

Canine viscerocutaneous leishmaniasis is mainly found in the Mediterranean basin, extending eastwards into central Asia. Its distribution is focalized within this range, with particular concentrations in southern Spain, southern France, western and southern Italy and certain Greek islands. The infection is also widespread in South and Central America, where it must have been imported from Europe. The detailed distribution of the infection must be determined by that of each of the several sand-fly vectors, which, in turn, are each associated with specific bioclimatic and vegetation zones.

Parasite

The parasite causing CanL is the same as that causing human infantile visceral leishmaniasis, *L. d. infantum*. The parasite in South America is identical; some authors insist on using the specific name *chagasi* for the New World parasite, but this is a junior synonym of *infantum*, and its use has no justification. Variants of this parasite have differential pathogenic potential in humans, but the spectrum of canine disease appears to be unrelated to parasite strain. The infectious process in the dog is such that the dog is an excellent source of parasites for transmission. This contrasts with humans, in whom parasites can rarely be found in the blood or skin. The dog is clearly the main vertebrate host in the ecological reservoir of infection, and so is the main reservoir host.

Clinical symptoms

Canine viscerocutaneous leishmaniasis affects dogs of all breeds, though it is more frequent in those which are selected for rural pursuits. The initial sign of infection may or not be a small ulcerating lesion at the site of the infective bite, usually on the muzzle or the ear. Alternatively, the first sign may be serological positivity. This is followed by a progressive disease, with swelling of the lymph nodes, intermittent pyrexia, wasting, depilation, which commences around the eyes, giving a spectacled appearance, and overgrowth of the claws. In the last stages, the animal presents a sorry sight of wasting and depilation, but none of the signs is diagnostic. The disease may resolve at any stage, but late resolution is exceptional. Even with treatment, complete resolution of advanced cases is unusual. Many animals apparently become infected and even infectious without showing any sign of disease.

Diagnosis

The signs and symptoms are reasonably pathognomonic when they all occur together in an otherwise healthy endemic area. However, many presentations are atypical, and demonstration of the parasite is desirable before embarking on a long and expensive course of treatment. Confirmation depends on the demonstration of parasites in aspirates, usually from bone marrow or lymph nodes; they may be seen in stained microscopic preparations or in culture medium. Asymptomatic dogs are frequently found by active case detection. These cases can only be diagnosed prospectively, usually by serology, followed by confirmatory parasitology.

Several serodiagnostic tests are routinely performed at specialized laboratories. It is preferable to duplicate the tests, as the results obtained by different methods are not always in agreement.

Transmission

As with human leishmaniasis, transmission is normally by the bite of a phlebotomine sand-fly. It may be that alternative methods occur exceptionally, as indicated by the rare infection of dogs in sand-fly-free areas. In many parts of southern Europe, the transmission rate is so high that it is difficult to keep dogs.

Treatment

This involves the use of the same antimony compounds as for humans, but is less effective and usually requires to be repeated annually. Good nutrition and lack of stress are important factors in maintaining the health of infected dogs.

Control

Control of transmission has two potential purposes: to reduce the likelihood of human disease and to protect the dogs themselves. The human disease is usually very rare and is closely dependent on age and nutritional state; improved lifestyles in southern Europe since the 1950s have almost eliminated the infantile disease. It is normally preferable, and even more economical, to alleviate human deprivation and to identify and treat patients than to control transmission. The most important action in the protection of people from this canine zoonosis is to ensure that all human infections can be correctly and rapidly diagnosed and treated. This is a far from trivial undertaking even in endemic areas and, in exotic areas, correct initial diagnosis is the exception rather than the rule.

In areas of high transmission, protection of individual dogs is very difficult, and protection of the dog population is out of the question. Elimination of sick dogs is ineffective, as many dogs are infectious before they show symptoms, and valuable working dogs or pets will be withheld.

The relaxation of quarantine restrictions on animals entering the UK is likely to lead to increasing numbers of dogs visiting endemic areas in southern Europe. Increased awareness among veterinary practitioners in UK is actively being promoted in advance of this problem.

Selected bibliography

Ashford, R.W. (1996) Leishmaniasis reservoirs and their significance in control. *Clinics in Dermatology* 14, 523–532.

Chang, K.P. and Bray, R.S. (eds) (1985) *Human Parasitic Diseases*, Vol. 1, *Leishmaniasis*. Elsevier, Amsterdam, 490 pp.

Corbet, G.B. and Hill, J.E. (1980) *A World List of Mammalian Species*. British Museum (Natural History), London, 226 pp.

Dedet, J.-P. (ed.) (1999) *Les Leishmanioses*. Ellipses, Paris, 253 pp.

Dowlati, Y. and Modabber, F. (eds) (1996) Cutaneous leishmaniasis. *Clinics in Dermatology* 14, 417–546.

Hart, D.T. (ed.) (1987) *Leishmaniasis. The Current Status and New Strategies for Control.* NATO ASI Series A, Life Sciences, Vol. 163. Plenum Press, New York, 1041 pp.

Killick-Kendrick, R. (ed.) (1999) *Canine Leishmaniasis: an Update. Proceedings of the International Canine Leishmaniasis Forum, Barcelona, Spain – 1999.* Hoechst Roussel Vet., 103 pp.

Molyneux, D.H. and Ashford, R.W. (1983) *The Biology of* Trypanosoma *and* Leishmania, *Parasites of Man and Domestic Animals.* Taylor & Francis, London, 294 pp.

Oumeish, O.Y. and Parish, L.C. (eds) (1999) Leishmaniasis. *Clinics in Dermatology* 17, 247–344

Peters, W. and Killick-Kendrick, R. (eds) (1987) *The Leishmaniases in Biology and Medicine,* Vol. 1. *Biology and Epidemiology.* Academic Press, London, pp. 1–551.

Peters, W. and Killick-Kendrick, R. (eds) (1987) *The Leishmaniases in Biology and Medicine,* Vol. 2. *Clinical Aspects and Control.* Academic Press, London, pp. 551 [*sic*]–941.

World Health Organization (1990) *Control of the Leishmaniases: Report of a WHO Expert Committee.* WHO, Geneva, 158 pp.

***Leptotrombidium* mites** *see* **Mites.**

Leucocytozoonosis

Ellis C. Greiner

Leucocytozoonosis is the infection of birds with blood-inhabiting protozoa of the genus *Leucocytozoon*. Five of 58 species of *Leucocytozoon* infect domesticated galliform and anseriform birds. Some of these are known to be pathogenic, but the impact on avian health of the others is unknown.

Leucocytozoon simondi infects waterfowl (Anatidae), *L. smithi* parasitizes turkeys and *L. caulleryi, L. macleani* and *L. schoutedeni* have chickens as their vertebrate hosts. Minor *Leucocytozoon* species which infect domesticated birds and about which very little is known include *L. marchouxi* of pigeons and doves (Columbidae), *L. neavei* in Guinea fowl (*Numida meleagris*) and *L. struthionis* in the Ostrich (*Struthio camelus*).

Distribution

Leucocytozoon simondi is Holarctic in its distribution. Because most free-ranging waterfowl species are migratory and this is a vector-borne pathogen, one must be cognizant of where transmission occurs. This is usually on the breeding grounds in the northern portions of their biological range. In the Nearctic, transmission has not been documented south of latitude 43°N, but whether this same distribution is present for the Old World is unknown. Most of the data we have on this species are from free-ranging birds, but domesticated waterfowl are equally susceptible. Therefore, people raising waterfowl in the regions where this parasite is transmitted could experience avian mortalities because of it.

The other relevant species of *Leucocytozoon* infect non-migratory domestic birds, which can be moved around by people. *Leucocytozoon smithi* is indigenous in North and Central America and occurs in western Europe and southern Africa where turkeys have been introduced. *Leucocytozoon schoutedeni* resides in chickens in sub-Saharan Africa. *Leucocytozoon macleani* infects chickens in southern and eastern Asia, as does *L. caulleryi*. The former species has been reported from chickens in Asia as *L. sabrasezi*, but it is now referable as *L. macleani*. Literature on *L. caulleryi* can be confusing for some people because many papers use the name *Akiba caulleryi*, but *Akiba* is now considered to be a subgenus of *Leucocytozoon*.

Parasite

Only gametocytes of *Leucocytozoon* are present in circulating blood cells. They develop in either erythrocytes or leucocytes and sometimes both, depending upon the species. They enlarge and distort the host cell so that it is no longer recognizable and they lack malarial pigment. Typically the parasites are round, filling most of the host cell cytoplasm, and the host cell nucleus forms a cap at the periphery of the parasite–host cell complex. Some species (*L. simondi*, *L. smithi* and *L. macleani*) have elongate gametocytes (Fig. 1) and induce the host cell to form clear, polar, wing-like extensions, and again the host cell nuclear cap is present. In two of these species (*L. smithi* and *L. macleani*) the host cell nucleus is typically split into two pieces, which are located along the sides of the elongate gametocyte. Both round and elongate gametocytes occur in some species, such as in *L. simondi* (Fig. 2) and *L. macleani*.

Most species are transmitted by species of black-flies (Simuliidae), but the vectors of *L. caulleryi* are biting midges of the genus *Culicoides* (Ceratopogonidae). The gametocytes of *L. caulleryi* are round and cause the erythrocyte nucleus to be eliminated from the parasite–host cell complex (Fig. 3). Host specificity of the genus is usually at the avian family level, but a few species appear to infect a single species of bird. Studies with *L. caulleryi* have shown that it is restricted to domestic chickens, and *L. smithi* does not infect other species of gallinaceous birds.

Once sporozoites are inoculated into birds by the feeding vector, they move via

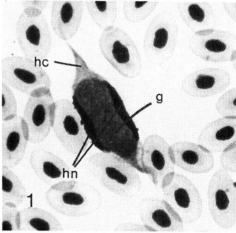

Fig. 1. *Leucocytozoon smithi*, typical elongate gametocyte from a turkey: hc, host cell cytoplasm; hn, host cell nucleus; g, gametocyte.

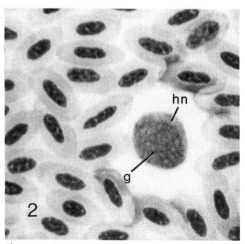

Fig. 2. *Leucocytozoon simondi*, round gametocyte from a mallard duck: hn, host cell nucleus; g, gametocyte.

the circulatory system throughout the body (Fig. 4). Most major organ systems may be involved and support development of the schizonts. The asexual replication (= schizogony) occurs in fixed cells, typically in the reticular endothelial system. Very large schizonts (= megaloschizonts) occur in most species of *Leucocytozoon*, at least in species in which they have been sought. They are evidently absent in chickens infected with *L. caulleryi*. However, a second round of schizogony in *L. caulleryi* is probably analogous, as these schizonts may cause severe haemorrhage when they mature and release their merozoites, which then enter the type of circulating blood cell used by that species for the production of gametocytes. If erythrocytes are infected, then infections with very high numbers of gametocytes may induce anaemia. The infection is now ready for acquisition by the vector.

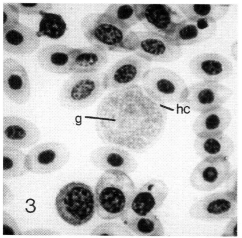

Fig. 3. *Leucocytozoon caulleryi* gametocyte from a chicken (note lack of a host cell nuclear remnant): hc, host cell cytoplasm; g, gametocyte.

Clinical signs

Disease is caused by *L. simondi* in anatids, *L. smithi* in turkeys and *L. caulleryi* in chickens. Sick poultry often assume a squatting posture with wings hanging loose. Signs of leucocytozoonosis include

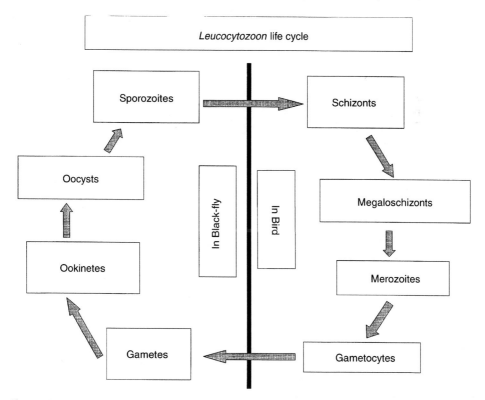

Fig. 4. Diagrammatic representation of a generalized life cycle of *Leucocytozoon*.

listlessness, anaemia, hepatomegaly, spleno-egaly, diarrhoea, anorexia, lethargy and dyspnoea. Some chicks infected with *L. caulleryi* will die within 13 days in cases where the eruption of the second round of schizonts causes haemorrhage. Leucocyto-zoonosis caused by *L. caulleryi* is referred to in parts of Asia as 'Bangkok haemorrhagic disease', as the afflicted birds haemorrhage and may lose sufficient blood to cause death. Chicks will continue to die as the infection progresses and other problems develop. In some cases growth of young birds is retarded and egg production in mature females may be curtailed. While younger birds are more prone to die, older birds may die as well if they have never been challenged and are inoculated with sporozoites as adults. The higher the number of sporozoites inoculated by the vectors, the more damage will be done and the shorter the time to death. Strains of *L. caulleryi* also vary in their degree of pathogenicity. Mortality may range from 20 to 80% of the birds infected with this disease.

In anatids, an autoimmune mechanism may contribute to anaemia rather than just erythrocyte destruction by the parasite. With *L. simondi* a relapse phenomenon occurs in which the parasitaemia is greatly enhanced at a time when young birds will be hatching and when vectors will be available to effect transmission. This is believed to occur with most species of *Leucocytozoon* and related genera (e.g. *Haemoproteus* and *Babesia* species) of blood parasites, but it evidently does not occur with *L. caulleryi*. Because of this, we do not know how this parasite overwinters.

Diagnosis

Most infections of *Leucocytozoon* are diag-nosed by blood smears, which are stained with Giemsa and scanned microscopically. In geographical regions where there is a his-tory of a particular species causing mortal-ity, signs and timing of events may support the blood smear diagnosis. Whereas with true malarial parasites one is able to subinoculate blood into another susceptible bird and produce a patent infection, this cannot be done with *Leucocytozoon* para-sites, because there is no asexual replication in the peripheral blood, as there is with *Plasmodium*. Serological procedures, such as indirect immunofluorescent antibody (IFA) and enzyme-linked immunosorbent assay (ELISA), are used in parts of Asia for the detection of *L. caulleryi* infections.

Transmission

Vectors are mainly simuliid black-flies for most species of *Leucocytozoon*, but, as mentioned earlier, *L. caulleryi* is transmit-ted by biting midges of the genus *Culicoides* (Ceratopogonidae). Both of these groups of vectors are pool-feeders and only females take blood meals.

When the vector feeds on birds with gametocytes circulating in the blood, the gametocytes leave their host cells, assume a roundish shape and undergo gametogenesis. There is one macrogamete formed per female gametocyte, whereas about eight micro-gametes are usually formed from one male gametocyte. The male gametes break free from the remaining residual body (remnants of the gametocyte not incorporated into the gametes) and search for a female gamete for fertilization to occur. This happens in the lumen of the gut of the vector. The resultant zygote becomes elongated and motile and moves to the limiting gut wall. It enters the wall and forms an oocyst just under the base-ment membrane of the gut. Asexual repro-duction occurs within the oocyst, resulting in the production of sporozoites, which rupture into the haemocoel of the vector. These move into the anterior portion of the body and enter the salivary glands. They are inoculated into a bird when the vector feeds on blood. These sporozoites are then carried by the circulatory system throughout the body, where they will enter cells to eventu-ally form the schizonts (another stage in which asexual reproduction occurs).

Different species of black-flies function as vectors of different species of *Leucocyto-zoon* and, for widely disseminated parasites, different species transmit the parasite in disparate geographical areas. *Simulium rugglesi* is the primary vector of *L. simondi* in the north-eastern Nearctic, but *Simulium anatinum, Simulium innocens, Simulium vittatum* and *Cnephia ornithophilia* are also reported to transmit the species in this region, whereas *Simulium fallisi* and *Simulium rendalense* are European vectors of the same parasite.

Leucocytozoon smithi is vectored by *Simulium meridionale, Simulium slossonae, Simulium congareenarum, Simulium aureum, Simulium croxtoni, Simulium jenningsi, Simulium pictipes* and *Prosimulium hirtipes* in the Nearctic region, where the turkey is indigenous. The relative efficacy of these species as vectors has not been compared. Vectors have not been identified in the Old World, into which the turkey has been exported.

Different species of vector become active at different times during the year, as is shown by the following example. Two species of black-flies are involved for the yearly perpetuation of *L. simondi* in Michigan, USA, and Ontario, Canada. In Michigan, *S. innocens* begins transmission, followed by *S. rugglesi*, while *S. anatinum* is the early vector in Ontario and again *S. rugglesi* is the vector later in the season. Such a switch in vector species may occur even when there is a severe winter. This contrasts with locations in the semi-tropics or tropics, where the same potential vectors may be present for most of the year.

The primary vector of *L. caulleryi* for much of South-East Asia is *Culicoides arakawae*. Two more species of biting midge support development of *L. caulleryi* to the sporozoite stage, namely *Culicoides circumscriptus* and *Culicoides odibilis*. As few as 100 sporozoites of some strains of the parasite are fatal to chicks. It is interesting to note that this form of leucocytozoonosis has not been demonstrated where there is an absence of *C. arakawae*.

Control

Treatment

Drug studies on these parasites have been primarily aimed at the parasite species in chickens, and drugs are being developed for preventive, not therapeutic, purposes. Drugs that have been used to prevent leucocytozoonosis in Asia include pyrimethamine, used for about 3 years before a resistant strain developed, when it was then used in combination with sulfonamides, such as sulfamethoxine and sulfaquinoxaline and others, and proved successful in preventing leucocytozoonosis. Other combinations of sulfa drugs have been used. A more recent combination is sulfamonomethoxine and ormetoprim, which, when introduced into feeds, were shown to be effective if given within 10 days of an infective inoculation of sporozoites. Clopidol has been used for prevention of *L. smithi* and *L. caulleryi* infections. In some instances a low level of parasitaemia developed, but disease did not ensue.

Vaccines

A killed vaccine is under development and initial studies indicate that partial protection is possible, but this appears more labour-intensive than using the medicated feeds.

Vectors

The likelihood of breaking the transmission cycle is remote because there are several vector species for *L. simondi* and *L. smithi* and the primary vector of *L. caulleryi* lives in rice-associated waters. Efforts to treat black-fly-producing streams with insecticides, such as temephos (Abate), or with *Bacillus thuringiensis* subsp. *israelensis* in South Carolina, USA, reduced the numbers of vectors, but did not preclude transmission of *L. smithi* to turkeys.

Selected bibliography

Akiba, K. (1970) Leucocytozoonosis of chickens. *National Institute of Animal Health Quarterly (Japan)* 10, 131–147.

Bennett, G.F., Earle, R.A., Peirce, M.A., Huchzermeyer, F.W. and Squires-Parsons, D. (1991) Avian Leucocytozoidae: the leucocytozoids of the Phasianidae *sensu lato*. *Journal of Natural History* 25, 1407–1428.

Desser, S.S. and Ryckman, A.K. (1976) The development and pathogenesis of *Leucocytozoon simondi* in Canada and domestic geese in Algonquin Park. *Canadian Journal of Zoology* 54, 634–643.

Greiner, E.C. (1991) Leucocytozoonosis in waterfowl and wild galliform birds. *Bulletin of the Society of Vector Ecologists* 16, 84–93.

Greiner, E,C. and Bennett, G.F. (1975) Avian Haematozoa. I. A color pictorial guide to species of *Haemoproteus, Leucoytozoon,* and *Trypanosoma. Wildlife Diseases* 66, 1–59. (Also on microfiche.)

Morii, T., Nakamura, K., Lee, Y.C., Iijima, T. and Hoji, K. (1986) Observations on the Taiwanese strain of *Leucocytozoon caulleryi* (Haemosporina) in chickens. *Journal of Protozoology* 33, 231–234.

Val' kiunas, G. (1997) Bird Haemosporida. In: *Acta Zoologica Lituanica*, Vols 3–5, Vilnius, Lithuania, 607 pp. (In Russian, English summary and index.)

Leucocytozoon **species** *see* **Leucocytozoonosis.**

Lice (Phthiraptera)

M.W. Service

There are over 3000 species of lice, belonging to three suborders, the Anoplura (sucking lice) and the Ischnocera and Amblycera (chewing lice). (Some specialists, however, consider the Anoplura as an order containing suborders Siphunculata (sucking lice) and Mallophaga (chewing lice)).

There are probably more than 1000 species of Anoplura, but only three are ectoparasites of humans and of medical importance, namely the body or clothes louse (*Pediculus humanus*), the head louse (*Pediculus capitis*) and the pubic or crab louse (*Pthirus pubis*). All three species have a more or less worldwide distribution, but body lice are often more common in temperate climates.

Polyplax species, such as the rat louse (*P. spinulosa*), are ectoparasites on animals, mainly Muridae.

Biology

Although head and pubic lice can cause considerable distress, the body louse is regarded as the principal vector transmitting infections among people; consequently only its biology is summarized here.

Both male and female lice bite and take several blood meals a day. Feeding occurs at any time of the 24 h day. Lice live permanently on people and cling to hairs of clothing or the body. The female glues about six to nine eggs (Fig. 1) a day to hairs of clothing and occasionally also to body hairs. During

her life, of about 2–4 weeks, a louse may lay 200–300 eggs. Eggs, often called nits, hatch within 7–10 days, although those on discarded clothing may not hatch until after 2–3 weeks, because of the lower temperatures away from the body. Eggs cannot survive for more than a month. Nymphs that hatch from the eggs resemble miniature editions of adult lice, take blood meals and pass through three nymphal instars. After about 7–12 days, they develop into adults, but the duration of the nymphal stages may be prolonged if the clothing to which they are attached is discarded at night or for longer periods.

Unfed lice die within a few days away from their human hosts, although blood-engorged individuals may survive for up to 10 days. Lice are temperature-sensitive and quickly leave a dead person and also sick people with high temperatures.

A heavily infested person may harbour several hundred or even thousands of lice, but there are usually fewer than 100 lice on any individual. Body lice are spread by close contact. Lice are particular common in situations where people are crowded together and wash infrequently, such as encountered in primitive jails, in refugee camps and in trenches during wars. People living in mountainous areas, such as in East Africa, Ethiopia, Burundi, Nepal and the Andean regions of South America, where, because of cold weather, they wear several layers of clothes, which may be rarely changed or

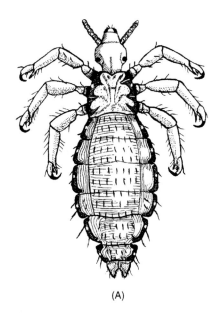

(A)

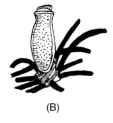

(B)

Fig. 1. (A) An adult (female) body louse (*Pediculus humanus*); (B) egg glued to fibres of clothing (modified from M.W. Service (2000) *Medical Entomology for Students*, Cambridge University Press, Cambridge).

washed, often have large lice populations. In more developed countries body lice are commonly found on homeless people, and infestations may reach a peak in winter, when more clothes are worn.

Species of *Polyplax* are ectoparasites of animals and are usually transmitted by close body contact. Mice and rats can have several hundred *P. spinulosa*, but grooming helps reduce the number of lice on their bodies. Surveys have shown that around 7% of mice were infested, but as many as 67% of larger murids, such as rats, were infested with lice. The incubation of the eggs is about a week and the time from egg laying to adult is about 2 weeks.

Diseases

Body lice are vectors of rickettsiae responsible for epidemic (louse-borne) typhus, *Bartonella quintana* (trench fever) and spirochaetes causing louse-borne relapsing fever (see entries). Head lice may also play a minor role in the transmission of louse-borne relapsing fever.

Species of *Polyplax*, such as *P. spinulosa* and *P. serrata*, are vectors of pathogens causing haemotrophic mycoplasmas (see entry). *Neohaematopinus sciuropteri* transmits *Rickettsia prowazekii*

to flying squirrels (*Glaucomys volans*) (see epidemic typhus).

Control

Washing clothing in water hotter than 60°C followed by ironing will get rid of lice. However, in epidemic situations this may not be practical; consequently insecticides are used, although in some areas lice have developed resistance to DDT, malathion and some pyrethroids. Insecticidal powders are usually applied between the body of a person and his/her clothing.

Selected bibliography

Burgess, I.F. (1995) Human lice and their management. *Advances in Parasitology* 36, 271–342.

Chetwyn, K.N. (1996) An overview of mass disinfestation procedures as a means to prevent epidemic typhus. In: Wildey, K.B. (ed.) *Proceedings of the 2nd International Conference on Insect Pests in the Urban Environment (ICIPUE)*. Organizing Committee of the ICIPUE, pp. 421–426.

Mumcuoglu, K.Y. (1996) Control of lice (Anoplura: Pediculidae) infestations: past and present. *American Entomologist* 42, 175–178.

Weidhaas, D.E. and Gratz, N.G. (1982) I. Lice. WHO/VBC/82.858, World Health Organization mimeographed document, Geneva, 10 pp.

Loa loa *see* **Loiasis.**

Loiasis

W. Crewe

Infections of humans and other primates with filarial worms of the genus *Loa*. There is only one species, *Loa loa*.

Loiasis, human

The disease is endemic in central Africa, from the Gulf of Guinea to the Great Lakes of East Africa, and it has been estimated that at least 13 million people are infected. Most infections with *Loa*, however, cause only relatively minor symptoms. The commonest signs are transient subcutaneous swellings, which are known as 'Calabar swellings' (after the Nigerian town of that name). Occasionally a young adult worm or a developing larva can be seen crossing the eye under the conjunctiva, and these have given rise to the common name 'eye-worm'. The name eye-worm has also been given to other helminth parasites – for example, the 'Oriental' eye-worm *Thelazia* and the 'Ugandan' eye-worm, which was originally thought to be *Loa* but is now considered to be *Mansonella*.

Distribution

Transmission of loiasis occurs only in Africa, and infection is confined to the equatorial rain forest from Sierra Leone to south-western Sudan (Bahr-el-Ghazal) and as far south as Gabon and Zaïre (Fig. 1). Possible, but unconfirmed, foci of loiasis have been reported from Uganda and Ethiopia. The known distribution of loiasis throughout this whole area is patchy, probably because of local topographical features but also because of a lack of information from some areas. Cases of loiasis have been recorded from many countries, and because the disease has a long incubation period these are sometimes erroneously recorded as new infections. Loiasis has repeatedly been introduced into the New World, but

has never become established outside Africa.

Parasite

Loa loa is a typical filarial worm, the adult female measuring 50–70 mm × 0.5 mm and the adult male 30–35 mm × 0.4 mm. Adult worms can live for up to 20 years. Microfilariae appear in the blood about 6 months after the infective bite of the vector. They are sheathed, 250–300 μm long and 6–8 μm wide, and they are diurnally periodic.

Clinical symptoms

Normally loiasis is not highly pathogenic, and individuals may be infected for many years without showing any definite signs or symptoms. The adult worms move actively through the connective tissues, and have been found during surgical operations in many parts of the body. When they are subcutaneous they may cause the non-pitting

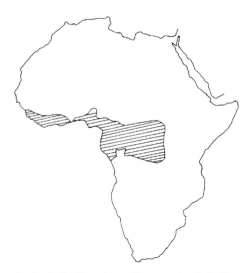

Fig. 1. Indication of overall geographical distribution of *Loa loa*.

oedematous Calabar swellings, which are probably local reactions to a worm's excretory products. Calabar swellings develop rapidly and may last for 2–3 days; they are most common on the back of the hand or the forearm (Fig. 2). They usually appear 1–2 years after infection, occur at irregular intervals for about a year, and then disappear. The disappearance may be associated with the worms' migration to deeper tissues. Occasionally young adult worms may be seen crossing the bridge of the nose under the skin or moving across the eye under the conjunctiva, when they may be accompanied by local itching and erythema and oedema of the eyelids. A somewhat similar painless oedema of the eyelids occurs in Uganda, where it is known as 'bung-eye'; it is, however, probably due to infection not with *Loa* but with *Mansonella* (see *M. perstans* under entry of Mansonelliasis). Infection with *Loa* is normally associated with a high eosinophilia (50–70%), and in endemic areas there may be very heavy infections (which are not uncommon because one *Chrysops*, the vector, can deposit up to 200 infective larvae), with over 50 microfilariae mm^{-3} of blood. In these cases the microfilariae may give rise to meningoencephalitis, which may be fatal. The risk of encephalitis is considerably increased by the administration of diethylcarbamazine (DEC) or ivermectin (see Treatment).

Diagnosis

Infection is usually first indicated by the occurrence of Calabar swellings or by the presence of moving adult worms in the subcutaneous tissues in an individual who has lived in or travelled to the equatorial rain-forest areas of Africa. The presence of a high eosinophilia or of microfilariae in blood taken between 1000 h and 1400 h is further evidence. Loiasis can be specifically diagnosed by examining (under oil immersion) the microfilariae in a thick blood film stained with haematoxylin. Microfilariae of *L. loa* measure 250–300 μm × 6–8 μm and are covered by a close-fitting sheath, which normally extends beyond the two extremes of the body; the tail is often bent back on the

body, and the nuclei extend right to the tip of the tail (Fig. 3). Occasionally a microfilaria may escape from its sheath while the blood film is drying, or the sheath may not have stained (which it will not do if the blood film is stained with Giemsa's stain), but the microfilaria can still be identified by the arrangement of the nuclei in the tail. Immunodiagnostic tests are not very

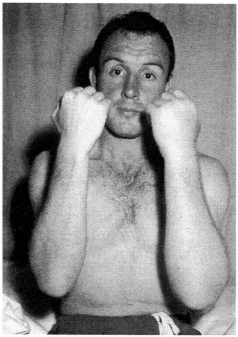

Fig. 2. Calabar swellings on the back of the patient's left hand and left forearm (with permission from the Liverpool School of Tropical Medicine).

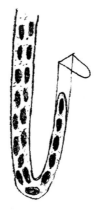

Fig. 3. Diagram of tail of microfilaria of *Loa loa*. Note nuclei extending to tip of tail and bent sheath extending beyond tail.

specific, and routine diagnosis is by examination of stained blood films.

Transmission

All the vectors of loiasis are members of the genus *Chrysops* (see Horse-flies). The most important vector in Nigeria and the Cameroun Republic is *C. silacea*, and this species is probably the major vector in most parts of the West African rain forest except where *C. dimidiata* is locally more common. *Chrysops zahrai* is a minor vector. In Bahr-el-Ghazal, Sudan, on the fringes of the forest, the most important vector is probably *C. distinctipennis*, although *C. longicornis* also acts as a vector. These flies are 'canopy dwellers', living mainly in sunlight above the forest canopy, but during daylight hours they will descend to ground level in cleared areas, along roadways or at the forest fringes. They are attracted down by movement of people or vehicles or by wood smoke. When biting, the flies repeatedly probe the skin and so rupture blood capillaries and produce a subcutaneous haemorrhage. The fly obtains its meal from this pool of blood and takes up any contained microfilariae. These microfilariae develop in the muscular and connective tissue of the fly, mainly in the abdomen but also in the thorax and head. The developing larvae moult twice, and the resulting third-stage infective larvae are 1800–2300 μm long and 30–45 μm wide. On about the tenth day (though development may take 7–15 days) the infective larvae congregate in the head of the fly, mainly near the root of the proboscis. When the fly bites again the larvae break out from the labium, swarm down the outside of the biting mouthparts and are deposited on the skin surface. As many as 200 larvae may be deposited during the short time that the fly is feeding. Most of the larvae die, as they are unable to penetrate unbroken skin, but many penetrate through the punctures made by the feeding fly or through other skin abrasions. The larvae develop in the connective tissue of the host, mainly subcutaneously, moving around the body as they do so, and become mature worms in about 3 months. Microfilariae appear in the

blood from about 6 months after the bite of the fly.

Treatment

For patients with few or no circulating microfilariae the drug of choice is diethylcarbamazine (DEC). This is curative in most cases, although multiple courses of therapy are often necessary, and relapses may occur up to 8 years after treatment. Mild side-effects, such as Calabar swellings, urticaria and fever, are common during the first few days of therapy, but these usually respond to antihistamines or corticosteroids. The risk of adverse side-effects can be reduced by commencing treatment with low dosages of DEC and gradually increasing the dosage as treatment continues. In patients with high microfilaraemias, however, DEC or ivermectin treatment may cause serious complications, including meningoencephalitis and renal failure. These side-effects are thought to be caused by allergic reactions to large numbers of dead and dying microfilariae in the capillaries. If treatment is considered necessary for such patients, it is important first to reduce the number of circulating microfilariae. Both mebendazole and albendazole have been shown to reduce microfilaraemia without adverse side-effects.

Control

The larvae of *Chrysops* live in mud and can be destroyed by insecticides, but the inaccessibility of the breeding sites in the forest renders this impracticable as a control method. Clearance of forest around houses and screening of houses against mosquitoes will reduce the risk of bites indoors. The wearing of light-coloured clothing and frequent application of insect repellents or wearing clothing impregnated with pyrethroid insecticides, such as permethrin, will reduce the risk of bites outdoors. Personal prophylaxis with DEC has been shown to be efficient in expatriates working in endemic areas.

Loiasis, animal

The only known animal hosts of loiasis are primates, particularly cercopithecid monkeys and drills, but it is unlikely that any of these act as reservoir hosts for the human infection, because the vectors of animal loiasis rarely bite humans (see Transmission). Infections with *Loa* have been recorded in monkeys, Drills (*Mandrillus leucophaeus*), baboons (*Papio* species), Chimpanzees (*Pan troglodytes*) and Gorillas (*Gorilla gorilla*) from various parts of the rain forest and gallery forests of Africa. The primate parasites show important differences from the human parasites, but little is known about their biology and at present they are all considered to be subspecies or strains of *L. loa*.

Distribution

Primate infections with *Loa* have been recorded from the Cameroon Republic, Uganda, Zaïre and Guinea, but there is little doubt that they are widespread throughout the equatorial forest belt of Africa. Possibly their distribution is coincident with that of human loiasis.

Parasite

The primate parasites are generally slightly larger than the human ones, the adult females measuring 50–75 mm and the adult males 35–40 mm. The important difference between the human and animal parasites is that the microfilariae of the animal parasites, which are morphologically similar to those of the human parasite, are nocturnally periodic. However, an apparently diurnally periodic strain has been observed in the Cameroon Republic in a Drill (*M. leucophaeus*), which, unlike most monkeys, spends much of its time during the day at ground level.

Transmission

Most of the studies on monkey loiasis have been carried out in the Cameroon Republic, where the vectors are *Chrysops langi* and *Chrysops centurionis*. Although all species of *Chrysops* found in the forest seem able to support the development of both human and monkey *Loa*, there can be very little transference of monkey loiasis to humans (or of human loiasis to monkeys). The only *Chrysops* which behave in a manner which

brings them into contact with humans – that is, which bite at ground level in daylight – are *C. silacea* and *C. dimidiata* (and occasionally *C. zahrai*). Although these species are also abundant at canopy level, they are exclusively diurnal in their biting habits there also. During the daytime, when they are active and alert, monkeys will catch and eat, or drive away, biting flies. At dusk, when the monkeys settle in the treetops to sleep, they may be successfully attacked by *Chrysops*, but at this time the vectors of human loiasis cease biting. On the other hand, the flies which behave in a manner which enables them to feed on monkeys – that is, which feed at canopy level at dusk and dawn – are *C. langi* and *C. centurionis*. These flies never descend to ground level and, even if they did, they would be unlikely to find human prey, for the human inhabitants of the rain forest rarely move outside their houses after dark. It is thus extremely unlikely that *C. langi* or *C. centurionis* could carry infections from monkeys to humans or vice versa. Occasionally *C. silacea* must succeed in biting monkeys during daylight hours, and so could possibly transmit larvae of human loiasis to monkeys, but transmission in the opposite direction is less likely because the microfilariae of monkey loiasis are nocturnally periodic and unlikely to be present in the monkeys' peripheral blood-vessels during daylight hours.

Selected bibliography

Beaver, P.C., Jung, R.C. and Cupp, E.W. (eds) (1984) *Clinical Parasitology*, 9th edn. Lea & Febiger, Philadelphia, pp. 377–380.

Cook, G.C. (ed.) (1996) *Manson's Tropical Diseases*, 20th edn. W.B. Saunders, London, pp. 1351–1354.

Duke, B.O.L. and Wijers, D.J.B. (1958) Studies on loiasis in monkeys. I – The relationship between human and simian *Loa* in the rain-forest zone of the British Cameroons. *Annals of Tropical Medicine and Parasitology* 52, 158–175.

Duke, B.O.L. (1963) Studies on the chemoprophylaxis of loiasis. II – Observations on diethylcarbamazine citrate (Banocide) as a prophylactic in man. *Annals of Tropical Medicine and Parasitology* 57, 82–96.

Gardon, J., Gardon-Wendall, N., Demanda-Ngangue, Kamgno, J., Chippaux, J.-P. and Boussinesq, M. (1997). Serious reactions after mass treatment of onchocerciasis with ivermectin in an area endemic for *Loa loa* infection. *The Lancet* 350, 18–22.

Strickland, G.T. (ed.) (2000) *Hunter's Tropical Medicine and Emerging Infectious Diseases*, 8th edn. Saunders, Philadelphia, pp. 754–756.

Warren, K.S. and Mahmoud, A.E.F. (1990) *Tropical and Geographical Medicine*, 2nd edn. McGraw-Hill, New York, pp. 420–423.

Louping ill, sheep

E.A. Gould

Louping ill (LI) virus is the aetiological agent of a sheep encephalomyelitic disease that has been recognized in the British Isles for at least 200 years. The verb 'to loup' describes one symptom of the disease, in which sheep leap or jump in an ungainly manner as their condition deteriorates. The virus is transmitted to sheep by infected ticks, *Ixodes ricinus*, as they take a blood meal. A wide variety of other animal species, including humans, are also susceptible to LI virus infection, but the frequency with which this is likely to occur and the outcome of infection are dependent upon a variety of factors that will be described later.

Distribution

Louping ill refers specifically to sheep encephalitis in the British Isles. However, a strikingly similar disease, also associated with *Ixodes ricinus*, is recognized in Spain, Norway, Greece, Turkey and Bulgaria. On the British mainland, the virus can be isolated from *Ixodes* species collected on hillsides and moorlands where sheep are grazed (Fig. 1). The moist undergrowth and rotting vegetation associated with upland rough pastures provide the necessary high humidity, i.e. close to saturation, for long-term survival of the tick. Overt disease in sheep and Red grouse (*Lagopus lagopus scoticus*) is most frequently observed on the moorlands of Scotland, northern England, Wales and south-west England. In Ireland, louping ill is often seen at lower elevations in horses and cattle as well as sheep, probably because the relatively higher moisture content in the lowland grasses provides conditions suitable for long-term survival of the ticks.

Virus

Louping ill virus is a tick-borne flavivirus. It is genetically closely related to a group of viruses known as the tick-borne encephalitis (TBE) virus complex in the genus *Flavivirus*, which also includes mosquito-transmitted viruses, as well as viruses with no known arthropod vector. Under the electron microscope, the flaviviruses appear

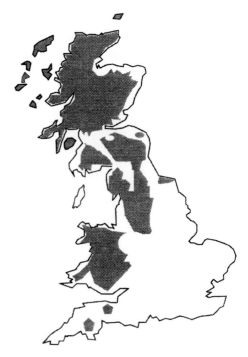

Fig. 1. Schematic representation of the regions on the British mainland where louping ill virus may be present (black shading).

spherical. They all contain a positive-sense, single-stranded RNA genome approximately 10.5 kb in length and encapsulated in a capsid (C) protein, which is enclosed by a lipid membrane containing glycosylated envelope (E) proteins, each intimately associated with a glycosylated membrane (M) protein. In addition to these three structural proteins, the viral RNA also encodes seven non-structural proteins, NS1, NS2A, NS2B, NS3, NS4A, NS4B and NS5, which are responsible for virus maturation, RNA translation, proteolytic processing of translated proteins and RNA replication (Fig. 2).

Virus replication
The infectious process starts when specific domains on the viral envelope protein attach to host cell receptors and the viruses become engulfed in endosomal vesicles. The relatively low pH of the vesicle leads to a conformational change in the envelope protein, which then fuses with the endosomal membrane, releasing the genomic RNA into the cytoplasm to initiate the translational and transcriptional processes. Due to its positive polarity, the incoming RNA acts as messenger RNA (mRNA) and is translated as a polyprotein, which is either concurrently or subsequently cleaved proteolytically by both virus-encoded and host cell proteases. The newly produced NS3 and NS5 non-structural proteins form a replication complex with the RNA, which is replicated, and the replicated molecules serve as both mRNA for translation of more proteins and progeny RNA to be incorporated into newly forming virions. The process of RNA encapsulation has not been adequately defined. During the virion maturation process, which occurs in association with the membranes of the endoplasmic reticulum, the precursor to the membrane protein (PrM) becomes intimately associated with envelope protein, which, in this form, remains inert to the relatively low pH of the endosomal membranes. As far as

is known, the pre-membrane protein is cleaved immediately prior to release of the virions from the cell, at which time the envelope protein attains its mature conformation on the virion surface as a pH-sensitive dimer.

Clinical symptoms in sheep
The severe form of disease is characteristically biphasic and in non-immune sheep is frequently fatal. Experimentally infected sheep develop a viraemia within 24 h lasting for up to 8 days. The first phase of illness usually presents as a fever with associated weakness. Neurological symptoms develop during the second phase. As the condition deteriorates, sheep develop cerebellar ataxia and hyperexcitability, followed by posterior paresis, complete flaccid paralysis and tremors. When the symptoms reach this stage, recovery is unlikely.

Clinical symptoms in humans
About 40 cases of louping ill have been recorded in humans, most of which were due to laboratory infections and none of which was fatal. The disease in humans is similar to the western European form of tick-borne encephalitis (see entry), although generally milder, and is typically biphasic. Onset of symptoms commences about 4–6 days post-exposure to the bite of an infected tick. The patient suffers excessive sweating and a general feeling of malaise, with a fever, sore throat, headache and photophobia, perhaps accompanied by puffy eyelids. Recovery from this first phase of illness takes about 1–2 weeks. A few days later, a more clinically severe form of the illness returns, with vomiting, fever, lymphadenopathy and meningoencephalitis, often accompanied by significant loss of coordination and memory. Complete recovery usually takes 10–12 weeks from the onset of illness.

C	pRM	E	NS1	NS2A	NS2B	NS3	NS4A	C	C

Fig. 2. Genome organization of flaviviruses. The virus proteins are shown in shaded boxes. The untranslated regions are depicted as solid black lines at the ends of the RNA genome.

Pathogenesis

Pathological examination reveals most or all of the following conditions: lymphadenopathy, leucopenia, subconjunctival haemorrhages, meningoencephalitis, Purkinje cell destruction, severe chromatolysis, reactive gliosis and astrocytosis.

Diagnosis

Although LI virus is antigenically closely related to the other viruses in the TBE virus complex, there is no geographical overlap between louping ill, which occurs almost exclusively on sheep-grazed moorlands, and tick-borne encephalitis, which is a forest-associated disease. Therefore, despite the antigenic cross-relationships between these viruses, serological diagnosis is a reliable indicator of LI virus infection. Comparison of acute and convalescent sera should show increasing antibody levels against LI virus. This seroconversion can be detected by haemagglutination inhibition, complement fixation, plaque reduction neutralization, enzyme-linked immunosorbent assay or fluorescent antibody titration.

A more definitive diagnosis can be carried out by isolation of the virus from the infected host, using cell culture methods, and virus identification, using either an appropriate monoclonal antibody that is specific for LI virus or by reverse transcription and polymerase chain reaction (RT-PCR) of a fraction of the envelope gene. Sequencing of this genomic RNA fragment not only identifies the virus but can also be used to identify the region of the British Isles in which the virus originated. It is now possible to identify the virus by RT-PCR-sequencing the RNA extracted directly from the infected tick or animal specimen, without the need for virus isolation in tissue culture cells.

Transmission

The hard (ixodid) tick *Ixodes ricinus* is the major vector of LI virus. Experimentally, both *Rhipicephalus appendiculatus* and *Hyalomma anatolicum* may also transmit the virus trans-stadially and most species of Ixodidae (hard ticks) are possible vectors, although there is little evidence that they

are involved in the epidemiology of louping ill. The tick may become infected at any of the feeding stages in its life cycle, i.e. larva, nymph or adult. The virus enters the tick via the mid-gut and then crosses this barrier before replicating in other parts of the tick, including the brain and the salivary glands. Once infected, the tick remains infected throughout the remainder of its life cycle, which may be as long as 3–5 years. The virus survives the trans-stadial changes that occur as the tick moults from larva to nymph and then to adult. However, although transovarial transmission has been reported with European and Far East Asian strains of TBE complex viruses, there is no direct evidence of transovarial transmission of LI virus. Conventionally, an uninfected tick – for example, a larva – becomes infected when it takes a blood meal from a viraemic host. Once this infected larva is fully engorged, it drops off the animal and, within a few weeks, under suitable environmental conditions, moults to the next stage in the life cycle, i.e. the nymphal stage. After a period of several months or even 1–2 years when the climatic conditions are suitable, the infected nymph will take a blood meal and transmit the virus to the host, which, if susceptible, becomes infected, develops a viraemia and transmits the virus to other non-infected ticks that take a blood meal during the viraemic period.

While the above transmission events undeniably take place, they do not adequately explain the persistence of LI virus in the natural environment. There is now good evidence to show that some animals that do not develop significant viraemia following exposure to the virus may nevertheless support virus transmission from infected ticks to non-infected ticks co-feeding on these insusceptible animals. Louping ill virus persistence in the British Isles can therefore be explained by a combination of the following factors: (i) the constant introduction of susceptible animals, such as sheep, into areas where infected ticks are present; (ii) the ability of ticks to become infected when feeding on viraemic animals; (iii) the ability of ticks to become infected on non-viraemic animals when co-feeding with infected ticks; (iv) the ability of ticks to remain infected for the entire life cycle; and (v) the presence of other animals, such as deer, which amplify the tick population without necessarily acting as hosts for the transmission of the virus.

A third mechanism of virus transmission has also been described that may also contribute to LI virus persistence in the environment. It has been shown that, in common with many other flaviviruses, LI virus may be transmitted orally to susceptible hosts. Thus, animals removing ticks from the skin of other animals or eating ticks present in the undergrowth may become infected. Alternatively, animals eating infected animals may also become infected.

In addition to infections in the laboratory, humans may become infected following tick bites obtained during walks on the moorlands and in areas with thick moist undergrowth on the upper hillsides, a favourite haunt for *I. ricinus*. A serological survey of abattoir workers indicated that about 8% had experienced infection, although few cases have been reported in the UK. Butchers, veterinarians and farmworkers also theoretically face an increased risk of infection from infected sheep, but there is little evidence that this is the case.

Epidemiology

Louping ill is a very rare disease in humans for two main reasons. Firstly, human exposure to *I. ricinus* is relatively uncommon in the UK and, secondly, the infection rate of ticks in the most active areas for louping ill disease is estimated to be less than 2%. On the other hand, annual outbreaks of sheep encephalitis occur in late spring and early summer on the upland sheep-grazing areas of Scotland, northern England, north Wales, Devon, Northern Ireland and Eire. Infected *I. ricinus* occur in abundance and feed predominantly on sheep, which are farmed intensively in these regions. Early records of louping ill-like disease suggest that epidemics occurred commonly on the uplands of southern Scotland, rather than in the Highlands north of the Forth–Clyde, where Red grouse prosper. The disease was subsequently introduced to the Highlands as sheep farming was intensified in this

region. Red grouse were therefore exposed to LI virus only relatively recently. Newborn lambs are theoretically protected by colostric antibody from mothers that have either been immunized or previously exposed to and survived virus infection. Otherwise, newborn and young lambs are highly susceptible to infection and need to be immunized and protected from tick bites, using acaricides, either before or soon after being introduced on to the hillsides containing infected ticks. The peak feeding period for ticks is the late spring and and early summer, which coincides with the peak period for young susceptible lambs. Classically, the high-titre viraemia detected in susceptible sheep when they develop clinical infection provides ideal conditions for transmission of the virus to feeding ticks. However, LI virus appears to be able to persist and cause fresh epidemics on moorlands where the sheep have been systematically immunized and treated with acaricides, implying that other wildlife species contribute to LI virus persistence in the natural environment.

The chicks of Red grouse, which nest in the Highland heather on the moorland and hatch in the spring, are highly susceptible to infection by LI virus, developing high-titre viraemias. However, the fact that louping ill was only recently introduced to the Highlands and mortality rates in Red grouse as high as 80% have been recorded implies that they probably do not play a major part in sustaining louping ill long-term.

Susceptibility of other animal species
The host preference of immature *I. ricinus* is catholic and they will take blood meals indiscriminately from any vertebrate that feeds or nests on the ground. The Red fox (*Vulpes vulpes crucigera*), a variety of rodents, the Blue mountain hare (*Lepus timidus scoticus*), and several species of birds, horses, pigs, cattle and dogs are also susceptible to infection by LI virus, but few of these animals occur in significant numbers on the moorlands and therefore exposure in mainland Britain is infrequent. In Northern Ireland and the more northern parts of Eire, however, the undergrowth has

a higher moisture content at lower altitudes, and the rainfall is quite regular throughout the year, favouring tick survival. For these reasons, louping ill is seen more commonly in horses, cattle, pigs and farm dogs.

Wild rabbits, deer and rodents are not considered to be highly susceptible to the virus and, although they may serve a role as amplification hosts for tick populations, they are unlikely to be significantly involved in spreading the disease. The Blue mountain hare, on the other hand, has been shown to be relatively efficient as a host for virus transmission between co-feeding ticks and is likely to have an important role in LI virus persistence in the natural environment. It was previously believed that, since transovarial transmission of LI virus does not occur, infected adults represented a dead-end stage for the virus, but, in view of the observation that transmission between ticks occurs as they co-feed, it now seems likely that infected adult ticks do contribute to LI virus persistence.

Treatment

There is no specific treatment for louping ill but, under some circumstances, hydrocortisone has been found to relieve the symptoms of encephalitis, possibly by reducing the oedema resulting from an inflammatory antigen/antibody reaction. Until recently, humans in mainland Europe suspected of being exposed to the related TBE virus were given human immunoglobulin known to contain antibody to the virus. It was believed that this might prevent the onset of disease and in most cases seemed to work. However, accumulating evidence suggested that some cases of encephalitis that did develop in the presence of the administered antibody were more severe than normal and the practice has now been discontinued.

Control

In the UK, humans are only at risk from infection by LI virus if they wander through tick-infested areas on the moorlands and hillsides identified earlier. Even under these circumstances, the risk of infection is very low if they wear appropriate clothing to prevent questing ticks from contacting exposed skin, i.e. good boots, socks over long trousers and/or use of chemical repellents. In the winter or late autumn, ticks do not quest and therefore the risk of infection becomes negligible.

There is no human vaccine for LI virus but it is generally believed that immunization with the inactivated vaccine for TBE virus will provide immune protection against LI virus. While this vaccine is not officially registered for use in the UK, it has been used extensively throughout Europe and is recommended for visitors to forested regions of Europe known to contain TBE virus. In theory the most effective form of control would be to eradicate the tick but this is totally impractical and attempts to achieve this might have other undesirable side-effects on the environment. A formalin-inactivated vaccine that protects sheep against LI virus has been used effectively and extensively throughout the UK. Acaricides are also effective deterrents but they have to be applied just before the most active questing period for ticks and they may need to be applied more than once.

Regardless of how effective the current control measures are, the annual reintroduction of susceptible sheep and the constant presence of other host species capable of supporting LI virus ensure that the control measures have to be repeated regularly.

Selected bibliography

Gould, E.A. (1998) Encephalitis viruses (*Flaviviridae*): tick-borne encephalitis and Wesselsbron. In: Webster, R.G. and Granoff, A. (eds) *Encyclopedia of Virology*. Academic Press, London, pp. 430–437.

McGuire, K., Holmes, E.C., Gao, G.F., Reid, H.W. and Gould, E.A. (1998) Tracing the origins of louping ill virus by molecular phylogenetic analysis. *Journal of General Virology* 79, 981–988.

Monath, T.P. and Heinz, F.X. (1996) Flaviviruses. In: Fields, B.N., Knipe, D.M. and Howley, P.M. (eds) *Virology*, Vol. 1. Lippincott-Raven, Philadelphia, New York, pp. 961–1034.

Reid, H.W. (1984) Epidemiology of louping ill. In: Mayo, M.A. and Harrap, K.A (eds) *Vector Biology*. Academic Press, London, pp. 161–178.

Rice, C.M. (1996) *Flaviviridae*: the viruses and their replication. In: Fields, B.N., Knipe, D.M. and Howley, P.M. (eds) *Virology*, Vol. 1. Lippincott-Raven, Philadelphia, pp. 931–960.

Louse-borne relapsing fever

David A. Warrell

This is an infection of humans with spirochaetes of *Borrelia recurrentis*.

War, famine and other disasters favour the spread of louse-borne infections, such as louse-borne relapsing fever and epidemic typhus (see entry). During the first half of the 20th century, there were at least 50 million cases of louse-borne relapsing fever with 10 million deaths in Europe, the Middle East and northern Africa. There is a continuing potential for epidemic spread of this disease from its current foci in the Horn of Africa.

Distribution

Currently, the main epidemic focus is in the highlands of Ethiopia, where there is an annual epidemic of at least 10,000 cases in the cool, rainy season. In recent years, cases have also occurred throughout the year. There have been outbreaks in Sudan and Somalia. In early 1999, an epidemic in Rumbek county, southern Sudan, killed hundreds of people in the course of a few weeks. The infection may still exist in Andean areas of Peru. There is no known animal reservoir host. Between epidemics, *B. recurrentis* persists as mild or asymptomatic human infections.

Aetiological agent

Borrelia recurrentis, first described by O.H.F. Obermeier in 1867, is one of the spirochaete phylum of bacteria, which also comprises treponemes, the cause of syphilis, yaws, bejel and pinta, as well as two other groups of *Borrelia*, which cause Lyme disease (see Lyme borreliosis) and tick-borne relapsing fever (see entry). The organisms are 12–18 μm long with a wavelength of 1.7 μm and a thickness of 0.4–0.5 μm. The ends are sharply pointed.

Fifteen to 20 flagella are inserted at each end and lie in the periplasmic space between the two cell membranes. Borrelia can be identified in blood films by Wright's, Giemsa's, Leishman's and Romanovsky's stains, and by dark-ground illumination and acridine orange fluorescence (QBC®). *Borrelia recurrentis* is microaerophilic and has been cultured in an artificial medium, BSKII, for growth of Lyme disease borreliae, and on chick chorioallantoic membrane and can be maintained in rodents. Culture requirements include serum, glucose, albumin, peptides, amino acids, vitamins, gelatin and *N*-acetylglucosamine.

The outer membrane contains variable major lipoproteins, which stimulate monocytes to produce tumour necrosis factor (TNF). There is no true endotoxin. *Borrelia recurrentis* is an extracellular pathogen, found predominantly in the blood but also in organs and tissues, such as spleen, liver, brain, eye and kidney.

Clinical symptoms

Poor, indigent, malnourished street-dwellers, beggars and prisoners seem most likely to become infected, especially young men. Pregnant women appear to be especially susceptible to severe disease and abortions are frequent.

After an incubation period of 4–18 (average 7) days, the illness starts suddenly with rigors and high fever. Early symptoms include headache, dizziness, nightmares, general aches and pains, especially affecting the lower back, knees and elbows, anorexia, nausea, vomiting and diarrhoea. Later there is upper abdominal pain, cough and epistaxis. Patients are usually prostrated and confused. Hepatic tenderness is found in about 60% of patients and hepatomegaly in about half. Splenic tenderness and enlargement are frequent. Jaundice occurs in 10–80% of patients. A petechial or ecchymotic rash is seen, especially on the trunk, in 10–60%.

Epistaxis (25%), haemoptysis and conjunctival and retinal bleeding are typical. Many patients have tender muscles. Neurological features include meningism (40%), cranial nerve lesions, monoplegias, flaccid paraplegia and focal convulsions. Severe manifestations include myocarditis, which may present as acute pulmonary oedema, liver failure and severe bleeding attributable to thrombocytopenia, liver damage and disseminated intravascular coagulation. Complicating secondary infections include bacillary dysentery, salmonellosis, typhoid, typhus, malaria and tuberculosis. Case fatality can be reduced to less than 5% with antibiotic treatment. During large epidemics, case fatalities of 40–70% have been reported. Survivors usually recover completely and enjoy persistent (sterile) immunity.

Relapses

In untreated cases, the first attack of fever resolves by crisis after 4–10 (average 5) days. There follows an afebrile remission of 5–9 days and then a series of up to five relapses. The relapses are less severe than the initial attack; there is no petechial rash but iritis or iridocyclitis and severe epistaxis may occur.

Immunological basis of the relapse phenomenon

Borrelia recurrentis exhibits antigenic variation of variable membrane proteins (Vmps), which are outer membrane lipo-proteins. The organism has a repertoire of many Vmps but, at any one time, only one is expressed and is immunodominant. The expressed Vmp gene is situated near the end of a linear plasmid and changes every 1000–10,000 cell divisions. Immunoglobulin M (IgM) is induced against the immunodominant Vmp, leading to selection of borreliae of the next, emerging serotype. This explains the relapse phenomenon and the successive appearance of borreliae

expressing different Vmps during the course of an untreated infection. These same Vmps are the principal TNF-inducing factors in louse-borne relapsing fever. Variable membrane proteins may differ in their potency as TNF inducers and may also determine the invasiveness of the borreliae, for example, into the central nervous system and they may affect virulence in other ways.

The spontaneous crisis and Jarisch–Herxheimer reaction

With or without treatment, the illness usually ends dramatically. On about the fifth day of the untreated illness, or 1–2 h after antibiotic treatment, the patient becomes restless and apprehensive and develops shaking chills lasting 10–30 min. Temperature, respiratory and pulse rates and blood pressure rise sharply. There is delirium, nausea, vomiting, diarrhoea, cough and limb pains. Some patients die of hyperpyrexia at the peak of the fever. The flush (vasodilatation) phase, which lasts several hours, is characterized by profuse sweating, a fall in blood pressure and a slow decline in temperature. Deaths during this phase follow intractable hypotension or the development of acute pulmonary oedema from myocarditis.

Pathology

The vast majority of spirochaetes are confined to the lumen of blood-vessels, but tangled masses of *B. recurrentis* are also found in splenic miliary abscesses, in infarcts and adjacent to haemorrhages in the central nervous system. Some strains of tick-borne borreliae can invade the central nervous system, aqueous humour and other tissues. In louse-borne relapsing fever, a perivascular, histiocytic, interstitial myocarditis has been described, which explains the conduction defects, arrhythmias and fatal myocardial failure observed in some patients. Splenic rupture with massive haemorrhage, cerebral haemorrhage and hepatic failure are other causes of death. Hepatitis is associated with patchy midzonal haemorrhages and necrosis. Other changes include meningitis, perisplenitis, petechial haemorrhages of serosal cavities and evidence of disseminated intravascular coagulation, such as the presence of thrombi in small blood-vessels.

Diagnosis

Spirochaetes can be seen in stained thin or thick blood films, except a few hours after spontaneous crisis or the Jarisch–Herxheimer reaction (J-HR) and during remissions. Motile spirochaetes can be seen by phase-contrast or dark-field microscopy. Serological methods are not necessary. False-positive reactions for *Proteus* OXK, OX19, OX2 and syphilis occur in 5–10% of patients, and false-positive Lyme borreliosis serology is common.

Differential diagnosis

In a febrile patient with jaundice, petechial rash, bleeding and hepatosplenomegaly, falciparum malaria, yellow fever, viral hepatitis, rickettsial infections (especially epidemic (louse-borne) typhus)), leptospirosis and a viral haemorrhagic fever should be considered, depending on the travel history. Mixed epidemics and mixed infections of louse-borne relapsing fever and epidemic typhus have been described. The possibility of a complicating infection, especially typhoid, should not be forgotten.

Differences between louse-borne and tick-borne relapsing fever

The tick-borne disease is generally milder and less protracted. The initial fever lasts only about 3 days, but there may be up to 13 relapses. Jaundice is less common but neurological signs are more frequent in tick-borne disease.

Laboratory findings

Common abnormalities include a moderate normochromic anaemia, neutrophil leucocytosis (with marked leucopenia during the spontaneous crisis or J-HR), thrombocytopenia, mild coagulopathy, evidence of hepatocellular damage and mild renal impairment. The cerebrospinal fluid shows a polymorph/lymphocyte pleocytosis without visible spirochaetes.

Transmission

Humans are probably the only reservoir of louse-borne relapsing fever. The vector is the human body louse, *Pediculus humanus*, and, to a lesser extent, the head louse, *Pediculus capitis*. *Borrelia recurrentis*, ingested by the louse during a blood meal, multiplies in its body cavity. Under conditions of crowding and poor hygiene, lice move from person to person. When the host's body surface temperature deviates far from 37°C, as a result of death, fever or exposure, or if infested clothing is discarded, the louse is forced to find a new host. A new person is infected when the infected louse is crushed and its body haemolymph is applied to mucous membranes, such as the conjunctiva by rubbing the eye, or to abraded skin, or inoculated through intact skin by scratching.

Transmission is also possible by blood transfusion, needle-stick injuries or even, in medical personnel, by contamination of broken skin, such as paronychia on the fingers, by infected patients' blood. Unlike the tick vectors of tick-borne relapsing fever, which are also reservoirs of the infection, lice cannot transmit the infection transovarially to their progeny.

Treatment

Antibiotic treatment

Borrelia recurrentis is highly sensitive to tetracyclines, chloramphenicol, erythromycin and other macrolides and cephalosporins; relatively resistant to quinolones and aminoglycosides; and completely resistant to rifampicin, metronidazole and sulfonamides. In patients who can swallow and retain tablets, the treatment of choice is a single oral dose of tetracycline, erythromycin or chloramphenicol – 500 mg for adults, 12.5 mg kg^{-1} for children. Erythromycin is the preferred treatment for pregnant women and children under the age of 8 years. The most effective parenteral treatment is tetracycline, 250–500 mg by slow intravenous injection. Single-dose benzylpenicillin (adult dose 500 mg by intramuscular or slow intravenous injection) or benzylpenicillin with procaine benzylpenicillin (adult dose 500 mg by intramuscular injection) may cause a milder but more prolonged J-HR reaction, but with delayed clearance of spirochaetaemia and the risk of relapses.

The Jarisch–Herxheimer reaction to antibiotic treatment

Severe J-HRs, with a case fatality of about 5%, complicate treatment in 30–90% of cases. There is no evidence, however, that the shorter and more intense reaction following tetracycline is more dangerous than the more prolonged but apparently milder reaction following penicillin. Corticosteroids and paracetamol do not prevent the reaction but meptazinol, an opioid antagonist with agonist properties, decreases the intensity of the J-HR. A polyclonal, ovine, Fab, anti-TNFα antibody infused for 30 min before treatment with penicillin or tetracycline reduces the incidence and severity of the J-HR.

Ancillary treatment

Patients must be nursed in bed for at least 24 h after treatment to prevent postural syncope, falls (with a risk of splenic rupture) and fatal cardiac arrhythmias. Hyperpyrexia should be prevented by vigorous tepid sponging and fanning and with antipyretics. Most patients with acute louse-borne relapsing fever are hypovolaemic. Adults may require 4 l or more of isotonic saline by intravenous infusion during the first 24 h. Infusion should be controlled by observing jugular venous pressure or monitoring central venous pressure. Myocardial failure may present as acute pulmonary oedema during the flush phase of the J-HR or spontaneous crisis. In adults, digoxin 1 mg has proved effective when given intravenously over 5–10 min. Diuretics may accentuate the circulatory failure by reducing circulating volume. Oxygen should be given during the reaction. Vitamin K is indicated in patients with prolonged prothrombin times. Heparin is not effective in controlling coagulopathy and should not be used. Complicating infections, such as typhoid, salmonellosis, bacillary dysentery, tuberculosis, typhus and malaria, must be identified and treated appropriately.

Control

Patients with louse-borne relapsing fever are infectious until their louse-infested clothing is disinfected by heat, such as washing in water hotter than 60°C, preferably followed by ironing. Because in heavy infestations lice may be attached to body hairs, it is sometimes good practice to shave off all body hairs and wash patients' bodies with soap and a 1% lysol (disinfectant) solution; however, it should be remembered that most lice will be attached to clothing, not body hairs. These simple approaches are impractical in epidemic situations; consequently insecticides are widely used for louse control. Ten per cent DDT powder can be blown by an insecticidal duster between the body and clothing. If DDT-resistant lice are present, then dusts of 1% malathion, 2% temephos (Abate), 1% propoxur or 0.5% permethrin can be used. Impregnation of clothing with a pyrethroid insecticide may give long-lasting protection against lice, and treated clothes may remain effective even after 6–8 washings.

No vaccine is available.

Selected bibliography

Barbour, A.G. (1987) Immunobiology of relapsing fever. *Contributions to Microbiological Immunology* 8, 125–137.

Bryceson, A.D.M., Parry, E.H.O., Perine, P.L., Warrell, D.A., Vukotich, D. and Leithead, C.S. (1970) Louse-borne relapsing fever: a clinical and laboratory study of 62 cases in Ethiopia and a reconsideration of the literature. *Quarterly Journal of Medicine* 153, 129–170.

Cutler, S.J., Fekade, D., Hussein, K., Knox, K.A., Melka, A., Cann, K., Emilianus, A.R., Warrell, D.A. and Wright, D.J.M. (1994) Successful in-vitro cultivation of *Borrelia recurrentis*. *The Lancet* 343, 242.

Fekade, D., Knox, K., Hussein, K., Melka, A., Lalloo, D.G., Coxon, R.E. and Warrell, D.A. (1996) Prevention of Jarisch–Herxheimer reactions by treatment with antibodies against tumor necrosis factor α. *New England Journal of Medicine* 335, 311–315.

Vidal, V., Scragg, I.G., Cutler, S.J., Rockett, K.A., Fekade, D., Warrell, D.A. and Wright D.J.M. (1998) Variable major lipoprotein is a principal TNF-inducing factor of louse-borne relapsing fever. *Nature Medicine* 4, 1416–1420.

Warrell, D.A., Pope, H.M., Parry, E.H.O., Perine, P.L. and Bryceson, A.D. (1970) Cardio-respiratory disturbances associated with infective fever in man: studies of Ethiopian louse-borne relapsing fever. *Clinical Science* 39, 123–145.

Louse-borne typhus *see* **Epidemic typhus.**

Lumbar paralysis *see* **Setariosis.**

Lyme borreliosis

Klaus Kurtenbach

Lyme borreliosis, or Lyme disease, is the most frequent tick-borne infection in humans. The disease, caused by the spirochaete *Borrelia burgdorferi* sensu lato (s.l.), has been named after the town of Old Lyme in Connecticut, USA, where a clustering of clinical cases was observed in the late 1970s. This prompted a large-scale epidemiological study, resulting in the identification of the causative agent by Dr Willy Burgdorfer in 1982.

Distribution

Lyme borreliosis occurs in temperate climates of the northern hemisphere, in both the New World and the Old World (Fig. 1). Its distribution is correlated with the prevalence of vector-competent hard (ixodid) ticks, most of which belong to the *Ixodes ricinus* species complex. Lyme borreliosis prevails in a large variety of different habitats, ranging from woodlands and urban parks to pastures (in maritime climates). As a general rule, moist woodland habitats usually harbour the highest numbers of infected ticks.

Lyme disease has become the commonest arthropod-transmitted infection to humans in the USA, with some 122,000 cases reported from 1990 to 1999, of which over 16,000 occurred in 1999.

Aetiological agent

Borrelia burgdorferi s.l. is a motile, two-membrane and spiral-shaped spirochaete with a diameter of around 0.2 μm and a length of up to 15 μm (Fig. 2). No free-living stages of this pathogen are known. In the vertebrate host it lives primarily extracellularly, but has been shown to occasionally survive in macrophages. Throughout the life cycle, the microenvironment alternates as the spirochaete is cyclically transmitted between the invertebrate vector (tick) and

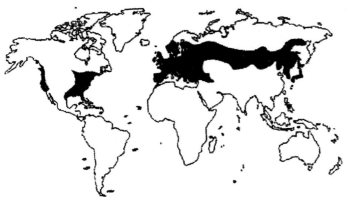

Fig. 1. Global distribution of Lyme borreliosis.

the vertebrate host. Motility is based on a set of periplasmic flagella, which allow the spirochaetes to move through viscous solutions. As chemotaxis genes have been identified, motility in the host is likely to be directed. The metabolic capacities of the microparasite are limited. Therefore, culturing of *B. burgdorferi* s.l. is fastidious and requires complex media and low oxygen tension.

The genome of one strain of *B. burgdorferi* sensu stricto (s.str.) has been sequenced recently, revealing a highly unusual genomic organization. The pathogen contains a linear chromosome and up to 20 linear and circular plamids ('minichromosomes'). About half of all proteins are encoded by genes located on such extrachromosomal elements – for example, the major outer surface lipoproteins OspA, OspB and OspC. Based on sequence information, approximately 40% of the open-reading frames (ORF) on the chromosome cannot yet be assigned a biological function. Only 16% of the plasmid ORFs could be identified, including the proteins OspA–D, the VisE lipoprotein recombination cassette and the decorin-binding proteins. Thus, the biological significance of many plasmid-encoded genes remains obscure. Another striking result of the genome project was that no virulence factors were recognized, and yet a subset of the bacteria causes disease in

humans and some domesticated and laboratory animals.

Genetic recombination by one or other mechanism occurs at a number of loci, generating antigenic diversity, a feature *B. burgdorferi* s.l. shares with relapsing fever spirochaetes (see Louse- and Tick-borne relapsing fevers). Furthermore, antigenic phase variation ('switch on–off') plays an important role in the biology of *B. burgdorferi* s.l. For example, OspA, OspB and OspC (and many other genes) are differentially expressed in the host and the tick vector. Antigenic phase variation is likely to be an important mechanism of immune evasion or immune avoidance. This finding has been exploited for the design of a transmission-blocking vaccine targeting a concealed antigen, the OspA, selectively expressed in the mid-gut of the infected tick. Vaccine-induced borreliacidal antibodies directed to OspA are taken up by the feeding tick and thus eradicate the spirochaetes before they are delivered to the host.

Phylogenetic analyses have revealed that *B. burgdorferi* s.l. is a genetically diverse species complex. At present, ten named *Borrelia* genospecies have been delineated and given Linnaean binomial species names, i.e. *B. burgdorferi* s.str., *B. afzelii*, *B. garinii*, *B. valaisiana*, *B. bissettii*, *B. japonica*, *B. lusitaniae*, *B. andersonii*, *B. turdae* and *B. tanukii*. The species complex also

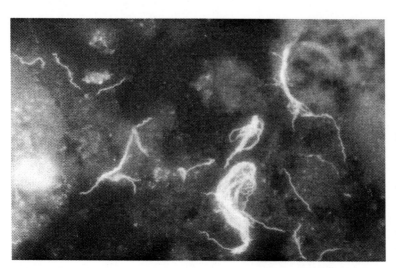

Fig. 2. *Borrelia burgdorferi* s.l. in the mid-gut of a questing *Ixodes ricinus* tick. The bacteria are probed with an immune serum to the outer surface protein A and visualized by immunofluorescence.

comprises a number of as yet unnamed genomic groups. The phylogenetic relationships of the various genospecies and genomic groups are not fully resolved. Multilocus genotyping methods are likely to clarify the evolutionary relationships in the near future.

Clinical symptoms

Human Lyme borreliosis comprises a large range of early and late (chronic) disease symptoms. Between 2 and 30 days after an infectious tick bite, the disease may set off with a typical skin rash, called erythema (chronicum) migrans (Fig. 3), or, more uncommonly, with borrelial lymphocytoma. Untreated, the disease may progress and become disseminated. The clinical features of early disseminated Lyme borreliosis (up to a year after initial infection) may include myalgia, arthralgia, radiculopathy, carditis and early neuroborreliosis (facial palsy, polyradiculitis, peripheral neuritis and mild encephalitis). Years post-infection, Lyme borreliosis may progress to late (chronic) disease, involving Lyme arthritis (frequent in North America), acrodermatitis chronica atrophicans (Fig. 4) (the most common manifestation of chronic Lyme borreliosis in Europe) or chronic neuroborreliosis (Eurasia). It is now accepted that the delineation of genospecies of *B. burgdorferi* s.l. is clinically relevant, in that the genospecies cause distinct symptoms of the disease. *Borrelia burgdorferi* s.str. is associated with Lyme arthritis, *B. afzelii* with dermatological symptoms and *B. garinii* with neuroborreliosis. The pathogenic potentials of the other genospecies are unknown.

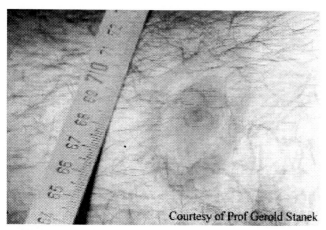

Courtesy of Prof Gerold Stanek

Fig. 3. Erythema chronicum migrans, an early skin manifestation of Lyme borreliosis.

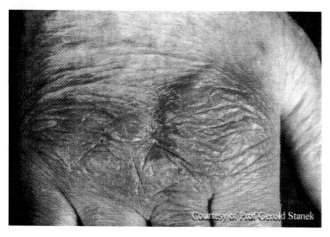

Courtesy of Prof Gerold Stanek

Fig. 4. Acrodermatitis chronica atrophicans, a late and chronic skin manifestation of Lyme borreliosis.

Diagnosis

Diagnosis of Lyme borreliosis in humans is based on a variety of non-microbiological, microbiological and serological methods.

Non-microbiological

Histopathological findings, in particular lymphocytic infiltrations, may be indicative for cutaneous manifestations of Lyme borreliosis, whereas lymphocytic pleocytosis in cerebrospinal fluid is an important indication of neuroborreliosis.

Microbiological

In recent years, the polymerase chain reaction (PCR), amplifying *Borrelia* DNA directly from tissue biopsies, cerebrospinal fluid or urine, has become an available technique, but it remains confined to specialized laboratories. Although PCR only detects spirochaetal DNA and not viable bacteria, it is recommended that positive results should prompt antibiotic treatment. Culturing of *B. burgdorferi* s.l. is widely regarded as the 'gold standard' in Lyme borreliosis diagnosis; however, it appears to be much less sensitive than PCR.

Serological

Serology remains the most important testing approach. It is based on the detection of specific antibodies to antigens of *B. burgdorferi* s.l. Antibodies can be detected using the immunofluorescence antibody assay (IFA), enzyme-linked immunosorbent assay (ELISA) and immuno- (Western) blot. Generally, IFA and ELISA tests are used in serodiagnostic screening, whereas the immunoblot is more specific and used as a confirmatory test. Recombinant antigens are now being used in ELISA and immunoblot assays, increasing sensitivity and specificity. Due to the antigenic heterogeneity of *Borrelia* strains, the correct source of antigen used is crucial in the interpretation of results. Standardization of criteria for interpretation of immunoblots is still incomplete.

Transmission

Ticks

All the genospecies of *B. burgdorferi* s.l. are transmitted by hard (ixodid) ticks belonging to the *Ixodes ricinus* species complex. In the north-east of the USA *Ixodes scapularis* (synonym *Ixodes dammini*) is the most abundant vector tick, whereas in the north-west of the USA (e.g. California) *Ixodes pacificus* prevails. *Ixodes ricinus* is the most important vector in many parts of Europe (Fig. 5). Towards the east of Europe, *I. ricinus* becomes rare, gradually being replaced by *Ixodes persulcatus*, a tick species adapted to more continental climates.

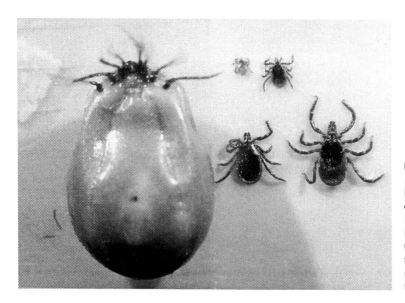

Fig. 5. *Ixodes ricinus* ticks. Upper lane from the left: questing larva, questing nymph. Lower lane from the left: fully engorged adult female, questing male, questing female.

The two tick species overlap geographically along a corridor in the east of Europe. Various other ixodid ticks play roles in the ecology of *B. burgdorferi* s.l., but many of these species do not bite humans. For example, *Ixodes spinipalpis* (= *neotomae*) or *Ixodes jellisoni* (in the USA) and *Ixodes hexagonus* and *Ixodes trianguliceps* (in Eurasia) maintain the spirochaetes in cryptic transmission cycles.

Ticks ingest spirochaetes during a blood meal on an infected animal. The spirochaetes then colonize the mid-gut of the tick and, under permissive conditions, are usually retained throughout the development to the next life stage (i.e. trans-stadial transmission), occasionally also involving transovarial transmission. Transmission of the pathogens from the tick to the host is a complex process. Stimulated by the blood meal, the spirochaetes multiply in the mid-gut of the tick. After penetration of the mid-gut epithelium, they migrate to the salivary glands, from where they are delivered to the host. During this process, which lasts several days and which involves the interaction of spirochaetes with host-derived factors, such as plasminogen, the bacteria undergo antigenic phase variation and become host-adapted. There seem to be critical steps in the process. For example, host complement poses selective contraints on the bacteria in the ticks' mid-gut (see below). In addition, transmission of *Borrelia* between ticks and hosts appears to be influenced by immunological processes at the tick–host interface. Tick saliva affects the hosts' haemostatic, immune and inflammatory responses. Immunomodulatory and immunogenic qualitites of tick saliva may either potentiate or inhibit transmission of *B. burgdorferi* s.l., depending on the particular combination of host and tick species in a density-dependent way. The precise mechanisms underlying these observations are unknown.

Reservoir hosts

Reservoir hosts are hosts upon which a feeding tick efficiently acquires *B. burgdorferi* s.l. Stable circulation of *B. burgdorferi* s.l. in nature (i.e. the basic reproduction number, R_0, is higher than 1) requires the coincidence of vector-competent ticks and reservoir hosts. Small rodents have always been regarded as the principal reservoir hosts, but accumulating evidence indicates that many bird species are highly reservoir-competent for *B. burgdorferi* s.l. Deer have been shown to be reservoir-incompetent for *B. burgdorferi* s.l.; however, they can play an important role as tick hosts and thus indirectly contribute to the circulation of Lyme disease spirochaetes.

Globally, more than 100 animal species have so far been recorded as reservoir hosts. In terms of biomass, small rodents, passerine birds and, at least locally, game birds are considered to be the most important reservoir hosts in sylvatic foci of Lyme borreliosis. Spirochaetes may persist for a long time in vertebrates (sometimes lifelong), despite the generation of specific antibodies. Reservoir hosts do not seem to develop disease, although minor symptoms may be confounded by other factors.

Reservoir competence seems to be species-specific. West European genotypes of *B. garinii* and *B. valaisiana*, for example, are preferentially transmitted to ticks by birds, whereas *B. afzelii* is maintained by rodent hosts. *Borrelia burgdorferi* s.str., in contrast, has a broader host range, involving both avian and mammalian species. The reservoir hosts of other *Borrelia* species, such as *B. lusitaniae*, are still unknown. A key determinant of reservoir competence is the complement system of the host, an important element of innate immunity. *Borrelia* strains differ in their sensitivity/resistance to complement of animal species. Complement-mediated lysis (i.e. selection) appears to take place in the mid-gut of the feeding tick rather than in the host, rendering the mid-gut of the tick a bottleneck in terms of transmission. Population genetic studies, furthermore, suggest the operation of frequency-dependent selection of *B. burgdorferi* s.l., probably mediated by adaptive immunity. Altogether, information on the genetic population structure of

B. burgdorferi s.l. and on the forces that shape this structure is highly relevant in our understanding of the ecology and evolution of the spirochaetes.

Consistent with the observation that the ecology of Lyme borreliosis is substantially influenced by the structure of the host community, the global distribution of the genospecies and subtypes of *B. burgdorferi* s.l. is not even. In the north of America, *B. burgdorferi* s.str. is the most prevalent strain, followed by *B. bissettii* and *B. andersonii*. In Eurasia, *B. afzelii*, *B. garinii* and *B. valaisiana* are the most frequent genospecies. Surprisingly, it emerged that *B. burgdorferi* s.str. is very rare in Europe and absent from Asia. High genospecies diversity and infection prevalences have been recorded for central parts of Eurasia, with 50% or more of questing adult ticks carrying borreliae. Data available so far indicate that genospecies diversity declines towards the south–west of the Old World geographical range of Lyme borreliosis. *Borrelia garinii*, the genetically most diverse genospecies of *B. burgdorferi* s.l., displays a pronounced geographical population structure. Most strains of this genospecies occurring in the west of Europe (type 20047) have been found to be maintained by avian hosts, while the strains detected towards the east of Eurasia (type NT 29) are adapted to mammalian–tick transmission systems. A few genospecies are geographically restricted. *Borrelia lusitaniae* mainly occurs on the Iberian Peninsula, while *B. japonica*, *B. turdi* and *B. tanukii* are confined to the Far East, including Japan.

Treatment

At present, treatment of Lyme borreliosis is based on antibiotics. As a guideline, all cases with clinical symptoms should receive antibiotic treatment in order to prevent disease progression.

The drugs of choice are as follows.

1. For erythema migrans and borrelia lymphocytoma: amoxicillin (3 × 500 mg, oral for 14–21 days), doxycycline (2 × 100 mg, oral for 14–21 days), penicillin V (3 × 1000 mg, oral for 14–21 days) and cefuroxime axetil (2 × 500 mg, oral for 14–21 days).

2. For Lyme arthritis: amoxicillin (4 × 500 mg, oral for 21–28 days), doxycycline 2 × 100 mg, oral for 21–28 days), ceftriaxone (1 × 2000 mg, i.v. for 14–21 days) and cefotaxime (3 × 2000 mg, i.v. for 14–21 days).

3. For neuroborreliosis: ceftriaxone (1 × 2000 mg, i.v. for 14–21 days), cefotaxime (3 × 2000 mg, i.v. for 14–21 days), penicillin G (3 × 3000 mg, i.v. for 14–21 days) and doxycycline (2 × 200 mg, oral for 14–21 days).

4. For acrodermatitis chronica atrophicans: amoxicillin (4 × 500 mg, oral for 21–28 days), doxycycline (2 × 100 mg, oral for 21–28 days), ceftriaxone (1 × 2000 mg, i.v. for 14–21 days), cefotaxime (3 × 2000 mg, i.v. for 14–21 days) and penicillin G (3 × 3000 mg, i.v. for 14–21 days).

5. For Lyme carditis: ceftriaxone (1 × 2000 mg, i.v. for 14 days), cefotaxime (3 × 2000 mg, i.v. for 14 days) and penicillin G (3 × 3000 mg, i.v. for 14 days).

Tetracyclines are contraindicated in children (of less than 12 or 8 years) and pregnant women. Jarisch–Herxheimer reactions sometimes occur during the first day of treatment and patients with heart block may require cardiac monitoring.

In the future, polyvalent therapeutic vaccines may become available. At present, preclinical developments are under way.

Prevention and control

Because tick control measures are not appropriate for the control of Lyme borreliosis, prevention largely relies on personal precautions against tick bites and prophylaxis.

Personal precautions take the biology of the tick and the life cycle of *B. burgdorferi* s.l. into consideration. Avoiding tick bites is possible either by staying away from tick habitats, especially in spring and summer, or by applying chemical repellents and the use of protective clothing, preferably impregnated with tick repellents or insecticides, such as the pyrethroids. Careful examination of clothes and body for ticks is recommended, because it usually takes at least 24 h after attachment before the spirochaetes are transmitted. Hence, early removal of attached ticks can be an effective preventive method.

Antibiotic treatment after a tick bite is a possible measure of prevention; however, it is not recommended in Europe. A vaccine is now commercially available in the USA (LYMErix, SmithKline Beecham). The OspA-based vaccine has been designed against *B. burgdorferi* s.str. and is not cross-protective against the most abundant pathogenic genospecies in Eurasia, *B. garinii* and *B. afzelii*. Although various preclinical studies are currently being carried out, a major obstacle in the development of vaccines against Eurasian *Borrelia* strains is the substantial allelic diversity of the proteins targeted.

Selected bibliography

Anderson, J.F. (1991) Epizootiology of Lyme borreliosis. *Scandinavian Journal of Infectious Diseases* 77, 23–34.

Barbour, A.G. and Hayes, S.F. (1986) Biology of *Borrelia* species. *Microbiological Reviews* 50, 381–400.

Burgdorfer, W., Barbour, A.G., Hayes, S.F., Benach, J.L., Grunwaldt, E. and Davis, J.P. (1982) Lyme disease – a tick-borne spirochetosis. *Science* 216, 1317–1319.

Coleman, J.L., Gebbia, J.A., Piesman, J., Degen, J.L., Bugge, T.H. and Benach, J.L. (1997) Plasminogen is required for efficient dissemination of *B. burgdorferi* in ticks and for enhancement of spirochetemia in mice. *Cell* 89, 1111–1119.

Fraser, C.M., Casjens, S., Huang, W.M., Sutton, G.G., Clayton, R., Lathigra, R., White, O., Ketchum, K.A., Dodson, R., Hickey, E.K., Gwinn, M., Dougherty, B., Tomb, J.-F., Fleishmann, R.D., Richardson, D., Peterson, J., Kerlavage, A.R., Quackenbush, J., Salzberg, S., Hanson, M., van Vugt, R., Palmer, N., Adams, M.D., Gocayne, J., Weidman, J., Utterback, T., Watthey, L., McDonald, L., Artriach, P., Bowman, C., Garland, S., Fujii, C., Cotton, M.D., Horst, K., Roberts, K., Hatch, B., Smith, H.O. and Venter, J. C. (1997) Genomic sequence of a Lyme disease spirochaete, *Borrelia burgdorferi*. *Nature* 390, 580–586.

Gylfe, Å., Bergström, S., Lunstrom, J. and Olsen, B. (2000) Epidemiology – reactivation of *Borrelia* infection in birds. *Nature* 403, 724–725.

Humair, P.F., Rais, O. and Gem, L. (1999) Transmission of *Borrelia afzelii* from *Apodemus* mice and *Clethrionomys* voles to *Ixodes ricinus* ticks: differential transmission pattern and overwintering maintenance. *Parasitology* 118, 33–42.

Kurtenbach, K., Sewell, H.-S., Ogden, N.H., Randolph, S.E. and Nuttall, P.A. (1998) Serum complement sensitivity as a key factor in Lyme disease ecology. *Infection and Immunity* 66, 1248–1251.

Qui, W.-G., Bosler, E., Campbell, J.R., Ugine, G.D., Wang, I.-N., Luft, B.J. and Dykhuizen, D.E. (1997) A population genetic study of *Borrelia burgdorferi* sensu stricto from eastern Long Island, New York, suggested frequency-dependent selection, gene flow and host adaptation. *Hereditas* 127, 203–216.

Randolph, S.E. (1998) Ticks are not insects: consequences of contrasting vector biology for transmission potential. *Parasitology Today* 14, 186–192.

Steere, A.C. (1989) Lyme disease. *New England Journal of Medicine* 321, 586–596.

Zhong, W.M., Stehle, T., Museteanu, C., Siebers, A., Gem, L., Kramer, M., Wallich, R. and Simon, M.M. (1997) Therapeutic passive vaccination against chronic Lyme disease in mice. *Proceedings of the National Academy of Sciences of the United States of America* 94, 12533–12538.

Lyme disease *see* **Lyme borreliosis.**

Lyperosia *see* **Horn-flies.**

Malaria, avian

Carter T. Atkinson

Avian malaria is a common mosquito-transmitted disease of wild birds that infects domestic fowl and 'cage birds' when suitable vectors and wild reservoir hosts are present. Infections are caused by a complex of more than 30 species of *Plasmodium*, which differ widely in host range, geographical distribution, vectors and pathogenicity. They are currently organized into five subgenera, which are distinguished by the morphological characteristics of the erythrocytic stages of the parasites, by the morphological changes in their host cells and by their preference for either mature erythrocytes or erythrocyte precursors. Species that infect domestic birds occur in four of these five subgenera and are separated further by host range, developmental characteristics and vectors. The avian species of *Plasmodium* share morphological and developmental features with closely related haemosporidian parasites in the genera *Haemoproteus* and *Leucocytozoon* (see Haemoproteosis and Leucocytozoonosis) but are distinguished from these parasites by the presence of schizogony in circulating erythrocytes.

Plasmodium relictum (subgenus Haemamoeba)

Distribution

Worldwide: *Plasmodium relictum* has one of the widest host ranges of the avian plasmodia, occurring naturally in 70 different avian families and 359 species of wild birds. This species can infect Canaries (*Serinus canaria*) and other 'cage birds' when suitable reservoir hosts and vectors are present.

Parasite

The life cycle (Fig. 1) begins when infective sporozoites are inoculated by a mosquito vector into a susceptible host. Sporozoites invade macrophages and fibroblasts near the site of the mosquito bite and undergo asexual schizogony as cryptozoites. These mature in approximately 36–48 h and release ovoid merozoites, which invade cells of the lymphoid–macrophage system in brain, spleen, kidney, lung and liver tissue to begin a second generation of asexual schizogony as metacryptozoites. The metacryptozoites mature and release merozoites, which are capable of invading circulating erythrocytes and capillary endothelial cells of the major organs. Merozoites that continue with a third generation of schizogony in fixed tissues of the host are called phanerozoites and produce merozoites that can either invade circulating erythrocytes or reinvade endothelial cells to continue additional generations of schizogony in fixed tissues. Merozoites that invade the circulating erythrocytes develop within 36 h into either mature segmenters, containing 8–32 ovoid merozoites, or gametocytes, which are infective to mosquito vectors. Schizogony can continue indefinitely in the peripheral circulation and evidence suggests that merozoites from some erythrocytic schizonts can reinvade fixed tissues and continue development as phanerozoites.

Birds typically undergo an acute phase of infection, where parasitaemia increases steadily to reach a peak approximately 9 days after parasites first appear in the blood. This is followed by a rapid decline in intensity of infection to chronic levels, which persist for the lifetime of infected individuals.

Plasmodium relictum can readily infect canaries, but occurs more rarely in ducks and does not develop in chickens or turkeys. The parasite has been reported rarely from Pheasants (*Tragopan satyra*) and Blue quail (*Coturnix chinensis*). Many different strains of the parasite have been described that differ slightly in morphological features, developmental characteristics and ability to be transmitted by different species of mosquitoes. Two subspecies of the parasite are

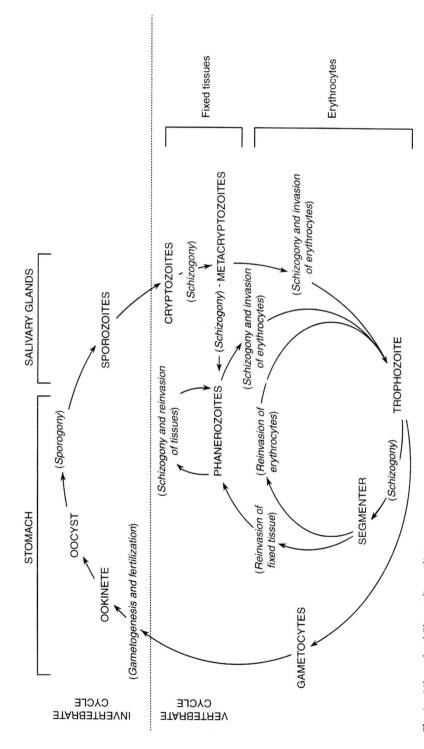

Fig. 1. Life cycle of *Plasmodium relictum*.

currently recognized – *P. relictum relictum* and *P. relictum capistranoae* – but their relationships with each other and to closely related species of *Plasmodium* are poorly defined.

Related species

Closely related Plasmodium species from non-galliform hosts include *P. matutinum* from pigeons and doves (*Columba* species) and *P. cathemerium* and *P. giovannolai* from passerine birds. They are distinguished from *P. relictum* by relatively minor morphological and developmental differences and variability in host range. It is likely that further work on this complex of closely related species will lead to taxonomic revisions.

Clinical symptoms

Plasmodium relictum can be highly pathogenic in canaries. Birds with acute infections are typically lethargic and anorexic, with ruffled feathers. Gross lesions include thin and watery blood and enlargement and discoloration of the liver and spleen by deposition of malarial pigment in tissue

macrophages (Fig. 2). Infected birds succumb to severe anaemia, caused by destruction of erythrocytes by developing schizonts. Birds that recover from acute infections are immune to reinfection with homologous strains of the parasite.

Diagnosis

Parasites can be detected in Giemsa-stained thin blood smears (Fig. 3). The presence of schizonts with 8–32 merozoites and round or oval gametocytes that displace the host cell nucleus is characteristic of passerine species of the subgenus *Haemamoeba*. *Plasmodium relictum* is differentiated from its closely related species by both host species and morphological and developmental differences.

Transmission

Culex species such as *C. quinquefasciatus*, *C. tarsalis* and *C. stigmatasoma* are proved natural vectors of *P. relictum* in Hawaii and California, but few detailed epidemiological studies of *P. relictum* have been done and natural vectors of the parasite in other parts of its range are unknown. More than 20

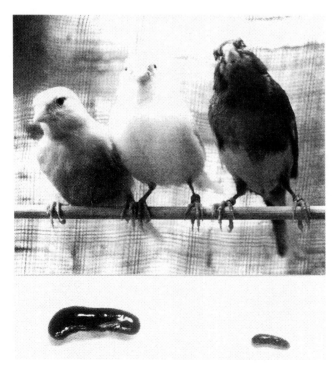

Fig. 2. Spleens from infected (left) and uninfected (right) canaries.

species of anopheline and culicine mosquitoes in four different genera (*Anopheles*, *Aedes*, *Culex* and *Culiseta*) are capable of transmitting *P. relictum* in the laboratory. Sporogony in developing oocysts is rapid at temperatures between 25 and 30°C and takes 5–8 days, eventually producing thousands of sporozoites, which bud from multiple sporoblasts (Fig. 4). Oocysts subsequently rupture, releasing sporozoites into the haemocoel of the mosquito. These invade the salivary glands and pass through the salivary ducts during the next blood meal.

Treatment
Both chloroquine phosphate and primaquine phosphate may be effective in treating canaries infected with *P. relictum*. However, detailed studies of the pharmacokinetics of these drugs in passerines have not been done. Appropriate dosages are not established.

Control
Reduction of populations of mosquito vectors could probably reduce transmission of *P. relictum*, but this method has not been tested for this parasite. More cost-effective measures include housing 'cage birds' in screened, mosquito-proof buildings, or locating birds in areas that are isolated from wild reservoir hosts.

Plasmodium gallinaceum (subgenus *Haemamoeba*)
Distribution
South-East Asia, Indonesia, Malaysia, Borneo, India and Sri Lanka. The natural host for *P. gallinaceum* is the wild Red jungle fowl (*Gallus gallus*). The distribution of the parasite in domestic chickens coincides with the geographical range of the natural host and has not expanded with the movement of domestic poultry to other parts of the world.

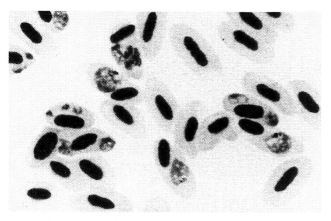

Fig. 3. Giemsa-stained blood smear from a canary infected with *Plasmodium relictum*.

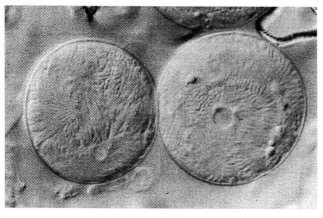

Fig. 4. Oocysts of *Plasmodium relictum* on the mid-gut wall of *Culex quinquefasciatus*. Both oocysts contain densely packed, slender sporozoites.

Parasite

The life cycle begins when infective sporozoites are inoculated by a mosquito vector into a susceptible host. Sporozoites invade macrophages near the site of the mosquito bite and undergo asexual schizogony as cryptozoites. These mature in approximately 36–48 h and release elongate merozoites, which spread via the circulation. These merozoites invade macrophages and begin a second generation of asexual schizogony as metacryptozoites. Metacryptozoites reach maturity at approximately 72 h and release merozoites that are capable of invading circulating erythrocytes, cells of the lymphoid–macrophage system in the skin, spleen and lungs and capillary endothelial cells of the major organs, with the exception of the brain and bone marrow. Merozoites that continue with a third generation of schizogony in fixed tissues of the host are called phanerozoites and produce merozoites that can either invade circulating erythrocytes or reinvade endothelial cells and macrophages to continue additional generations of schizogony in fixed tissues. Merozoites that invade the circulating erythrocytes develop within 36 h into either mature schizonts, containing 16–20 ovoid merozoites, or gametocytes, which are infective to mosquito vectors. Schizogony can continue indefinitely in the peripheral circulation.

Birds typically undergo an acute phase of infection, where parasitaemia increases steadily to reach a peak approximately 9 days after parasites first appear in the blood. This peak is followed by a rapid decline in intensity to chronic levels, which persist for years.

Plasmodium gallinaceum can infect geese, ducks, pheasants (*Tragopan satyra*), turkeys, Partridges (*Perdix perdix*) and Guinea fowl (*Numida meleagris*) in the laboratory, but the susceptibility of these hosts to the parasite is low and they probably do not acquire infections under natural conditions of transmission.

Closely related species

Closely related *Plasmodium* species from galliform hosts include *P. griffithsi* from domestic turkeys in South-East Asia, *P. tejerai* from domestic turkeys in South America and *P. coturnixi* from quail (*Coturnix coturnix*) in Pakistan. *Plasmodium griffithsi* can cause fatal infections in adult domestic turkeys.

Clinical symptoms

Plasmodium gallinaceum can be highly pathogenic in domestic chickens, particularly when European breeds are introduced into endemic areas where the cycle is maintained in wild Red jungle fowl (*G. gallus*). Young chicks are more susceptible than adult birds. Birds with acute infections may be lethargic, have pale combs and suffer from diarrhoea and partial or total paralysis. Anaemia, caused by destruction of circulating erythrocytes by developing schizonts, and neurological complications, caused by obstruction of capillaries in the brain by exoerythrocytic schizonts, are the primary causes of death.

Diagnosis

Parasites can be seen in Giemsa-stained thin blood smears. The presence of schizonts with numerous merozoites and round gametocytes that displace the host cell nucleus are distinctive for *P. gallinaceum*. The only other malarial parasite known to occur in domestic chickens is *P. juxtanucleare*, which can be distinguished by its smaller size and more elongate gametocytes.

Transmission

Mansonia crassipes is a proved natural vector of *P. gallinaceum* in Sri Lanka, but detailed epidemiological studies of *P. gallinaceum* have not been done and vectors of the parasite in other parts of its range are unknown. More than 40 different species of anopheline and culicine mosquitoes in six different genera (*Anopheles*, *Aedes*, *Armigeres*, *Culex*, *Culiseta* and *Mansonia*) are capable of transmitting *P. gallinaceum* in the laboratory (*Aedes aegypti* is a convenient laboratory host for transferring infections from bird to bird by mosquito bite). Sporogony in developing oocysts takes about 10 days, eventually producing thousands of sporozoites, which bud from multiple sporoblasts. Oocysts subsequently rupture, releasing sporozoites into the haemocoel of the mosquito. These invade the salivary glands and pass down the salivary ducts during the next blood meal and are injected into a new avian host.

Treatment

Plasmodium gallinaceum is a common laboratory model for screening the efficacy of experimental antimalarial drugs for humans, but little work has gone into adapting these compounds for veterinary use. The anti-coccidial drugs sulfamonomethoxine, sulfa-chloropyrazine and halofuginone are some-what effective in treating *Plasmodium durae* in domestic turkeys and may also be effective against *P. gallinaceum*.

Control

Reduction of populations of mosquito vectors can in theory probably reduce transmission of *P. gallinaceum*, but this method has not been tested for this parasite. More cost-effective measures may be to move poultry operations into screened, mosquito-proof buildings, or to locate birds in areas that are isolated from wild reservoir hosts.

Plasmodium durae (subgenus *Giovannolaia*)

Distribution

Sub-Saharan Africa, with reports from Kenya, Nigeria, Zimbabwe and South Africa. *Plasmodium durae* is a parasite of wild francolins (*Francolinus leucoscepus* and *Francolinus levaillantii levaillantii*) that infects domestic turkeys when wild reservoir hosts and vectors are present.

Parasite

The detailed life cycle of *P. durae* has not been described.

Exoerythrocytic schizonts have been found in capillary endothelial cells of lung, liver, spleen and brain tissue, but are especially numerous in the brain, where their large size can occlude blood flow. When infections in domestic turkeys are initiated by subinoculation of infected blood, parasitaemias peak between 15 and 25 days post-inoculation and subsequently decline to subpatent levels. The erythrocytic cycle

requires 24 h for merozoites to mature into schizonts or gametocytes. Mature gameto-cytes are most numerous in the peripheral circulation after peak parasitaemia.

Plasmodium durae can be transmitted by blood inoculation to Japanese quail (*Coturnix japonica*) and Lady Amherst pheasants (*Chrysolophus amherstiae*), but domestic chickens, ducks, Guinea fowl (*Numida meleagris*) and Canaries (*Serinus canaria*) are refractory to infection.

Related species

Closely related species in the subgenus *Giovannolaia* that can occur in domestic birds include *P. fallax*, *P. circumflexum*, *P. polare*, *P. lophurae*, *P. gabaldoni*, *P. pinotti*, *P. pediocettii*, *P. formosanum*, *P. anasum* and *P. hegneri*. These parasites have been reported from ducks, geese, turkeys, francolins, Guinea fowl, quail (*Coturnix* species), Partridges (*Perdix perdix*) and pigeons (*Columba* species) from around the world. Little is known about their pathogenicity under conditions of natural transmission.

Clinical symptoms

Plasmodium durae is highly pathogenic in domestic turkeys. Depending on geographical origin and strain of the parasite, mortalities can be up to 90% in young poults. Young turkeys exhibit few clinical signs until immediately before death, when severe convulsions may occur. Adult turkeys typically become lethargic and anorexic and often develop right pulmonary hypertension as a consequence of hypoxic pulmonary arterial hypertension. Adult birds may also develop oedematous legs and gangrene of the wattles. Cerebral capillaries may be blocked by developing exoerythrocytic schizonts and infected birds may exhibit neurological signs and paralysis before death.

Diagnosis

Giemsa-stained thin blood smears will identify the presence of parasites. The presence of small round schizonts and elongate gametocytes that do not curve around the host erythrocyte nucleus separate *P. durae* from *P. fallax*, *P. lophurae* and *P. circumf-lexum*. *Plasmodium formosanum*, *P. ana-sum*, *P. pinotti*, *P. pediocettii* and *P. hegneri* have not been reported from Africa. Neither *P. gabaldoni* nor *P. polare* has been reported in galliform hosts, but could potentially be confused with *P. durae*.

Transmission

Neither natural nor experimental mosquito vectors have been identified for *P. durae* and nothing is known about the sporogonic stages or epidemiology of the parasite. Out-breaks of the disease in domestic turkeys and pheasants have been documented in Kenya and Zimbabwe.

Treatment

The anticoccidial drugs sulfamono-methoxine, sulfachloropyrazine and halofuginone are somewhat effective in treating *P. durae* in domestic turkeys. Sulfamonomethoxine suppresses para-sitaemia, but does not provide full protec-tion from mortality when given after the appearance of circulating parasites. Sulfa-chloropyrazine reduces mortality, but has no effect on parasitaemia, suggesting that it has some efficacy against exoerythrocytic schizonts. Halofuginone delays para-sitaemia, but suppresses it to only a minor extent.

Control

As the mosquito species that transmit this parasite are unknown, vector control meth-ods are inappropriate. More cost-effective approaches to control may be to move poultry operations into screened, mosquito-proof buildings or to locate birds in areas that are isolated from wild reservoir hosts.

Plasmodium juxtanucleare (subgenus *Novyella*)
Distribution

Mexico, Brazil, Uruguay, Sri Lanka, Philip-pines, Taiwan, Japan, Malaysia, South Africa and Tanzania. *Plasmodium juxta-nucleare* is a parasite of wild birds that infects domestic chickens when wild reservoir hosts and vectors are present.

Parasite

Details about the pre-erythrocytic develop-ment of *P. juxtanucleare* have not been described. Exoerythrocytic schizonts have been reported in lymphoid–macrophage cells of the spleen, liver, kidney, heart, lung, bone marrow, testes, pancreas and brain, but are most common in the spleen. In sporozoite-induced experimental infec-tions, parasitaemia peaks 6–8 days after infection and then declines to chronic lev-els. The erythrocytic cycle requires approxi-mately 24 h for merozoites to mature into schizonts or gametocytes.

Proved wild reservoir hosts of infection in Sri Lanka, South Africa and Taiwan, respectively, are Red jungle fowl (*Gallus gallus*), Greywing francolins (*Francolinus africanus*) and Bamboo partridges (*Bam-busicola thoracica*), but natural hosts are not known for other parts of its range. *Plasmodium juxtanucleare* can be transmit-ted to domestic chickens and turkeys, but pigeons (*Columba* species), ducks, Guinea fowl (*Numida meleagris*), Canaries (*Seri-nus canaria*) and sparrows (*Passer* species) are not susceptible to the parasite.

Related species

Closely related species in the subgenus *Novyella* that can occur in 'cage birds', pigeons, waterfowl, Guinea fowl, Pheasants (*Tragopan satyra*), quail (*Coturnix* species) and turkeys include *P. vaughani*, *P. rouxi*, *P. nucleophilum*, *P. kempi*, *P. leanucleus* and *P. dissanaikei*. Little is known about their pathogenicity under conditions of natural transmission.

Clinical symptoms

Infected chickens appear healthy until shortly before death, when they become lethargic and anaemic and often develop diarrhoea. New World strains of the parasite are believed to be more pathogenic in domestic chickens than isolates from other parts of the world.

Diagnosis

Parasites can be seen in Giemsa-stained thin blood smears. *Plasmodium juxtanucleare* is one of only two malarial parasites that have been described in domestic chickens. This species can be distinguished from *P. gallinaceum* by its more elongate gametocytes and by the tendency of its asexual stages to cling closely to the host cell nucleus.

Transmission

Proved natural vectors include *Culex* species, such as *C. sitiens*, *C. annulus*, *C. gelidus* and *C. tritaeniorhynchus* in Malaysia and *Culex saltanensis* in Brazil. Natural vectors in other parts of its range remain unknown and detailed epidemiological studies of the parasite have not been undertaken.

Unusual pedunculated or stalked oocysts have been described during sporogonic development of the parasite on the outer midgut wall of its culicine vectors.

Treatment

Specific treatments for *P. juxtanucleare* have not been developed. As the anticoccidial drugs sulfamonomethoxine, sulfachloropyrazine and halofuginone are somewhat effective in treating *P. durae* in domestic turkeys, they may also be effective against *P. juxtanucleare*.

Control

Reduction of populations of mosquito vectors can reduce transmission of *P. juxtanucleare*, but this method has not been tested for this parasite and may not be practical in areas where the vectors are unknown. More cost-effective measures may be to move poultry operations into screened, mosquito-proof buildings or to locate birds in areas that are isolated from wild reservoir hosts.

Plasmodium elongatum (subgenus *Huffia*)

Distribution

North and South America, Europe and Africa. *Plasmodium elongatum* has a wide host range, occurring naturally in 21 different families and 59 species of birds. It infects 'cage birds', pigeons (*Columba* species) and ducks when wild reservoir hosts and suitable vectors are present.

Parasite

Details about the early pre-erythrocytic development of *P. elongatum* are unknown. After the parasite invades erythrocytes, exoerythrocytic schizonts are found primarily in haemocytoblasts and other erythrocyte precursors in bone marrow. *Plasmodium elongatum* and other species in the subgenus *Huffia* do not develop in capillary endothelial cells of the major organs, but instead undergo exoerythrocytic schizogony in haematopoietic tissues of the host. Merozoites from both erythrocytic and exoerythrocytic schizonts preferentially invade reticulocytes and complete asexual schizogony in 24 h. Gametocytes are long and narrow in shape, with irregular margins, and are found in mature erythrocytes. After parasites appear in circulating erythrocytes, parasitaemia increases steadily, peaks in intensity between 8 and 10 days and then declines.

Related species

Closely related species in the subgenus *Huffia* include *P. hermani* from Wild turkeys (*Meleagris gallopavo*) in the southeastern USA. This parasite does not cause high mortality in domestic turkeys.

Clinical symptoms

Plasmodium elongatum is highly pathogenic in canaries. Birds with acute infections are typically lethargic and anorexic, with ruffled feathers. Gross lesions include thin and watery blood and enlargement and discoloration of the liver and spleen by deposition of malarial pigment in tissue macrophages. Infected birds succumb to severe anaemia caused by destruction of haematopoietic tissue in the bone marrow and other organs. Birds that recover spontaneously from acute infections do not develop immunity to reinfection.

Diagnosis

Giemsa-stained thin blood smears will identify the parasites. *Plasmodium elongatum* and other members of the subgenus *Huffia* develop preferentially in reticulocytes. This characteristic, plus the presence of elongate, thin gametocytes, is diagnostic for this species.

Transmission

Proved natural vectors of *P. elongatum* are *Culex* mosquitoes and include *C. pipiens* and *C. restuans* in the eastern USA. *Culex nigripalpus*, *C. restuans* and *C. salinarius* are probable natural vectors in the south-eastern USA, based on their ability to transmit the parasite in the laboratory. Natural vectors in other parts of the world remain unknown.

Treatment

Both chloroquine phosphate and primaquine phosphate may be effective in treating canaries infected with *P. elongatum*, but detailed studies of the pharmacokinetics of these drugs in passerines have not been done. Appropriate dosages have not been established.

Control

Reduction of populations of mosquito vectors can reduce transmission of *P. elongatum*, but this method has not been tested for this parasite. More cost-effective measures may be to keep small cage birds in screened, mosquito-proof buildings or to locate birds in areas that are isolated from wild reservoir hosts.

Selected bibliography

Bennett, G.F. and Warren, M. (1966) Biology of the Malaysian strain of *Plasmodium juxtanucleare* Versiani and Gomes, 1941. III. Life cycle of the erythrocytic parasite in the avian host. *Journal of Parasitology* 52, 653–659.

Bennett, G.F., Bishop, M.A. and Peirce, M.A. (1993) Checklist of the avian species of *Plasmodium* Marchiafava & Celli, 1885 (Apicomplexa) and their distribution by avian family and Wallacean life zones. *Systematic Parasitology* 26, 171–179.

Garnham, P.C.C. (1966) *Malaria Parasites and Other Haemosporidia.* Blackwell Scientific Publications, Oxford, 1114 pp.

Huchzermeyer, F.W. (1993) Pathogenicity and chemotherapy of *Plasmodium durae* in experimentally infected domestic turkeys. *Onderstepoort Journal of Veterinary Research* 60, 103–110.

Huchzermeyer, F.W. (1996) Host range, survival in dead hosts, cryopreservation, periodicity and morphology of *Plasmodium durae* Herman in experimental infections. *Onderstepoort Journal of Veterinary Research* 63, 227–238.

Laird, M. (1998) *Avian Malaria in the Asian Tropical Subregion.* Springer-Verlag, Singapore, 130 pp.

Peirce, M.A. and Bennett, G.F. (1996) A revised key to the avian subgenera of *Plasmodium* Marchiafava & Celli, 1885 (Apicomplexa). *Systematic Parasitology* 33, 31–32.

Van Riper, C., III, Atkinson, C.T. and Seed, T.M. (1994) Plasmodia of birds. In: Kreier, J.P. (ed.) *Parasitic Protozoa*, Vol. 7. Academic Press, New York, pp. 73–140.

Malaria, human

M. Renshaw and J.B. Silver

Human malaria involves the infection of humans with four species of *Plasmodium*:

- *Plasmodium falciparum*;
- *Plasmodium malariae*;
- *Plasmodium ovale*;
- *Plasmodium vivax*.

Plasmodium falciparum is the most dangerous species of malaria parasite, as it may lead to the death of the patient, particularly if diagnosis and treatment are delayed. The greater severity of falciparum malaria is related to the sequestration of red blood cells containing dividing forms of the parasite in the deep capillaries of major organs. The other three species of malaria may also cause severe illness, but they are rarely fatal. The malaria parasite is transmitted to humans by mosquitoes of the genus *Anopheles*.

Distribution

Malaria is endemic in more than 100 countries and territories worldwide (Fig. 1), and current estimates put the number of people at risk at more than 2000 million, or 40% of

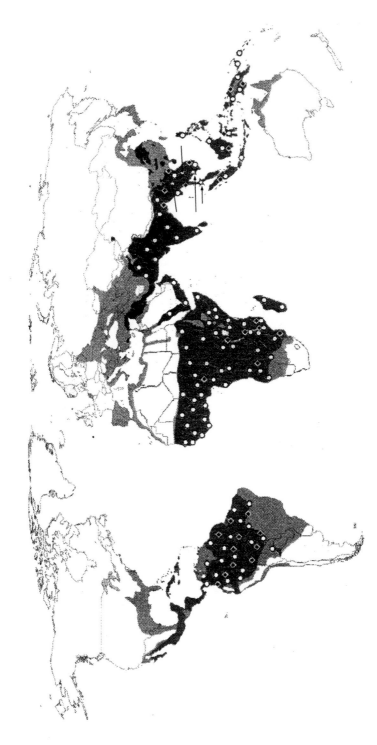

Fig. 1. Worldwide distribution of malaria transmission and drug resistance. Key: ■ Malaria transmission areas. ▦ Areas where malaria has been largely eliminated. ○ Resistance to chloroquine. ◆ Resistance to sulfadoxine–pyrimethamine reported. ☆ (and arrowed) Resistance to several antimalarial drugs, including chloroquine, sulfadoxine–pyrimethamine and mefloquine. Drawing by courtesy of UNICEF, adapted from an original by WHO.

the world's population. More than 90% of malaria cases occur in sub-Saharan Africa, where as many as three-quarters of a million people, mostly children under 5 years of age, die from the disease each year. Malaria also occurs in tropical regions of South America and Central and South-East Asia. *Plasmodium vivax* malaria is the most widespread species, occurring in both temperate and tropical regions. This species was formerly endemic in much of Europe, but has been largely eliminated through a combination of land drainage, socio-economic development, housing improvements, changes in animal husbandry practices and large-scale eradication campaigns. *Plasmodium falciparum* is the most common species in tropical Africa and much of South-East Asia, whilst *P. ovale* and *P. malariae* also occur in Africa, but at much lower frequencies. *Plasmodium falciparum* accounts for more than 95% of cases in many African countries.

As a result of increasing air traffic between temperate and tropical countries, the number of cases of falciparum malaria being imported into western Europe and North America is increasing. Malaria is currently undergoing an expansion into areas where it was previously absent, such as North and South Korea, or where it was previously under control, including Azerbaijan, northern Iraq and eastern Turkey. Changes in land use linked to development activities, such as road construction, agricultural and irrigation projects, mining and logging, have also led to a resurgence in malaria. Armed conflicts, mass movement of refugees and deterioration of health services have all contributed to reported increases in the disease. The worsening malaria situation globally has been exacerbated by the spread of *P. falciparum* resistance to chloroquine, an affordable drug with few side-effects, and the emergence of multi-drug-resistant strains of the parasite in parts of South-East Asia.

Parasite

Intracellular protozoan parasites in the phylum Apicomplexa, genus *Plasmodium*. *Plasmodium* species have a life cycle which includes both sexual and asexual phases (Fig. 2). Asexual phases occur in vertebrate animals, while the sexual phase of development takes place in vector mosquitoes.

Clinical symptoms

Symptoms of malaria vary between children and adults and will be considered separately (Table 1). Malaria illness (all species) should be suspected in any child exposed to malaria presenting with an acute fever of any periodicity. Symptoms of uncomplicated, non-severe malaria are highly variable and clinical presentation may mimic other infections and diseases, including septicaemia, acute respiratory infection, meningitis, typhoid, influenza and dengue. It is particularly difficult to distinguish between malaria and acute respiratory infection in children, as both are characterized by coughing, rapid and shallow breathing and fever. Diagnosis of malaria infection is important, as falciparum malaria can rapidly develop into a severe and complicated, life-threatening disease, particularly in small children, pregnant women and non-immune travellers. In practical terms, children in endemic areas presenting with fever should be treated with antimalarials unless malaria can be specifically excluded. A case of malaria is classified by the World Health Organization (WHO) as severe or complicated when there are parasites in the blood and one or more of the following symptoms are present: coma (cerebral malaria), respiratory distress, low blood sugar (hypoglycaemia), severe anaemia, repeated generalized convulsions, metabolic acidosis or shock. Other symptoms that support a diagnosis of severe malaria in children but are not definitive are: impaired consciousness, prostration and extreme weakness, high parasite loads, jaundice and a rectal temperature above 40°C. Signs of cerebral malaria or respiratory distress are important from a clinical perspective, as they are most commonly associated with death of the child.

Adults with uncomplicated malaria also present with acute fever, plus one or more of the following: headache, malaise, chills and sweats, abdominal and muscle

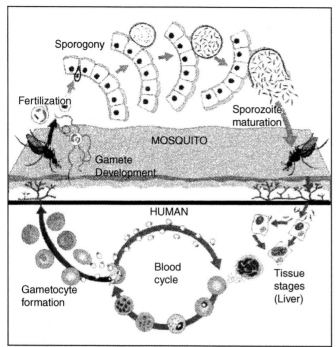

Fig. 2. Malaria parasite life cycle in the mosquito and in humans. Reproduced by courtesy of the Wellcome Trust.

pain, vomiting and watery diarrhoea. Adults do not usually present with a cough, rapid and shallow breathing or febrile convulsions. The most dangerous signs of severe and complicated malaria in adults are: coma, renal failure and pulmonary oedema.

Immunity to malaria

In areas of year-round, stable malaria transmission, repeated exposure to malaria parasites through frequent bites from infected mosquitoes leads to the acquisition of specific immunity. This specific acquired immunity largely restricts severe disease and death to children under 5 years of age and pregnant women. Malaria in older children and adults tends to be less severe and is rarely life-threatening, although attacks with fever and headache still occur. Infants under the age of 3 months are largely protected from severe malaria by antibodies obtained from the mother through the placenta and in breast milk. Young children are particularly at risk of cerebral malaria and severe anaemia, with the incidence of cerebral malaria peaking at around 3 years

of age, while severe anaemia is most common in children up to 18 months old. The severity of clinical attacks begins to decline in the fourth year, with the acquisition of immunity, although parasite densities can remain high. Malaria deaths become less common in children of more than 5 years of age and clinical attacks become less frequent and less severe. Immunity to malaria does not develop under conditions of low transmission intensity and, in countries where malaria is at the limit of its range of distribution, both adults and children are susceptible to severe disease and death. Immunity to malaria is not stable and may be lost in the absence of repeated bites from infected mosquitoes.

Diagnosis

A definitive diagnosis of malaria can only be obtained by demonstration of parasites in stained finger-prick blood smears examined under a microscope at high magnification (×1000). Thick films are prepared by placing a single drop of blood on to the centre of a glass slide. This drop of blood is

Table 1. Characteristics and symptoms of non-severe and uncomplicated and severe and complicated malaria in children and adults.

Children		Adults	
Non-severe, uncomplicated	Severe and complicated	Non-severe, uncomplicated	Severe and complicated
Acute fever (temperature > 37°C)	Cerebral malaria (impairment of consciousness or convulsions)	Acute fever (temperature > 37.5°C)	Cerebral malaria (impairment of consciousness or convulsions)
Headache	Respiratory distress	Headache	Acute renal failure
Muscle pain (myalgia)	Repeated generalized convulsions	Muscle pain (myalgia)	Pulmonary oedema
Vomiting	Severe anaemia	Vomiting	Severe anaemia
Watery diarrhoea	Hypoglycaemia (low blood sugar)	Watery diarrhoea	Hypoglycaemia (low blood sugar)
Rapid, shallow breathing (tachypnoea)	Fluid, electrolyte and acid–base disturbances	Malaise	Repeated generalized convulsions
Cough	Shock	Chills and sweats	Fluid, electrolyte and acid–base disturbances
Febrile convulsions (less than 30 min duration)	High parasite count	Abdominal pain	Spontaneous bleeding
Chronic anaemia	Liver dysfunction and jaundice		Impaired consciousness
	Hyperpyrexia (temperature > 40°C)		Extreme weakness
			High parasite count
			Jaundice
			Hyperpyrexia (temperature > 40°C)

then spread out to a thickness that allows printed text to be read through the smear. Thin films are prepared by placing a drop of blood towards one end of a glass slide and then spreading this drop of blood along the slide to form a layer one cell thick. Blood smears are dried and then stained with Leishman's, Field's or Giemsa's stains prior to examination under a microscope. Facilities for laboratory diagnosis are often absent at peripheral health services in malaria-endemic countries and in this situation clinical assessment of fever or a recent history of fever, after the exclusion of other major causes, remains the only practical method of diagnosis. In non-endemic areas, malaria should be suspected, whatever the clinical presentation, if the patient has travelled to a malarious area or has recently received a blood transfusion. Several commercial, rapid, malaria test kits have been developed that do not require the use of a microscope, relying instead on detection of parasite proteins or nucleic acids by production of a line or other visual indication of the presence of these molecules. These tests are sensitive, but are generally not suitable for use in malaria-endemic areas, as a large proportion of adults in highly endemic areas will have malaria parasites in their blood but will not be ill. In addition, a patient may continue to produce a positive result for several weeks after parasites have been cleared from the body, due to circulating parasite molecules. Patients with malaria must be carefully evaluated to determine whether they have uncomplicated malaria, which can be treated on an out-patient basis, or severe and complicated disease, which requires intensive management and different therapy and carries a risk of death.

Symptoms of severe malaria have been listed in Table 1.

Transmission

Malaria is transmitted to humans and other mammals by certain species of mosquitoes of the genus *Anopheles* (see Mosquitoes). Of the approximately 3200 species of mosquito so far described, some 430 belong to the genus *Anopheles*, of which 70 species are known to transmit human malaria and about 40 species are important vectors. Several species of mosquito, including vectors of malaria, are in fact groups of closely related species, which are difficult or impossible to distinguish morphologically, but differ in their ecological and behavioural characteristics and hence their importance for malaria transmission. Perhaps the most important mosquito species complex is the *Anopheles gambiae* complex, which consists of six named species (*A. gambiae* sensu stricto, *A. arabiensis*, *A. melas*, *A. merus*, *A. quadriannulatus* and *A. bwambae*), plus a seventh as yet unnamed species, recently discovered in Ethiopia. *Anopheles gambiae* sensu stricto and *A. arabiensis* are the two most important malaria vectors in sub-Saharan Africa. In contrast, *A. quadriannulatus* bites cattle rather than humans and is not a malaria vector.

Other species complexes within the genus *Anopheles* include: *A. nuneztovari* (Neotropical, four species), *A. culicifacies* (Oriental, five species) and *A. punctulatus* (Australasian, 11 species). Individual members of species complexes can often only be distinguished by examining banding patterns on polytene chromosomes or by applying biochemical or molecular genetic techniques, such as polymerase chain reaction (PCR).

When the female mosquito (definitive host) feeds on a human (intermediate host) with malaria, it ingests blood that may contain gametocytes, the infective stages of the *Plasmodium* parasite (Fig. 2). After ingestion by the mosquito, the male and female gametocytes escape from the red blood cells to become free gametes, which undergo sexual reproduction in the blood meal to form a zygote. The zygote develops into an invasive ookinete, which migrates through the blood meal and burrows into the mosquito gut wall, forming oocysts on its outside surface. Within the oocysts the parasites undergo asexual reproduction to produce large numbers of sporozoites. When the oocyst bursts, sporozoites are released into the body cavity of the mosquito, from where they migrate to the head and enter the salivary glands. The female mosquito is now infective.

Different species of mosquito differ in the proportion of individuals that typically contain infective sporozoites in their salivary glands, the sporozoite rate. An efficient vector, such as *A. gambiae* sensu stricto may have a sporozoite rate as high as 5–10%, while *A. culicifacies* in Asia and most Neotropical vectors typically have sporozoite rates of 0.01–0.1%. When a mosquito with sporozoites in its salivary glands feeds on a human, it first injects a small amount of saliva into the blood to prevent it clotting and blocking the insect's mouthparts. Contained in this saliva are the sporozoites, the stage in the malaria parasite's life cycle that is infective to humans. The process of parasite development within the mosquito takes approximately 10–12 days, but is highly dependent on temperature and the species of malaria parasite. On entering into the bloodstream of a human host, the parasites invade liver cells, where they develop first into hepatic trophozoites, which grow and divide by asexual multiplication into invasive merozoites. When the liver cells burst, merozoites are released into the blood. (In *P. vivax* some sporozoites may become hypnozoites, which lie dormant within liver cells for months or even years, before developing and causing relapses of disease.) The merozoites then enter red blood cells and begin to feed and grow, becoming trophozoites. Trophozoites develop into schizonts, which divide internally to form new merozoites, which emerge into the bloodstream when the red blood cell bursts. Merozoites may infect further red blood cells to form new trophozoites or they may develop into separate male and female gametocytes, the stage which is infective to the mosquito.

Treatment of uncomplicated malaria
Chloroquine
Chloroquine is available as tablets containing 50 mg, 100 mg or 150 mg of base (diphosphate or sulphate) and syrup containing 50 mg base in 5 ml. The full treatment dose for adults and children is 25 mg base kg⁻¹ body weight up to a maximum

total dose of 1500 mg, given over 3 days in the ratio 10 : 10 : 5. Chloroquine is a 4-aminoquinoline drug, which functions as a blood schizonticide, but has no effect on liver stages of the parasites. It is effective against *P. malariae* and *P. ovale*, as well as chloroquine-sensitive parasites of *P. falciparum* and *P. vivax*. Chloroquine remains the first-line drug of choice in many African countries, despite high and increasing levels of parasite resistance. Malawi, Tanzania and Kenya have switched their first-line drug to sulfadoxine-pyrimethamine, while other countries in the region are evaluating their resistance situation, with a view to changing policy in the future. Although severe adverse effects are rare at normal doses, pruritus (itching) does occur, especially in darker-skinned individuals. Chloroquine is safe for use in pregnancy.

Amodiaquine
Amodiaquine is available as tablets containing 200 mg and 600 mg base (hydrochloride) or 153.1 mg base (chlorohydrate) and a suspension containing 10 mg base per ml. Amodiaquine is also a 4-aminoquinoline, which is more palatable and achieves more rapid parasite clearance than chloroquine. Use of amodiaquine has declined since the 1980s, when a number of fatal adverse reactions (agranulocytosis or toxic hepatitis) were seen in travellers taking the drug as prophylaxis, and it is no longer recommended for this purpose. For treatment, amodiaquine is administered at 25–35 mg base kg⁻¹ body weight over 3 days. Amodiaquine may cause less skin itching than chloroquine. There is no evidence to suggest that amodiaquine cannot safely be used for treatment during pregnancy.

Sulfadoxine/pyrimethamine and sulfalene/pyrimethamine
Sulfadoxine/pyrimethamine and sulfalene/pyrimethamine are both available as tablets containing 500 mg sulfa drug plus 25 mg pyrimethamine. Sulfadoxine/pyrimethamine is also available as 2.5 ml ampoules of injectable solution. Sulfa drug/pyrimethamine combinations are antifolate drugs, which are highly effective

against schizonts of *P. falciparum*, but less active against other *Plasmodium* species. As the antifolates show no cross-resistance with the 4-aminoquinolines, they have been used very successfully in areas where *P. falciparum* is chloroquine-resistant. However, sulfa drug/pyrimethamine combinations have relatively long half-lives, which can accelerate selection of drug-resistant parasites. Evidence of parasite resistance to these drugs is beginning to emerge in Africa, while in most of Asia and South America these drugs are no longer effective treatments. The recommended treatment dosage for adults is 1500 mg sulfa drug, plus 75 mg pyrimethamine in total, administered as a single dose of three tablets. These drugs are not recommended for prophylaxis as they may cause severe skin reactions, including the fatal Stevens–Johnson syndrome. Although there is no evidence of adverse reactions in the human fetus, the drug manufacturers do not recommend its use in pregnancy, except when benefits outweigh the risks – for instance, in highly endemic chloroquine-resistant *P. falciparum* areas. Currently, administration of a full treatment dose at antenatal clinic attendance at the beginning of the second and third trimesters is used in some African countries to protect the mother and fetus from the potentially life-threatening effects of malaria infection.

Mefloquine

This drug should only be used when microscopical or careful clinical diagnosis of chloroquine- and sulfadoxine/pyrimethamine-resistant *P. falciparum* has been made or is strongly suspected. Mefloquine is available as tablets of 274 mg mefloquine hydrochloride, equivalent to 250 mg base (in the USA 250 mg mefloquine hydrochloride, 228 mg base). The curative dose for adults is five tablets, administered orally, in a single dose. Children should receive 20 mg kg^{-1} up to a maximum dose of 1250 mg, preferably split into two equal doses. Mefloquine may cause nausea, vomiting, abdominal pain, diarrhoea, headache, heart conduction abnormalities, dizziness

and psychiatric problems. It should not be administered to women during the first trimester of pregnancy, or to people suffering from pre-existing neurological or psychiatric problems, persons undertaking fine coordination and spatial discrimination (air crew, construction workers operating at height, etc.), persons taking quinine, quinidine or halofantrine treatment and those who received mefloquine treatment in the previous 4 weeks.

Quinine

This drug is usually effective against *P. falciparum* parasites that are resistant to chloroquine and sulfa drug/pyrimethamine combinations. Quinine is primarily used for the treatment of severe and complicated malaria cases. It should ordinarily only be used for the treatment of uncomplicated cases when the parasites exhibit multi-drug resistance (e.g. in border areas of South-East Asia) and should be used in combination with another drug if there is evidence of reduced quinine efficacy. An intravenous infusion (or alternatively an intramuscular injection) of quinine is often used to treat patients with uncomplicated malaria who are unable to take oral medication due to vomiting. Oral administration should be resumed as soon as possible. Quinine may also be used to treat patients who are allergic to sulfonamides or who fail to respond to first-line treatments. Quinine is available as several salts, including quinine hydrochloride (82% base), quinine dihydrochloride (82% base) and quinine sulfate (82.6% base). In areas where parasites are sensitive to quinine the dose is 8 mg kg^{-1} base three times a day for 7 days. In areas where parasites are sensitive to both quinine and sulfa drug/pyrimethamine, but compliance may be a problem, quinine should be administered at a dosage of 8 mg kg^{-1} each day for 3 days, plus 1500 mg sulfa drug, 75 mg pyrimethamine on day 1 of quinine treatment. Quinine is safe for use in pregnancy, but there is an increased risk of quinine-induced hypoglycaemia compared with non-pregnant patients and so blood glucose must be monitored carefully.

Quinine can cause tinnitus, muffled hearing, dizziness and vertigo (symptoms collectively referred to as cinchonism), which are generally reversible. There may be an increased risk of cardiac toxicity in patients who have previously taken mefloquine as prophylaxis.

Halofantrine

Halofantrine is a phenanthrene methanol drug which is effective against parasites resistant to chloroquine and sulfa drug/pyrimethamine, but has been associated with fatal cardiotoxicity under normal treatment regimens. In addition, it exhibits cross-resistance with mefloquine. Halofantrine should only be used on an individual basis in patients known to have a normal electrocardiogram and in areas where parasites are known to be resistant. Halofantrine is available as tablets containing 250 mg hydrochloride (233 mg base) and a paediatric suspension of 100 mg hydrochloride (93.2 mg base) per 5 ml and acts as a blood schizontocide. The dose for both adults and children is 8 mg base kg^{-1} in three doses at 6-hourly intervals. It should not be used in pregnant or lactating women except where there is no alternative.

Artemisinin (quinghaosu)

Artemisinin is a sesquiterpene lactone extracted from the annual plant *Artemisia annua* and is available in a number of formulations, including artemisinin (250 mg tablets), artesunate (50 mg tablets), artemether (50 mg capsule) and dihydroartemisinin (20 mg tablets). Use of artemisinin and its derivatives is associated with rapid parasite clearance and relief of symptoms, but the incidence of recrudescence is high, unless used in combination with other drugs, e.g. mefloquine. Use of artemisinin should be restricted to patients with severe malaria in areas where *P. falciparum* exhibits multi-drug resistance.

Tetracycline, doxycycline and clindamycin

These three compounds are broad-spectrum antimicrobial agents with activity against asexual stages of malaria parasites. They should be used in combination with other drugs, for the treatment of malaria, as they are all relatively slow-acting. Tetracycline is available as tetracycline hydrochloride tablets or capsules containing 250 mg salt (231 mg base). The dose, in combination with 8 mg kg^{-1} quinine for 3 days, is 250 mg four times per day for 5 days. Doxycycline is available as capsules or tablets containing 100 mg salt, given at a daily dosage of 200 mg salt for 5 days, in combination with mefloquine or artesunate. Tetracycline and doxycycline should not be used in children under 8 years of age or pregnant women. Clindamycin is used at a dosage of 300 mg base four times per day for 5 days in combination with quinine. Clindamycin can be used in pregnancy. All three compounds can cause gastrointestinal irritation, but the effects are reduced if taken with copious amounts of water and a meal.

Primaquine

Primaquine is an 8-aminoquinoline developed during the Second World War (1939–1945). It is primarily used in combination with chloroquine to treat patients with *P. vivax* or *P. ovale* infections in order to prevent relapses from persistent hypnozoites in the liver. Primaquine has no effect on erythrocytic stages. The adult dose is 15 mg base daily for 14 days or 45 mg base weekly for 8 weeks. The paediatric dose is 0.25 mg kg^{-1} daily for 14 days or 0.75 mg kg^{-1} weekly for 8 weeks. Primaquine can cause haemolytic anaemia in individuals with glucose-6-phosphate dehydrogenase (G6PD) deficiency. Patients with the Mediterranean and Canton variants of G6PD deficiency are at greater risk of haemolysis and should be treated with chloroquine for each relapse. The incidence of side-effects is lower with weekly, compared with daily, doses.

People with falciparum malaria who do not die usually recover within weeks or months unless re-infected, but with vivax malaria attacks may recur at intervals over the next 1–13 years as the liver forms (hypnozoites) develop and reinfect the blood. These relapses can be prevented by treatment with primaquine after the initial treatment with chloroquine or another schizonticide.

Treatment of severe and complicated malaria

Severe and complicated malaria is largely a characteristic of malaria caused by *P. falciparum*, although *P. vivax* can occasionally be fatal, usually as a result of rupture of the spleen. Symptoms of severe and complicated malaria in adults and children are shown in Table 1. Treatment of severe and complicated malaria is a specialized field, beyond the scope of this encyclopedia.

Prophylaxis

Chemoprophylaxis is recommended for all persons travelling to malaria-endemic regions from non-endemic areas. Chemoprophylaxis (or intermittent treatment) may also be recommended for pregnant women. Chloroquine is the drug of choice in areas where malaria parasites are sensitive to it. The recommended dose for adults is 500 mg chloroquine (300 mg base) in a single weekly dose, begun 1 week before travel and continued weekly until 4 weeks after leaving the malarious area. Children should receive a weekly dose of 5 mg kg^{-1}. Weekly chloroquine may be combined with a daily dose (200 mg) of proguanil, which should also be taken for 1 week before entering and 4 weeks after leaving a malaria-endemic zone. Chloroquine–proguanil is safe in pregnancy. In regions where there is chloroquine resistance, mefloquine is the drug of choice and is taken weekly at an adult dose of 250 mg (one tablet), again commencing 1 week prior to travel and continuing for 4 weeks after leaving a malarious area. Mefloquine should not be taken by patients with liver abnormalities, heart conditions, pyschiatric disorders or epilepsy. Doxycycline, an antibiotic, is an alternative to mefloquine and is taken at an adult dose of 100 mg daily, commencing 2 days before departure and continuing for 4 weeks after leaving a malarious area. Doxycycline should not be used by pregnant women or children under 8 years of age.

Sulfadoxine/pyrimethamine is not recommended for prophylaxis due to the rare occurrence of severe and occasionally fatal skin reactions.

Drug resistance

Malaria parasite resistance to proguanil and pyrimethamine was first reported in the early 1950s, followed by resistance to the 4-aminoquinolines (chloroquine and amodiaquine), which was first reported from Thailand in 1957, reaching Africa in 1978. Chloroquine resistance is now present in most African countries (Fig. 1). Chloroquine-resistant *P. vivax* has been reported from Papua New Guinea, Solomon Islands, Indonesia, Brazil and Colombia. In border areas of Asia, *P. falciparum* has become resistant to chloroquine, sulfadoxine–pyrimethamine, mefloquine and even quinine. Chloroquine resistance is due to a mutation in a gene on the parasite's chromosome 7, while resistance to pyrimethamine results from a mutation in the gene coding for the enzyme dihydrofolate reductase (DHFR).

The use of antimalarial drug combinations has recently been proposed as a method to prevent the development of drug resistance, thus prolonging the useful life of the cheaper antimalarials. Artemisinin or its derivatives are used to rapidly reduce the parasite population, and the remaining parasites are then exposed to the full concentration of a second, slower-acting drug, such as mefloquine or sulfadoxine–pyrimethamine. It is highly unlikely that a parasite will simultaneously develop resistance to two drugs with different modes of action.

Malaria in pregnancy

Malaria in pregnancy is a serious disease, which results in underweight babies (less than 2.5 kg at birth), who as a consequence suffer impaired physical and mental development, which may disadvantage them for the rest of their lives. In addition, malaria during pregnancy can lead to abortion or stillbirth, severe anaemia in the mother and even death of the mother. During pregnancy, a woman's immunity is decreased compared with that of a non-pregnant woman, and this reduction in immunity is greater during the first pregnancy. Methods to protect móthers and babies during pregnancy currently include intermittent malaria treatment (usually with sulphadoxine–pyrimethamine) during the second and third trimesters, plus promotion of the use of insecticide-treated mosquito nets.

Control

House spraying

Early attempts at malaria control largely relied on environmental management, such as draining of swamps, clearing of ditches, filling ponds and other water bodies to prevent mosquito breeding, and this proved successful in parts of southern Europe, including Italy. A large variety of toxic chemicals (e.g. Paris green) and oils were also applied to water bodies to kill mosquito larvae and control malaria, particularly during the first half of the 20th century, before the invention of modern insecticides. Following the Second World War (1939–1945), with the discovery of synthetic insecticides, such as DDT, the focus of malaria control activities changed and the adult mosquito became the target (although the natural insecticide pyrethrum had been used successfully against adult anophelines in South Africa in 1932–1933). Residual insecticides (Table 2), when applied to the interior surfaces of houses and other structures, can be highly effective against adult *Anopheles* vectors of malaria (Fig. 3).

The effectiveness of residual insecticides is due to the habit of many species of malaria vector of resting indoors on walls and ceilings during the day. This behaviour brings the mosquito into contact with insecticide deposits applied to the surfaces, and a lethal dose is taken up. Early successes with DDT encouraged the initiation of a Global Malaria Eradication Campaign, which began in 1957, under the management of WHO. By 1968, malaria had been eradicated from 36 countries and territories, protecting as many as 650 million people from the disease. However, malaria eradication was ultimately unsuccessful for several reasons: application of residual insecticides to large numbers of homes is time-consuming,

Table 2. Recommended target dosages (active ingredient) for insecticides commonly used in indoor residual spraying and for insecticide-treated mosquito nets (ITNs).

| Insecticide | Target dosage (g m^{-2}) | |
	ITNs	Residual spraying
Alphacypermethrin	0.02–0.04	
Bendiocarb		0.4
Cyfluthrin	0.03–0.05	
Cypermethrin		
DDT		2.0
Deltamethrin	0.015–0.025	0.05
Fenitrothion		2.0
Lambdacyhalothrin	0.01–0.02	0.025
Malathion		2.0
Permethrin	0.2–0.5	0.5

labour-intensive and expensive and many developing countries found it to be non-sustainable in the long term. The development of mosquito resistance to the residual insecticides, environmental concerns relating to DDT, dieldrin and other insecticides and the fact that not all malaria vector species rest indoors contributed to the lack of success. The African continent was always considered to be a special case epidemiologically and eradication of malaria was never seriously attempted in Africa. Residual spraying of houses for malaria control is currently used predominantly in southern Africa, but also in South America and parts of Asia. It remains a recommended strategy for epidemic prevention and control and may also be used in specific situations, such as refugee camps.

Personal protection measures against the bites of mosquitoes

Mosquito nets provide a barrier against the attacks of indoor, night-biting mosquitoes, including most vector *Anopheles*, as well as common nuisance biters (Fig. 4). The protective effects of mosquito nets are enhanced by treating them with insecticides, primarily synthetic pyrethroids (Table 2). Insecticide-treated nets (ITNs) can provide protection at both individual and family levels and may even reduce

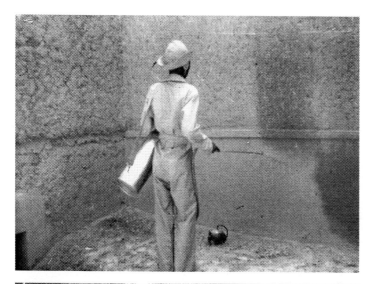

Fig. 3. Spraying the wall of a house with a residual insecticide. Reproduced by courtesy of the Wellcome Trust.

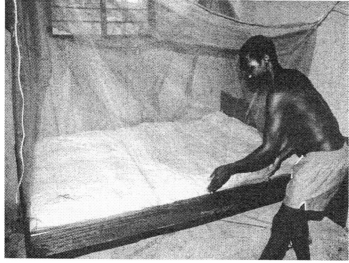

Fig. 4. Tucking an insecticide-treated mosquito net under the mattress of a bed. Reproduced by courtesy of the Wellcome Trust.

transmission if used on a large scale, due to the mass killing of mosquitoes. Insecticide-treated nets are recommended for use in a variety of epidemiological settings, including intense perennial transmission, and have proved successful in preventing morbidity and reducing all-cause child mortality by 17–63% in field research trials carried out in The Gambia, Tanzania, Burkina Faso (insecticide-treated curtains) and Kenya. Nets require treatment with insecticide every 6–12 months, depending on the insecticide and frequency of washing. Nets should be washed as little as possible between retreatments. When implemented outside rigidly controlled scientific trials, ITN coverage and retreatment rates are lower, with the consequence that they tend to be less effective in reducing mortality. The challenge remains to develop effective methods for the introduction of ITNs on a large scale, while continuing to achieve the high levels of protection shown to be possible. Insecticide-treated nets are currently used on a large scale in Sichuan, China (3.85 million treated nets by the late 1990s), and Vietnam; however, in both these countries, existing net use was already high due to the high biting densities of nuisance mosquitoes.

Other methods of personal protection

Individuals can protect themselves against biting mosquitoes, including those that transmit malaria, by using repellents (those that include diethyltoluamide (DEET) are best), burning insecticide coils or local leaves and herbs, screening doors and windows, taking antimalarial prophylactics, wearing long-sleeved shirts and long trousers and staying indoors between dusk and dawn, when mosquito biting is most frequent.

Biological control

Natural enemies of mosquitoes, such as fish, crustaceans, nematode worms, predatory mosquito larvae and fungi, have all been used for control, with limited success. Perhaps the most successful example of biological control has been the use of species of cyprinodontid fish (e.g. *Gambusia affinis*, *Poecillia reticulata* and species of *Nothobranchius* and *Cynolebias*). This method of control was first suggested as early as 1900, with the first trials being carried out in the mid-1920s. Larvivorous fish may represent a useful additional control measure in certain situations – for example, against mosquito larvae in cisterns, small ponds and streams.

The bacterium *Bacillus thuringiensis* serotype H14 (= *B. thuringiensis* subsp. *israelensis* or *Bti*) contains a toxin which is fatal to mosquito larvae when ingested, while being biodegradable and harmless to fish, other animals and humans. There is no evidence of resistance to the toxin in mosquitoes in nature. The toxin contained in *Bti* is now produced industrially in a number of formulations, which need to be frequently applied to breeding sites. A second species, *Bacillus sphaericus*, produces a more potent and long-lasting toxin, but has not been used so widely.

Malaria vaccines

Exposure to malaria infection leads to the natural development of partial immunity in humans, and so the potential exists for the development of a vaccine. There are three types of vaccine currently under development: pre-erythrocytic vaccines, which prevent the sporozoite stage from invading liver cells, asexual blood-stage vaccines, which prevent the merozoite stage from invading red blood cells, and transmission-blocking vaccines, which work by inhibiting the sexual development of the parasite within the mosquito. The most well-known malaria vaccine is SPf66, a synthetic multicomponent peptide vaccine. Unfortunately, this vaccine has not yielded consistent results in field trials and is still under development. There are a number of transmission-blocking candidate vaccines, which are undergoing safety and immunogenicity trials in the USA. The search for an effective anti-malaria vaccine is hampered by several factors. First, the malaria parasite expresses different antigens at different stages of its life cycle and can even change these antigens to evade the host's immune responses. Secondly, malaria parasites are notoriously difficult to cultivate in sufficient quantities to develop vaccines based on attenuated parasites or their antigens. A further difficulty is that testing requires expensive and time-consuming animal-model systems. Perhaps the real challenge for any successful vaccine is to achieve sufficiently high coverage rates among the people most at risk from the disease – that is, the poor in underdeveloped countries with limited health resources. It is unlikely that an effective malaria vaccine will be available for widespread use in endemic countries before the second decade of the 21st century.

Roll Back Malaria Programme

Roll Back Malaria (RBM), a joint initiative between WHO, the United Nations Development Programme (UNDP), the United Nations Children's Fund (UNICEF) and the World Bank, was launched in November 1998 to reinforce the global malaria control efforts. The RBM partnership advocates the use of an integrated approach to malaria control, utilizing existing tools, such as ITNs, and prompt and effective treatment at community level, as well as encouraging development of new control methods, including drug combinations and vaccines. Roll Back Malaria has set a goal of 50% reduction in mortality due to malaria by the year 2010.

Selected bibliography

Bradley, D.J. and Warhurst, D.C. (1997) Guidelines for the prevention of malaria in travellers from the United Kingdom. *CDC Review 7*, R138–R151.

Busvine, J.R. (1993) *Disease Transmission by Insects: Its Discovery and 90 Years of Effort to Prevent it.* Springer-Verlag, Berlin, 361 pp.

Coluzzi, M. and Bradley, S. (eds) (1999) The malaria challenge after one hundred years of malariology. *Parassitologia* 41 (1–3), 528 pp.

Gilles, H.M. and Warrell, D.A. (1993) *Bruce-Chwatt's Essential Malariology*, 3rd edn. Edward Arnold, London, 340 pp. (4th edn in press.)

Knell, A.J. (ed.) (1991) *Malaria.* Oxford University Press, Oxford, 94 pp.

Nájera, J.A. (1999) *Malaria Control. Achievements, Problems and Strategies.* WHO/MAL/99.1087, and WHO/CDS/RBM/99.10, WHO, Geneva, 126 pp.

Nájera, J.A., Kouznetsov, R.L. and Delacollette, C. (1998) *Malaria Epidemics. Detection and control. Forecasting and Prevention.* WHO/MAL/98.1084 and 1084 Corr. 1, WHO, Geneva, 81 pp.

Newton, P. and White, N. (1999) Malaria: new developments in treatment and prevention. *Annual Review of Medicine* 50, 179–192.

Pasvol, G. (ed.) (1995) Baillière's Clinical Infectious Diseases: *International Practice and Research*, Vol. 2. Ballière, London, 408 pp.

Service, M.W. (1993) Mosquitoes (Culicidae). In: Lane, R.P. and Crosskey, R.W. (eds) *Medical Insects and Arachnids.* Chapman & Hall, London, pp. 120–240.

The Wellcome Trust (1998) *Malaria* CD-Rom. Topics in International Health. The Wellcome Trust, London.

Wernsdorfer, W.H. and McGregor, I.A. (eds) (1998) *Malaria. Principles and Practice of Malariology*, Vol. 1, pp. 1–912, Vol. 2, pp. 913–1818. Churchill Livingstone, Edinburgh, 1818 pp.

White, N.J., Nosten, F., Looareesuwan, S., Watkins, W.M., Marsh, K., Snow, R.W., Kokwaro, G., Ouma, J., Hien, T.T., Molyneux, M.E., Taylor, T.E., Newbold, C.I. Ruebush, T.K., II, Danis, M., Greenwood, B.M., Anderson, R.M. and Olliaro, P. (1999) Averting a malaria disaster. *The Lancet* 353, 1965–1967.

WHO/UNDP/UNICEF/World Bank (1999) *Roll Back Malaria. Proposed Strategy and Workplan.* World Health Organization, Geneva, 85 pp.

World Health Organization (1995) *Vector Control for Malaria and Other Vector-borne Diseases.* WHO Technical Report Series 857, Geneva, 91 pp.

World Health Organization (1997) *Management of Uncomplicated Malaria and the use of Antimalarial Drugs for the Protection of Travellers.* WHO/MAL/96.1075 Rev. 1, WHO, Geneva, 101 pp.

World Health Organization (2000) *International Travel and Health: Vaccination Requirements and Health Advice.* WHO, Geneva, 108 pp.

World Health Organization (2000) Severe and complicated malaria. *Transactions of the Royal Society of Tropical Medicine and Hygiene* 94 (suppl.), S1–S90.

Mansonella species *see* **Mansonelliasis.**

Mansonelliasis

W. Crewe

Infections of humans and other animals with filarial worms of the genus *Mansonella.* Certain species now included in the genus *Mansonella* have in the past been regarded as species of *Acanthocheilonema* or *Dipetalonema*, and may be recorded under these names in older publications.

Mansonelliasis, human

Relatively little work has been carried out on some species of *Mansonella*, and information on their biology is rather scant. Most infections with *Mansonella* are non-pathogenic, with no clearly defined symptoms, but sometimes infections are associated with cutaneous itching and inflammation, pruritus and general signs of allergic reactions, including eosinophilia. Four species have been recorded as parasitic in humans, but only three are of major importance. The fourth species, *Mansonella rodhaini*, has been recorded on only one occasion, when it was found in 14 people during a study in Gabon.

Mansonella ozzardi

This parasite has been recorded only from humans, but it has been experimentally transmitted to Patas monkeys (*Erythrocebus patas*).

Distribution

Mansonella ozzardi is widespread through Central and South America, from Panama to northern Argentina, and in the eastern Caribbean (Fig. 1). Throughout the whole of this area the distribution is patchy, and infections are usually found in isolated communities. Infection rates increase with age, and prevalences above 70% have been observed in adults in some localities.

Parasite

The only complete worms recovered from humans have been female, but worms of both sexes have been obtained from experimentally infected Patas monkeys. The female worms from humans measure 65–81 mm × 0.2–0.25 mm; the female worms from monkeys are 32–62 mm × 0.13–0.16 mm, and the male worms from monkeys are 24–28 mm × 0.07–0.08 mm. The microfilariae in humans are aperiodic; they are usually seen in blood films, but they may be present in skin biopsies.

Clinical symptoms

Infected individuals normally show no obvious signs of infection, but in some areas of South America infection has been associated with non-specific symptoms. Hydrocoel, enlarged lymph glands, headaches, pruritus and chronic arthritis have been recorded, but none of these has been shown to be directly caused by *Mansonella* infection. Eosinophilia is common.

Diagnosis

Infections are recognized by the recovery of microfilariae in blood films or in skin biopsies that are taken during surveys for onchocerciasis. The microfilariae of *M. ozzardi* are 200–225 µm long and 3–4 µm wide and do not have a sheath. The nuclei do not extend into the tail, which is long and tapering (Fig. 2(1)).

Transmission

In different parts of its range *M. ozzardi* is transmitted by species of either *Culicoides* or *Simulium*. For example, in the Caribbean islands and in Trinidad, Surinam and Argentina the vectors are *Culicoides*, mainly *C. furens* and *C. phlebotomus*; in Brazil, Colombia and Guyana the vectors are *Simulium*, mainly *S. amazonicum* and *S. sanguineum*. It is not known whether two different forms of *M. ozzardi* are involved. After the microfilariae are taken up by the feeding fly, development to the infective stage, whether in *Culicoides* or in *Simulium*, takes place in the thoracic muscles. The first larval moult takes place after 4–5

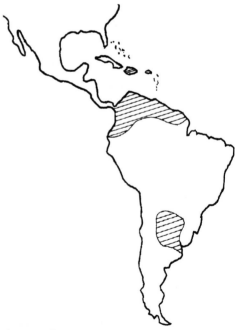

Fig. 1. Indication of overall geographical distribution of *Mansonella ozzardi*.

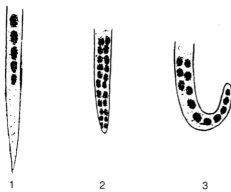

Fig. 2. Diagram of tails of unsheathed microfilariae of *Mansonella* species. 1. *M. ozzardi*; 2. *M. perstans*; 3. *M. streptocerca*. Note whether nuclei extend to end of tail and whether tail is straight or bent.

days, and the second after 5–7 days. The fly becomes infective 7–8 days after feeding, and the infective larvae are injected subcutaneously when the fly next bites. The pre-patent period in humans is not known, but in experimentally infected monkeys it is 5–6 months.

Treatment

There is at present no effective treatment for *M. ozzardi*. Diethylcarbamazine (DEC) has no effect on the microfilariae, but may have some slight effect on the adult worms. There have been reports from workers in Mexico that DEC can kill the adults, but studies in Trinidad showed no response to DEC treatment. In another investigation, ivermectin has been reported as effective in one patient.

Control

Although in some isolated areas the infection rate in adults has been found to be 96%, *M. ozzardi* is not considered a major public health problem and no large-scale control programmes exist. Small-scale local control measures are not at present feasible because the vectors breed in small and widely scattered bodies of water.

Mansonella perstans

Until recently this species was known as *Dipetalonema perstans*. Humans are the

important definitive hosts, but the parasite also occurs in Chimpanzees (*Pan troglodytes*) and Gorillas (*Gorilla gorilla*), which in some areas may perhaps be reservoir hosts.

Distribution

Mansonella perstans is widely distributed in tropical Africa, particularly throughout the rain-forest belt of Central and West Africa, and it is found in sylvatic foci as far south as Zimbabwe (Fig. 3). It has been recorded in islands in the Caribbean, and in Central and South America there are limited foci among Amerindian communities in the rain forests.

Parasite

Adult worms have only rarely been recovered from humans; they live in the serous cavities, mainly the peritoneal, pleural and pericardial cavities. *Mansonella perstans* has also been found in Chimpanzees and Gorillas, but it is widespread in humans in areas where there are no great apes. The adult female worms measure 60–80 mm × 0.1–0.15 mm, and the adult males are 35–45 mm × 0.05–0.07 mm. The microfilariae are unsheathed and aperiodic. They are usually 190–200 μm long and 4–5 μm wide, but small forms, 100 μm × 4 μm, have been described.

Clinical symptoms

The pathology is not well defined, because little pathological material has been available for study. Most infected individuals show few or no signs, but in some individuals there may be a variety of symptoms, including oedematous swelling of the arms, face and other parts of the body (similar to Calabar swellings (see Loiasis)), pruritus, fever, headaches, pains in the bursae or joints and exhaustion. Eosinophilia is usually present, and severe abdominal pain, especially in the liver region, has been reported. Signs are more common and prominent in individuals coming from non-endemic areas. There are also records of individuals in Uganda suffering from 'bung-eye' caused by *M. perstans*. However, individuals infected with *M. perstans*

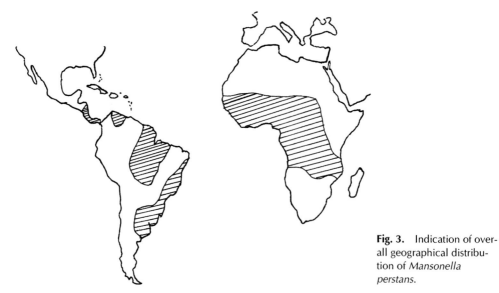

Fig. 3. Indication of overall geographical distribution of *Mansonella perstans*.

are frequently also infected with *Loa loa* or other filariae, so the aetiology of the symptoms may be doubtful; in some communities infection rates of over 50% occur without any symptoms being present.

Diagnosis

In the absence of any specific clinical signs, diagnosis is made by finding microfilariae in blood films taken during the day or the night. The microfilariae are 190–200 μm long and have a rounded tail, with the nuclei extending to the tip of the tail (Fig. 2 (2)).

Transmission

The only known vectors of *M. perstans* are species of *Culicoides*. The main vector in Africa is *C. grahami*, but *C. austeni* and other species are also involved. The species of *Culicoides* transmitting *M. perstans* in the New World have not been identified. *Culicoides* larvae feed mainly on decaying vegetable matter and live in many different types of habitat, including wet soil, leaf litter, humus and manure, on plants submerged in water and in tree holes. In West Africa they are often found in the rotting stems of cut banana plants. The adult flies bite at any time of the day or night, especially in shady localities, and some species are particularly active in the evenings and early mornings. Microfilariae of *M. perstans* are taken up by the feeding midges, and after 5 days they have developed into first-stage larvae in the fly's thorax. Thereafter rapid development occurs, and by the ninth day infective third-stage larvae are present in the head. These infective larvae are injected subcutaneously when the fly next bites.

Treatment

Although DEC and ivermectin have little effect on the adult worms and no obvious effect on the microfilariae, treatment with DEC may cause adverse side-reactions in individuals with high microfilaraemia. However, mebendazole has been shown to be capable of eliminating microfilariae, and two Swedish patients have been successfully treated with mebendazole.

Control

In view of the low pathogenicity of *M. perstans*, no large-scale attempt has been made to control this infection. The *Culicoides* breeding sites are small, numerous and spread over a wide area, so control of the vectors is at present impracticable.

Mansonella streptocerca

Until recently, this species was known as *Dipetalonema streptocerca*. It has been found in Chimpanzees (*Pan troglodytes*) as well as in humans, but it is not known whether Chimpanzees act as reservoir hosts.

Distribution

Mansonella streptocerca has a limited distribution in West and Central Africa, from Ghana to Zaire and north-western Angola (Fig. 4). It is most abundant in areas of rain forest, and in some localities in Zaire up to 90% of inhabitants are infected.

Parasite

Adult worms have rarely been recovered, and little is known of their morphology. They are found in the skin of both humans and Chimpanzees, and are relatively small, the female worms measuring 27 mm × 0.075 mm and the males 17 mm × 0.05 mm. In humans they live in the dermis of the shoulders and upper thorax, usually less than 1 mm below the skin surface. The microfilariae, which are also found in the skin, are unsheathed, aperiodic and about 200 μm long.

Clinical symptoms

Most patients show few signs of infection, the most common being chronic itching over the thorax and shoulders. Less frequently there may be pruritus, hypopigmented macules, oedema and thickening of the skin, changes that could be confused with the skin changes caused by onchocerciasis or leprosy.

Diagnosis

As the clinical signs are not specific, diagnosis must be made by examining the microfilariae, which are found in skin-snips. The microfilariae measure 180–240 μm × 3–5 μm and do not possess a sheath. The tail is markedly curved into a 'shepherd's crook' shape, and the nuclei extend in a single column to the tip of the tail (Fig. 2(3)).

Transmission

The vectors are species of *Culicoides*, the commonest probably being *C. grahami*. The

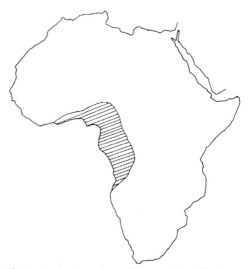

Fig. 4. Indication of overall geographical distribution of *Mansonella streptocerca*.

flies may feed at any time of the day or night and take up microfilariae from the skin. Complete development in the vector has been shown experimentally to take 9 days. Little is known about development from infective larva to adult in humans, and the pre-patent period is not known,

Treatment

Streptocerciasis can be effectively treated with DEC, which kills both the microfilariae and the adult worms. However, in most patients, even at a relatively low dosage level, treatment causes intense pruritus and the development of cutaneous papules, in which dead and decomposing adult worms can be found. In some patients more severe side-reactions, similar to the Mazzotti reaction following DEC treatment of onchocerciasis, may occur, but these are not common.

Control

As with all the species of *Mansonella* infecting humans, control of the *Culicoides* vectors is not feasible because the breeding sites are small and mainly inaccessible. There have been no attempts at large-scale control, and no information on possible chemoprophylaxis is available.

Mansonelliasis, animal

A number of species of *Mansonella* have been recorded from animals. *Mansonella evansi*, which is parasitic in camels (*Camelus* species), may cause arteriosclerosis and heart insufficiency, but other species appear to be non-pathogenic and so have not been studied extensively. *Mansonella dracunculoides* is parasitic in dogs and Hyaenas (*Crocuta crocuta*) in Kenya, *Mansonella grassi* in dogs in Kenya and Italy and *Mansonella reconditum* in dogs in Africa, Italy, Brazil and the USA. These records are probably reflections of the distribution of investigators rather than of the overall distribution of the parasites. *Mansonella reconditum* has been the subject of several studies because its microfilariae can be confused with those of the pathogenic dog heartworm *Dirofilaria immitis* (see Dirofilariasis), and must be differentiated for the diagnosis of dirofilariasis in domestic dogs.

Mansonella reconditum

It has been pointed out by previous workers that 'the canine parasite *M. reconditum* has, as its species name suggests, been seen by few human beings'. For this reason, relatively little is known about its biology.

Distribution

Most of the available information comes from America, where the parasite is widely distributed. It is particularly common in the eastern, south-eastern and southern states of the USA. It has also been recorded in Italy and parts of Africa, so its overall distribution is probably very wide.

Parasite

The adults are small slender worms, the females being 17–32 mm in length and the males 9–17 mm. They have been observed in the body cavity, subcutaneous connective tissue and perirenal tissue in dogs and wild canines, but usually in small numbers. The microfilariae, which occur in the blood and measure about 270 μm × 5 μm, are more commonly seen.

Clinical symptoms

No specific pathogenic effects have been associated with *M. reconditum*, but eosinophilia and occasionally subcutaneous abcesses and ulcerations have been recorded in infected dogs.

Diagnosis

In the absence of clinical signs, diagnosis depends on finding the unsheathed microfilariae in the blood, and distinguishing them from the commoner and larger microfilariae of *D. immitis*. Microfilariae of *M. reconditum* are unsheathed, 264–278 μm × 4.7–5.8 μm and, when alive, they move progressively in a definite direction. Their diagnostic features are that the tail of the microfilaria is curved into a 'button-hook' shape and the anterior end bears a cephalic hook, which can be seen with the ordinary high power of a standard microscope (Fig. 5).

Transmission

The known vectors are fleas (*Ctenocephalides canis*, *Ctenocephalides felis* and *Pulex irritans*), lice (*Heterodoxus spiniger*) and ticks (*Rhipicephalus sanguineus*). Development to the infective stage takes 7–10 days in fleas, but periods up to 19 days have been recorded in other vectors, which are possibly less suitable intermediate hosts. The pre-patent period in dogs is 61–68 days.

Treatment

Because the parasite is not markedly pathogenic, treatment is not normally required. It is not known whether anthelmintics have

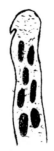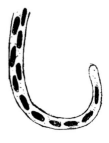

Fig. 5. Diagram of head with cephalic hook and curved tail of unsheathed microfilaria of *Mansonella reconditum*.

any effect on the adult worms, but a single dose of ivermectin has been shown to kill the microfilariae.

Control

Little has been done to investigate possible methods of control, as this is considered unnecessary. However, control of the arthropod parasites of dogs would obviously be beneficial.

Selected bibliography

Anderson, R.C. (2000) *Nematode Parasites of Vertebrates*, 2nd edn. CAB International, Wallingford, UK, 650 pp.

Baird, K.J., Neafie, R.C. and Connor, D.H. (1988) Nodules in the conjunctiva, Bung-eye, and Bulge-eye in Africa caused by *Mansonella perstans*. *American Journal of Tropical Medicine and Hygiene* 38, 553–557.

Beaver, P.C., Jung, R.C. and Cupp, E.W. (eds) (1984) *Clinical Parasitology*, 9th edn. Lea & Febiger, Philadelphia, pp. 380–385.

Cook, G.C. (ed.) (1996) *Manson's Tropical Diseases*, 20th edn. Saunders, London, pp. 1354–1357.

Lindsey, J.R. (1962) Diagnosis of filarial infections in dogs. II. Confirmation of microfilarial identification. *Journal of Parasitology* 48, 321–326.

Soulsby, E.J.L. (1982) *Helminths, Arthropods and Protozoa of Domesticated Animals*, 7th edn. Baillière-Tindall, London, 809 pp.

Strickland, G.T. (ed.) (2000) *Hunter's Tropical Medicine and Emerging Infectious Disease*, 8th edn. Saunders, Philadelphia, pp. 769–773.

Tidwell, M.A., Tidwell, M.A. and de Hoyos, P.M. (1980) Development of *Mansonella ozzardi* in a black fly species of the *Simulium sanguineum* group from Eastern Vaupes, Colombia. *American Journal of Tropical Medicine and Hygiene* 29, 1209–1214.

Wahlgren, M. (1982) The successful treatment of *Dipetalonema perstans* filariasis with mebendazole. *Annals of Tropical Medicine and Parasitology* 76, 557–559.

Warren, K.S. and Mahmoud, A.E.F. (1990) *Tropical and Geographical Medicine*, 2nd edn. McGraw-Hill, New York, pp. 423–427.

Marseilles fever *see* **Tick-borne typhuses.**

Mastitis

J. Eric Hillerton

Mastitis is inflammation of the mammary gland of dairy animals usually induced by various bacteria. It results from infection of the mammary gland of any mammal and, although a significant problem of well-being, is economically important in animals used to produce milk for human consumption. It may be caused by any of at least 135 different microorganisms and affect the mammary gland at any age of the animal and at any stage of its development. 'Summer mastitis' is one particular form of infection that affects only non-lactating glands, primarily of cows, and is associated with the muscid fly *Hydrotaea irritans*. The disease affects up to 10% of animals at risk, primarily in July to October, coincident with the occurrence of adult flies visiting cattle.

Distribution

The disease is endemic in the temperate dairy areas of northern Europe but similar problems have also been reported from North America, South America, parts of Africa and Australasia, where the supposed vector is absent but its niche is filled by other muscids.

Pathogens

The predominant bacterium isolated from cases is *Arcanobacterium pyogenes* (previously known as *Corynebacterium pyogenes*), which is commonly found in cutaneous lesions. The anaerobe *Peptococcus indolicus* is also regarded as a key component of the clinical disease. Other pathogens, including *Streptococcus dysgalactiae*, other anaerobes and an unspeciated

Stuart–Schwann coccus, are often isolated. The complexity of the bacterial flora is likely to be indicative of the quality of samples, the laboratory methodology and the amount of environmental exposure to infection.

Clinical symptoms

Summer mastitis usually presents as an acute or peracute multifactorial infection of the non-lactating mammary gland. It is also seen in male calves. Initially there is swelling and pain in the mammary tissue and a markedly purulent discharge. Progression of the disease may lead to extensive necrosis, including external rupturing of abscesses, systemic involvement from toxins elaborated, pyrexia, lameness and even death. Abortion or impaired fetal development are common in pregnant animals. There is usually permanent loss of secretory activity from affected tissue.

Diagnosis

Primary detection is by herdsman observation and is easy in later stages when there is a distended udder, separation of the affected animal from the herd, inappetence and a high infestation of flies on the affected teat. Early stages are only obvious if there is close monitoring of animals at risk and this is rare in these non-producing animals. Confirmation usually only extends to observation of a purulent, creamy discharge, indicative of the involvement of a complex of bacteria. Laboratory confirmation is rarely obtained. Confounding infections occur, usually caused by *Streptococcus uberis*, but lack the extensive clinical signs and poor prognosis.

Transmission

The disease occurs at a low frequency wherever and whenever dairy animals are maintained, indoors and outdoors. It occurs only at high incidence when the primarily univoltine fly *Hydrotaea irritans* (see entry) is abundant on cows. This is the only confirmed vector and infection is transferred mechanically to teat skin tissue. Female flies visit animals to obtain protein meals, usually achieved by sucking blood from wounds. When foraging on unaffected animals they may enlarge previous teat skin damage, often created by biting Stomoxinae (see Stable-flies), or abrade teat orifice tissue when feeding on intramammary secretions. The initial cutaneous wounds may be infected or the meal may be taken from a mastitic gland, the secretion of which contains chemoattractants, mostly organic acids, produced by the anaerobic bacteria. On subsequent feeding visits, up to 3 or 4 days later, the flies regurgitate their contaminated crop contents, to maintain blood flow, and thus infect and colonize the wound. The disease of the mammary tissue probably results from an ascending infection via the streak canal. The role of any other vector, especially in geographical areas other than Europe, is only speculation.

Treatment

All pathogens involved are sensitive to penicillins but systemic or intramammary application is rarely very effective because of poor distribution through the grossly affected tissue, which can be an extensive mass. In severe cases euthanasia is recommended. In some Scandinavian countries the teat is amputated to drain the abscess. Usually the affected part of the udder atrophies and may continue to be infected. In highly productive dairy areas the animals are diverted to beef enterprises or culled early. It is important to quarantine affected animals indoors to minimize subsequent transmission.

Control

The degree of control attempted is related to season and local incidence of summer mastitis. Limitation of exposure to infection is attempted by minimizing the number of animals at risk, especially by manipulating calving pattern and then by grazing animals at risk on pastures away from flies. This is done by avoiding wooded areas and using exposed grazing where wind speeds limit fly dispersal. Various insecticides, fly repellents and barriers applied to teats have been of limited use in prevention of summer mastitis. Since the mid-1980s the introduction of pyrethroid-impregnated ear-tags and then 'pour-on' formulations of synthetic pyrethroids has made fly control on animals kept on more remote pastures highly effective. A noticeable decline in incidence of summer mastitis has occurred since these techniques became available. Previously the only truly effective method was prophylactic infusion of long-acting antibiotic formulations into the mammary gland. These achieved a reduction of incidence of summer mastitis from approximately 10% to 2% of animals at risk. However, this method is inappropriate for animals prior to first calving. It has become unpopular in some countries as this use of antibiotic to treat uninfected animals is considered an unnecessary overuse of antibiotics in food animals, despite its effectiveness in improving animal welfare.

Selected bibliography

Chirico, J.P., Jonsson, P., Kjellberg, S. and Thomas, G. (1997) Summer mastitis experimentally induced by *Hydrotaea irritans* exposed to bacteria. *Medical and Veterinary Entomology* 11, 187–192.

Hillerton, J.E., Bramley, A.J. and Watson, C.A. (1987) The epidemiology of summer mastitis: a survey of clinical cases. *British Veterinary Journal* 143, 520–530.

Thomas, G., Over, H.J., Vecht, U. and Nansen, P. (1987) *Summer Mastitis*. Martinus Nijhoff, Dordrecht, 224 pp.

Mayaro virus

Charles H. Calisher

Mayaro (MAY) virus causes a non-fatal illness characterized by sudden onset, fever, chills, headache, myalgias and arthralgias of the small joints of the hands and feet. Two to 5 days after onset, fever begins to resolve and a maculopapular rash appears, lasting 3–5 days. Arthralgias may persist for many months. This virus has been isolated from haematophagous arthropods and vertebrates from South America and from people and birds who have departed from there recently.

Distribution

Mayaro virus was isolated for the first time from the serum of a human in Mayaro County, south-eastern Trinidad, in 1954; although not febrile at the time the serum was collected, the person became febrile the next day. In 1955, MAY virus was isolated from quarry and forest workers during an epidemic near Belém, Brazil, and, also during an epidemic, from recent settlers from Okinawa who were living in a rain forest in eastern Bolivia. Mayaro virus continues to cause periodic outbreaks of disease, including Brazilian outbreaks in 1991–1993. This virus was isolated in 1994 in Peru for the first time. Additional cases occurred in Peru in 1997, further suggesting the endemic nature of this virus in Amazonia.

Mayaro virus has also been isolated from humans in Suriname, French Guiana, Colombia and, in 2001, Venezuela, and antibody to it has been detected in Howler monkeys (*Alouatta pigra* (= *villosa*) and Agoutis (*Dasyprocta punctata*) in Panama and in humans and monkeys in French Guiana. Mayaro virus has also been isolated from two species of lizards (*Tropidurus torquatus hispidus* and *Ameiva ameiva ameiva*) in Brazil and a single isolation of MAY virus was made from a northbound migrant bird in Louisiana in April 1967.

Aetiological agent
Taxonomy
The taxonomic placement of MAY virus is in the family Togaviridae, genus *Alphavirus*. The virion diameter is 60–65 nm (cores are 40 nm), and the nucleocapsid is surrounded by a lipid envelope, which is apparently derived from host cell membrane during budding. Originally classified by antigenic means, the togaviruses were designated 'Group A' arboviruses, along with eastern equine encephalitis, western equine encephalitis, Venezuelan equine

encephalitis, Getah, Ross River, Sindbis, Semliki Forest (see entries), Sagiyama and others. The two envelope glycoproteins, E1 and E2, compose the external surface of the virion and take part in attachment of virions to cell surfaces, haemagglutination and neutralization. Antigenic subtypes and varieties are numerous for most viruses of this genus.

Genetics

Increasingly, genetic information is becoming available for MAY virus, and this virus has been used as a model for detailed studies of alphavirus replication and pathogenesis. Alphavirus genomes contain about 12,000 nucleotides arranged as single, non-segmented, positive-sense strands of RNA. The genomes are polyadenylated at the 3′ end and capped with 7-methylguanosine at the 5′ end. Phylogenetic relationships among isolates of MAY virus are being investigated by reverse transcription–polymerase chain reaction but results are not yet complete.

Genome transfer into the cytoplasm of the infected cell precedes three sequential stages of viral amplification, i.e. translation, transcription and replication of genomic RNA. Subgenomic messenger RNA (mRNA) (referred to as 26S RNA) is formed during replication and contains about 4100 nucleotides, the sequence of which is identical to the 3′ terminal third of the genomic RNA. This RNA is also polyadenylated and capped and is the template for the four viral structural proteins; the 49S RNA non-structural region serves as the template for four non-structural proteins and the capsid. Alphavirus genomes can accept mutations in the conserved regions without destroying biological activity. Only sequences at the 3′ and 5′ termini are indispensable for the genome to be amplified and packaged. In the region of the junction of non-structural and structural genes, 19 nucleotides upstream from the beginning of the 26S RNA sequence and five downstream from it are needed for production of 26S RNA.

Evolution

Although both structural and non-structural proteins of alphaviruses are conserved to some extent, the latter are more conserved than the former. Because amino acid sequences of various alphaviruses are encoded by different codons, alphavirus replication may allow use of different paths to the finished product but retention of similar requirements to accomplish fundamentals. Indeed, the original antigenic classification of the alphaviruses depended on the phenotypic expression (antigens) of the gene sequences (genotype). Because the protein structure of Sindbis virus corresponds with (is conserved among) protein structures of certain plant viruses that have genomic organizations dissimilar from that of the alphaviruses, because all alphaviruses and many plant viruses are arthropod-borne at some stage in their natural cycle and because mosquitoes belonging to some of the species that transmit alphaviruses typically feed on plant secretions as well as on vertebrates, alphaviruses and plant viruses may have had common ancestors. Highly conserved regions of alphavirus genomes may provide insight into more recent phylogeny. Relatively minor differences between viruses and virus variants may indicate relatively recent evolutionary drifts, and relatively major differences between viruses may indicate more remote genetic shifts.

Clinical symptoms

Human infections with MAY virus occur primarily in the rainy season, when mosquito populations are highest. Patients infected with MAY virus do not usually die from it; therefore, tissues from these patients are not readily available for histological examination. Treatment of MAY virus infections consists primarily of supportive therapy. Symptoms respond partially to non-steroidal anti-inflammatory drugs. Development of viraemia does not necessarily correlate with production of disease in experimentally infected animals. Antibody to MAY virus has been detected in various primates and domestic animals and in other vertebrates. Field strains of virus are non-pathogenic for adult mice but are pathogenic for suckling mice inoculated intracranially.

Diagnosis

Alphaviruses have common antigenic determinants, as shown by many serological tests, including haemagglutination inhibition, complement fixation, enzyme-linked immunosorbent assay (ELISA) and immunofluorescence. These viruses have been classified as belonging to one of six antigenic complexes; viruses in such complexes are more closely related to each other than they are to other viruses within the serogroup ('Group A' arboviruses). The six complexes are: (i) eastern equine encephalitis; (ii) Middelburg; (iii) Ndumu; (iv) Semliki Forest; (v) Venezuelan equine encephalitis; and (vi) western equine encephalitis. Mayaro virus belongs to the Semliki Forest complex, which also includes Semliki Forest, chikungunya, o'nyong-nyong, Getah, Sagiyama, Bebaru, Ross River and Una viruses. These viruses can be distinguished from one another by use of virus- or strain-specific monoclonal antibodies employed in haemagglutination inhibition, neutralization, ELISA and other tests. Because no two virus isolates are exactly the same, the definition and identification of an alphavirus depends on generalities as to placement in the serogroup, specific identification as to its nearest antigenic neighbour, and final placement with regard to type, subtype or variety. When type-specific antigens (polypeptides) and antibodies (against glycoproteins E1 and E2 and against nucleocapsids) become available, they can be used as reagents for rapid determination of serogroup, complex and virus type and for serodiagnosis of alphavirus infections.

Various cell cultures from vertebrates (VERO, LLC-MK2, BHK-21, hamster kidney, chicken embryo, duck embryo) and invertebrates (C6/36 cells from *Aedes albopictus* mosquitoes) are susceptible to MAY virus and useful for virus isolation and characterization. These cells can be used as substrates for ELISA or for tests to detect neutralizing antibodies to MAY virus, in which this virus forms plaques and causes cytopathic effects. Virus isolation is the test of choice for laboratory diagnosis of MAY virus infection. The virus can be isolated either in cell cultures or in suckling mice, which are slightly more sensitive than are cell cultures.

Infection with MAY virus leads to production of immunoglobulin M (IgM), IgG and, probably, IgA antibodies. As detected by IgM-capture ELISA, antibody to these viruses cross-reacts with heterologous alphaviruses but is most reactive with other viruses of the same antigenic complex. That is, IgM antibody from patients with MAY virus may have the highest titres to MAY virus but high titres to others of the Semliki Forest complex. Immunoglobulin M antibody peaks 2–3 weeks after onset and persists for about 2 months. Immunoglobulin G antibody also appears relatively soon after onset but, unlike IgM, persists for many months or years after the illness. Haemagglutination inhibition, complement fixation, immunofluorescence and neutralization tests simply detect IgM and IgG antibodies in other configurations. Immunoglobulin M antibody is haemagglutinin-inhibiting, immunofluorescing and neutralizing; IgG antibody reacts in these tests and in complement fixation tests as well. Thus, IgM ELISA is the diagnostic test of choice for determining recent infections (if confirmed by neutralization tests) and may be applied to single serum samples in some instances. The presence of IgG antibody to any of these viruses is simply an indication of past infection and, without demonstration of a significant (fourfold or greater) increase or decrease in titre between paired acute-phase and convalescent-phase serum samples, cannot be used to implicate the virus in the aetiology of the illness; usefulness of IgG assays is limited because of cross-reactivity. Clinical signs and symptoms cause confusion between infections with MAY virus and with dengue viruses.

Transmission and tissue tropism

Mayaro virus has been isolated principally from *Haemagogus janthinomys* mosquitoes, but a few isolates have been made from mosquitoes belonging to other genera, such as *Psorophora*, *Mansonia*, *Culex* and *Sabethes*. Experimentally infected marmosets (*Callithrix* species) and other primates develop high-titre viraemia. Little else is known about the natural history of this virus. This virus is transmitted to humans by the bite of transmission-competent, infected mosquitoes. When human viraemic titres reach such levels that mosquitoes subsequently feeding on them become infected, these mosquitoes can then transmit virus to the people on whom they next feed. If an infected human does not develop a high viraemia titre, that person cannot serve as a virus reservoir and becomes a dead-end host. The target tissues for these viruses are unknown but may include circulatory, synovial and epidermal cells. Intact *Aedes albopictus* mosquitoes have also been used for laboratory studies of MAY virus replication and transmission.

Treatment

There is no specific treatment for MAY virus infection. Treatment is entirely symptomatic.

Prevention and control

Because mosquitoes transmit MAY virus, prevention of human infection requires reduction of contact between the susceptible human and the vector. This can be effected by mosquito control operations, using larvicide or adulticide techniques, either on a large (e.g. aerial applications of insecticides) or a small (ground-based applications) scale. Public education projects (with ongoing publicity) and legal means are often used to direct intervention. Ongoing clinical, virological, serological and arthropod surveillance techniques should be used to ascertain the presence and prevalence of these viruses. In certain countries, this often requires considerable political will.

For preventing contact of mosquito vectors with humans, the use of mosquito nets and screening windows and doors with plastic mesh are recommended. Removing and subsequently destroying mosquito breeding sites (source reduction), providing piped water, maintaining liquid waste systems and managing irrigation systems have been successful ways of reducing populations of both maintenance and amplification vectors.

If measures taken to control arthropod vectors of MAY virus are not effective or are not possible because of economic, political or geographical considerations, vaccines hold some potential for prevention of disease in humans at risk of infection. With rapid air transport, an increasing number of tourists are exposed to potential infection (human infection with MAY virus has been diagnosed in the USA in a patient who had travelled to eastern Peru). Whether any travellers return home in the incubation (viraemic) period of MAY virus infection and can infect local mosquito populations is unknown.

Selected bibliography

American Committee on Arthropod-Borne Viruses (1985) *International Catalogue of Arboviruses Including Certain Other Viruses of Vertebrates*, 3rd edn, Karabatsos, N. (ed.). American Society of Tropical Medicine and Hygiene, San Antonia, Texas, 1147 pp.

Calisher, C.H., Shope, R.E., Brandt, W., Casals, J., Karabatsos, N., Murphy, F.A., Tesh, R.B. and Wiebe, M.E. (1980) Proposed antigenic classification of registered arboviruses. I. Togaviridae, *Alphavirus*. *Intervirology* 14, 229–232.

Calisher, C.H., El-Kafrawi, A.O., Mahmud, M.I. Al-D., Travassos da Rosa, A.P.A., Bartz, C.R., Brummer-Korvenkontio, M., Haksohusodo, S. and Suharyono, W. (1986) Complex-specific immunoglobulin M antibody patterns in humans infected with alphaviruses. *Journal of Clinical Microbiology* 23, 155–159.

Peters, C.J. and Dalrymple, J.M. (1990) Alphaviruses. In: Fields, B.N., Knipe, D.M. and Howley, P.M. (eds) *Virology*, Vol. 1, 2nd edn. Raven Press, New York, pp. 713–761.

Schlesinger, S. and Schlesinger, M.J. (1990) Replication of Togaviridae and Flaviviridae. In: Fields, B.N., Knipe, D.M. and Howley, P.M. (eds) *Virology*, Vol. 1, 2nd edn. Raven Press, New York, pp. 697–711.

Talarmin, A., Chandler, L.J., Kazanji, M., de Thoisy, B., Debon, P., Lelarge, J., Labeau, B., Bourreau, E., Vie, J.C., Shope, R.E. and Sarthou, J.L. (1998) Mayaro virus fever in French Guiana: isolation, identification, and seroprevalence. *American Journal of Tropical Medicine and Hygiene* 59, 452–456.

Tesh, R.B., Watts, D.M., Russell, K.L., Damodaran, C., Calampa, C., Cabezas, C., Ramirez, G.,

Vasquez, B., Hayes, C.G., Rossi, C.A., Powers, A.M., Hice, C.L., Chandler, L.J., Cropp, C.B., Karabatsos, N., Roehrig, J.T. and Gubler, D.J. (1999) Mayaro virus disease: an emerging mosquito-borne zoonosis in tropical South

America. *Clinical Infectious Diseases* 28, 67–73.

Theiler, M. and Downs, W.G. (1973) *The Arthropod-borne Viruses of Vertebrates.* Yale University Press, New Haven, Connecticut, 578 pp.

Mediterranean coast fever *see* **Theilerioses.**

Mediterranean spotted fever *see* **Tick-borne typhuses.**

Middelburg virus

Oyewale Tomori

Distribution

Middelburg (MID) virus was first isolated in 1957 from a pool of *Ochlerotatus*[1] *caballus* sensu lato mosquitoes, collected with human bait in Conway, Middelburg, in the Cape Province of South Africa. Additional isolates were later recovered from pools of *Aedes lineatopennis* and *Aedes albothorax* mosquitoes, also collected in Middelburg. Since then, numerous isolations of MID virus have been obtained from mosquitoes of various species in several African countries, such as South Africa, Zimbabwe, Kenya, Central African Republic, Cameroon, Senegal and Côte d'Ivoire. Serological surveys have revealed low prevalence of neutralizing antibodies to MID virus in human populations in South Africa, Mozambique and Angola. In addition, MID virus neutralizing antibodies have been detected in the sera of South African sheep, cattle, goats and horses.

Virus

Middelburg virus is a single-stranded RNA enveloped virus, belonging to the *Alphavirus* genus of the Togaviridae family. Under the electron microscope, the spherical virions measure 62–80 nm in diameter. In cross-plaque reduction neutralization tests, there was a low (1/10) neutralization of MID virus by antisera to Ross River and Ndumu viruses. Middelburg virus shows no significant serological relationship with more than 30 alphaviruses from Africa and the Americas. Although MID virus is not antigenically closely related to any other alphavirus, it has been placed in the western equine encephalitis (WEE) virus antigenic complex (see entry).

Middelburg virus is similar to other enveloped alphaviruses in physical and chemical characteristics. The virus is unstable at room temperature, but more stable at lower temperatures. It is inactivated by lipid solvents, such as chloroform, ether and sodium deoxycholate.

Clinical symptoms, pathogenesis and pathology

Suckling mice inoculated intracerebrally (i.c.) or intraperitoneally (i.p.) with MID virus die within 2 days of inoculation. High virus titres (as much as $10^{9.4}$ ml^{-1}) develop in the brains of these mice. Histopathology in mice infected i.c. reveals evidence of generalized infection, with encephalitis, myositis, myocarditis, necrosis of connective tissues in subcutis, periosteum and arteries. Weanling mice (from 3–4 weeks) are not susceptible to MID virus infection when inoculated i.p. or by the subcutaneous (s.c.) route. Day-old chicks, lambs and various species of wild rodents develop viraemia following experimental infection with MID virus, while adult guinea-pigs, Vervet (Green) monkeys (*Chlorocebus aethiops*[2]) and Red-billed teal (*Anas erythrorhynchos*) develop only antibodies. Middelburg virus is readily cultured in a variety of cell lines, with cytopathic effects and plaque development in baby hamster kidney (BHK-21) cells, but only plaque development in chick embryo, vervet monkey (VERO) African green monkey (LLC-MK2) and human diploid (MA-111) cells. Plaque variants (s and 1) of MID virus replicate in *Aedes aegypti* mosquitoes. Following infection, *Ochlerotatus caballus* successfully transmitted MID virus to lambs on days 4, 10 and 19 post-infection, with the lambs developing viraemia and a stiff gait. It is speculated that sheep and *O. caballus* may be involved in incidental transmission cycles of MID virus. No human disease has been associated with MID virus.

Diagnosis
The virus can be isolated by inoculation of laboratory animals and tissue cultures and identified by serological methods.

Treatment
There is no human disease associated with the virus and no treatments have been developed for disease in livestock.

Transmission
Numerous isolations of MID virus have been made from mosquitoes, in particular *Aedes* species, including *Aedes circumluteolus*, pools of *A. lineatopennis* and *A. albothorax*, and *Aedes* (*Aedimorphus*) species, and *O. caballus* sensu lato (Natal, South Africa); *Aedes cumminsii* (Cameroon, Kenya and Senegal); *Aedes dalzieli* (Senegal); *Aedes simulans* (Central African Republic); *A. lineatopennis* (Zimbabwe); and *Aedes palpalis* group (Côte d'Ivoire). In addition there have

been isolations from *Mansonia uniformis* (Central African Republic) and *Mansonia africana* (Cameroon and Central African Republic).

Although MID virus has been successfully transmitted by *O. caballus* and antibodies to it detected in livestock, the vertebrate hosts involved in the natural transmission cycle remain unknown.

Control
Because the vertebrate hosts are not known and human and livestock diseases have not been recognized, control measures are inappropriate.

Notes
[1] *Ochlerotatus* was formerly a subgenus of *Aedes*.
[2] This monkey was formerly in the *genus Cercopithecus*.

Selected bibliography
Karabatsos, N. (1975) Antigenic relationships of group A arboviruses by plaque reduction neutralization testing. *American Journal of Tropical Medicine and Hygiene* 24, 527–532.

Karabatsos, N. (ed.) (1985) *International Catalogue of Arboviruses Including Certain Other Viruses of Vertebrates*, 3rd edn. American Society of Tropical Medicine and Hygiene, San Antonio, Texas, 1147 pp.

Kokernot, R.H., De Meillon B., Paterson, H.E., Heymann, C. and Smithburn, K.D. (1957) Middelburg virus. A hitherto unknown agent isolated from *Aedes* mosquitoes during an epizootic in sheep in the Eastern Cape Province. *South African Journal of Medical Science* 22, 145–153.

Midges *see* **Biting midges.**

Mite-borne typhus *see* **Scrub typhus.**

Mites (Prostigmata and Mesostigmata)

M.W. Service

There are about 30,000 species of mites. Their classification into orders and families

is both complex and controversial. No attempt will be made to enter into such a debate. The mites that can transmit infections to humans and animals are the scrub typhus mites belonging to the genus *Leptotrombidium* and dermanyssid mites in the genera *Liponyssoides* and *Dermanyssus*.

Scrub typhus mites (chiggers, itch mites, leptotrombiculid mites, red bugs, trombiculid mites)

These mites are usually placed in the order Prostigmata and family Trombiculidae. There are some 3000 species of mites in this family belonging to several genera, but only about 20 species in the genus *Leptotrombidium* are of medical importance as disease vectors. They occur mainly in Asia.

Biology

Trombiculid mites have a complex life cycle. Adults are free-living and feed on a variety of soil-inhabiting arthropods. Eggs are laid on leaf litter or on the surface of soil that is damp but well drained, such as in pastures, scrub jungle and along riverbanks. In hot weather, egg laying continues throughout the year, but in cooler regions, including Japan, oviposition seems to cease during the cooler months, with adults entering partial hibernation. Eggs hatch within about a week, but the six-legged larva remains in the eggshell and is called a deutovum. After about a further week the larva emerges from the eggshell and becomes very active, climbing up grasses and other ground vegetation. Larvae are parasitic and attach themselves to mammals, especially rodents, but also to humans and birds. They congregate on areas of the skin that are soft and moist, such as in the ears and on or around the genitalia and anus of rodents; on people larvae seek out areas where clothing is tight, such as around the ankles and waist. On the host larvae pierce the skin and inject saliva, which causes disintegration of cells and a skin reaction in the host, in which a vertical tube-like structure (stylostome, histiosiphon) is formed. Larvae do not usually suck up blood but feed on lymph, other fluids and semi-digested materials. Larvae of *Lepto-*

trombidium species that transmit scrub typhus usually remain on people for 2–10 days, after which the engorged larvae drop to the ground and bury themselves under leaves or just below the soil.

The buried and inactive larva is called a protonymph (Fig. 1). After 7–10 days, the protonymph moults to become an eight-legged reddish deutonymph, which feeds on soil-living arthropods. A few days or 1–2 weeks later, the deutonymph stops feeding, becomes inactive and is called a tritonymph. After a further 2 weeks, this moults to become an adult. The only stage in the life cycle that is parasitic is the larva.

The ecological requirements for the life cycle can be complex. For example, larval mites need areas in which there is a plentiful supply of small mammals on which to feed, whereas the free-living nymphal stages and adults require moist conditions and a good supply of soil arthropods on which to feed. Areas that satisfy these needs and support mite populations are called 'mite islands', which can comprise just a few square metres to several kilometres.

The complete life cycle (Fig. 1) usually lasts 6–12 weeks, but may be prolonged to about 9 months.

Diseases

Certain species of the genus *Leptotrombidium*, such as *L. deliense* and *L. akamushi*, are vectors of scrub typhus (see entry). Some species are also involved in the transmission of haemorrhagic fever with renal syndrome (see entry).

Control

The chance of being attacked by larval mites can be reduced by applying chemical repellents, especially around the ankles and lower parts of the legs. Clothing, such as socks, can be impregnated with repellents or pyrethroid insecticides, such as permethrin. The wide and patchy distribution of trombiculid mites and the difficulty of identifying mite islands can make their control with insecticides difficult.

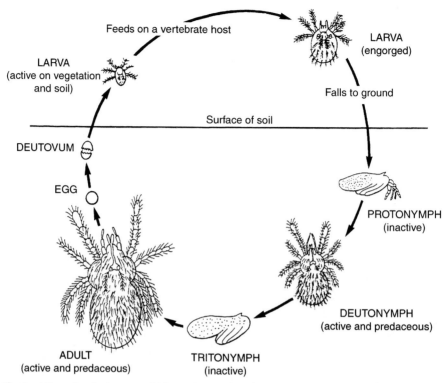

Fig. 1. Life cycle of a *Leptotrombidium* mite (scrub typhus mite) (courtesy of the Natural History Museum, London).

Liponyssoid mites (house-mouse mite)

These mites are usually placed in the order Mesostigmata. They belong to the family Dermanyssidae, and the only species of medical importance is *Liponyssoides sanguineus*, which has a localized but almost worldwide distribution.

Biology

The preferred host is the House mouse (*Mus musculus*), but other rodents, including rats, are commonly attacked, and also humans. Mites only occur on their hosts to feed; at other times they shelter in cracks and crevices in or near the hosts' nests or burrows, where they lay their eggs. Larvae, which hatch from the eggs after 4–5 days, are non-parasitic, but the two nymphal stages (protonymph and deutonymph) and adults take blood meals. Adult mites (Fig. 2), especially the females, take several

blood meals before reaching repletion, and engorged mites can withstand starvation for about 2 months and starved ones for about 6 weeks. The life cycle from egg to adult lasts 17–23 days.

Diseases

Liponyssoides sanguieneus is a vector of rickettsialpox to humans (see entry), and *Dermanyssus gallinae* is a vector of fowl pox (see entry).

Control

Rodenticides can be used to kill the reservoir rodent hosts, such as mice and rats, while residual insecticides can be sprayed in places harbouring the mites.

Selected bibliography

Audy, J.R. (1968) *Red Mites and Typhus*. The Athlone Press, London, 191 pp.

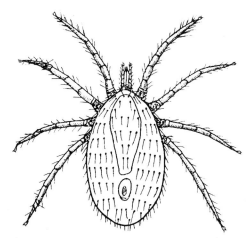

Fig. 2. An adult house-mouse mite (*Liponyssoides sanguineus*).

Baker, A.S. (1999) *Mites and Ticks of Domestic Animals. An Identification Guide and Information Source.* The Stationery Office, London, 240 pp.

Baker, E.W., Evans, T.M., Gould, D.J., Hull, W.B. and Keegan, H.L. (1956) *A Manual of Parasitic Mites of Medical or Economic Importance.* National Pest Control Association, New York, 170 pp.

Roberts, S.H. and Zimmerman, J.H. (1980) Chigger mites: efficacy of control with two pyrethroids. *Journal of Economic Entomology* 73, 811–812.

Sasa, M. (1961) Biology of chiggers. *Annual Review of Entomology* 6, 221–244.

Traub, R. and Wisseman, C.I. (1974) The ecology of chigger-borne rickettsiosis (scrub-typhus). *Journal of Medical Entomology* 11, 237–303.

Monkey disease *see* **Kyasanur Forest disease**.

Mosquitoes (Culicidae)

M.W. Service

There are some 3200 species and subspecies of mosquitoes belonging to 42 genera, all within the family Culicidae. Mosquitoes have a worldwide distribution. Although they can be common in tropical countries, the greatest numbers biting humans and animals are often encountered in subarctic areas. The species most concerned with the transmission of infections to humans and animals are contained in the genera *Anopheles, Culex, Aedes, Ochlerotatus* (formerly this was a subgenus of *Aedes*) and *Mansonia*. Mosquitoes are the major vectors of diseases to humans; they also transmit a few infections to animals, but ticks (see entry) are of greater importance in the transmission of animal infections.

The Culicidae are divided into three subfamilies, the principal two being the Anophelinae (anophelines) containing the genus *Anopheles* (and two other genera of no medical importance) and the Culicinae (culicines) containing *Aedes, Ochlerotatus, Culex, Mansonia, Coquillettidia, Culiseta, Haemagogus, Sabethes* and another 30 genera. The third subfamily, Toxorhyn-

chitinae, has just one genus, *Toxorhynchites*, species of which are incapable of blood-feeding and consequently are not disease vectors.

Identification

Useful taxonomic characters for distinguishing anopheline from culicine mosquitoes are as follows.

Anophelines

Eggs are laid singly on the water surface; they are not stuck together. They have a pair of air-filled lateral floats. Larvae lack a respiratory siphon and lie parallel to the water surface when breathing and feeding. Adults have black and whitish scales on the wings, which are arranged in blocks. They rest on surfaces with the body at an angle. Both males and females have palps about as long as the proboscis.

Culicines

Eggs are laid singly or formed into an egg raft or sticky mass and they never have floats. Larvae have a respiratory siphon and subtend at an angle to the water surface. Adults usually have brownish scales on the wing veins and sometimes also a scattering of white scales, but their dark and white scales are not arranged in blocks. They rest with the body more or less parallel to the surface. In males the palps are about as long as the proboscis, but in females they are much shorter than the proboscis.

Biology

It is convenient to describe the general biology of mosquitoes and then consider separately differences in the biology of anopheline and culicine mosquitoes.

Mosquitoes in general

Eggs are brown or blackish and are laid: (i) on the water surface of a diverse collection of waters, ranging from pools to puddles water-filled animal hoofprints, borrow pits, wells, discarded tin cans, clay or metal water-storage containers, grassy ditches, marshes, including sometimes salt-water ones, rice-fields, septic tanks, cesspools, water-filled tree holes, cut bamboo stumps and leaf axils of plants; (ii) on wet mud, leaf litter, damp walls of containers, such as tree holes or water-storage pots, or other damp substrates near the water's edge; and (iii) on the undersides of floating vegetation, to which they are 'glued'.

In the tropics, eggs hatch within 1–2 days, but in cooler climates hatching may not occur until after 1–2 weeks. Some mosquitoes (e.g. *Aedes* and *Ochlerotatus* species) have eggs that can withstand desiccation and may remain viable for months or years in a 'dry' state.

All mosquito larvae are aquatic, but they do not usually occur in large expanses of open water, such as lakes, or in the running water of streams, although they may live at the edges, where water flow is minimal and where they can shelter in vegetation, such as grasses. They feed on a variety of aquatic microorganisms and pass through four larval instars. With the exception of species of *Mansonia* and *Coquillettidia*, larvae have to come to the water surface to breathe. In tropical countries the larval period can be as short as 7–10 days,

but it is longer in cooler weather and in temperate regions may extend to weeks or months, and several species overwinter as larvae. The pupae are aquatic, do not feed and, with the exception of *Mansonia* and *Coquillettidia* species, remain at the water surface, where they breathe. However, if disturbed they rapidly swim up and down, as also do the larvae. Pupal life is commonly 2–3 days in tropical countries, but may be a week or more in temperate areas.

Only female adult mosquitoes bite; males feed on naturally occurring sugary secretions including nectar. Some species feed predominantly or exclusively on mammals, others may bite birds. Mosquitoes biting humans are termed anthropophagic (or anthropophilic), while those biting livestock and other animals are referred to as being zoophagic (zoophilic). Biting may occur in the evenings or at night (e.g. anophelines) or during the daytime (e.g. many culicines). Some species bite mainly inside houses (endophagic), while others bite out of doors (exophagic). After blood-feeding some species rest indoors while the blood meal is being digested and the eggs mature (endophilic), while others rest out of doors (exophilic) in various man-made or natural shelters. Many species exhibit a mix of these behavioural patterns, with species not being exclusively exophilic or exophagic or even anthropophagic. Speed of blood digestion is temperature-dependent and in tropical countries usually takes 2–3 days, after which the female is ready to lay her eggs, and she is referred to as being gravid. In temperate climates blood digestion may take 1–2 weeks. After egg laying females take another blood meal and develop a further batch of eggs, this process of feeding and oviposition is repeated several times during her life and is called the gonotrophic cycle. Some individuals of some species (e.g. *Aedes aegypti*) may take multiple blood meals before they become gravid.

Adult mosquitoes generally disperse just a few hundred metres from their emergence sites, and in control programmes and epidemiological studies it is usually assumed, for practical purposes, that mosquitoes do not fly further than 2 km.

However, there are records of mosquitoes being dispersed 100 km or more, usually assisted by the wind. Sometimes they get carried considerable distances in railway carriages or even further in aircraft. In tropical countries female adults probably live on average 1–2 weeks, but in temperate regions they commonly live for 1–2 months and sometimes fertilized females remain in hibernation for up to 9 months. Males usually have a much shorter life.

Anophelines

Anopheles eggs are black, have lateral floats (Fig. 1) and are laid on the water surface, not on damp substrates. They cannot withstand desiccation and hatch within 2–3 days, but in colder temperate regions eggs may not hatch until after 2–3 weeks. The larvae lack a siphon and lie parallel to the water surface, where they both breathe and feed. Like the pupae they only descend when disturbed. Larval habitats range from animal hoofprints, puddles, pools and wells, to rice-fields and marshy areas, including salt-water marshes and mangrove swamps. A very few species are found in water-filled tree holes and, in the southern USA and Central and South America, some species, including malaria vectors, breed in leaf axils of bromeliad plants that grow on trees. In general anophelines prefer clean water that is not polluted with animal and vegetable matter.

Anopheles adults feed mainly in the evenings and at night. Some species, such as *Anopheles albimanus* of Central America, bite mainly before midnight, whereas others such as *Anopheles gambiae* in sub-Saharan Africa, feed mostly after midnight. The times of biting, the degree of anthropophagy and whether adults rest indoors or outdoors are all of considerable importance in the epidemiology of disease transmission and control.

Culicines

Eggs of *Aedes* and *Ochlerotatus* species are black and are usually laid on damp substrates just beyond the water-line. They can withstand varying degrees of desiccation, and dry eggs may remain viable for many months and in some species even for a few years. Eggs hatch when they become flooded. *Culex* and also *Coquillettidia* mosquitoes have brownish eggs, which are laid upright and placed together to form an egg raft that floats on the water surface (Fig. 1), while female *Mansonia* lay their eggs in a sticky mass that is glued to the undersides of floating vegetation, such as leaves of the Water lettuce (*Pistia stratiotes*).

Culicine larvae have a short or long siphon, which most species use to breathe at the water surface. Larvae hang down from the surface, and thus do not lie parallel to it as do anophelines. However, larvae of *Mansonia* and *Coquillettidia* insert their modified siphons into aquatic plants to obtain oxygen via plant tissues; larvae do not surface but remain submerged and attached to plants. (Pupae of these two genera also remain submerged, obtaining oxygen from plants by inserting into them their specialized respiratory trumpets.) Larvae of some species feed predominantly near the water surface while others feed on the debris and detritus at the bottom of larval habitats. Culicine larvae are found in a great variety of waters, ranging from puddles and ponds to swamps. Some species, especially of the genera *Aedes* and *Ochlerotatus*, breed in natural and man-made container-type habitats, such as water-filled tree holes, cut bamboo stems, plant axils, rock pools, water-storage pots, discarded tin cans and motor vehicle tyres. In subarctic areas *Aedes* and *Ochlerotatus* species are often found in snow-melt pools. They are also sometimes found in snow-melt waters at high elevation in temperate zones and, in the eastern USA and northern Europe, even at low elevations. Larvae of most *Culex* species are found in ground collections of water, such as pools, ponds, ditches and borrow pits. Some *Culex* species (e.g. *Culex tritaeniorhynchus*) breed in rice-fields, while larvae of *Culex quinquefasciatus* tolerate high levels of organic pollution and can be found in latrines, septic tanks and soak-away pits. Larvae of *Mansonia* and *Coquillettidia* are found only in waters in which there are aquatic plants to which their larvae and pupae can attach themselves.

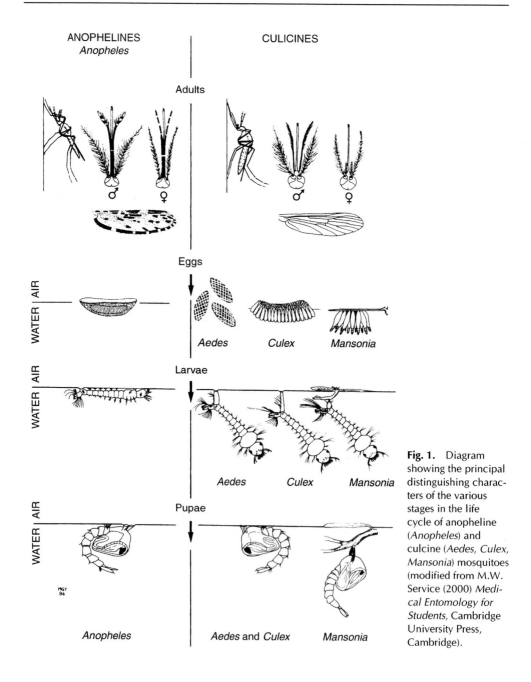

Fig. 1. Diagram showing the principal distinguishing characters of the various stages in the life cycle of anopheline (*Anopheles*) and culcine (*Aedes, Culex, Mansonia*) mosquitoes (modified from M.W. Service (2000) *Medical Entomology for Students,* Cambridge University Press, Cambridge).

Adults of many, but not all, *Aedes* and *Ochlerotatus* species bite during the day or early evening, while adults of many *Culex* species and most *Mansonia* and *Coquillettidia* bite at night. Most culicines feed and rest out of doors, but *C. quinquefasciatus* bites inside houses as well as outside, and commonly rests in houses after blood-feeding.

Diseases

Mosquitoes transmit more pathogens to humans than do any other arthropods and, in addition, are the vectors of some pathogens to domesticated animals. For example, anophelines transmit human malaria parasites, bancroftian and brugian filariae and o'nyong nyong and a few other arboviruses, while culicine mosquitoes transmit avian malaria parasites, bancroftian and brugian filariae, dirofilariae, *Setaria* species and numerous arboviruses, including those causing yellow fever, dengue, Rift Valley fever, fowl pox and the encephalitides (see entries under names of these infections).

Control

Mosquitoes can be controlled by directing efforts either at the larvae or at the adults.

Larval control

Larval habitats can sometimes be drained or filled in to eradicate breeding places. Environmental modifications, such as digging out marshy areas to create impoundments containing uninterrupted standing water, which is unsuitable as a larval habitat for many species, is sometimes practised on a small or large scale. Covers and screens can sometimes be placed on domestic water containers and cisterns to prevent egg laying occurring. Alternatively chemicals, such as oils, Paris green (copper aceto-arsenite), organophosphate and carbamate insecticides, or microbial insecticides, such as *Bacillus thuringiensis* subsp. *israelensis* (*Bti* or serotype H-14) can be applied to many breeding places to kill the larvae. Sometime insect growth regulators (IGRs) such as Dimilin (diflurobenzuron) or Altosid (methoprene) can be applied. All these chemicals have to be repeatedly sprayed because they have little, if any, long-lasting effect. Biological control, using fish and other agents, has not generally proved very effective in reducing biting densities of mosquitoes or reducing disease transmission.

Adult control

Mosquito screening over windows and doors of houses and hospitals may assist in reducing the likelihood of being bitten by mosquitoes. Better personal protection against night-biting species (e.g.

anophelines and *C. quinquefasciatus*) is provided by mosquito bed nets, especially if they are impregnated with pyrethroid insecticides. Insect repellents may also provide some degree of protection against biting. Ground or aerial applications of insecticides, especially ultra-low-volume (ULV) spraying, can often give rapid, albeit usually temporary, relief over relatively small areas. This approach is usually best suited to achieving a rapid kill of mosquitoes, included infective ones, in epidemics such as dengue outbreaks.

The application of residual insecticides to the inside surfaces of walls, ceilings or roofs of buildings, mainly houses, can often give effective control of endophilic mosquitoes, such as some anophelines, for 3–6 months. At present, there are no genetic methods that can be routinely advocated for mosquito control.

Selected bibliography

Clements, A.N. (1992) *The Biology of Mosquitoes*, Vol. 1, *Development, Nutrition and Reproduction*. Chapman & Hall, London, 509 pp.

Clements, A.N. (1999) *The Biology of Mosquitoes*, Vol. 2, *Sensory Reception and Behaviour*. CAB International, Wallingford, UK, 740 pp.

Gillett, J.D. (1971) *Mosquitos*. Weidenfeld & Nicolson, London, 274 pp.

Harbach, R. and Sandlast, G. (1997) CABIKEY: *Mosquito Genera of the World*. CD-ROM for Windows 3x or Windows 95 on a 486PC with 8 MB RAM. CAB International, Wallingford, UK.

Lacey, L.A. and Lacey, C.M. (1990) The medical importance of riceland mosquitoes and their control using alternatives to chemical insecticides. *Journal of the American Mosquito Control Association* 6 (suppl. 2), 1–93.

Service, M.W. (1993) Mosquitoes (Culicidae). In: Lane, R.P. and Crosskey, R.W. (eds) *Medical Insects and Arachnids*. Chapman & Hall, London, pp. 120–140.

Service, M.W. (2000) [Chapters 1–3 on mosquitoes.] In: Service, M.W. *Medical Entomology for Students*. Cambridge University Press, Cambridge, pp. 1–78.

Service, M.W. and Townson, H. (2001) The *Anopheles* vector. In: Gilles, H.M. and Warrell, D.A. (eds) *Bruce-Chwatt's Essential Malariology*, 4th edn. Edward Arnold, London.

World Health Organization (1997) *Vector Control. Methods for Use by Individuals and Communities*, prepared by J.A. Rozendaal. World Health Organization, Geneva, 412 pp.

Murine typhus *see* **Endemic typhus.**

Murray Valley encephalitis

Ian D. Marshall

Murray Valley encephalitis (MVE) virus is a mosquito-borne, single-stranded RNA arbovirus of the Flaviviridae family.

Distribution

Murray Valley encephalitis virus has been recovered from mosquitoes collected at latitudes ranging from about 4°S on the Sepik River, Papua New Guinea (PNG), to about 37°S in the Murray River basin (Fig. 1). In New Guinea the virus is enzootic and endemic on the coastal plains and foothills north and south of the high central mountain range. Overt disease is extremely rare. In continental Australia, MVE virus seems now to be enzootic and endemic on much of the north coast and immediate hinterland, with rare epidemic activity in the Murray–Darling river system. The first of the endemic cases occurred in the Kimberley region in 1978, 4 years after the 1974 epidemic, which involved all states. There were four Murray Valley encephalitis cases on this occasion and a further 25 cases in 10 of the following 18 years. Over the same time period, there were 14 cases in the 'Top End' of the Northern Territory (NT) and four cases on Cape York Peninsula, but there were no cases in the Murray–Darling Basin or in South Australia (SA). The damming of the Ord River and the introduction of irrigated farming in the Kimberley region might explain the altered behaviour of MVE virus in this formerly seasonally arid region. Perhaps increased population and the resultant 'development' have influenced the behaviour of the virus in the NT and northern Queensland.

Aetiological agent

Murray Valley encephalitis virus grown in mosquito cell culture was found to be 40 nm in diameter. In common with all flaviviruses, the virions contain a nucleocapsid core composed of a single-strand, positive-sense RNA genome complexed with a single species of capsid protein. The nucleocapsid is composed of a lipid bilayer and two proteins: a membrane (M) protein and the envelope (E) protein.

The nucleotide sequences of the gene encoding the E protein from 11 MVE virus isolates from Australia and PNG have been compared. The isolates were from four fatal human cases, a heron (Ardeidae) and six pools of mosquitoes collected over a period of 25 years. The nucleotide sequences of Australian strains were remarkably stable, showing not more than 1.7% divergence in pairwise comparisons. However, there was 6.8% divergence in the E gene between the two PNG strains and 9–10% divergence between a PNG strain and the Australian prototype.

Murray Valley encephalitis virus is closely related to Japanese encephalitis (JE) virus (from Japan to India and recently in PNG, the Torres Strait Islands and Cape York), St Louis encephalitis (SLE) virus (USA), West Nile (WN) virus (Africa, Europe, Israel and recently the north-eastern USA) and Kunjin (KUN) virus (Australia). See entries on all these arboviruses.

Clinical symptoms

As with other arboviral encephalitides, the morbidity rate is very low – perhaps one clinical case for every 800–1000 seroconversions.

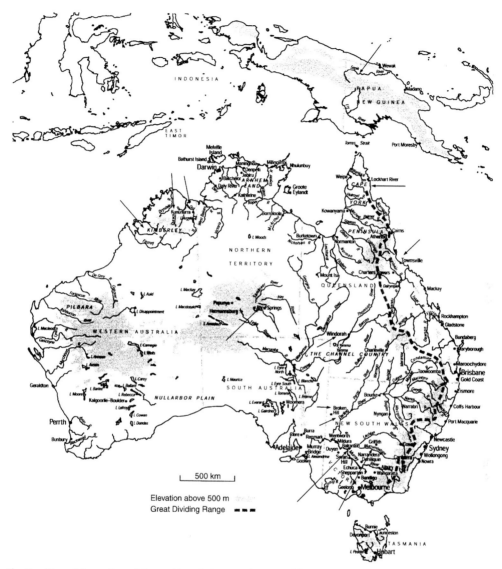

Fig. 1. Map of Australia and Papua New Guinea, with some of the main foci of human infections of Murray Valley encephalitis arrowed.

Based on published reports by physicians attending a total of 48 cases during the 1951 and 1974 outbreaks:

onset was sudden, fever invariable, with daily peaks of up to 40.6°C, anorexia and severe frontal headache common, and about half the patients suffered nausea, vomiting and diarrhoea. Some had an early vague sensation of dizziness. The first indication of disturbed brain function usually

appeared 2–5 days after onset with lethargy, drowsiness, irritability, a dullness deepening into confusion, disorientation and ataxia. About one-third of the patients had convulsions and fits.

The 1974 patients at one hospital were divided into mild (11 patients), severe (seven) and fatal (four) groups. In the 'mild' group, neurological involvement stabilized between the fifth and tenth day of illness but all had frank encephalitis. All had neck stiffness and one lapsed into a coma, responding only to painful stimuli. They were discharged after 2 weeks to 3 months and, at review 16 months later, seven had completely recovered and four had mild degrees of impaired coordination or emotional problems. In the 'severe' group, all lapsed into coma. Pharyngeal paralysis developed in two and respiratory failure in the other five. The latter would have died without the use of artificial respiration and all seven had severe residual disabilities. In 1951, 19/45 (42%) reported cases were fatal and, in 1974, 13/58 (22%). If the five saved by artificial respiration are included, the percentage would be 40%.

Diagnosis

Early diagnosis can only be by clinical symptoms, tempered by awareness of the season, the location of the patient at and before onset, the intensity of mosquito activity and perhaps the movement of water-birds, such as the Nankeen night heron (*Nycticorax caledonicus*), into the region. Of course, diagnosis of the first case in an impending epidemic is the most challenging one. The virus is rarely isolated from blood, but small samples should be taken daily for serological testing, particularly for the presence of immunoglobulin M (IgM) antibody.

Treatment

Treatment can only be symptomatic as the individual case progresses or regresses, and, except in the mildest cases, the prognosis is not good.

Physiography relevant to epidemiology

The Great Dividing Range follows the east coast of Australia from near the tip of Cape York down to the south-east corner of Victoria and then runs west roughly parallel to the southern coast and almost to the border of South Australia (SA). The cities of Brisbane, Sydney and Melbourne and a large proportion of the population of Australia are on the relatively narrow coastal plains. The highest mountains in the range, and the only reliable winter snowfields, are in the

south-east corner of the continent and give rise to two major rivers, the Murray and the Murrumbidgee, which meander through the high country before heading west. The Murrumbidgee receives water from the Lachlan River and other smaller tributaries before it flows into the Murray. Several substantial tributaries flow northward from the Victorian Alps to the Murray River and its ana-branches, billabongs and swamps receive a final offering from the Darling River before crossing into SA, where it is diverted south to Lake Alexandrina and the Southern Ocean. This vast drainage network has but one mouth and, because the rivers in the network have been so used and abused, its final passage across the sand-dunes has to be periodically opened artificially.

South of the Tropic of Capricorn (Rockhampton on the east coast, northern tip of Lake Macloud on the west coast), the Queensland rivers rising on the western slopes of the Great Dividing Range flow south and west. The Barwon, Culgoa, Bogan, Macquarie, Namoi, Warrego and several other streams amalgamate as they approach the north-western New South Wales (NSW) town of Bourke and leave the town as the Darling River. The Darling and a maze of short tributaries sluggishly enter and leave extensive water-bird-breeding marshes during the slow journey south to the Murray River. Other, mostly non-perennial, streams flow through the 'channel country' into the also non-perennial North and South Lakes Eyre in the deserts of South Australia. When full, they too are utilized for opportunistic breeding by water-birds.

North of the Tropic of Capricorn, from the rugged coast of Western Australia across the 'Top End' to the east coast of Cape York, all life is governed by the monsoonal wet and dry seasons. The highly variable wet season starts in December and continues to April and the dry season extends from May to November. The wet season annually activates the northern streams and rivers, frequently to excess. Most of those on Cape York flow west from the Great Divide into the Gulf of Carpentaria.

The Ord River, one of the ephemeral streams in northern Western Australia has been harnessed to form the large Lake Argyle and a small 'diversionary' dam regulates the flow of water to an irrigation area. This has greatly increased human activities in the immediate area and provides the opportunity for year-round mosquito and water-bird breeding in what was previously a seasonally arid region, exacerbating the persistence and activity of MVE and other arboviruses.

With no 'dividing range' to channel the rivers inland, the great bulging west coast of Western Australia has numerous independently flowing short streams, backed by rugged broken plateaux rich in mineral deposits, semi-deserts and deserts. Agricultural and forest industries and most of the population of this huge state are located in the relatively verdant south-west corner, where, in recent years, Ross River and Barmah Forest viruses have caused concern but not Murray Valley encephalitis. Ross River virus and Barmah Forest virus (see entries) are hosted, probably exclusively, by animals and were probably unwittingly introduced to the area by humans, whereas MVE virus is hosted primarily, but certainly not exclusively, by birds and particularly by water-birds. Many northern NSW kangaroos and feral pigs have antibodies to MVE virus.

History of epidemics
1917 and 1918
Epidemics of a severe, highly lethal encephalitis were reported in eastern Australia during the summers of 1917 and 1918. Early in the first epidemic, a virus was recovered from the brain of a fatal case in Townsville, a tropical Queensland coastal town, which caused a similar lethal encephalitis when inoculated into monkeys. A second strain was isolated in the following year and the disease was given the sobriquet of 'Australian X disease'. During these years, there were scattered localized outbreaks of encephalitis, extending from Townsville to the Murray Valley. By the end of 1918, 172 cases had been reported in NSW, 118 of them fatal, and 13 cases in northern Victoria and at least 20 cases in and near Townsville, most of them fatal.

1922–1925
In a poorly reported outbreak in and near Brisbane in 1922, it was stated that 49 of 79 cases of Australian X disease were fatal. Between January and April 1925, nine cases were reported at Broken Hill in the far west of NSW and one at Tibooburra, 322 km to the north; six of these died. In April and May of the same year, at least 11 cases again occurred in Townsville; all were children under 8 years and ten died. This was the last appearance of the virus on the east coast of Australia.

1950–1951
It was not until the southern hemisphere summer of 1950–1951 that cases similar to Australian X disease were again seen in Australia. The first of 45 cases occurred in late December 1950 near Wentworth and Mildura at the confluence of the Darling and Murray Rivers (Fig. 1). An early fatal case occurred in dryland farming country west of the Murray River in SA and the last of the series in April 1951 at Narrabri in central NSW on the Namoi River, a tributary of the Darling River. All other cases occurred in the broadly defined Murray Valley of northern Victoria and southern NSW. The age of patients ranged from 7 weeks to 69 years, 62% were less than 15 years and 69% were male.

A presumptive virus was recovered from the brain of the young SA girl by intracerebral inoculation into both infant and adult mice: this was the method used in the successful establishment of JE and SLE viruses. Investigators at the Walter and Eliza Hall Institute in Melbourne used embryonated eggs, a technique largely developed at that institute. Virus was recovered from each of four fatal cases: the SA case, the Narrabri, NSW, case and two cases from northern Victoria. All isolates produced small focal lesions 3 days after direct inoculation on the chorioallantoic membrane of developing chicken embryos; specific antisera were produced against the four strains and cross-reaction was absolute in complement fixation titrations and in neutralization tests in suckling and weaned mice. American collaborators demonstrated that the virus is closely related to, but not identical with, JE, WN and SLE viruses (see entries). As all except the Narrabri case occurred in the Murray Basin, the virus was named Murray Valley encephalitis virus.

Australian X disease and Murray Valley encephalitis

Not surprisingly, when MVE virus was isolated in 1950, there was no virus or tissue from Australian X disease patients available for direct comparison with Murray Valley encephalitis. However, from the recorded descriptions of the earlier outbreaks, Murray Valley encephalitis seemed indistinguishable from Australian X disease. In particular, the clinical picture, the morbid anatomy and histology, the age incidence, the sex distribution and the seasonal incidence were closely comparable.

As mentioned earlier, nine cases were identified at Broken Hill in 1925. There were no overt cases in Broken Hill in 1951. A serological survey of Broken Hill residents was carried out in 1952 and the sera tested for the presence of a neutralizing antibody to the newly isolated MVE virus. A higher proportion of residents born before 1919 (19 of 92) had antibody to MVE virus than did people under 34 years of age (2 of 69). This finding is consistent with the similarity of the clinical symptoms of Australian X disease and Murray Valley encephalitis and is perhaps the most objective and convincing evidence that the causative agent is the same. The antigenic relationship to SLE and JE viruses (see entries) also implied that it was almost certainly mosquito-borne. The summer of 1950–1951 is significant for another reason: a section of the Murray Valley was the site of yet another attempt to create an epidemic of myxomatosis (see entry) in introduced European wild rabbits (*Oryctolagus cuniculus*), which had reached disastrous levels during the Second World War (1939–1945). On this occasion, the plague of mosquitoes responsible for the Murray Valley encephalitis epidemic was instrumental in permanently establishing myxomatosis in the Australian rabbit population.

The 1951 Murray Valley encephalitis epidemic tapered off during the autumn and plans were made to mount a major effort in the following spring, summer and autumn to detect some pattern in the waxing and waning of this elusive virus. A team of virologists, epidemiologists, entomologists and physicians was mustered for work in the field, laboratory and hospital. Several medical entomologists in Australia with wartime experience in malaria and dengue fever took the opportunity to work with a Californian medical entomologist experienced in arbovirology, particularly St Louis encephalitis and western equine encephalitis.

Large numbers of mosquitoes were collected in and around Mildura on the banks of the Murray River, rapidly processed and inoculated into chick embryos. Blood samples were taken from blood donors, birds and other wildlife. However, no cases were seen in hospitals or by general practitioners throughout Australia in 1952. The mosquito pools yielded only the recently introduced myxoma virus and a bird-pox virus, both of which are transmitted 'mechanically' on the proboscis of probing insects, such as mosquitoes and fleas. On the positive side, Murray Valley encephalitis and myxomatosis stimulated continuing research on mosquitoes as vectors of disease and theories based on rainfall patterns and seasonal distribution were developed to anticipate the next outbreak of Murray Valley encephalitis. A highly successful search for arthropod-borne viruses was undertaken in tropical northern Queensland and extensive serological surveys were carried out in temperate and tropical Australia aimed at plotting the distribution of MVE virus during and between epidemics. An unexpected episode occurred in March 1956 when two cases of Murray Valley encephalitis were serologically confirmed on the Murray River upstream from Mildura and seroepidemiological studies indicated a patchy distribution of the virus in a small area close to the two cases. This had not been predicted by rainfall patterns and in the following year, when an outbreak was anticipated, no activity was detected. Similarly, in 1971 minor MVE virus activity occurred in the Murray–Darling Basin, with a serologically confirmed case of severe encephalitis in a child at

Charleville, on the Warrego River in southern Queensland at the northern extremity of the basin, and another at Henty between the Murrumbidgee and Murray Rivers in southern NSW. Antibody was detected in domestic fowls at some localities and in horses with 'nervous disease' in the Murray Valley.

1974

The first substantial epidemic since 1951 occurred in 1974 and eventually involved every mainland state and the NT. As in 1951, there were almost simultaneous infections scattered over a large area of the Murray Valley. The first eight cases, with onset in January 1974, extended from Albury, NSW, to Goolwa at the mouth of the Murray River in South Australia. There had been 21 cases in the Murray Valley by 19 February 1974 when the first case occurred outside the valley at Windorah in the 'channel country' of south-western Queensland. The last of the 39 cases in the Murray Valley had an onset of symptoms on 15 April and the final case of the series of 58 occurred at Kununurra, northern Western Australia, on 9 May – the only case to occur in that state. There were ten cases scattered through Queensland, all on the western slopes or inland of the Great Divide and the five in the NT included two in Alice Springs, near the geographical centre of the continent. The ten in SA included two in the arid Musgrave Ranges near the NT border south-west of Alice Springs. There were 13 deaths and, unlike the epidemic of 1951, there was a double peak of age prevalence, one peak under 10 years and a second over 50 years. Retrospectively, several of the 1974 cases might have been due to KUN virus rather than MVE virus. Rather more ominous were two fatal cases where low-titre KUN virus antibody was detected when the patients were first admitted to hospital but this was replaced by MVE antibody before death. These might have been examples of virus replication enhanced by low titre or imprecisely matched antibody, as is seen with another group of flaviviruses, the four dengue viruses and dengue haemorrhagic fever.

1975–1997

During this period, 14 Murray Valley encephalitis cases were diagnosed in the NT and Queensland and 18 cases in northern Western Australia. Ten of these 32 infections were fatal.

The development of the water impoundment and agricultural irrigation area on the Ord River at Kununurra has increased the population of people, water-birds and mosquitoes in the Kimberley area. This has resulted in increased arbovirus activity and has converted a Murray Valley encephalitis enzootic area with very rare overt disease into an enzootic-endemic area with disease incidence mainly during the transition from the wet to the dry season. The majority of sentinel chicken seroconversions to flaviviruses in the Kimberley region are to MVE virus, but those in the Pilbara region have been mostly to KUN virus (see entry). As in southern epidemic regions, *Culex annulirostris* is the main vector of both viruses. Although viraemic water-birds may play a role in reintroducing MVE and KUN viruses in these tropical areas, there is increasing evidence that the viruses are reactivated through vertical transmission in dormant *Ochlerotatus*[1] *normanensis* and *Ochlerotatus tremulus* eggs.

In contrast to the Ord River development, the dams built on two more tributaries of the Murray River since 1974 and more dams on the Darling River further upstream have contributed to increased salting in the Murray Valley and natural seasonal flooding is now a rare event. The few remaining River redgum (*Eucalyptus camaldulensis*) forests are under threat of extinction.

Transmission and vertebrate hosts

The 1974 epidemic and several preceding and succeeding years provided an opportunity to contemporaneously observe the generation and decline of an epidemic of Murray Valley encephalitis. A lengthy drought in eastern Australia was broken in April 1973 and, from northern NSW down the Paroo River to the Murrumbidgee and Murray, mosquitoes were far more plentiful than is usual in autumn. Later in the year, water-birds moved in large numbers to the flooded feeding and breeding grounds of the Murray–Darling system. Ducks and other herbivores were the first of the birds to benefit from the exuberant plant growth but, as the numbers of crustaceans, fish, insects and their larvae, tadpoles, frogs, small marsupials, lizards, placental mice and the nestlings of other birds proliferated, so did the carnivores and omnivores: herons (Ardeidae), cormorants (*Phalacrocorax* species), grebes (Podicipedidae), pelicans (Pelecanidae) and ibis (Threskiornithidae). Waters began receding from the flood plains in late November 1973 and an abnormally large hatching of spring *Aedes* species tormented residents of the river towns. *Culex annulirostris* are summer night-feeding mosquitoes, which overwinter as adults and prefer warm, shallow, grassy pools for egg laying. By mid-December, floodwater had receded sufficiently for *C. annulirostris* to swarm through the overcrowded colonies of nesting water-birds in the Barmah, Moira and other redgum forests. At the height of the epidemic, a total of 136,077 *C. annulirostris* yielded 238 isolates of 11 antigenically distinct viruses, including 38 strains of MVE virus and 111 strains of KUN virus. *Culex australicus* yielded one isolate of MVE virus and there were no isolates of any viruses from 917 culicine mosquitoes of other species, or from 1184 *Anopheles annulipes*. There seems no doubt that *C. annulirostris* is the major epidemic vector for both MVE and KUN viruses.

Water-birds were suspected as being important in the transmission cycle from the time that the virus was first identified in 1951. Serological surveys during the 1974 epidemic indicated a high incidence of MVE antibodies in the families Ardeidae (55%) and Phalacrocoracidae (41%). Within Ardeidae the highest incidence of MVE antibodies was 22/25 Nankeen night herons (*Nycticorax caledonicus*), followed by 4/10 Sacred ibis or White ibis (*Threshkiornis molucca*), 3/9 Pacific herons or White-necked herons (*Ardea pacifica*) and 6/18 White-faced herons (*Ardea novaehollandiae*). Additionally, MVE virus was recovered from the blood of a White-faced heron.

Within the families Phalacrocoracidae (cormorants, shags) and Anhingidae (darters), 1/3 Great cormorants (*Phalacrocorax carbo*), 11/26 Little-black cormorants (*Phalacrocorax sulcirostris*), 18/46 Little-pied cormorants (*Phalacrocorax melanoleucos*) and 2/4 Darters (*Anhinga melanogaster*) had MVE antibodies.

The family Anatidae (geese, swans and ducks) was of particular interest because it was thought that, as ducks were capable of rapid long-distance flight, they might be responsible for transferring virus from the tropics to the temperate region. In Black swans (*Cygnus atratus*) 2/9 had antibodies to MVE virus. Of a total of 222 ducks, 158 were Grey teal (*Anas gibberifrons*), only nine of which tested positive, and 20 Pacific black ducks (*Anas superciliosis*), one of which tested positive. All sera were also tested for antibodies to Sindbis virus, an alphavirus active on all continents except the Americas. As with MVE virus, the highest prevalence of Sindbis antibody was in herons and cormorants (46% and 56% positive), but 70/222 ducks (32%) also had Sindbis antibodies. Anatidae are clearly susceptible to mosquito attack but presumably require a larger dose of MVE virus than Sindbis virus to raise an antibody response.

Although percentage prevalence and antibody titres in Nankeen night herons continued to be high during the first summer after the epidemic, persistent flooding prevented breeding of *C. annulirostris* at levels sufficient to continue transmission of the virus to the human population. The mosquito catch was less than 10% that of the previous year.

The mechanism by which the virus survives between epidemics has not been satisfactorily established. There is no evidence that the virus persists in *C. annulirostris*. It has been shown in the laboratory and in field studies in the Kimberley area that MVE virus is maintained in the eggs of *Aedes* species and it may be that in non-epidemic years this allows limited transmission to vertebrates in winter and spring. Or it may simply be that the recirculation of virus in the bloodstream of a persistently infected vertebrate is sufficient to infect a few mosquitoes in spring. If conditions are favourable, as they were in 1950 and 1973, for an explosion in the populations of *C. annulirostris* and susceptible vertebrates, an epidemic ensues.

Control

The recent incursion of JE virus into the Torres Strait Islands and western Cape York Peninsula brings the number of flaviviruses isolated in Australia to 14. Whether or not JE virus persists, the use in Australia of currently available vaccines against JE virus or the development and use of an MVE vaccine could be hazardous. The four dengue viruses are flaviviruses, and dengue haemorrhagic fever, the severe and frequently lethal manifestation of a second infection with a non-matching dengue virus, is the classic example of antibody enhancement of virus replication. The four arboviral encephalitides are antigenically related and pose a similar problem in the design and application of vaccines. Japanese encephalitis vaccine is currently being used only where JE is the only endemic encephalitic flavivirus.

The 1951 epidemic in Australia was followed by several years of adequately funded research, which was orientated towards the characterization of the abundant arboviruses in Australia, their epidemiology and effect on health and important fundamental aspects of viral replication. In the wake of the 1974 outbreak, the Commonwealth Department of Health encouraged the states to develop strategies for cooperative ventures in anticipating epidemics and coordinating control measures. This cooperation has been sustained, partly because other arboviruses, such as Ross River, Barmah and KUN viruses have attracted public health attention. The sentinel fowl programme designed primarily to anticipate epidemics of Murray Valley encephalitis is still functioning in NSW, Victoria and Western Australia, but the very successful annual training schools for health inspectors, Shire engineers, Armed Services personnel and Pacific Islanders were terminated for lack of funds. However, there remains a core of trained personnel, familiar with the basics of mosquito control strategies and techniques, who are involved in public education programmes.

Note

[1] *Ochlerotatus* was formerly a subgenus of *Aedes.*

Selected bibliography

Broom, A.K., Lindsay, M.D.A., Johansen, C.A., Wright, A.E. (Tony) and Mackenzie, J.S. (1995) Two possible mechanisms for survival and initiation of Murray Valley encephalitis virus activity in the Kimberley region of Western Australia. *American Journal of Tropical Medicine and Hygiene* 53, 95–99.

Lobigs, M., Marshall, I.D., Weir, R.C. and Dalgarno, L. (1988) Murray Valley encephalitis virus field strains from Australia and Papua New Guinea: studies on the sequence of the major envelope protein gene and virulence for mice. *Virology* 165, 245–255.

Mackenzie, J.S., Coelen, R.J., Lawson, M.A., Sammels, L., Howard, M., Hall, R.A. and Broom, A.K. (1991) Molecular approaches to the study of the epidemiology of two Australian flaviviruses: Murray Valley encephalitis and Kunjin viruses. *Proceedings of the Australian Physiological and Pharmacological Society* 22, 121–131.

Marshall, I.D. (1988) Murray Valley and Kunjin Encephalitis. In: Monath, T.P. (ed.) *The Arboviruses: Epidemiology and Ecology*, Vol. III. CRC Press, Boca Raton, Florida, pp. 151–189.

Nicholls, N. (1986) A method for predicting Murray Valley encephalitis in southeast Australia using the Southern Oscillation. *Australian Journal of Experimental Biology and Medical Science* 64, 587–594.

Russell, R.C. (1998) Vectors vs. humans in Australia – who is on top Down Under? An update on vector-borne disease and research on vectors in Australia. *Journal of Vector Ecology* 23, 1–46.

Mycoplasma species *see* **Haemotrophic mycoplasmas.**

Myxomatosis

Frank Fenner

Disease of European rabbits (*Oryctolagus cuniculus*) caused by a virus of the genus *Leporipoxvirus*.

Distribution

In the Americas, myxomatosis may occur wherever, within the distributions of *Sylvilagus bachmani* (Brush rabbit) or *Sylvilagus brasiliensis* (Forest rabbit), European rabbits are farmed or kept as pets (Fig. 1). In addition, it is enzootic in Tierra del Fuego, where it was introduced to control wild European rabbits in 1954. It seems likely that the presence of foci of infection in *S. bachmani* or *S. brasiliensis* played a major role in preventing European rabbits from becoming a wild animal pest in the many suitable habitats that occur in the Americas. Elsewhere, the disease is enzootic in areas into which it was introduced to control wild rabbits, i.e. in Australia and many countries of Europe, except on small islands, where it was sometimes introduced for rabbit control but died out.

Aetiological agent

The viral genus *Leporipoxvirus* is one of eight genera in the subfamily Chordopox-virinae, family Poxviridae. It contains five species, four of which occur naturally in leporids and squirrels in the Americas. The species of greatest importance are myxoma virus, of which there are two subspecies, and the immunologically related fibroma virus.

Natural history

Myxoma virus was one of the first animal viruses to be recognized as such, when it was recovered from laboratory (European) rabbits suffering from a disfiguring and invariably fatal disease by Guiseppe Sanarelli, working in Montevideo, Uruguay. Several years later the disease was found in farmed and laboratory European rabbits in the Oswaldo Cruz Institute in Rio de Janeiro (Fig. 1). In 1943 H.B. Aragão showed that in Brazil, and indeed throughout South America, its natural host was *S. brasiliensis* (Fig. 2), in which it produced a small localized fibroma, very like that seen in *S. bachmani* (Fig. 3A). He also showed that it could be transmitted mechanically from one rabbit to another by bites of cat fleas or mosquitoes. The virus is highly specific for a limited range of species of leporid.

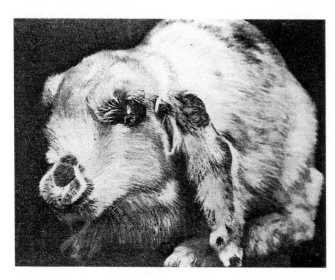

Fig. 1. Myxomatosis in a spontaneously infected laboratory rabbit, at an advanced stage of the disease. This is the first published photograph of a rabbit with myxomatosis, produced by Aragão in 1927. (From Fenner and Fantini (1999), *The History of Myxomatosis – an Experiment in Evolution*, CAB International, Wallingford, UK.)

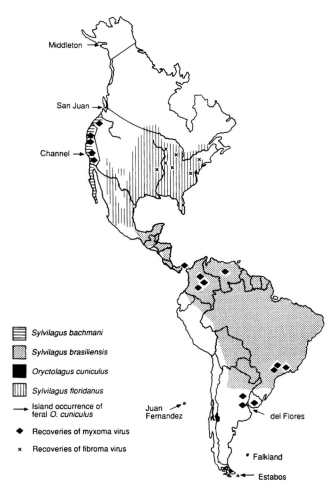

Sylvilagus bachmani

Sylvilagus brasiliensis

Oryctolagus cuniculus

Sylvilagus floridanus

Island occurrence of feral O. cuniculus

◆ Recoveries of myxoma virus

× Recoveries of fibroma virus

Fig. 2. Map of the Americas, showing the distributions of the reservoir hosts of fibroma virus (*Sylvilagus floridanus*), South American myxoma virus (*Sylvilagus brasiliensis*) and Californian myxoma virus (*Sylvilagus bachmani*) and of feral *Oryctolagus cuniculus* in the Americas. Symbols indicate some of the sites from which the different leporipoxviruses have been isolated from their natural hosts. (From Fenner and Fantini (1999), *The History of Myxomatosis – an Experiment in Evolution*, CAB International, Wallingford, UK.)

Myxomatosis was a worry to persons farming European rabbits in California in the 1930s, but it was not until 1960 that I.D. Marshall and D.C. Regnery showed that the natural host in California was the Brush rabbit, *S. bachmani* (Fig. 2). The lesions in this species were again small localized fibromas, but in European rabbits it produced a lethal disease, which often killed very quickly (7–8 days after probing by an infective mosquito) but occasionally caused a disease similar to that produced by the Brazilian strain (Fig. 3).

Fibroma virus was recognized by Richard E. Shope as a disease causing a localized lump in the skin of *Sylvilagus floridanus*, the Eastern cottontail rabbit, found in the eastern states of the USA (Fig. 2). It was also transmissible by mosquito bite, but, unlike the myxoma viruses, it produced only a localized fibroma in European rabbits.

Clinical features in European rabbits

As derived from their respective reservoir hosts, the South American and Californian subspecies of myxoma virus are highly lethal for the European rabbit, *O. cuniculus*. However, the signs produced in infected rabbits are sometimes strikingly different (compare Figs 1 and 3B). After an incubation period of 4–5 days, all recently isolated South American strains produce florid lesions with large protuberant tumours at the inoculation site and elsewhere on the body. Virtually all inoculated rabbits die, with survival times of 9–16 days. On the other hand, many Californian strains, as

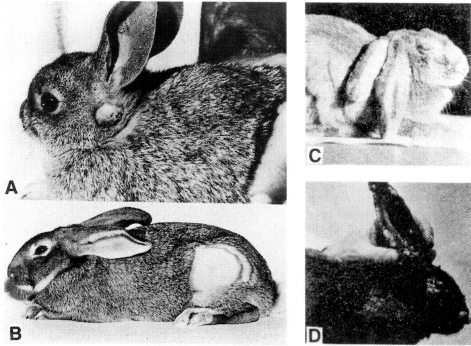

Fig. 3. (A) Myxoma virus infection in the reservoir host in California, the Brush rabbit, *Sylvilagus bachmani*, showing the fibroma produced by the bite of a mosquito which had probed a similar lesion in another *Sylvilagus bachmani*. (B) Myxomatosis in *Oryctolagus cuniculus* due to infection with the Californian strain of myxoma virus. Disease with few obvious lesions 7 days after the intradermal inoculation of a small dose of virus; the rabbit died the next day. (C) Acute disease and (D) advanced disease, as observed with virus recovered in California in 1930; both cases were fatal. (From Fenner and Fantini (1999), *The History of Myxomatosis – an Experiment in Evolution*, CAB International, Wallingford, UK.)

derived from their natural host, produce a hyperacute infection that kills laboratory rabbits in 7–10 days, often before extensive skin lesions develop (Fig. 3B). However, in some parts of the range of *S. bachmani* (Fig. 2), a disease with more obvious skin and eye lesions develops, very like that seen after infection with South American strains (Fig. 3C, D).

Diagnosis

Diagnosis can usually be made clinically. If necessary, virus can be isolated from skin lesions in rabbits, in cultured cells or on the chorioallantoic membrane of the developing egg. Recovered rabbits can be recognized by tests for antibody by any of several methods, enzyme-linked immunosorbent assay (ELISA) being the preferred method.

Myxomatosis for the control of wild European rabbits

Myxomatosis occurred only as an occasional nuisance to rabbit farmers or pet owners in Brazil and eastern USA until the early 1950s, when it was successfully introduced to control wild European rabbits in Australia and France.

In Australia the introduction of wild European rabbits by English settlers in 1859 was a major disaster. Within 10 years of their introduction they were recognized to be a major agricultural pest. In 1918 H.B. Aragão proposed to the Australian Government that myxoma virus should be used to control this pest, but the quarantine authorities refused its entry. However, between 1937 and 1943, preliminary trials were carried out in Australia on its host specificity and ability to be spread by mosquitoes and fleas. Preliminary field trials were conducted, but further work was deferred because of pressures of the Second World War (1939–1945). In 1949 a special Wildlife Survey Section was established, its first task being to make a thorough trial of myxomatosis. In late 1950 it spread far beyond the trial sites, producing enormous mortalities among the very numerous wild rabbits. Enthused by this demonstration, a French paediatrician obtained a Brazilian strain of the virus to control rabbits on his estate; inoculation of two rabbits in June 1952 led to its spread over the greater part of Europe, among both wild and farmed rabbits. Subsequently extensive laboratory and field studies of the disease in European rabbits were carried out in Australia, France and Great Britain.

Transmission

Aragão in Brazil and L.B. Bull in Australia had shown that myxomatosis could be transmitted mechanically by mosquitoes and fleas. Infection can also occur by close contact between diseased and healthy animals, or by exposure to artificially produced aerosols containing virus. However, mechanical transmission by mosquitoes in Australia (until introduced in 1966, rabbit fleas (*Spilopsyllus cuniculi*) did not occur there), and fleas and mosquitoes in Europe, is by far the most important mechanism of transmission.

Mosquito transmission

In the early 1950s F. Fenner and M.F. Day of CSIRO Entomology, Australia, demonstrated several important aspects of mosquito transmission. Female *Aedes aegypti* mosquitoes and sharp pins were used to determine the source of virus and the period over which transmission could occur. Mosquitoes were fed (or pinpricks made) on the rabbit's ear in places where there were no skin lesions and through a skin tumour at various times after the rabbit was infected with myxomatosis. Six days after inoculation the rabbit was viraemic and a local lesion had developed at the inoculation site. Titration of the heads (including proboscis) and the abdomens of the mosquitoes showed that immediately after a blood feed

on the ear the abdomens always yielded virus but the heads were negative, whereas after feeding through the tumour both head and abdomen were positive, although due to the amount of blood it contained the titre of virus was much higher in the abdomen.

Mosquitoes that had obtained a blood feed on the ear never transmitted myxomatosis, even after 4 weeks had elapsed to allow for replication of virus in the mosquito (if it occurred), whereas many of those that had fed through the tumour transmitted immediately after feeding and at intervals over the next 3 weeks. Pinpricks gave similar results. Electron micrographs of a mosquito's mouthparts showed that virions were attached to the maxillae of a mosquito that had probed through a tumour (Fig. 4). Thus transmission depended on contamination of the mouthparts not with viraemic blood but with virus from epidermal cells over the skin lesion (Fig. 5).

The infectivity for probing mosquitoes of various accessible parts of the body of advanced cases of myxomatosis showed that 100% of mosquitoes became infective after probing through the skin over the primary lesion, 78% after probing the swollen eyelids, 58% by probing the swollen base of the ears and 15% after probing secondary skin lesions. Probing in unaffected skin gave negative results. When mosquitoes were allowed to probe through tumours at times ranging from 5 to 10 days after inoculation (the last in a dead rabbit) and then tested by probing on susceptible rabbits, positives rose from 38% on day 5 to 71% on day 9, and to 92% on the dead rabbit (probably because they probed repeatedly in an attempt to obtain blood).

At about this time scientists in the USA and Europe suggested that, although mechanical transmission of leporipoxviruses occurred, these viruses might multiply in the mosquito. The problem was therefore re-examined, paying particular attention to the possibility of replication of the virus in the mosquito. Using rabbits surviving after infection with slightly attenuated strains of virus, groups of individually housed mosquitoes were allowed to probe repeatedly on susceptible rabbits at various times from 2

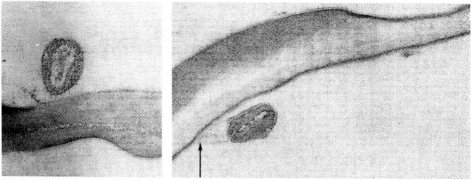

Fig. 4. Electron micrograph of myxoma virions on the maxilla of an *Aedes aegypti* mosquito after probing through a skin tumour. (From Fenner and Fantini (1999), *The History of Myxomatosis – an Experiment in Evolution*, CAB International, Wallingford, UK.)

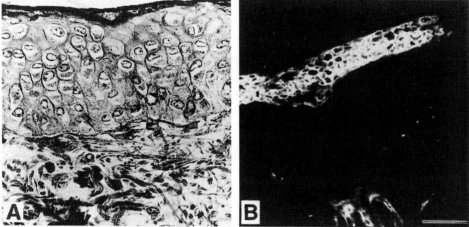

Fig. 5. Sections of skin lesion produced by intradermal inoculation of a domestic rabbit with the Moses (later called Standard laboratory) strain of myxoma virus. (A) Stained with haematoxylin and eosin (× 270), showing hyperplasia of epithelial cells and numerous cytoplasmic inclusions. (B) Stained with immunofluorescent antibody. The abundance of virus in these cells explains why insect vectors contaminate their mouthparts during probing through these lesions. (From Fenner and Fantini (1999), *The History of Myxomatosis – an Experiment in Evolution*, CAB International, Wallingford, UK.)

to 18 days after probing through a tumour, whereas the 18-day controls had not probed on the infected rabbit until that day. The steady fall in positive results in the test mosquitoes suggested that virus on the proboscis was eventually 'wiped off' and that there was no enhancement of infectivity by replication. In another experiment large numbers of *Aedes aegypti* and *Anopheles annulipes* mosquitoes were fed through skin lesions containing high titres of virus and individually tested for virus at intervals after the acquisition feed. There was a progressive diminution in the virus titre of the mosquito

suspensions and no evidence whatever of a rise after a latent interval.

Flea transmission

The European rabbit flea (*Spilopsyllus cuniculi*) did not occur in Australia, and it was not until some time after myxomatosis had spread in Britain that detailed research was carried out on its role in transmission. Transmission by these fleas was shown to be mechanical, positive results being obtained immediately after removal from a diseased rabbit and after several days of starvation. The piercing mouthparts of a flea are about 300 μm long, about one-tenth as long as the proboscis of a mosquito, so fleas are capable only of relatively shallow probing. However, the highly developed cutting plates of the laciniae of fleas are better adapted for retaining large numbers of virus particles than the scanty teeth on the maxillae of mosquitoes and, as Fig. 5 indicates, there are numerous infected epithelial cells in the epidermis over a myxomatous skin lesion.

The year-round occurrence of cases of myxomatosis in Britain focused attention on the European rabbit flea as an important vector. The rabbit flea is well-suited for maintaining infection through the winter. For example, rabbits released in deserted burrows 50 days after the inhabitants had died of myxomatosis became infested with fleas and died of myxomatosis, suggesting that fleas could act as a reservoir of infection for several months after rabbits had deserted a burrow. The potential prolonged infectivity of fleas was confirmed by the observation that some fleas that had fed through lesions of a rabbit with myxomatosis and were then buried in the ground in glass tubes were infective for as long as 112 days. In France, mosquitoes were responsible for summer epizootics among wild rabbits and for introducing the virus into rabbitries, but fleas were important in maintaining chains of infection in the cooler months. Following autumn outbreaks, quiescent rabbit fleas were recovered from soil scrapings from deep burrows that had been abandoned by rabbits 10 weeks earlier and myxoma virus was recovered from these fleas.

Reproductive biology of Spilopsyllus cuniculi
Although other fleas parasitize rabbits, *S. cuniculi* is unique in that egg maturation in the female is dependent on hormones found only in female rabbits at the late stages of pregnancy; for successful reproduction male fleas also need to have probing contact with a rabbit in the final stages of pregnancy or with a newborn nestling (Fig. 6). This complicated life cycle is peculiar to *S. cuniculi* and is not found in the Spanish rabbit flea, *Xenopsylla cunicularis*; its elucidation was crucial to the success

of the importation and distribution of *S. cuniculi* in Australia.

Efficiency of transmission of strains of low virulence
In the field, in both Australia and Europe, it was found that over a period of some years the virulence of the virus diminished such that most field strains killed 70–90% of rabbits instead of over 99%, as initially observed. It was noted earlier that the important virus from the point of view of mosquito (or flea) transmission was that in the superficial layers of skin through which the mosquito probed in search of a blood meal. The titres of virus in skin slices taken at different times from rabbits that had been infected with strains of myxoma virus of differing virulence were compared with the numbers of infections resulting from 20 successive probes on marked sites on the back of susceptible rabbits (Fig. 7). Highly virulent strains produced sufficiently high titres of virus in the skin for effective transmission from about the fourth day after infection until the rabbit died on the tenth or eleventh day. Even the highest skin titre of a highly attenuated laboratory variant (neuromyxoma) was almost two logs lower than that of highly virulent strains, and mosquito transmission was correspondingly poor – only 12 out of 136 positive probes compared with 53 out of 88 for a virulent strain. Another significant result was that skin titres in rabbits infected with somewhat attenuated strains, with longer survival times, remained high as long as the rabbits survived, sometimes for over 20 days after infection. These results proved of great value in interpreting the evolution of virus in the field in Australia.

Transmission by other arthropods
Since transmission is mechanical, any arthropod that probes through a skin tumour of an infected rabbit and then bites another rabbit is potentially a vector of myxomatosis. Data collected in Australia over the period 1944–1958 and summarized by F. Fenner and F.N. Ratcliffe (see Selected bibliography) support this view. The critical features are the extent to which the

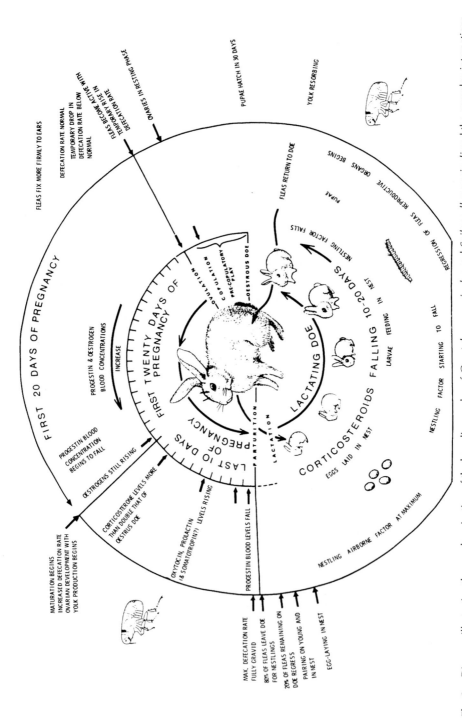

Fig. 6. Diagram illustrating the synchronization of the breeding cycles of *Oryctolagus cuniculus* and *Spilopsyllus cuniculi* and the complex interactions between host hormonal activity and the breeding of the flea. (From Fenner and Fantini (1999), *The History of Myxomatosis – an Experiment in Evolution*, CAB International, Wallingford, UK.)

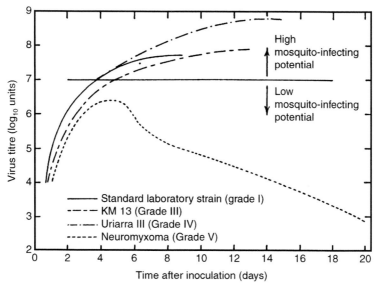

Fig. 7. Changes with time in the titre of virus in skin slices taken from the surface of lesions produced by the intradermal inoculation of rabbits with large doses of various strains of myxoma virus. Standard laboratory strain: highly virulent strain used to initiate myxomatosis in Australian wild rabbits; neuromyxoma: laboratory strain of very low virulence; KM 13 and Uriarra III: Australian field strains of moderate virulence. Lesions produced by highly attenuated strains rarely reach concentrations high enough to contaminate the proboscis of a probing mosquito; lesions produced by moderately or highly virulent strains reach high skin titres, but rabbits infected with highly virulent strains die soon after. Lesions caused by moderately virulent viruses may have highly infectious skin lesions for many days after infection, especially in the 10% or more animals that survive. (From Fenner and Fantini (1999), *The History of Myxomatosis – an Experiment in Evolution*, CAB International, Wallingford, UK.)

arthropod concerned feeds on rabbits and moves from one rabbit to another. In an effort to enhance the efficacy of myxomatosis in arid parts of Australia, the Spanish rabbit flea (*X. cunicularis*), which is a vector of myxomatosis in drier parts of Spain and France and proved easy to breed in the laboratory, was introduced in many sites in inland Australia, and appears to be relatively effective.

Prevention

When first introduced in Europe, myxomatosis was a serious threat to the large-scale rabbit farming common in many countries, notably France and Italy. There is no treatment, but initially vaccination with the related fibroma virus was used as a control measure; then an attenuated strain of myxoma virus was developed as a vaccine and now it is common to vaccinate first with fibroma virus and then with the attenuated myxoma virus vaccine.

Selected bibliography

Fenner, F. and Fantini, B. (1999) *Biological Control of Vertebrate Pests. The History of Myxomatosis – an Experiment in Evolution.* CAB International, Wallingford, UK, 339 pp.

Fenner, F. and Ratcliffe, F.N. (1965) *Myxomatosis.* Cambridge University Press, Cambridge, 371 pp.

Fenner, F. and Ross, J. (1994) Myxomatosis. In: Thompson, H.V. and King, C.M. (eds) *The European Rabbit.* Oxford University Press, Oxford, pp. 205–239.

Mead-Briggs, A.R. (1977) The European rabbit, the European rabbit flea and myxomatosis. *Applied Biology* 2, 183–261.

Nagana *see* **Animal trypanosomiasis.**

Nairobi sheep disease

J.S.M. Peiris

Nairobi sheep disease was first recognized in 1910, following an outbreak of a fatal disease in sheep brought into Nairobi. Soon afterwards, experimental transmission studies in sheep established that the causative agent was a filterable agent transmitted by the ixodid (hard) tick, *Rhipicephalus appendiculatus*. These studies also established that the agent was transmitted transovarially in the tick.

Distribution

Nairobi sheep disease outbreaks have been documented in Kenya, Uganda, Rwanda, Tanzania and the highlands of western Somalia. Serological evidence of virus activity has also been found in eastern Ethiopia. Nairobi sheep diease (NSD) virus (Ganjam strain) has also been isolated in India (states of Orissa, Karnataka, Andhra Pradesh and Tamil Nadu) and in Sri Lanka.

Virus

Nairobi sheep disease virus is an enveloped, single-stranded RNA virus. It is classified in the genus *Nairovirus* within the family Bunyaviridae. The *Nairovirus* genus contains seven antigenic groups and over 33 viruses, including Crimean–Congo haemorrhagic fever virus (see entry). Nairobi sheep disease and Dugbe viruses form an antigenic group (NSD virus group) within this genus.

The virus is spherical or pleomorphic and between 80 and 120 nm in size. Nairoviruses have three surface glycoproteins (in contrast to other Bunyaviridae, which have two) and a nucleocapsid with helical symmetry. The RNA genome is in three segments, RNA-L, RNA-M and RNA-S, containing 11,000–14,400, 4400–6300 and 1700–2100 nucleotides, respectively.

There are no discernible differences between African NSD virus strains, either antigenically or in cross-protection experiments. Ganjam, a virus isolated in south India, is now known to be antigenically indistinguishable from NSD virus by complement fixation and immunofluorescence tests and is considered to be a strain of NSD virus. However, these immunological tests are broadly reactive and do not detect subtle antigenic differences. Genetic or virus cross-protection studies comparing these two virus strains are yet to be done. In order to keep data from these two geographical strains distinguishable for the purposes of this review, the terms NSD and NSD (Ganjam strain) will be used to denote the African and South Asian viruses, respectively.

Clinical symptoms in animals

Nairobi sheep disease can cause severe and fatal disease in sheep and goats, typically following the introduction of non-immune animals into an endemic region. In outbreaks in sheep, mortality can exceed 90%. The disease is characterized by high fever (41.5°C), collapse and diarrhoea. Fever follows an incubation period of 2–4 days and lasts for 2–8 days. The animals are depressed and anorexic and have conjunctival injection and a serosanguinous nasal discharge. Diarrhoea may appear 2–4 days after the onset of fever and is watery initially but subsequently becomes mucoid and bloody. Infection in pregnant animals can lead to abortion. Prescapular and precrural lymph nodes may be palpable. The white cell blood count is low in the early stage of the illness.

In fatal sheep or goat infections, death usually occurs in the early stage of the illness. At this time post-mortem may be unremarkable but a high awareness of the possibility of Nairobi sheep disease should be maintained in endemic areas. Mesenteric lymph nodes are usually enlarged and serve as ideal specimens for virus isolation. Animals dying later in the course of the illness may have evidence of a mucoid or haemorrhagic ulcerative enteritis in the abomasum, duodenum, caecum and colon, and a tubular nephritis.

East African hair sheep varieties are highly susceptible and high (75–95%) rates of mortality have been observed in non-immune field populations. Breeds of imported wool sheep, such as Romney and Corriedale, appear less susceptible to overt disease. Cattle are not susceptible to NSD virus, even though this is the preferred host of the tick vector, *Rhipicephalus appendiculatus*. There is neither evidence of disease nor serological evidence of infection in other domestic livestock or wild ruminants. However, the death of two Grey (common) duiker (*Sylvicapra grimmia*) in the Entebbe zoo has been attributed to Nairobi sheep disease.

The Asian NSD (Ganjam strain) virus has been reported to cause a similar illness and fatality but outbreaks on the scale of that reported in Africa have not been reported. In contrast to the situation in Africa, local breeds of sheep were infected asymptomatically, while imported breeds or cross-breeds were more likely to develop clinically overt disease. Experimental infection of Langur monkeys (*Semnopithecus entellus*[1]) with NSD (Ganjam strain) virus resulted in viraemia without clinically overt disease, and infection of Bonnet monkeys (*Macaca radiata*) resulted in seroconversion without detectable viraemia.

Clinical symptoms in humans

Human infection with NSD virus is rare but has been reported both with the African and the Asian (Ganjam) strains of the virus. Clinical features were those of a self-limited febrile illness, with shivering, abdominal pain, back pain, headache, nausea and vomiting. Conjunctival injection and a temperature–pulse deficit were noted in some patients. In Kenya, no serological evidence of infection was found in humans.

Laboratory workers handling this virus or infected animals, even those who had accidental needle-stick exposure to potentially infectious material, failed to seroconvert or become ill. However, serological evidence of infection was found in laboratory workers and in the general population in Uganda and India and in workers on a goat farm in Sri Lanka. A number of presumed laboratory-acquired infections (confirmed by virus isolation from the serum), leading to disease, have been reported in India. These infections were not attributable to needle-stick injury. However, some of the infected laboratory workers were involved in washing contaminated glassware. Percutaneous transmission via non-intact skin through pre-existing skin damage or disease or injury acquired during the washing procedure remains a possibility.

Diagnosis

Serum (1/10 dilution), plasma or 10% homogenates of post-mortem mesenteric lymph node, liver or spleen tissues are suitable specimens for virus isolation. Virus isolation from the blood is only successful in the acute stage of the illness.

Laboratory-reared sheep, newborn (2–4-day-old) mice or cell culture (e.g. baby hamster kidney (BHK-21C-13) cells) can be used for primary virus isolation. Inoculation of Nairobi sheep disease-susceptible sheep held in isolation, though inconvenient, is the most sensitive method for virus isolation. This is especially useful when the original field samples may have been exposed to adverse transport conditions, with associated loss of viable virus titre. Pyrexia and clinical symptoms in the animal allow a tentative diagnosis of Nairobi sheep disease and provide specimens for virological confirmation of the diagnosis.

Mice injected by the intracerebral route develop neurological signs and die within 5–9 days of inoculation. Ideally, two litters of mice are used for each sample. Homogenates of mouse brain diluted 1/100 are used for further passage in mice or in cell culture.

Virus-containing specimens inoculated on to BHK-21C-13 cells will result in cytopathic effect in 3–6 days. Immuno-fluorescent staining for virus antigen can lead to a diagnosis sooner (1–3 days). Though marginally less sensitive than mouse inoculation, the latter approach has the advantage of providing relatively rapid virological diagnosis and is a useful routine diagnostic method. Other cell lines known to be useful for primary isolation of NSD virus from field isolates include primary or secondary lamb or hamster kidney cells. African green monkey kidney (VERO) and pig kidney (PS) cells can be used for sub-culturing NSD viruses but are not ideal for primary isolation from clinical specimens.

Virus can be isolated from infected ticks by intracerebral inoculation of 10% homo-genates of infected ticks or pools of ticks into newborn mice. Baby hamster kidney cells have also been used for this purpose, although comparative sensitivity studies with mouse inoculation have not been done.

Once isolated, the virus can be identi-fied by complement fixation or enzyme-linked immunosorbent assay (ELISA) tests done on mouse brain suspensions or cell cul-ture fluids using specific immune sera or by immunofluorescence tests on infected cell culture monolayers. Some cross-reaction may occur with hyperimmune sera raised to other nairoviruses, but these viruses are not usually associated with disease in sheep or goats.

Antiviral antibody can be detected by indirect immunofluorescence, comple-ment fixation, ELISA, immunodiffusion or haemagglutination inhibition tests. Signifi-cant rises in titre between acute and convalescent sera will establish the diag-nosis. Antibody tests also provide useful seroepidemiological data on the distribution of the infection. The indirect immunofluo-rescence test is the most suitable test for serology. However, one should be aware that cross-reactions occur with other nairovir-uses, including Dugbe and Crimean–Congo haemorrhagic fever viruses.

Transmission

Ixodid (hard) ticks are the vectors of natural NSD virus infection in animals, and direct transmission by aerosol, fomites or contact is not documented. *Rhipicephalus appendi-culatus* is the main vector in the enzootic areas of Africa. Experimental transmission of the virus to sheep and goats by infected ticks has been documented. The virus has been shown to persist and be transmitted from an infected tick for as long as 871 days. In the tick, the virus is transmitted transovarially and trans-stadially. Feeding upon immune hosts does not result in the 'sterilization' of the virus within the tick, and such ticks continue to transmit the virus through subsequent feeds at the adult stage. Transovarial transmission, however, appears to require an infective feed at the adult stage.

Not all populations of *R. appendicula-tus* are able to transmit the virus efficiently. Thus different populations of this species have differing levels of vectorial capability for NSD virus. *Rhipicephalus appendicula-tus* primarily feeds on wild Bovidae, e.g. Buffalo (*Syncerus caffer*) and Waterbuck (*Kobus ellipsiprymnus*), and on domestic cattle. Sheep and goats are less preferred hosts. In Africa, changes in climate, such as heavy rainfall, increased cloud cover and humidity, favour the extension of the 'Eco-climatic Zone IV' and thereby the geograph-ical range of *R. appendiculatus* and of NSD virus. These climatic changes occur in 5–15 year cycles and may persist for 1–3 years.

Rhipicephalus pulchellus may be an important vector in Somalia and Ethiopia and *Amblyomma variegatum* and other *Rhipicephalus* species may also be occa-sional vectors. Epidemiological data of Nairobi sheep disease outbreaks in Somalia occurring in the absence of either *R. appen-diculatus* or *Amblyomma* species suggested that *R. pulchellus* was a possible vector. Though Kenyan populations of *R. pul-chellus* are unable to transmit NSD virus experimentally, the Somali population of the tick can. The virus has been isolated from *A. variegatum* in the lake basin of western Kenya and this tick can transmit the virus in experimental studies.

The NSD (Ganjam strain) virus has been isolated frequently from *Haemaphysalis intermedia* collected in India and Sri Lanka. Occasional isolates of the virus have also been obtained from *Haemaphysalis welling-toni*, and from *Culex vishnui* mosquitoes in India.

Prevention and control

In enzootic areas, the majority of sheep and goats have serological evidence of infection without significant disease. Young animals probably get infected early in life while they are partially protected by maternal antibody, leading to asymptomatic infection and subsequent lifelong immunity. Epidemics are usually associated with the introduction of susceptible animals from non-enzootic areas to areas where the disease is enzootic or when climatic changes lead to the extension of the range of the vector (and the virus) to areas where the hosts have hitherto been non-immune.

In enzootic areas where virus infection is nearly universal, vector control measures are not thought to offer significant benefit. This is because they may lead to temporary and partial reduction in the vector population and virus transmission, which leads to the increase of a population of susceptible animals that eventually get infected and diseased. Thus naturally acquired 'herd' immunity is probably best left undisturbed.

Remote-sensing data from satellites may provide information of ecological changes that may lead to the extension of the range of the vector (and of the virus) and provide early warning of impending outbreaks of disease. In 'extension zones', i.e. those areas in which the vector (and consequently the disease) emerges from time to time due to ecological change, aggressive tick control measures may be a short-term option to reduce the impact from the disease. Local application of acaricides by dipping animals or spraying them has been attempted but resistance in the vector, the toxic effects of the compounds on the livestock and the potential for residual acaricides in meat used for human consumption limit their usefulness. Pyrethrum-based grease preparations or 'pour-on' lotions are an alternative option. However, vector control measures are not likely to be of benefit in the long term.

Nairobi sheep disease is on list B of the Office International des Epizooties. It is important that control measures are taken to prevent the importation of the vector and virus into areas where they are currently not present.

Both killed and attenuated experimental vaccines against Nairobi sheep disease have been developed. But, with the realization that naturally acquired immunity early in life in enzootic areas provides efficient and cheap 'natural' protection, the role for a vaccine is unclear. Potentially, vaccines may have usefulness when climatic changes produce increased risk of the spread of the disease to adjacent geographical areas with non-immune populations of livestock. However, vaccine efficacy in such a situation has not yet been demonstrated.

Note

[1] This monkey was formerly in the genus *Presbytis*.

Selected bibliography

Banerjee, K. (1984) Emerging arboviruses of zoonotic and human importance in India. In: Misra, A. and Polasa, H. (eds) *Virus Ecology*. (Based on a symposium organized at the University of Warwick.) South Asian Publishers, New Delhi, pp. 109–121.

Davies, F.G. (1989) Nairobi sheep disease. In: Monath, T.P. (ed.) *The Arboviruses: Epidemiology and Ecology*, Vol. III. CRC Press, Boca Raton, Florida, pp. 191–203.

Davies, F.G. (1997) Nairobi sheep disease. *Parassitologia* 39, 95–98.

Davies, F.G., Mungai, J.N. and Taylor, M. (1977) The laboratory diagnosis of Nairobi sheep disease. *Tropical Animal Health and Production* 9, 75–80.

Ghalsasi, G.R., Rodrigues, F.M., Dandawate, C.N., Gupta, N.P., Khasnis, C.G., Pinto, B.D. and George, S. (1981) Investigation of febrile illness in exotic and cross-bred sheep from sheep farm, Palamner in Andrha Pradesh. *Indian Journal of Medical Research* 74, 325–331.

Karabatsos, N. (ed.) (1985) *International Catalogue of Arboviruses Including Certain Other Viruses of Vertebrates*, 3rd edn. American Society of Tropical Medicine and Hygiene, San Antonio, Texas, 1147 pp.

Mohan Rao, C.V.R., Dandawate, C.N., Rodrigues, J.J., Prasada Rao, G.L.N., Mandke, V.B., Ghalsasi, G.R. and Pinto, B.D. (1981) Laboratory infections with Ganjam virus. *Indian Journal of Medical Research* 74, 319–324.

Office International des Epizooties (2000) Nairobi sheep disease. Http://www.oie.int

Perera, L.P., Peiris, J.S.M., Weilgama, D.J., Calisher, C.H. and Shope, R.E. (1996) Nairobi sheep disease virus isolated from *Haemaphysalis intermedia* ticks collected in Sri Lanka. *Annals of Tropical Medicine and Parasitology* 90, 91–93.

Nematoda

M.W. Service

Nematodes are generally regarded as constituting a phylum that contains at least 40,000 species arranged in about 2271 genera in 256 families. Many species occur in the soil, marine and freshwater habitats, others parasitize arthropods, such as insects and mites, while about a third of the genera have species parasitizing a broad spectrum of vertebrates. Of these, several infections are transmitted by arthropods.

Adult nematodes are unsegmented roundworms, usually cylindrical but tapering at the anterior and posterior ends. They range in size from 250 μm to 9 m in length! Nearly all species are dioecious. Fertilized females usually lay eggs which hatch into larvae, of which there are four growth stages. Usually, but not invariably, the third-stage larva is responsible for infecting a new host. In the filarioid nematodes the first-stage larvae are called microfilariae. The hierarchical classification used here is that adopted by R. Anderson (see Selected bibliography) but only the orders and families containing arthropod-transmitted nematodes are considered.

The Nematoda are divided into two classes: the Adenophorea and the Secernentea; only the latter contains arthropod-transmitted nematodes.

Class: Secernentea. Contains monoxenous species (i.e. those that infect the host directly without involving intermediate stages in vectors, such as *Ascaris* and *Strongyloides* species – not considered in the encyclopedia) and heteroxenous species, which have intermediate hosts involved in transmission. Frequently transmission requires ingestion of larval nematodes in the tissues of vertebrate hosts by non-biting intermediate hosts, but some, such as those belonging to the superfamily Filarioidea are transmitted by blood-sucking arthropods, usually insects. The stages that occur in the invertebrate hosts are the first- to early third-stage larvae.

Order: Spirurida. Most species produce eggs containing a fully developed first-stage larva, which can only develop to the third stage in an arthropod intermediate host.

1. Superfamily: Thelazioidea. There are three families but only the Thelaziidae are of medical or veterinary importance.

Family: Thelaziidae. The so-called eyeworms. Species in the genus *Thelazia* infect eyes of birds and mammals and are transmitted by non-biting flies, such as species of *Fannia* and *Musca* (see Thelaziasis).

2. Superfamily: Habronematoidea. A biologically diverse family with species parasitizing birds, mammals and fish.

Family: Habronematidae. Of three genera the most important economically are *Habronema* and *Draschia*, species of which occur in the stomachs of horses and certain ruminants (see Habronemiasis). Transmission is by non-biting muscid flies, such as species of *Musca*.

3. Superfamily: Filarioidea. The filarioids occur in all types of vertebrates except fish, and are usually transmitted by haematophagous arthropods.

Family: Filariidae. Contain subcutaneous parasites of mammals having dipteran intermediate hosts.

Subfamily: Filariinae. Contains four genera, of which the genus *Parafilaria* parasitizes cattle and horses (see Parafilariasis). Transmission is by non-biting flies, such as *Musca* species.

Subfamily: Stephanofilariinae. This subfamily contains a single genus, *Stephanofilaria*, species of which parasitize cattle (see Stephanofilariasis). Vectors include non-biting flies, such as *Musca* species, and blood-sucking flies, such as species of *Haematobia*.

Family: Onchocercidae. A very diverse collection of nematodes belonging to numerous genera. Larvae are usually found in the definitive vertebrate host. The immature larvae, called microfilariae, occur in the host's blood (e.g. species of *Wuchereria*, *Brugia*, *Loa*) or the skin (e.g. *Onchocerca* species).

Subfamily: Setariinae. The genus *Setaria* has species that infect artiodactyles, especially Bovidae, but also equines (see Setariosis). Transmission is by mosquitoes of several genera.

Subfamily: Dirofilariinae. Several genera occurring in birds, reptiles and mammals. The genus, *Dirofilaria*, has species that infect carnivores and primates. Infections which occur in dogs and humans are transmitted by various mosquito species in several genera (see Dirofilariasis). Genus *Loa*, the species *L. loa* (see Loiasis) is a parasite of humans in Africa transmitted by tabanids (horse-flies).

Subfamily: Onchocercinae. Several species which have blood-inhabiting microfilariae exhibit marked circadian periodicity in the peripheral blood system of their vertebrate hosts (e.g. *Wuchereria bancrofti*). The subfamily contains the medically most important nematodes transmitted by arthropods to humans. Species in the genus *Mansonella* infect humans and other primates (see Mansonelliasis). Transmission is by *Culicoides* flies (biting midges). *Elaerophora schneideri* (see entry) occurs in cattle and deer and is transmitted by tabanids (horse-flies).

Species of the genera *Brugia* and *Wuchereria* cause lymphatic filariasis in humans and are transmitted by several mosquitoes in various genera. The genus *Onchocerca* contains species that cause onchocerciasis (see entry) in humans, often termed river blindness; vectors are *Simulium* species. Animal onchocerciasis (see Onchocerciasis, animal) is transmitted by species of *Simulium* and *Culicoides* and infects equines, cattle and other domesticated livestock.

Subfamily: Splendidofilariinae. Contains the genus *Splendidofilaria*, a parasite of birds, such as quail (*Coturnix* species) and ducks (see Splendidofilariasis). Parasites are transmitted by species of *Simulium* and *Culicoides*.

Selected bibliography

Anderson, R.C. (2000) *Nematode Parasites of Vertebrates: Their Development and Transmission*, 2nd edn. CAB International, Wallingford, UK, 650 pp.

Muller, R. (2001) *Worms and Disease. A Manual of Medical Helminthology*, 2nd edn. CAB International, Wallingford, UK.

Ockelbo disease *see* **Sindbis virus.**

Omsk haemorrhagic fever

Irina N. Gavrilovskaya

Omsk haemorrhagic fever is an infectious disease of humans and other mammals caused by Omsk haemorrhagic fever (OHF) virus. The virus is transmitted to people through bites of *Dermacentor* ticks or by direct contact with infected Muskrats (*Ondatra zibethicus*), or with their carcasses. Outbreaks and sporadic cases of Omsk haemorrhagic fever are observed in the Omsk region of western Siberia, and now in adjacent regions (Russia). Genetically and antigenically OHF virus is very similar to tick-borne encephalitis (TBE) virus (see entry), but it causes a different clinical picture: acute febrile disease with haemorrhagic symptoms in patients and a relatively benign course. The mortality rate is about 1%.

Distribution

In wet grasslands of the Barabin forest steppe in the Omsk and Novosibirsk regions of western Siberia (Russia). Originally (1944–1949), Omsk haemorrhagic fever cases were observed in three districts in the north of the Omsk region and, since 1950, in adjacent districts of Novosibirsk and Tyumen regions. Omsk haemorrhagic fever is endemic to the following areas only: Bolsherechensk, Sargatsk, Soldatsk and Tyukalinsk (Omsk region); Barabinsk, Vengerovsk, Zdvinsk, Ust-Tarsk and Chanovsk (Novosibirsk region). All these areas are situated át the same latitude and have the same landscape characteristics, i.e. northern forest steppe with small areas of birch–aspen forests and many lakes.

Virus

Omsk haemorrhagic fever virus is an arthropod-borne virus and a member of the family Flaviviridae, genus *Flavivirus*. Omsk haemorrhagic fever virus is serologically related (based on cross-neutralization tests with polyclonal hyperimmune mouse ascitic fluids prepared against each of the viruses) to other members of the genus, which include: TBE, including European and Far Eastern subtypes, Kyasanur Forest disease (KFD), louping ill (LI), Powassan (POW), Langat (LGT) (see entries), Negishi, Royal Farm, Carey Island and Phnom Penh bat viruses. Two antigenic types of OHF virus have been determined by agar precipitation and immunoadsorption methods.

Omsk haemorrhagic fever virus is a spherical or slightly polygonal enveloped virus, with a diameter of approximately 37 nm and a membrane layer approximately 6 nm thick. The electron-dense nucleocapsid is 25 nm in diameter, with icosahedral symmetry. The virus localizes in reservoirs of the endoplasmic reticulum and in vesicles and vacuoles of the Golgi complex. Omsk haemorrhagic fever virus causes cytolysis in pig embryo kidney cells. The virions contain about 17% lipid and 9% carbohydrate within the viral membrane. The virus is sensitive to lipid solvents. Omsk haemorrhagic fever virus has a positive-sense genome of 10 kb single-stranded RNA. The viral proteins are encoded in one open-reading frame containing both structural and non-structural (NS) proteins. The core proteins include the premembrane (prM), membrane (M) and envelope (E) proteins. There are seven NS proteins: NS1, NS2a, NS2b, NS3, NS4a, NS4b and NS5. The viral E protein is glycosylated and agglutinates goose erythrocytes at pH 6.8. The E protein antigenically induces cross-reactive neutralizing and protective antibodies in infected animals. Genetically, OHF virus is most closely related to TBE virus (81% nucleotide identity and 93% amino acid identity). About 20 amino acid substitutions between

OHF and TBE virus have been described. It is possible that more than one domain within the viral E protein determines Omsk haemorrhagic fever pathogenesis. Omsk haemorrhagic fever virus is pathogenic for experimentally infected adult and newborn white mice, in which it is neurotropic. In naturally and experimentally infected Muskrats, the virus causes a lethal haemorrhagic disease. This animal is an ideal model for studying the pathogenesis of the human disease, while differentiating OHF virus from TBE, which is non-pathogenic for Muskrats. In nature, OHF virus may be isolated from ticks (*Dermacentor reticulatus*). Rare isolations have been obtained from *Dermacentor marginatus* or from the blood of patients taken during the acute period of infection.

Clinical symptoms

The incubation period of Omsk haemorrhagic fever is short (2–4 days). The prodromal period lasts about 12 h and is manifested by fatigue, myalgias and headache. The prodromal phase is followed by the febrile phase (5–15 days) and finally the convalescent phase (2–4 weeks). In approximately half of all cases a second febrile phase occurs. Clinical manifestations during the second febrile phase are typically milder than in the first. Usually the disease begins abruptly, with a brief chill followed by high fever (39–40°C). The fever lasts for 3–4 days at this level and then decreases to 37.5–38.5°C. Later, 9–15 days after onset of the disease, the fever slowly abates. On the first day after the onset of fever, headache, myalgia and flushing of the face and neck are typical. Sclerae are usually bright red. These symptoms increase for 3–5 days after the onset of fever and then slowly disappear. Complete absence of these symptoms coincides with abatement of the fever. The haemorrhagic manifestations occur at the beginning of the febrile phase. Haemorrhages may occur in oral mucous membranes, pharynx or conjunctivae (up to 47% of cases). Petechial skin rash is seen in 82% of cases. Massive nasal (43%), uteral (23%), gum (15%) or lung (9%) haemorrhage may occur. Enhancement of vessel fragility in the febrile phase of the disease is observed in virtually all cases.

Physical findings

These include a temperature of 39–40°C, bradycardia (30% of cases) and, in some cases, tachycardia. The most common manifestations of Omsk haemorrhagic fever are associated with lung injury. Bronchitis can occur during the first day of the onset of fever in most cases. Pneumonia develops in 31% of cases, usually in the right lung (59%). Chest X-rays reveal light infiltration of lung tissue. Signs of upper respiratory tract disease, including sore throat, rhinorrhea, sinusitis and ear pain, are absent, though a non-productive cough can be observed. Pulmonary onset usually occurs 3–5 days after the onset of fever, lasts for 1–1.5 weeks and then disappears towards the end of the febrile phase. Hepatomegaly is seen in 29–67% of cases. An enlarged spleen is detected by palpation in only 9.5% of cases. Involvement of kidneys is insignificant and is manifested by slight proteinuria in 90% of patients.

Laboratory findings

Elevation of haemoglobin and haematocrit is observed during the first days after the onset of fever. During the early febrile phase a prominent leucopenia develops. White blood cell counts of less than 3000 mm^{-3} are observed in 51.4% of patients (in some cases, as low as 1200 mm^{-3}). Other haematological observations include slight enhancement of neutrophils (two-thirds of cases), lymphocytes comprising nearly 40% of total white cell count, and mild thrombocytopenia. A lumbar puncture during the febrile phase shows a myeloid reaction with a shift to the left. The level of this shift corresponds to the severity of the disease. Erythropoiesis in the febrile stage is suppressed. Biochemical findings are not significant and are manifested in slight proteinuria.

After the temperature decreases (normally 5–10 days after onset of the disease) the convalescent phase begins. During this period all symptoms disappear. Headache and myalgia resolve quickly but fatigue and weakness last up to 1 month. Flushing of face and neck, haemorrhages and bradycardia disappear. Hypotension may be observed for 2–3 weeks. After normalization of the temperature the clinical symptoms of pneumonia also vanish. In 50% of cases the convalescent phase is interrupted with a second febrile phase of Omsk haemorrhagic fever. In cases with a severe course of the disease, the second wave of fever begins after 3–9 days of apyrexia. In cases with a moderate course, the second wave is observed after 10–18 days of normal temperature. The prolongation of the second febrile phase is 3–12 days.

All the symptoms described above for the febrile phase recur, but in a less manifest form, and then disappear after the temperature returns to normal. During the convalescent phase, patients may complain of persistent weakness. Transient hair loss in convalescence is frequently seen. After the convalescent phase, complete recovery occurs; there are no sequelae. Case-fatality rate is variable, but is generally low – 0.4% to a maximum of 2.5%.

Pathogenesis and pathophysiology

There are no morphological changes typical for Omsk haemorrhagic fever. Its characteristics, in common with other haemorrhagic fevers, are: a generalized increase in vascular permeability, extravasation and perivascular infiltration, with thrombi in small vessels. The pathogenesis is determined by the degree of vascular damage, thrombocytopenia and bleeding in the brain, kidney, endocardium, myocardium, stomach and intestines. Oedema of the brain causes sensory changes. Hypotonia can lead to collapse and shock in serious or fatal cases, particularly in the first week of illness. Haemosiderin deposits are found in the Kupffer cells of the liver.

Diagnosis

Clinical manifestation of Omsk haemorrhagic fever in its febrile stage has a typical course, which makes the diagnosis straightforward. Such symptoms as sudden onset of high fever, chills, myalgia, complete absence of appetite, flushing of face and neck, haemorrhages, haemoptysis, pneumonia, hypotension, leucopenia, enlargement of the liver, and often a second febrile phase allow a diagnosis to be made from clinical evidence. In milder cases, diagnostic mistakes may be made.

Omsk haemorrhagic fever must be differentiated from other acute diseases, such as bronchopneumonia, pseudotuberculosis, leptospirosis and tick-borne encephalitis. With regard to bronchopneumonia caused by meningococcaemia, Omsk haemorrhagic fever is characterized by leucopenia, which is not typical for bronchopneumonia of different aetiology. Enlargement of the liver is an important symptom, since this is not typical for microbial pneumonias. Leucopenia, which is an important sign of Omsk haemorrhagic fever, does not occur in pseudotuberculosis and leptospirosis. In years of Omsk haemorrhagic fever epidemic outbreaks, clinical diagnosis is simpler. In years following epidemics, with only sporadic cases, diagnosis should be based on laboratory investigation, including isolation of the virus from blood taken during the acute phase of illness and seroconversion detected in paired serum samples by virus neutralization. Newer techniques, such as immunofluorescence tests and enzyme-linked immunosorbent assay (ELISA), are also available. The close antigenic relationship of OHF and TBE viruses makes it necessary to differentiate between them for a correct diagnosis. In Omsk haemorrhagic fever, antibody titres to OHF antigens are four or more times higher than titres to TBE virus, and absence of typical neurological symptoms in a patient suggests a diagnosis of Omsk haemorrhagic fever.

Transmission

The first description of a new disease, later called Omsk haemorrhagic fever, was made in 1944–1945 by A. Gavrilovskaya and G. Sizemova. Winter outbreaks among Muskrat hunters were recorded in the Omsk region (western Siberia). In 1946–1948, spring–autumn outbreaks of the disease were recorded. During this period 1344 cases of Omsk haemorrhagic fever were registered. Omsk haemorrhagic fever cases appear mainly from April to October (with occasional single cases in November and December). The seasonal morbidity curve has two peaks, in May and in August–September, which correlate with the seasonal dynamics of ticks (*D. reticulatus*) (formerly called *Dermacentor pictus*). In April, when the first cases of Omsk haemorrhagic fever were described, only *D. reticulatus* could be found in nature in the active state. Mosquitoes and horse-flies arrive in May and July. Their activity increases in June–July, when Omsk haemorrhagic fever morbidity decreases or disappears. The number of Omsk haemorrhagic fever cases correlates with the size and activity of the *D. reticulatus* population. The main role of *D. reticulatus* in the transmission of the causative agent of Omsk haemorrhagic fever was confirmed by M.P. Chumakov and colleagues with the isolation of OHF virus strains from *D. reticulatus*. An additional reservoir host of virus in the endemic areas is *D. marginatus*, from which a strain of OHF virus has also been isolated. Nevertheless, *D. reticulatus* is the principal reservoir and vector of OHF virus.

Virus is transmitted between vertebrates via the bite of infected ticks. In ticks, transmission may be transovarial and trans-stadial. There is apparently no direct human-to-human transmission, and no hospital outbreaks have been observed.

Contacts of humans with ticks may occur during field work, visits to the forest or gardening. The possibility of such contacts is very high. *Dermacentor reticulatus* has a wide spectrum of hosts, e.g. 37 species of mammals and birds. However, the main ones are cattle and Narrow-head voles (*Microtus gregalis*). Attempts to isolate OHF virus from these animals have been unsuccessful, even though the antibody to the virus is frequently found, and voles are sensitive to experimental infection with OHF virus. It could be explained by a short period of virus circulation in the blood and a fast immune response, which results in complete virus elimination. An exception to this is the Muskrat (*Ondatra zibethicus*), which is highly sensitive to OHF virus in nature. Epizootics among Muskrat populations are frequent, and many isolates of OHF virus strains have been obtained from these animals. Muskrats were introduced into the Barabin steppe from Canada 70 years ago for hunting. Muskrats successfully adapted to the Siberian environment and became involved in OHF virus circulation as an additional host for *D. reticulatus*. Muskrats play an important role in direct transmission of OHF virus to humans (Fig. 1).

All cases of Omsk haemorrhagic fever observed in the winter months occur in persons who have been hunting Muskrats and treating their carcasses. After the great outbreaks in 1946–1948 caused by transmission

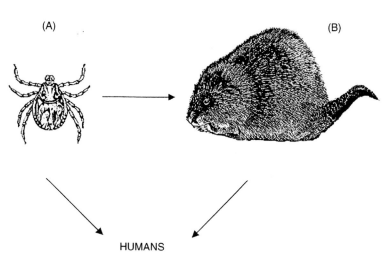

(A)

(B)

Fig. 1. Main reservoir host of OHF virus in nature and routes of transmission. (A) By bite of the tick, *Dermacentor reticulatus*. (B) By direct human contact with Muskrats (*Ondatra zibethicus*).

HUMANS

through ticks, the morbidity of Omsk haemorrhagic fever has decreased to just sporadic cases. Although Omsk haemorrhagic fever cases have not been officially recorded for more than 20 years, in the last 10 years an increase of OHF virus infections in endemic areas has been apparent. Sporadic cases have been recorded in Tyumen (1987), Omsk (1988) and Kurgan (1992) regions. Outbreaks of Omsk haemorrhagic fever have occurred in the Novosibirsk region (1989, 1998). All 155 cases of Omsk haemorrhagic fever recorded in recent years were connected with an OHF virus epizootic among Muskrats. More than 20 strains of virus were isolated from these animals, but, at the same time, all the attempts to isolate the virus from *D. reticulatus ticks* were unsuccessful.

A few virus isolations have been made from mosquitoes, such as *Coquillettidia richiardii, Ochlerotatus[1] flavescens* and *Ochlerotatus excrucians*, and it is possible they transmit the virus to Muskrats in certain regions. But mosquitoes play a very minor role, if any, in the epidemiology of Omsk haemorrhagic fever; ticks are the principal vectors.

Treatment

There is no specific treatment for Omsk haemorrhagic fever. The management of the patient must be supportive and based on the understanding of the pathogenesis of the disease. Although clinical management depends on each phase of the disease, important points in general management are as follows: (i) early diagnosis, early hospitalization, early rest; (ii) close observation, especially during the first week after normalized temperature, when recurrence of the disease could occur; (iii) careful handling of the patient; (iv) supportive treatment; and (v) prevention of complications. Strict maintenance of fluid balance is necessary. The goal during the hypotensive state is to maintain cardiovascular stability. In the case of a secondary infection, administration of antibiotics is strongly recommended.

Control

Since the disease has not been very active in recent years, there is no need for special surveillance programmes, but medical authorities should be vigilant, especially for any increase in morbidity suggestive of an outbreak of Omsk haemorrhagic fever. Anti-tick control measures, such as spraying acaricides, are not justified at present. However, workers in endemic areas should wear specially designed nylon-net-like protective clothes or clothing impregnated with acaricides or repellents for general protection when exposure to ticks is particularly likely. Muskrat hunters should avoid contact with sick animals.

Note

[1]   *Ochlerotatus* was formerly in the subgenus *Aedes*.

Selected bibliography

Anon. (1991) Classification and nomenclature of viruses. *Archives of Virology* 2 (suppl.), 223–227.

Belov, G.F., Topanyuk, E.V., Kurzhukov, G.P. and Kuznetsova, V.G. (1995) Clinical–epidemiological characterization of Omsk hemorrhagic fever at the period of 1988–1992. *Journal of Microbiology, Epidemiology and Immunology* 4, 88–90. (In Russian.)

Busygin, F.F. (2000) Omsk hemorrhagic fever. Up-to-date state of problem. *Voprosy Virulsologii* 45, 4–9. (In Russian, English summary.)

Gritsun, T.S., Lashkevich, V.A. and Gould, E.A. (1993) Nucleotide and deduced amino acid sequence of the envelope glycoprotein of Omsk haemorrhagic fever virus: comparison with other flaviviruses. *Journal of General Virology* 74, 287–291.

Smorodintsev, A.A., Kazbintsev, L.I. and Chudakov, V.G. (1963) *Virus Hemorrhagic Fevers*. State Publisher House of Medical Literature, Leningrad, 292 pp.

World Health Organization (1985) *Viral Haemorrhagic Fevers*. WHO Technical Report Series 721, 53–57.

***Onchocerca* species** *see* **Onchocerciasis.**

Onchocerciasis, animal

Alfons Renz

Distribution

There are about 27 species of *Onchocerca* infecting animals other than humans. Onchocercal infections occur worldwide and are very common in cattle, horses, donkeys, Dromedary camels (*Camelus dromedarius*), deer (e.g. *Cervus elaphus* and *Rangifer tarandus*), antelopes and pigs, including the Warthog (*Phacochoerus aethiopicus*), mainly in the tropics but also in temperate zones up to the polar circle. Although their prevalence often exceeds 90% and simultaneous infections by several species are frequent, they are often overlooked, because they do not usually cause any great pathological changes.

Parasite

Adult worms, so-called 'macrofilariae', live in nodules either in or under the skin, where they can be palpated on the living animal (these nodules must be distinguished from *Demodex* cysts and swellings caused by tick bites) or are attached to the fasciae of the muscles. However, there are other *Onchocerca* species that live more or less free in the surrounding connective tissue of the ligamentum nuchae or gastrolienale or along the tendons of the joints of the legs. These are only seen at slaughter. *Onchocerca armillata* lives in the intima of the aorta wall of ruminants, but also forms nodules attached to the outer wall.

The skin-dwelling microfilariae are only occasionally seen in the blood (cf. *Setaria* species (see Setariosis)). Transmission is restricted to areas where the vectors, zoophagic and especially boophagic species (e.g. bovid feeders) of the genus *Simulium* and *Culicoides*, prevail. These insects do not usually enter animal quarters and stables, but bite out of doors. Onchocerciasis therefore mainly affects animals kept in pastures and declines increasingly with keeping animals indoors.

Bovine onchocerciasis

Ten *Onchocerca* species have been described worldwide from cattle (Table 1 and Fig. 1), and co-infections of up to four or more species can occur in the same host. Adult worms are either located in well-developed nodules in and under the skin (often attached to fasciae of the thoracic or dorsal muscles) or lie more loosely in the connective tissue surrounding the ligaments and tendons of the neck, the lower legs or the intestine. Other species live in flat nodules attached to bones (tibiotarsal joints) or in the aorta wall (Fig. 2).

In contrast to human onchocerciasis, most bovine *Onchocerca* species seem better adapted and cause very few pathological changes in their natural hosts. Large numbers of microfilariae in the skin (>10 mg⁻¹) may lead to inflammation (mostly when they die), but skin irritation is also caused by the bites of the vectors; in fact, *Simulium* toxicosis can be severe and even lethal to cattle.

Aorta lesions are frequent in old cattle infected with *O. armillata* and are usually associated with calcifications and nodulations, involving arteriosclerosis, arteritis and aneurism formation.

Nodules of *Onchocerca ochengi* (Fig. 2A–C) and *Onchocerca gibsoni* in the skin decrease the value of hides for tanning. Their presence in large numbers on the carcasses of slaughtered animals (e.g. *Onchocerca dukei* in cattle, *Onchocerca fasciata* in camels) or nodular lumps on the lower legs are considered unsightly. However, there is no risk for human consumption. Although *Onchocerca* nodules are easy to differentiate from tuberculosis nodules (at least when cut open), they may be incorrectly diagnosed by inexperienced meat inspectors, so that carcasses are unnecessarily condemned.

Table 1. Some *Onchocerca* species of domesticated animals and location of their adult worms. Frequent species, characteristic for the host genus, are in bold characters.

Host	*Onchocerca* species, location	Vector	Distribution
Cattle	**O. gutturosa**, LN, TTL	*Culicoides* species *Simulium* (?)	Worldwide
	O. armillata, AW	?	Africa, Asia
Bos taurus Humpless cattle	**O. lienalis**, LGL, SJ	*Simulium ornatum*	Europe, Australia
	O. stilesi, J&B	?	North America
	O. gibsoni, SCN, brisket	*Culicoides*	South-East Asia, Australia
	O. denkei, SCN, dorsal	?	Afrotropical (Senegal, Ndama cattle)
	O. suzukii	*Simulium bidentatum*	Japan
Bos indicus Zebu cattle	**O. ochengi** (syn. *dermata*), IDN, SCN, inguinal, pectoral	*Simulium damnosum* s.l.	Afrotropical
	O. dukei, SCN, pectoral	*Simulium bovis*	Afrotropical (savannah)
Bubalus bubalis Water buffalo	**O. cebei** (syn. *sweetei*), SCN, IDN, pectoral	*Culicoides*	Asia, Australia
Horse	**O. reticulata**, TTL, forelegs	*Culicoides*	America, Europe
	O. cervicalis, LN	*Culicoides*	America, Europe
	O. bohmi, in arteries and veins	?	Europa (Austria)
	O. gutturosa, LN	*Culicoides variipennis*	America, Europe
Donkey	**O. raillieti**, SCN, LN	*Culicoides* ?	
	O. cervicalis, LN	*Culicoides*	
	O. gutturosa, LN	*Culicoides* or *Simulium*	Tropical Africa

Host	*Onchocerca* species, location	Vector	Geographic distribution
Camel *Camelus dromedarius*	**O. fasciata**, SCN, neck, shoulder	?	Arabia, south-west Asia, Australia,
	O. gutturosa, LN	Culicoides	Africa, Asia
Sheep	O. gutturosa, LN	Culicoides	Worldwide
	O. armillata, AW	?	Tropical Africa, Asia
	O. gibsoni, SCN, brisket, stiffle, hip	Culicoides	Australia
Suidae *Sus scrofa jubatus*	**O. dewittei**, TTL	?	Malaysia
Phacochoerus aethiopicus	O. ramachandrini, TTL	Simulium damnosum s.l.	Cameroon, savannah (warthog)
Goat	O. armillata, AW	?	Asia

AW, aorta wall (posterior part of female in the intima, anterior part in nodule attached to aorta outer wall); LN, ligamentum nuchae; LGL, attached to the ligamentum gastrolienale; SCN, subcutaneous; IDN, intradermal nodules containing a single female and, on average, one male worm; SJ, in thin capsule attached to the stiffle joint; TTL, tibia-tarsal ligaments; J&B, nodules attached to joints and bones on lower legs.

Equine onchocerciasis (horse and donkey)

The pathology caused by microfilariae and adult worms is more frequently seen in horses and has been described from North America, Britain, Central Europe and Australia. Microfilariae of *Onchocerca cervicalis* are the cause of remittent dermatitis in the head and nuchal region (sweet itch). Equine periodic ophthalmia, moon-blindness and conjunctivitis have been attributed (not unanimously) to the presence of microfilariae in the eyes.

Inflammatory reactions around nodules in the ligamentum nuchae lead to fistulous withers and, more rarely, to poll-evil (possibly in connection with brucellosis). Stiffness of the joints has been reported and is likely to be due to the calcification of nodules (e.g. *Onchocerca reticulata*) inside the joint capsules or along the tendons of the lower leg.

Other animals

Although bovids and equines remain the most common animals to be infected with onchocercal worms, camels, sheep, rarely goats (Table 1) and wild animals are sometimes infected.

Zoonosis

The accidental infection of humans by an animal *Onchocerca* species (most probably *O. gutturosa*) has been reported from North America, Europe and Japan, but never from any of the tropical areas, endemic for human filariae, where such infections must certainly also occur but are more difficult to recognize.

Differential diagnosis

Onchocerca infections of living animals are identified to species by the morphology of the microfilariae from the skin (Fig. 3) rather than by examination of adult worms (as only nodules in the skin can be removed surgically). Multiple infections by several filaria species are very common. The location of microfilariae and adult worms in the skin and body is more or less species-specific (Fig. 1), but may vary with the biting behaviour of the local vector and also depends on the adult worm load. In very heavy infections worms also invade less characteristic areas on the body. Microfilariae usually accumulate in those body sites that are favoured feeding sites of the vectors. Moreover, maximum microfilarial numbers are observed at times, seasonally and diurnally, when maximum numbers of black-flies bite. Skin microfilarial densities peak in young or middle-aged animals when transmission is high, while the adult worm load continues to increase. Newborn calves can carry a few maternal microfilariae, but their own new infections can

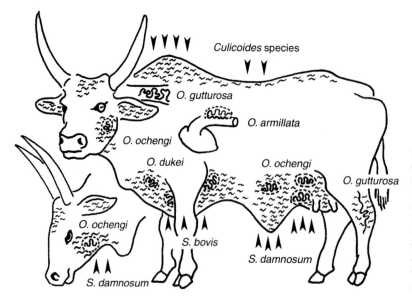

Fig. 1. Location of *Onchocerca* adult worms (ᴧᴧ), microfilariae (~) and biting behaviour of *Simulium* and *Culicoides* vectors (ᴧᵞ) on cattle. Nodule-forming species are encircled.

become patent after only 6–9 months. *Onchocerca armillata* microfilariae are often difficult to find in older cattle, though the prevalence can be over 90%. The life expectancy of adult worms is high (up to 10 years, or longer).

Microfilariae differ morphologically in their length, diameter, shape (Fig. 3) and

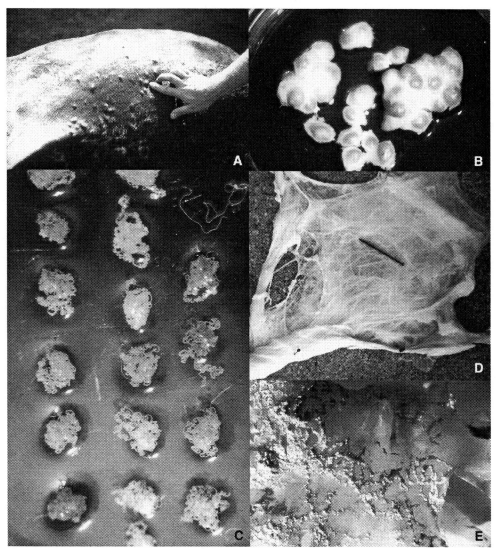

Fig. 2. (A) Intradermal nodules of *O. ochengi* in the ventral skin of a heavily infected cow in Cameroon. (B) Freshly isolated nodules of *O. ochengi* from the slaughter-house: subcutaneous lumps of nodules (diameter 3–8 mm) occur in the udder, but, regardless of population density, each nodule is clearly separated and contains just one female worm. (C) Collagenase-digested nodules of *O. ochengi*; each nodule contains one female and on average one male worm. Young worms are whitish, transparent and later turn yellow to brownish before they calcify. (D) Ligamentum nuchae from cattle with *O. gutturosa* (at tip of needle). Worms are best recognized with transparent or reflected light, when the cuticular striae are visible at 10× magnification. (E) Air-dried aorta wall from cattle with *O. armillata* (partially calcified). Parts of worm (total length of female 20–60 cm) and calcifications are easily visible when the aorta is left in the sun to dry so that it becomes transparent.

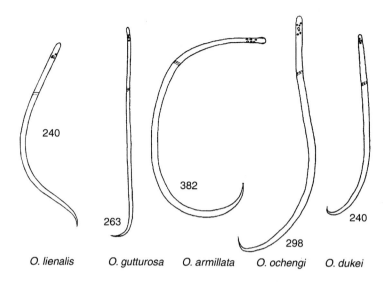

Fig. 3. Identification of microfilariae. Typical shape of freshly heat-inactivated or dead microfilaria in water. Note the length of larvae (lengths given in µm), the diameter and shape of the anterior and posterior ends and the bend of the body and tail.

240
263
O. lienalis

382
O. gutturosa

O. armillata

298
O. ochengi

240
O. dukei

movements. Adult worms are distinguished by their cuticular structures, form and dilatation of the anterior end (*O. gutturosa*, for example, is characterized by a swelling in the anterior part of the body). Male worms typically carry spiculae and papillae at the posterior end. Live adult filariae can be isolated from their nodules by collagenase digestion (0.5% collagenase A in Rosewell Parc Memorial Institute tissue culture medium (RPMI) for 24 h at 35°C, under aerobic conditions) or squeezed out mechanically – this works well with males, but females usually break into pieces, although the intrauterine microfilariae can be collected from them for identification. Old nodules often contain only debris of degenerate and calcified worms.

Skin biopsies

These can be taken from the live animal or at the slaughter-house. From the shaved skin, small superficial biopsies (3–5 mm², 5–30 mg weight) are taken with a scalpel blade. They are incubated in a drop of water, saline or tissue culture medium and kept for up to 24 h at 35°C. Microfilariae start wriggling out within a few minutes and are easily recognized at low magnification (×20–100) under a compound, or preferably a dissecting, microscope. Under optimum conditions, about 80% of the larvae leave the biopsy within 24 h. Larger

skin biopsies (6 mm punches have often been used) should be avoided because most of the microfilariae will fail to emerge. Several snips should be taken from various body parts of each animal (inguinal region, head, ears, back, thorax, legs), both because of the highly aggregated distribution of skin microfilariae and to account for the species-specific location of microfilariae (Fig. 1).

Live microfilariae show characteristic species-specific movements, which vary from strong and quick entanglements to slow bendings. Their length and morphology are studied after heat inactivation (e.g. by gently heating up a slide with microfilariae with a gas-lighter), and this is best done with specimens in water, not saline, so as to avoid shrinkage. Staining with Giemsa or haemalum should be done on single microfilariae transferred to a small drop of water on a microscope slide and left to dry quickly. The head of the microfilariae (shape, diameter and hook), as well as the shape of the tail (length, form of tip, nuclei), should be examined at high magnification (×500–1000).

Treatment

It is usually unnecessary to treat infected animals, because the microfilariae do not cause much harm and the adult worms cannot be killed without risking the life of the animal. Avermectins (ivermectin, doramectin or moxidectin) are highly efficient against microfilariae, but, as in the treatment of human onchocerciasis (see Onchocerciasis, human), there is a potential risk of dangerous reactions when other concomitant filarial infections are present. Nodules in the ligamentum nuchae or in the lower legs of horses can be removed surgically.

Control of transmission

Vector control is rarely possible or even necessary, except in the tropics, where *Simulium* also transmits human onchocerciasis (see Onchocerciasis, human). Keeping animals in shelters or dark stables into which simuliid vectors will not enter is highly effective in reducing transmission, but is less so against *Culicoides* species.

Insect repellents, such as diethyltoluamide (DEET), applied to the skin give some protection against biting, but only for a few hours.

Selected bibliography

Bain, O. (1981) Le genre *Onchocerca*: hypothèses sur son évolution et clé dichotomique des espèces. *Annales de Parasitologie (Paris)* 56, 503–526.

Ottley, M.L., Moorhouse, D.E. and Holdsworth, P.A. (1985) Equine and bovine onchocerciases. *Veterinary Bulletin* 55, 571–588.

Renz, A., Enyong, P. and Wahl, G. (1994) Cattle, worms and zooprophylaxis. *Parasite* 1 (suppl.), 4–6.

Wahl, G., Achu-Kwi, M.D., Mbah, D., Dawa, O. and Renz, A. (1994) Bovine onchocercosis in North Cameroon. *Veterinary Parasitology* 52, 297–311.

Onchocerciasis, human

John B. Davies

Commonly known as 'river blindness' because the disease is associated with river valleys, where the simuliid (black-fly) vectors breed, and the disease can cause blindness. Also known as 'onchocercose' (French) and 'oncocercosis' (Spanish). Sometimes known in Africa as craw craw, a West African name describing an itchy skin. The disease remains endemic in 34 countries and an estimated 17.7 million people are infected, of which 270,000 are blind and another 500,000 have severely impaired vision.

Distribution

About 95% of all cases occur in Africa, mostly in West and Central Africa, with limited foci in East Africa from Ethiopia to Tanzania and with isolated pockets in Malawi, Sudan and southern Yemen, possibly extending into Saudi Arabia. In the Americas onchocerciasis is found in localized areas of southern Mexico, Guatemala, Brazil, Venezuela, Ecuador and Colombia (Fig. 1). (There is evidence that the disease was probably introduced into the Americas during the slave trade.)

Parasite

Onchocerca volvulus (Nematoda: Onchocercidae). Male (3–5 cm long, 0.13–0.2 mm diameter) and female (30–50 cm long, 0.25–0.4 mm diameter) worms live in subcutaneous tissues, often forming tangled masses of threadlike worms in fibrous nodules. Adult females can live for up to 17 years, the mean being about 10 years. The female worm is ovoviviparous and from maturity she produces large numbers of minute sheathless microfilariae (200–300 μm × 10 μm), which migrate to the host's skin. The appearance of microfilariae in the skin occurs about 15–18 months after infection, and their presence is usually accompanied by clinical symptoms. Microfilariae live free in the skin for about 2 years.

Onchocerciasis is not a zoonotic disease, although natural infections with *O. volvulus* have been reported once in a Spider monkey (*Ateles geoffroyi*) in Central America and in a Gorilla (*Gorilla gorilla*) in Africa. Chimpanzees (*Pan troglodytes*) can be infected experimentally.

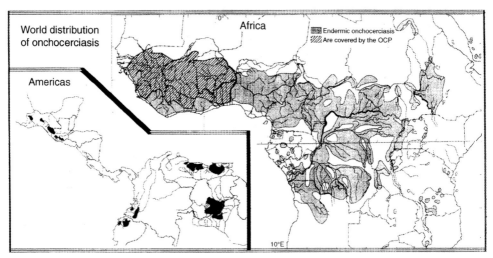

Fig. 1. World distribution of onchocerciasis and the area covered by the Onchocerciasis Control Programme (OCP) (adapted from maps published by the World Health Organization (1995), Technical Report Series 852).

Clinical symptoms

The disease is accumulative, requiring repeated infection over several years to produce serious symptoms. When infection is light, there may be no obvious clinical symptoms. There is often a period of 1–3 years between infection and symptoms, which are caused by the microfilariae. The most obvious and distressing symptom is severe itching of the skin. Adult worms are of secondary importance and the subcutaneous nodules which contain them present no more than cosmetic blemishes. In chronic infections these fibrous, but well-vasculated, nodules, varying in size from a pea to a golf ball and containing one or many adult worms, can be felt and seen over bony prominences. In Africa nodules are found mainly around the pelvic region, knees, lateral chest and spine (Fig. 2). In Central America nodules more commonly occur on upper parts of the body, especially on the head. It is believed that the location of the nodules reflects areas most commonly bitten by the simuliid vectors, but it could also be due to differences in the geographical race of the parasite. Other bundles of worms may be found in deep connective tissue between the muscles, where they cannot be detected by palpitation. In light

or early infections there may be few skin reactions, but in most patients pruritus, with skin lesions, occurs, accompanied by a persistent itchy rash (filarial itch) consisting of papules, the severity and extent of which can be very variable, with some persons appearing to be more tolerant than others. There may be lymphadenopathy in the axilla or groin. Onchodermatitis (sowda) can lead to thickening of the skin, caused by intradermal oedema, and also to pachydermia (crocodile skin). Loss of skin elasticity may lead to 'hanging groin' – that is, pendulous sacs containing inguinal glands – or to hernias. In advanced chronic infections loss of skin elasticity can present a prematurely aged appearance (presbydermia) and paper-thin skin forming folds on the knees and buttocks. Mottled depigmentation ('leopard skin') is common, particularly on the shins (Fig. 2).

The most important sequela of infection is deteriorating eyesight, which can result in total blindness. In Africa, blindness is more common in savannah areas, where over 10% of a population may be completely blind and another 20% have impaired vision. There are two types of eye lesions, one occurring in the anterior part of the eye and the other in the posterior segment. Anterior lesions are caused by microfilariae entering the cornea through the conjunctiva. When they die in the cornea, they cause a punctate keratitis with many fluffy (snowflake) opacities,

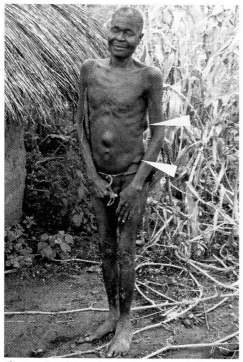

Fig. 2. An advanced case of onchocerciasis. Note nodules on lower ribs and waist (arrowed), depigmentation of shins, thickened skin on the knees and eyes closed due to photophobia. (Reproduced from an original photograph by B.O.L. Duke.)

which are often symptomless, involving no corneal scarring, but there may be photophobia and watering of the eyes, with chronic conjunctivitis. The more severe pathology involves vascularization of the cornea, usually starting in the lower half of the cornea and spreading upwards and inwards to eventually obscure the pupil. This sclerosing keratitis (Fig. 3), often associated with iritis due to dead microfilariae in the iris muscle, is the major cause of blindness. The aetiology of the posterior lesions is less clear and is usually associated with heavy infections. Retinal damage occurs, with or without optic atrophy, and can lead to complete blindness or tunnel vision. This in turn can lead to increased risk of trauma, a dependency on the community for food, malnutrition and a reduction in life expectancy.

Diagnosis

There are a number of methods available, such as those outlined below.

1.   The simplest and most commonly used diagnostic procedure is the biopsy (skin-snip). This entails removing a small, shallow, bloodless snip of skin (approx. 2 mm²), from the thighs, buttocks and iliac crests in African patients, but from the scapula and outer canthus in those in Central America. Preferably, a Walser corneoscleral punch should be used, but alternatively a razor blade or scalpel and a sharp needle will suffice. The skin-snip is placed on a microscope

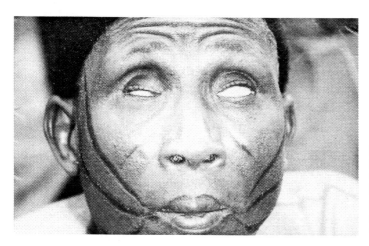

Fig. 3. Onchocercal blindness. The final stage, with eyes totally obscured by sclerosing keratitis. (Reproduced with permission from a World Health Organization publication.)

slide in physiological saline or water and after about 20–30 min examined under a microscope for actively writhing microfilariae. Only about 20% of the microfilariae may emerge at this stage, which may be sufficient for diagnosis, but, if the skin-snip is incubated in saline in a covered microtitre plate for 12–24 h, emergence will increase to about 80%, which is better for assessing intensity or detecting light infections. In parts of West Africa the parasites must be distinguished from those of another filarial skin parasite, *Mansonella streptocerca* (see Mansonelliasis). In the Amazon area confusion with *Mansonella ozzardi* (see Mansonelliasis) is possible.

2. The presence of palpable subcutaneous nodules 0.5–10 cm in diameter. Further confirmation can be obtained by surgical excision and removal of the nodule, from which fragments of adult worms may be obtained by dissection.

3. Slit-lamp examination of the eyes under ×16 magnification after the patient has been seated with the head bent down for about 2 min, this allowing microfilariae in the anterior chamber and dead corneal microfilariae to be detected and counted. With ×25 magnification and retroillumination live corneal microfilariae can be observed.

4. Oral administration of 50–100 mg of diethylcarbamazine (DEC) and observation for up to 24 h (Mazotti test). This drug causes skin microfilariae to die, which results in intense itching and a rash and so indicates infection. The severity of the reaction depends on microfilarial density, so this test should be used only when parasites cannot be demonstrated in multiple skin-snips or in the eyes. This test is potentially dangerous and can result in oedema of the limbs and face, postural hypertension, vomiting, adenitis, ocular discomfort and loss of visual acuity.

5. Serological tests for antibodies (e.g. enzyme-linked immunosorbent assay (ELISA), fluorescent antibody test (FAT)) and DNA probes on skin-snips can be useful in diagnosis when microfilarial loads are low. These techniques are 'high tech' requiring skilled personnel, and are expensive for use in mass surveys, but they are claimed to improve sensitivity by as much as 50%.

Transmission

Vectors are certain species of simuliid black-flies (see Black-flies). Only adult female black-flies take blood and they normally feed during daylight, usually in the open in strong sunlight. The fly uses its mouthparts to tear and rasp the host's skin to rupture blood capillaries so that it can suck blood (and microfilariae of *O. volvulus*, if present) from the wound.

Most of the ingested microfilariae die in the blood meal (over 1000 may be present), but some penetrate the fly's stomach wall and migrate to the thoracic muscles (Fig. 4), where they develop into a sausage-shaped stage (referred to as L_1) and moult to an intermediate stage (L_2). Some survive a second moult and elongate into thinner worms (L_3), which pass through the head and down the short proboscis. There is no multiplication of the parasite in the vector. The infective third-stage larva (about 660 µm in length) leaves the proboscis and penetrates the host's skin via the wound when the fly feeds again. Two moults later, it develops into an adult male or female *O. volvulus*. The development interval between the ingestion of microfilariae to infective L_3 depends on temperature and vector species (usually 6–8 days with the African vector *Simulium damnosum*, but 10–12 days with the Central American vector *Simulium ochraceum*). An infective fly rarely carries more than four infective larvae, although ten or more have occasionally been recorded. Not all larvae are necessarily transmitted at a single feed. As a fly usually feeds every 3–4 days, it cannot become infective until the second or third blood meal after ingesting microfilariae.

In Africa, vectors may fly 15–30 km from their emergence sites to obtain blood meals and may also be further dispersed long distances on the wind (adult *S. damnosum* may be found biting 60–100 km from their nearest breeding sites, and in West Africa there is strong evidence that seasonal monsoon winds can carry adults 400–600 km). In the forested mountain valleys of Central

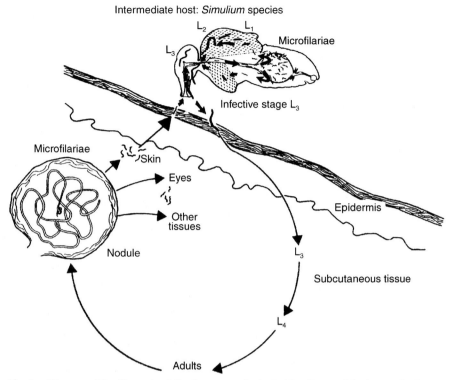

Intermediate host: *Simulium* species

Fig. 4. Diagram of the life cycle of *Onchocerca volvulus* in *Simulium* and the human host (original by G.S. Nelson, reproduced from the *Annals of Tropical Medicine and Parasitology* (1991) 85, with the permission of the Liverpool School of Tropical Medicine).

America dispersal of *S. ochraceum* is of the order of 2–10 km between valleys.

The principal vectors in Africa are species within the *S. damnosum* complex, which contains about 40 almost morphologically identical cytoforms, many of which are recognized as formal species. The main *Simulium* vectors are *S. damnosum* sensu stricto, *S. sirbanum*, *S. sanctipauli* and *S. leonense*. Other but less important vectors include *Simulium neavei*, which is responsible for transmission in parts of the Congo, Zaire and Uganda, and formerly Kenya. *Simulium neavei* is an unusual phoretic species, as larvae and pupae are attached to freshwater crabs of the genus *Potamonautes*. The immature stages of all other vector species are found attached to submerged vegetation, rocks and debris in rivers and streams (see Black-flies).

Simulium ochraceum sensu lato is the principal vector in southern Mexico and Guatemala, while *Simulium metallicum* sensu lato is the main vector in northern Venezuela, but in other Central American countries it is considered of minor importance. In Colombia the only known vector is *Simulium exiguum* sensu lato, a species which is also a primary vector in Ecuador and a secondary one in Venezuela. Above 150 m above sea level in the Brazil/Venezuela Amazon focus the main vector is *Simulium guinense* sensu lato, while below this altitude the vectors belong to the *Simulium oyapockense* species complex.

Epidemiology

The impact of onchocerciasis on a community is usually expressed as the prevalence of persons having demonstrable microfilariae in skin-snips. The following four categories of endemicity are generally used: sporadic, below 10%; hypoendemic, 10–29%; mesoendemic, 30–59%; and hyperendemic, over 59%. The prevalence by age group (Fig. 5) demonstrates the cumulative nature of the disease, in which there is little or no acquired immunity. In hyperendemic communities almost everybody over the age of 30 years is infected. In older persons with thickened skin, skin-snips may not always reveal microfilariae; thus such surveys may not always show a 100% infection in the older age groups.

Treatment

The drug of choice is ivermectin (Mectizan®), which was approved for mass distribution in 1987. A single oral dose of 150 µg kg^{-1} body weight given once or twice a year reduces the numbers of skin microfilariae to low levels for up to a year, thus alleviating many symptoms and making the recipient less infective to the vector. It is now used for mass treatment, as in the Onchocerciasis Control Programme (OCP) in West Africa, but should not be given to children under 5 years of age or weighing less than 15 kg, pregnant women and a few other categories specified in the manufacturer's exclusion criteria. It does not kill the adult worms, but seems to reduce fecundity. Formerly, the more toxic drug DEC was given, at a dose of 2 mg kg^{-1} body weight three times a day for 7 days, but it also does not kill the adult worms and, because it produces severe side-effects, is no longer recommended. Suramin given intravenously is the only drug currently available that kills adult worms. Although it has been used in a few past campaigns, it is potentially dangerous and is no longer recommended.

Control

Insect repellents, such as diethyltoluamide (DEET) and dimethylphthalate (DIMP), can give protection against simuliid bites for about 2 h, but are not practical for constant use in endemic areas.

Prior to the release of Mectizan®, vector control, to break the transmission cycle, was the only option to control the disease. Insecticidal fogging or spraying of vegetation harbouring adult flies results in very temporary and localized control. The only practical method available is the application of insecticides to rivers in which black-flies breed so as to kill the larvae. Insecticides need be applied to only a few selected sites on a watercourse, because the water carries the insecticide a relatively long way downstream (as far as 50 km in large, swift rivers). Because larvicides are only effective against larvae and these have a short development time in the tropics (6–10 days) applications have to be repeated every 7–10 days. The quantity of insecticide needed is calculated

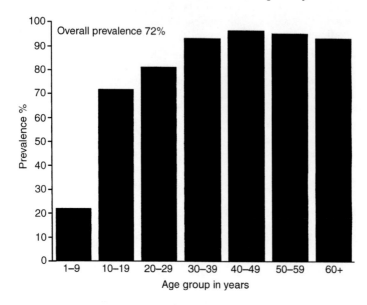

Fig. 5. Age prevalence of positive skin-snips in a West African community with an overall prevalence of 72% (compiled from data published in Davies, J.B. (1993) *Annals of Tropical Medicine and Parasitology* 87, 41–63).

from water depth and flow rates at dosages of the order of 0.05 mg l⁻¹.

Since D.B. Blacklock discovered the vector of onchocerciasis in 1926, there have been many attempts at controlling the vector by larviciding. The use of DDT gave good control of *S. damnosum* sensu lato in Nigeria and Uganda, and helped to eradicate *S. neavei* from Kenya, but this insecticide is no longer environmentally acceptable. Acceptable insecticides with very low vertebrate toxicity include the organophosphates, such as temephos (Abate®), and microbial ones, such as *Bacillus thuringiensis* subsp. *israelensis*. In many areas ground application is difficult, either because of the enormous size of the rivers requiring treatment or the distance from roads and bridges, or because breeding occurs in a large network of small rivers and watercourses. Under these conditions aerial application from small aircraft or helicopters is essential (Fig. 6). Helicopters are almost indispensable for prospection and follow-up surveys.

The world's most ambitious and largest control programme against any vector was initiated in 1974 by the World Health Organization (funded by a consortium of donor countries and international agencies through the World Bank), and is called the Onchocerciasis Control Programme (OCP). By 1986 there were 11 participating countries, namely Benin, Burkina Faso, Côte d'Ivoire, Ghana, Guinea, Guinea Bissau, Mali, Niger, Senegal, Sierra Leone and Togo (Fig. 1). Some 50,000 km of rivers over an area of 1.3 million km² were dosed weekly with temephos, which was dropped from helicopters or light aircraft (Fig. 6). Resistance to temephos appeared in 1980 in some populations and species of the *S. damnosum* complex. Consequently affected rivers were treated with other insecticides or with *B. thuringiensis* subsp. *israelensis*. Larviciding is planned to continue until the reservoir of adult parasites in the human population has died of old age, and in the last remaining parts of the OCP area this should occur in the year 2002. Since 1988 the OCP has been undertaking the large-scale distribution of Mectizan®. Results of both regimes have been spectacular, and transmission of river blindness has ceased over most of the OCP area. At the end of 2002, responsibility for surveillance and control will be devolved to the individual participating countries.

In 1995 the African Programme for Onchocerciasis Control (APOC) was created to cover populations at risk in 19 countries outside the OCP area. The objective is to establish, within 12 years, a sustainable community-based ivermectin treatment regimen, backed up with focal larviciding. Because ivermectin does not kill the adult worms, control needs to continue for about 20 years – that is, until the reservoir of

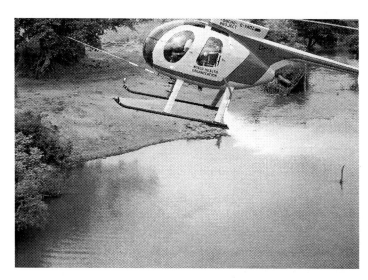

Fig. 6. Helicopter applying larvicide to a river in Burkina Faso (original photograph by J.B. Davies).

infection in the human population (i.e. adult *Onchocerca* worms) dies out. But, if the regime is interrupted locally for any reason before all female worms have died, there is a danger that transmission could recommence, requiring the programme to continue for yet another 20 years. Mectizan® is provided free of charge to the port of entry via the Mectizan® Donation Programme by its manufacturer. In 1998 about 30 million treatments were distributed.

Mass nodulectomy to remove adult worms has been practised routinely in Mexico and parts of Guatemala for many years. This has reduced the incidence of severe ocular complications and prevented blindness, but patients from which all palpable nodules have been regularly removed may still have large numbers of microfilariae in the skin and develop fresh nodules. This shows that, while the regime has reduced microfilarial levels and morbidity, transmission, albeit at a lower level, is still continuing.

Selected bibliography

Anon. (1990) O-Now. Proceedings of the symposium on onchocerciasis, September 20–22 1989, Leiden. *Acta Leidensia* 59 (1 and 2), 483 pp.

Anon. (1998) Mectizan and onchocerciasis; a decade of accomplishment and prospects for the future: the evolution of a drug into a development concept. *Annals of Tropical Medicine and Parasitology* 92 (suppl.), 179 pp.

Blacklock, D.B. (1926) The development of *Onchocerca volvulus* in *Simulium damnosum. Annals of Tropical Medicine and Parasitology* 20, 1–48.

Cook, G.C. (1996) *Manson's Tropical Diseases*, 20th edn. W.B. Saunders, London, 1779 pp.

Crosskey, R.W. (1990) *The Natural History of Blackflies.* John Wiley & Sons, Chichester, UK, 711 pp.

Davies, J.B. (1994) Sixty years of onchocerciasis vector control: a chronological summary with comments on eradication, reinvasion and insecticide resistance. *Annual Review of Entomology* 39, 23–45.

Molyneux, D.H. and Davies, J.B. (1997) Onchocerciasis control: moving towards the Millennium. *Parasitology Today* 13, 418–425.

Samba, E.M. (1994) The onchocerciasis control programme in West Africa. An example of effective public health management. *World Health Organization Public Health in Action* 1, 1–107.

World Health Organization (1987) *WHO Expert Committee on Onchocerciasis.* World Health Organization Technical Report Series 752, Geneva, 167 pp.

World Health Organization (1995) *Onchocerciasis and its Control.* WHO Technical Report Series 852, WHO, Geneva, 103 pp.

World Health Organization (1997) *Twenty Years of Onchocerciasis Control. Review of the Work on the Onchocerciasis Control Programme in West Africa from 1974 to 1994.* WHO, Geneva, 178 pp. (In English or French.)

O'nyong-nyong virus

Jack Woodall

This is an infection of humans. O'nyong-nyong (ONN) virus was first isolated in 1959 from the serum of a 40-year-old febrile woman with severe joint pains during an epidemic affecting 90% of the population in the rural district of Acholi, Uganda. The name comes from that given to the disease by the Acholi people, and means 'joint-breaker', reminiscent of the name 'bone-breaker' for dengue fever, which it resembles. It is a descriptor, not a place name like most other arboviral names, so, like dengue and yellow fever, it does not begin with a capital letter. (Some early publications refer to the virus as 'Gulu'; this was another strain, isolated from mosquitoes, named for the town where the mosquitoes were collected.) Many other local names were given to the epidemic as it subsequently spread through Uganda to Kenya, Tanzania, Zambia, Malawi and Mozambique, involving several million people – the largest recorded mosquito-borne virus epidemic in history. The epidemic died out in 1962, but sporadic cases were seen in Nigeria in 1966 and 1969, where the virus isolated was initially considered to be different and was named Igbo-Ora; a small outbreak was also identified in Côte d'Ivoire in 1984–1985. In 1996 it reappeared in epidemic form in Uganda after a 35-year absence, although serological studies of febrile patients in Kenya in 1994 and 1995 suggested that the virus might have been circulating there earlier.

Distribution

The epidemic of o'nyong-nyong spread from Uganda to Kenya, southern Sudan, Congo, Tanzania, Zambia, Malawi and Mozambique, as shown by virus isolation or antibody detection. In addition, ONN virus has been isolated from sentinel mice in Senegal, where a serosurvey showed that up to 55% of the populations surveyed had haemagglutination inhibiting (HI) antibody, and from three patients in Nigeria and an outbreak involving 33 people in Côte d'Ivoire (the Igbo-Ora strain in both countries).

Domestic animals

O'nyong-nyong virus has not been isolated from any domestic animal, although it produces viraemia when inoculated into newly hatched ('wet') chicks. The antibody found in serosurveys, such as complement fixation (CF) antibody in 11% of 62 horses tested in Nigeria with the Igbo-Ora strain, could have been due to cross-reactions with antibody elicited by infections with chikungunya (CHIK) virus (see entry).

Virus

O'nyong-nyong virus is an RNA virus that has been placed in the genus *Alphavirus* of the family Togaviridae. Alphaviruses have been classified as belonging to one of six antigenic complexes; viruses in such complexes are more closely related to each other than they are to other viruses within the serogroup. O'nyong-nyong virus belongs to the Semliki Forest complex, which includes four viruses: Semliki Forest, CHIK (subtypes CHIK (several varieties) and ONN), Getah (subtypes Getah, Sagiyama, Bebaru and Ross River) and Mayaro (subtypes Mayaro and Una) (see entries on all these

viral infections except for Sagiyama, Bebaru and Una).

The genome is constructed in the same way as that of CHIK virus, to which ONN virus is closely related. Phylogenetic studies indicate that CHIK and ONN viruses occupy anciently distinct evolutionary lineages, and therefore that o'nyong-nyong outbreaks do not result from repeated mutation of African CHIK viruses. Sequence data show that the 1959 epidemic strain of ONN virus is closely related to the 1996–1997 epidemic strain, and that Igbo-Ora virus is clearly a strain of ONN virus.

O'nyong-nyong virus has been isolated only from humans, mosquitoes and sentinel mice. It produces antibodies in hamsters and viraemia in newly hatched ('wet') chicks. Various cell cultures are susceptible to ONN virus (see entry on chikungunya virus).

Clinical symptoms

The virus causes illness characterized by sudden onset, fever, severe chills, severe headache, eye pain, myalgia, symmetrical arthralgia, dry cough and coryza in some cases, leucopenia and often a rash. The clinical syndrome caused by ONN virus is similar to that caused by CHIK virus (see entry). After at least an 8-day incubation period the patient experiences sudden onset of joint pain, particularly in the knees, elbows, wrists, fingers and ankles, in that order. An itching morbilliform rash, often accompanied by resolution of the illness, occurs about 4 days later in most patients and lasts 4–7 days. It begins at the face and descends. Postcervical, axilla and groin lymph nodes are enlarged. The itching rash and joint pain distinguish the infection from measles and rubella (but not from dengue), and the marked lymphadenitis distinguishes it from CHIK infection. As determined by coordinated serological and clinical surveys, most infections produce typical symptoms. Haemorrhagic signs have not been seen. Recovery is complete; no deaths or sequelae due to ONN virus infection have been recorded, and a post-epidemic survey in the area of presumed origin in Africa showed no increase in the incidence of congenital birth defects.

Diagnosis

Virus isolation is the test of choice for laboratory diagnosis. Field strains of ONN virus are non-pathogenic to adult mice but are pathogenic for suckling mice inoculated intracranially; however, the only sign on initial passage may be runting and/or a patchy alopecia in the newly emerging hairy coat. Although alphavirus antigens participating in haemagglutination and neutralization appear to be conserved, plaque-reduction neutralization tests to distinguish CHIK and ONN viruses are successful when single-dose (infection-immune) antisera are used.

Transmission

The virus is transmitted by mosquitoes; the vectors of ONN virus are the malaria vectors *Anopheles funestus* and *Anopheles gambiae* and probably others of the complex; consequently the virus can spread to wherever malaria is found in Africa. This is in contrast to the closely related CHIK virus and most other mosquito-borne viruses, which are transmitted by culicine mosquitoes. Attempts to infect the North American *Anopheles quadrimaculatus* and *Aedes aegypti* in the laboratory were unsuccessful. Primate and other vertebrate hosts of ONN virus are unknown.

Treatment

In the absence of a specific antiviral drug, this consists primarily of supportive therapy. Symptoms respond partially to non-steroidal anti-inflammatory drugs.

Control

Prevention of human infection involves reducing contact between humans and mosquitoes by avoidance behaviour, and mosquito control operations. Clothing that covers the arms and legs, applying insect repellents to exposed skin, staying indoors in mosquito-screened houses after dark and using mosquito bed nets, preferably insecticide-impregnated, can all be effective.

Routine malaria control measures involving spraying houses with residual insecticides, draining swamps and managing irrigation systems, and providing piped water can be effective in reducing the transmission potential. Community education and media publicity are essential to engage the general public in cleaning up the environment to get rid of mosquito breeding places.

A live, attenuated CHIK vaccine has been developed by the US military; tests in humans show that it blocks conversion to subsequent Venezuelan equine encephalitis (see entry) vaccination, meaning that it might cross-protect against other alphaviruses, including ONN virus.

Selected bibliography

Lanciotti, R.S., Ludwig, M.L., Rwaguma, E.B., Lutwama, J.J., Kram, T.M., Karabatsos, N., Cropp, B.C. and Miller, B.R. (1998) Emergence of epidemic O'nyong-nyong fever in Uganda after a 35-year absence: genetic characterization of the virus. *Virology* 252, 258–268.

McClain, D.J., Pittman, P.R., Ramsburg, H.H., Nelson, G.O., Rossi, C.A., Mangiafico, J.A., Schmaljohn, A.L. and Malinoski, F.J. (1998) Immunologic interference from sequential administration of live attenuated alphavirus vaccines. *Journal of Infectious Diseases* 177, 634–641.

Moore, D.L., Causey, O.R., Carey, D.E., Reddy, S., Cooke, A.R., Akinkugbe, F.M., David-West T.S. and Kemp, G.E. (1975) Arthropod-borne viral infections of man in Nigeria, 1964–1970. *Annals of Tropical Medicine and Parasitology* 69, 49–64.

Powers, A.M., Brault, A.C., Tesh, R.B. and Weaver, S.C. (2000) Re-emergence of chikungunya and o'nyong-nyong viruses: evidence for distinct geographical lineages and distant evolutionary relationships. *Journal of General Virology* 81, 471–479.

Rwaguma, E.B., Lutwama, J.J., Sempala, S.D.K., Kiwanuka, N., Kamugisha, J., Okware, S., Bagambisa, G., Lanciotti, R., Roehrig, J.T. and Gubler, D.J. (1997) Emergence of epidemic o'nyong-nyong fever in southwestern Uganda, after an absence of 35 years. *Emerging Infectious Diseases* 3, 77.

Williams, M.C. and Woodall, J.P. (1961) O'nyong-nyong fever: an epidemic virus disease in East Africa. *Transactions of the Royal Society of Tropical Medicine and Hygiene* 55, 135–141.

Oriental sore *see* **Leishmaniasis.**

Oriental spotted fever *see* **Tick-borne typhuses.**

Orientia tsutsugamushi see **Scrub typhus.**

Oropouche virus

P.S. Mellor

Oropouche (ORO) virus is the cause of one of the most important arboviral diseases in the Americas. It was first isolated in 1955 from a febrile forest worker, a resident of Vega de Oropouche in Trinidad. Since that time the virus has caused at least 27 epidemics and many thousands of clinical cases in Central and South America. Serological surveys suggest that up to half a million people may have been infected since the beginning of the 1960s in Brazil alone.

Distribution

Oropouche virus is Central and South American in distribution and cases of fever caused by this virus have been recorded from Brazil, Panama, Peru and Trinidad. Antibodies to the virus have also been detected, in non-human primates, in Colombia – a finding that suggests the virus is probably present in most countries in the region. By far the greatest number of epidemics have been in the Brazilian Amazon region, which is the only part of Brazil to be affected.

Most occurrences of Oropouche fever have been in the form of urban epidemics and have involved such centres as Belém and Manaus, the largest cities of the Brazilian Amazon, and the city of Iquitos in the Peruvian Amazon region. Elsewhere, antibodies to ORO virus have been detected in the residents of villages scattered across virtually the entire Amazon region.

Aetiological agent

Oropouche virus is a member of the genus *Bunyavirus*, family Bunyaviridae, and is included in the Simbu serogroup of bunyaviruses. The virion is spherical and 90–100 nm in diameter and displays surface glycoprotein projections, which are embedded in a lipid bilayered envelope. Four structural proteins have been identified and surround the three segments of single-stranded RNA (ssRNA).

Clinical symptoms

Oropouche fever is characterized by an abrupt onset and fever, headache, myalgia, arthralgia, anorexia, dizziness, chills and photophobia. Nausea, vomiting, diarrhoea, epigastric pain, retrobulbar pain, conjunctivitis and meningitis have also been reported. The acute phase of the illness usually lasts for 2–5 days, but recurrence of the original symptoms over the next 10 days is common in patients who resume strenuous activities too quickly. Reinfection with ORO virus has not been documented, so a single infection seems to provide lifelong immunity. To date, no fatalities have been attributed to Oropouche fever.

Oropouche virus is not known to cause overt disease or death in any domestic species of animal or in wildlife.

Diagnosis

Oropouche fever in humans may be diagnosed by isolation and identification of the virus from serum during the febrile phase of the disease or, subsequently, by the demonstration of ORO virus-specific antibodies.

Virus may be isolated by intracerebral (i.c.) and intraperitoneal (i.p.) inoculation of suckling mice, by i.c., i.p. and subcutaneous (s.c.) inoculation of adult hamsters or by the inoculation of a range of cell cultures. Virus identification is by indirect immunofluorescence antibody (IFA) or virus neutralization (VN). A range of assays can be used to demonstrate the presence of ORO virus-specific antibodies including, haemagglutination inhibition (HI), complement fixation (CF), VN and enzyme-linked immunosorbent assay (ELISA).

Transmission

In the field ORO virus has been isolated occasionally from mosquitoes and frequently from the biting midge, *Culicoides paraensis*. This species is typically found at high density during epidemics of Oropouche fever and bites humans both inside houses and outside. Biological transmission has been demonstrated via *C. paraensis* from infected to susceptible hamsters and from infected humans to susceptible hamsters, with transmission rates as high as 83%. Transmission of ORO virus between hamsters has also been demonstrated using the mosquito *Culex quinquefasciatus*, although this is much less efficient. Concentrations of virus higher than those usually occurring in humans were necessary to initiate an infection in mosquitoes and even then transmission rates never exceeded 5%. These findings strongly suggest that *C. paraensis* is the major biological vector of ORO virus between humans during urban epidemics of the disease. However, the vector(s) of the virus in its 'silent' sylvatic cycle remain unknown.

Epidemics of Oropouche fever tend to be explosive in nature, rapidly affecting large numbers of people, with prevalence rates as high as 60%, and, as a consequence of this, have had a significant social and economic impact. In general, epidemics of Oropouche fever begin during the rainy season and tend to decline with the onset of the dry period, though in some locations virus transmission has been detected for as long as 6 months. This seasonal incidence of the disease is linked to the population densities of the major vector, *C. paraensis*, which peak during months with high levels of rainfall. The predominant risk factor for Oropouche fever, therefore, is proximity to large populations of the vector. Individually *C. paraensis* seems to be an inefficient

vector, but it is able to compensate for this by being widely distributed in both urban and rural environments and by being extremely abundant during the high-rainfall periods. It is most active during the late afternoon and early evening, when people are likely to be relaxing out of doors and are therefore more easily accessible. Agricultural occupations, such as cultivating cacao or banana plants around houses, activities that provide ideal breeding sites for the vector, are important risk factors. All ages and both sexes appear to be equally susceptible to ORO virus. Female cases have predominated in some localized outbreaks, though not in others, and this probably represents differential exposure to the vector.

Oropouche virus is the only *Culicoides*-borne virus that is a major cause of disease in humans; all other viruses transmitted by *Culicoides*, if they cause disease at all, do so in non-human animals.

Vertebrate hosts

Humans seem to be the main host of ORO virus, at least during the dissemination of the virus in urban (epidemic) situations. During the long interepidemic periods, however, it is postulated that the virus is maintained in a 'silent', sylvatic cycle. This secondary cycle is poorly understood but, on the basis of antibody detection, the vertebrate hosts or reservoirs are suspected to be non-human primates, sloths and birds of the family Formicariidae. However, apart from humans, the virus itself has only been isolated on four occasions, all from Three-toed sloths (*Bradypus tridactylus*).

Treatment

Apart from supportive treatment, there is no specific therapy for Oropouche fever. Patients should refrain from strenuous activities, retire to bed and consult their physician.

Prevention and control

The most effective way to prevent or curb the impact of epidemics of Oropouche fever is to attempt to control the vector, *C. paraensis*. Such measures could involve insecticidal fogging to kill adult midges during their activity periods, though this is likely to be of short-term benefit only. Destruction or removal of the vector's larval habitats (decomposing trunks of felled banana plants, rotting cacao husks) may offer a more permanent control strategy. Individuals may also acquire short-term protection against attacks of the vector by applying insect repellents directly to the skin.

At present, there is no vaccine available against Oropouche fever and, in the light of the relatively benign nature of the disease, it is unlikely that one will be developed in the near future.

Selected bibliography

Dixon, K.E., Travassos da Rosa, A.P.A., Travassos da Rosa, J.F.S. and Llewellyn, C.H. (1981) Oropouche virus, II. Epidemiological observations during an epidemic in Santarem, Pará, Brazil in 1975. *American Journal of Tropical Medicine and Hygiene* 30, 161–164.

LeDuc, J.W. and Pinheiro, F.P. (1988) Oropouche fever. In: Monath, T.P. (ed.) *The Arboviruses: Epidemiology and Ecology*, Vol. IV. CRC Press, Boca Raton, Florida, pp. 1–14.

Pinheiro, F.P., Hoch, A.L., de Lourdes, M., Gomes, C. and Roberts, D.R. (1981) Oropouche virus, IV. Laboratory transmission by *Culicoides paraensis. American Journal of Tropical Medicine and Hygiene* 30, 172–176.

Pinheiro, F.P., Travassos da Rosa, A.P.A., Travassos da Rosa, J.F.S., Ishak, R., Freitas, R.B., Gomes, M.L.C., LeDuc, J.W. and Oliva, O.F.P. (1981) Oropouche virus, I. A review of clinical, epidemiological and ecological findings. *American Journal of Tropical Medicine and Hygiene* 30, 149–160.

Roberts, D.R., Hoch, A.L., Dixon, K.E. and Llewellyn, C.H. (1981) Oropouche virus, III. Entomological observations from three epidemics in Pará, Brazil, 1975. *American Journal of Tropical Medicine and Hygiene* 30, 165–171.

Travassos da Rosa, A.P.A., Vasconcelos, P.F.C. and Travassos da Rosa, J.F.S. (1998) *An Overview of Arbovirology in Brazil and Neighbouring Countries.* Instituto Evandro Chagas, Belém, 296 pp.

Watts, D.M., Phillips, I., Callahan, J.D., Griebenow, W., Hyams, K.C. and Hayes, C.G. (1997) Oropouche virus transmission in the Amazon River basin of Peru. *American Journal of Tropical Medicine and Hygiene* 56, 148–152.

Oroya fever *see* **Carrión's disease.**

Papataci fever *see* **Phlebotomus fevers**.

Parafilariasis

R.C. Anderson

Infection of horses and cattle with nematodes of the genus *Parafilaria*, which live in subcutaneous tissues and pierce the skin to release eggs in blood ingested by muscid flies, which act as intermediate hosts. The vulva is beside the oral opening (Fig. 1).

Parasites
Parafilaria bovicola

Moderately sized, whitish nematodes in subcutaneous nodules. Males are 2–3 cm and females 4–5 cm in length. Eggs are 40–55 μm × 23–33 μm in size and oval, with smooth shells. Mature larvae are 215–230 μm in length.

DISTRIBUTION   In cattle and Water buffalo (*Bubalus bubalis*) in Europe, Africa, India, Pakistan and the Philippines.

CLINICAL SIGNS   Focal cutaneous haemorrhages, mainly along the back, which bleed on to the surface of the skin, usually in the spring and early summer. If severe, lesions may impair the working ability of bullocks. The lesions give the carcass a bruised appearance, which make superficial parts of it unacceptable for human consumption.

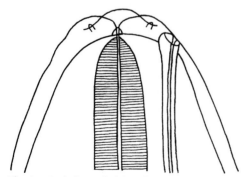

Fig. 1.   Cephalic end of *Parafilaria multipapillosa* (female) showing 'anterior' vulva.

DIAGNOSIS   Examination of blood in the lesions for the presence of the eggs by microscopic examination in water (if necessary, after centrifugation).

TRANSMISSION   Intermediate hosts attracted to the bleeding lesions are *Musca autumnalis* in Europe and *Musca lusoria* and *Musca xanthomelis* in South Africa. Flies ingest eggs together with blood. The eggs hatch and the larvae invade the tissues of the fly and develop to third-stage larvae (2.0–4.3 mm in length), which move to the mouthparts of the fly and enter the host while the latter is feeding on a lesion or on the orbit. Cattle have been infected experimentally by allowing infected flies to feed on fresh incisions, or when inoculated subcutaneously or into the jugular or the orbit. The nematodes may move some distance from the site of introduction. The pre-patent period is reported as 242–319 days. In South Africa the main period for transmission is summer from August to February. In Sweden the main period of transmission is in June.

CONTROL   According to the Merck Veterinary Manual (see Anon., 1991), ivermectin (200 μg kg^{-1}) or nitroxynil (20 μg kg^{-1}) given subcutaneously reduced the number and extent of the lesions. In Sweden pyrethroid-impregnated ear tags on cattle reduced the vector population and the lesions (by 75%).

Parafilaria multipapillosa

Similar to *P. bovicola*. Males are 2.8 cm and females 4–7 cm in length. Eggs are about 50–58 μm × 24–33 μm in size. Larvae are 220–230 μm in length.

DISTRIBUTION   In subcutaneous tissues of equines (horse, donkey and mule) in Asia, the Commonwealth of Independent States (CIS), Europe, South America and North Africa.

CLINICAL SIGNS   Skin nodules occur mainly on the head and upper forequarters. The female worm pierces the nodule and the nodules bleed to the outside, usually in the summer, resulting in the condition being termed 'bloody sweat' or 'summer bleeding'. Lesions may suppurate and also interfere with harnesses. Lesions are seasonal (spring and summer) and disappear in winter in temperate regions.

DIAGNOSIS   Discovery is by microscopic examination for eggs in the blood leaving bleeding nodules (see above).

TRANSMISSION   The known vector in the CIS is the biting dipteran *Haematobia atripalpis*. The fly ingests eggs while feeding on the blood from a lesion. The eggs hatch in the gut of the fly and larvae develop in the haemocoel and fat body in 10–15 days at 20–36°C. Infective larvae are 1.67–2.67 mm in length. Horses presumably become infected when flies break the skin of the definitive host while feeding, thus allowing the infective larvae to invade the subcutaneous tissues. The pre-patent period was 281 and 387 days in horses naturally infected by the bites of *H. altripalpis*. The nematodes may migrate extensively from the point of infection, and sunlight may be a stimulus for the lesions to bleed because of increased activity of the ovipositing female nematodes.

CONTROL   Nothing has been reported, but presumably the same treatment as that used in infections of *P. bovicola* would be effective, as well as similar vector control measures.

Selected bibliography

Anderson, R.C. (2000) *Nematode Parasites of Vertebrates: their Development and Transmission*, 2nd edn. CAB International, Wallingford, UK, 650 pp.

Anon (1991) *The Merck Veterinary Manual*, 7th edn. Merck and Company Inc., Rahway, New Jersey, 1831 pp.

Baumann, R. (1946) Beobachtungen beim parasitären Sommerbluten der Pferde. *Wiener Tierärztliche Monatsschrift* 33, 52–55.

Bech-Nielsen, S., Bornstein, S., Christensson, D., Wallgren, T.B., Zakrisson, G. and Chirico, J. (1982) *Parafilaria bovicola* (Tubangui, 1934) in cattle: epizootiology–vector study and experimental transmission of *Parafilaria bovicola* to cattle. *American Journal of Veterinary Research* 43, 948–954.

Gnedina, M.P. and Osipov, A.N. (1960) Contribution to the biology of *Parafilaria multipapillosa* (Condamine and Drouilly, 1878) parasitic in the horse. *Helminthologia, Bratislava* 2, 13–16. (In Russian with English, French and German summaries.)

Nevill, E.M. (1975) Preliminary report on the transmission of *Parafilaria bovicola* in South Africa. *Onderstepoort Journal of Veterinary Research* 42, 41–48.

Nevill, E.M. (1979) The experimental transmission of *Parafilaria bovicola* to cattle in South Africa using *Musca* species (subgenus *Eumusca*) as intermediate hosts. *Onderstepoort Journal of Veterinary Research* 46, 51–57.

Parafilaria species *see* **Parafilariasis.**

Phlebotomine sand-flies (Phlebotominae)

M.W. Service

There are about 700 species of phlebotomine sand-flies (often just called sand-flies) in six or more genera (the number depends on the hierachical classification adopted); but species in three main genera, *Phlebotomus*, *Lutzomyia* and *Sergentomyia*, blood-feed on vertebrate hosts. The former two genera contain species that transmit disease pathogens to humans and animals and are therefore of economic importance.

Phlebotomine sand-flies occur in tropical countries and warmer regions of temperate countries. The genus *Phlebotomus* is found only in the Old World, such as in Mediterranean countries, the Middle East, Africa, India and China. Most species inhabit semi-arid or arid regions in preference to forests. *Lutzomyia* species are found in the New World tropics, being especially common in forested areas of Central and South America.

Biology

Eggs are supposedly deposited in cracks and crevices in the ground, among leaf litter, between buttress roots of trees, at the bases of termite mounds, in masonry, on stable floors and in poultry sheds. The type of habitat depends on the species. Eggs require a moist microenvironment and, under optimum conditions, hatch in 6–17 days, but after longer periods in cooler conditions. Larvae are mainly scavengers, feeding, at least in the laboratory, on semi-rotting vegetable matter and decomposing arthropod bodies. There are four larval instars and development takes about 16–90 days, duration depending on species and environmental conditions. In arid and temperate regions, larvae may remain in a state of diapause for many months. The final-instar larva sheds its skin and the pupa is formed (Fig. 1). After about 5–10 days adults emerge from the pupae. The life cycle, from egg laying to adult emergence, may be 30–60 days, but extends to several months in some species having diapausing larvae. In temperate areas adults die off in late summer or autumn, but in tropical areas breeding continues throughout the year. However, little is known of the breeding of sand-flies in nature; larvae have been found only rarely.

Adults of both sexes feed on sugary secretions, including plant juices. Only females in addition suck blood from humans and a wide spectrum of hosts, which includes domestic livestock, dogs and urban and wild rodents, as well as reptiles and amphibia. Feeding usually occurs at night or late in the evenings and most species bite out of doors. A few species,

however, enter houses to feed and/or rest and are commonly referred to as domestic or peridomestic species; examples are *Phlebotomus papatasi* in the Mediterranean region and the *Lutzomyia longipalpis* complex in South America. Being very small (1.3–3.5 mm long) and delicate insects, adults do not usually disperse more than a few hundred metres from their breeding places, but they have occasionally been reported as dispersing up to about 2 km.

Diseases

Phlebotomine sand-flies are of the greatest medical and veterinary importance in transmitting the protozoan parasites causing leishmaniasis in humans and in animals, such as dogs. They also transmit viruses responsible for phlebotomus (sandfly) fevers and bacteria causing Carrión's disease to humans (see entries).

Control

Personal protection can be obtained by using suitable insect repellents and/or bed nets (sand-fly nets), in which the holes are smaller than those found in mosquito bed nets. However, small ventilation holes are unnecessary if nets are regularly impregnated with pyrethroid insecticides. Spraying the interior surfaces of walls and ceilings or roofs of houses with residual insecticides can reduce the numbers of those species that enter houses to feed or rest. If out-of-door resting sites are known, these can also be sprayed.

Most leishmaniasis involves animal reservoir hosts, and these, such as dogs and rodents, have sometimes been destroyed in attempts to reduce disease transmission. Occasionally vegetation around villages has been cleared to reduce Gerbil (e.g. *Psammomys obesis*) populations.

Selected bibliography

Killick-Kendrick, R. (1990) The biology of phlebotomine sandflies. *Clinics in Dermatology* 17, 278–289.

Lane, R.P. (1993) Sandflies (Phlebotominae). In: Lane, R.P. and Crosskey, R.W. (eds) *Medical Insects and Arachnids*. Chapman & Hall, London, pp. 78–119.

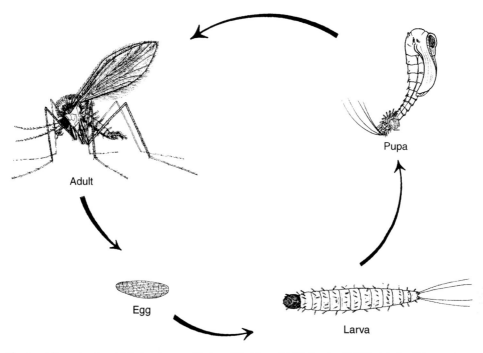

Fig. 1.   Life cycle of a phlebotomine sandfly (modified from M.W. Service (2000), *Medical Entomology for Students,* Cambridge University Press, Cambridge).

Ward, R.D. (1990) Some aspects of the biology of phlebotomine sandfly vectors. *Advances in Disease Vector Research* 6, 1–126. (Reprints and chapters are incorrectly dated 1989.)

Phlebotomus fevers

R.W. Ashford

Otherwise known as sandfly fevers, papataci fever or three-day fever. This is a febrile disease caused by viruses transmitted by phlebotomine sand-flies (Psychodidae: Phlebotominae). The prototype virus of this group is sandfly fever (Sicilian) (SFS), but various other types cause classical sandfly fever, and further related viruses cause occasional fever in the Americas.

In addition to the sandfly fever viruses, phlebotomine sand-flies are responsible for the transmission of ten of the 16 vesiculoviruses, as well as certain flaviviruses and orbiviruses.

Distribution

Classical sandfly fever occurs throughout the Mediterranean basin, including most of the islands, extending through south-west Asia to northern India. The initial isolation came from American troops in Sicily in the Second World War (1939–1945). Sandfly fever used to be a well-recognized occupational hazard among British troops stationed in the Middle East. In the 1980s, Russian troops became infected when they entered a previously unrecognized focus in Afghanistan, as did UN troops in Cyprus. The occurrence of related fevers, with associated meningitis and meningoencephalitis, has been recognized recently in central Italy, where 155 cases were identified in two regions in a 10-year survey.

This distribution coincides closely with that of the main vector, *Phlebotomus papatasi*, and, in Europe, with that of *Phlebotomus perniciosus*. *Phlebotomus papatasi* occurs in semi-arid, low-lying, sandy areas from western Europe and Africa to Central Asia and north-east India, while *P. perniciosus* is found in more humid areas, usually on calcareous substrates, throughout the Mediterranean littoral. The fever occurs focally within the overall distribution of the vectors. This focality is sometimes attributed to the short flight range of sand-flies but, in fact, sand-flies are known to fly considerable distances. While short 'hopping' flights are commonly observed, these are associated with the final approach to blood meal or sugar-meal sources. In fact, mark–release–recapture experiments show that these insects normally fly hundreds of metres between resting and feeding sites and can travel several kilometres.

In the Americas, related viruses capable of causing sandfly fever are widely but sporadically distributed between Panama and Brazil, but human cases are uncommonly recognized.

The diversity of phlebovirus species in the Americas conforms with the great diversity of sand-flies in that region. No phlebovirus species is known from South-East Asia or Australasia, where the fauna of mammal-biting sand-flies is poor.

Aetiological agent

Sandfly fever viruses belong to the family Bunyaviridae and the genus *Phlebovirus*. Thirty-eight viruses were listed in the genus *Phlebovirus* in 1988, 24 of which are transmitted by phlebotomine sand-flies. Since that time the number has reached over 50. The most important virus in the group, Rift Valley fever virus (see entry), is normally transmitted by mosquitoes, but there is some evidence that sand-flies may also be able to serve as vectors. At least nine strains of phlebovirus can cause human disease,

seven of which are transmitted by sand-flies (Table 1). The causes of classical sandfly fever are SFS and sandfly fever (Neapolitan) (SFN) viruses. The strain causing meningitis in Italy is known as Toscana (TOS) strain, and has recently been recognized in Portugal and Spain. This is transmitted by *P. perniciosus* and possibly *Phlebotomus perfiliewi*, both of which may occur in high densities.

Sandfly fever viruses replicate in their sand-fly hosts, with an extrinsic cycle of 7–10 days, which corresponds to a single gonotrophic cycle. They can be cultured in African green monkey (VERO) cells or in mosquito cells.

Clinical symptoms

The fever caused by these viruses is a self-limiting influenza-like disease. Following an incubation period of 2–6 days, the fever usually lasts 2–4 days. After resolution of the fever, there is complete immunity to the homologous strain, and there is no mortality. The disease is usually unnoticed in infants and children, and the high prevalence of antibodies in people with no history of disease indicates that it is frequently asymptomatic or overlooked. It is normally only when outbreaks occur in groups of travellers or visitors to endemic areas that the disease is recognized. In a series of volunteer infections the fever lasted between 6 and 74 h and was associated with headache, anorexia, myalgia, photophobia and lower back and retro-orbital pain.

The disease in South and Central America is similar, but is only known sporadically among people entering forested areas.

Diagnosis

This is usually presumptive, based on circumstantial evidence, and many cases go undiagnosed. It was estimated retrospectively that only 20% of SFS virus cases in Swedish tourists who had visited Mediterranean countries had been correctly diagnosed. For confirmation, serology is required, by haemagglutination inhibition, confirmed by neutralizing antibody tests.

Table 1. The serotypes of *Phlebovirus* (from Tesh, 1988; Kolakofsky, 1991).

Virus name	Prototype strain	Distribution	Arthropod associations	Vertebrate associations
Aguacate	VP-175A	Panama	*Lutzomyia* species	–
Alenquer	BeYH 30101	Brazil	–	Human
Ambe	BeAr 407981	S. America	*Lutzomyia* species	–
Anhanga	BeAn 46852	Brazil	–	Sloth (*Choloepus* species)
Arbia	ISS. Phl. 18	Italy	*Phlebotomus perniciosus, Phlebotomus perfiliewi*	–
Arboledas	CoAr 170152	Colombia	*Lutzomyia* species	Human? Opossum?
Armero	CoAr 171096	S. America	*Lutzomyia* species	–
Arumowot	Ar 1284-64	Africa	Culicidae	Rodents, birds, etc.
Belterra	BeAn 356637	Brazil		Spiny rat (*Proechimys* species)
Buenaventura	CoAr 3319	Colombia	*Lutzomyia* species	–
Bujaru	BeAn 47693	Brazil	–	Rodents
Cacao	VP-437R	Panama	*Lutzomyia trapidoi*	–
Caimito	VP-488A	Panama	*Lutzomyia ylephiletor*	–
Candiru	BeH 22511	Brazil	–	Human
Chagres	JW-10	Panama, Colombia	*L. trapidoi, L. ylephiletor*	Human
Chilibre	VP-118D	Panama	*Lutzomyia* species	–
Corfou	PaAr 814	Greece	*Phlebotomus major*	–
Durania	CoAr 171162	Colombia	*Lutzomyia* species	Human?
Frijoles	VP-161A	Panama	*Lutzomyia* species	–
Gabek Forest	Sud An 754-61	Africa	Possibly none	Rodents
Gordil	Dak An BR 496d	Central African Republic	–	Rodents
Icoaraci	BeAn 24262	Brazil	Culicidae, *Lutzomyia* species	Rodents, birds
Ixcanal	CAAr 170897	Guatemala	*Lutzomyia* species	–
Itaituba	BeAn 213452	Brazil	–	Opossum (*Didelphis marsupialis*)
Itaporanga	–	S. America	Culicidae	–
Joa	BeAr 371637	Brazil	*Lutzomyia* species	–
Karimabad	I-58	Iran	*Phlebotomus* species	Human, gerbils?
Mariquita	Mariquita A	Colombia	*Lutzomyia* species	–
Munguba	BeAr 389707	Brazil	*Lutzomyia umbratilis*	–
Nique	Nique-9C	Panama	*Lutzomyia panamensis*	–
Odrenisou	–	Africa	Culicidae	–
Oriximina	BeAr 385309	Brazil	*Lutzomyia* species	–
Pacui	BeAn 27326	Brazil	*Lutzomyia flaviscutellata*	Rodents
Punta Toro	D-4021A	Panama	*Lutzomyia trapidoi, Lutzomyia ylephiletor*	Human, sloth (*Bradypus* species), primates? Carnivores? Rodents?
Rift Valley fever	–	Africa	Culicidae, *Culicoides* species	Human, sheep, cattle, goat
Rio Grande	TBM3-24	USA (Texas)	–	Rodents
Saint Floris	DakAn BR 512d	Central African Republic	–	Rodents
Salehabad	I-81	Iran	*Phlebotomus* species	–

Continued

Table 1.   *Continued.*

Virus name	Prototype strain	Distribution	Arthropod associations	Vertebrate associations
Sandfly fever (Naples)	Sabin	N. Africa, S. Europe, C. Asia	*Phlebotomus papatasi*, *Phlebotomus perfiliewi*	Human
Sandfly fever (Sicilian)	Sabin	N. Africa, S. Europe, C. Asia	*Phlebotomus papatasi*	Human, sheep? gerbil (*Rhombomys opimus*)?
Tehran	I-47	Iran	*Phlebotomus papatasi*	–
Toscana	ISS.Phl.3	Italy, Portugal, Spain	*Phlebotomus perniciosus*	Human, bat (*Pipistrellus kuhlii*)
Tunis	–	Tunisia	*Argas reflexus* (tick)	–
Turuna	BeAr 352492	Brazil	*Lutzomyia* species	–
Urucuri	BeAn 100049	Brazil	–	Spiny rat (*Proechimys* species)

Question marks indicate serological evidence only.

Transmission

The virus is maintained by transovarial transmission in the sand-fly population, and humans can probably act as amplifier hosts, infecting further lines of sand-flies. The TOS strain has been maintained through 13 generations of *P. perniciosus* by transovarial transmission. Although it is usually stated that there is no reservoir host for sandfly fever, sheep in Sicily are seropositive, TOS has been isolated from the brain of a Kuhl's bat (*Pipistrellus kuhlii*) in Italy and, in Iran, 13 of 38 Great gerbils (*Rhombomys opimus*) were seropositive for SFS virus and 12 for the related Karimabad (KAR) virus. This suggests that a wildlife cycle exists, but this has not yet been demonstrated. Transovarial transmission is unlikely to be able to maintain a virus indefinitely, so it is probable that some horizontal transmission between sand-flies is essential to the maintenance of a focus.

The finding that TOS virus circulates in Tuscany with another phlebovirus, Arbia (ARB) virus, which seems not to infect humans, shows that different sandfly fever viruses can circulate sympatrically.

Treatment

There is no specific treatment, nor any real need for treatment of these short-lived, self-limiting diseases. A combination of interferon-alpha and ribavirin has been suggested on the basis of *in vitro* experimental results.

Control

Serological evidence demonstrated that, in Athens, the incidence of sandfly fever was greatly reduced coincidentally with the introduction of insecticides against mosquitoes. In the mid-1970s it was found that seropositivity was greatly reduced in people aged less than 35 years. The reasonable assumption is that the two events were linked, and that sand-flies were controlled incidentally with the mosquitoes. *Phlebotomus perniciosus*, the main vector in Europe, is not particularly synanthropic, so it is surprising that domestic use of insecticides should have controlled this species. More probably it was the widespread use of insecticides on the land that led to a reduction in sand-fly numbers. Nevertheless, insecticides were apparently successful in eliminating the infection from hotels in Cyprus, where there had been a problem. *Phlebotomus papatasi*, the main vector outside Europe, is both endophilic and sylvatic. Synanthropic populations can easily be controlled by insecticides, but it is not known whether these or the sylvatic populations, which are less accessible for control, are more responsible for the transmission of sandfly fever virus.

Personal protection against the bites of phlebotomine sand-flies is possible by avoiding being in the open at night or by the use of insect repellents, fine-mesh-screened windows or fine-mesh bed nets, preferably impregnated with pyrethroid insecticides.

It should be emphasized that this is not a sufficiently serious complaint for control measures to be relevant other than in exceptional circumstances.

Selected bibliography

Comer, J.A. and Tesh, R.B. (1991) Phlebotomine sand flies as vectors of vesiculovirus: a review. *Parassitologia* 33 (suppl.), 143–150.

Gonzalez-Scarano, F. and Nathanson, N. (1996) *Bunyaviridae*. In: Fields, B.N., Knipe, D.M. and Howley, P.M. (eds) *Fields Virology*, Vol. 1, 3rd edn. Lippincott-Raven, Philadelphia, pp. 1473–1495.

Kolakofsky, D. (ed.) (1991) *Bunyaviridae*. Current Topics in Microbiology and Immunology 169, Springer, New York, 256 pp.

Tesh, R.B. (1988) The genus *Phlebovirus* and its vectors. *Annual Review of Entomology* 33, 169–181.

Pigeon-fly *see* **Hippoboscids.**

Piroplasmosis

The term piroplasmosis has in the past been used to refer to infections with the parasites of the genera *Babesia* and *Theileria* – that is, for diseases in which piroplasms are found in the red blood cells. See Babesiosis and Theileriosis.

Plague

Thomas Butler

Infection of humans and other animals with the bacterium *Yersinià pestis*.

bloody sputum and can be transmitted directly by coughing near other persons.

Plague, human

The most common disease form is called bubonic plague, which starts suddenly with fever and a painful enlargement of one or more lymph nodes (the bubo), usually in the groin, axilla or neck. Disease progresses to severe sepsis and death in a few days if patients are not treated with antibiotics. Known as the 'Black Death' since the Middle Ages in Europe, because victims sometimes develop skin haemorrhages or gangrene before death, plague was estimated to have killed a quarter of Europe's population. Plague is transmitted by bites of fleas, which carry the infection from reservoir rodents, including domestic rats, squirrels (Sciuridae) and Prairie dogs (*Cynomys* species). A less common form is pneumonic plague, which causes fever, cough and

Distribution

Plague occurs worldwide, with most of the human cases reported from developing countries of Africa and Asia. During the decade of the 1990s through 1996, there were 16,005 cases of plague and 1214 deaths (7.6%) reported to the World Health Organization. The countries that reported more than 100 cases were, in the order from greatest to least: Tanzania, Madagascar, Vietnam, Congo, Peru, India, Myanmar, Zimbabwe, China and Uganda. In the USA, all the 64 plague cases occurred in the south-western states of New Mexico, Arizona, Colorado, Utah and California. Most of the American cases occur during the months of May to October, when people are outdoors and coming into contact with rodents and their fleas. Each endemic region has a specific season when plague tends to occur.

Parasite

Yersinia pestis is a Gram-negative, bipolar-staining bacillus that belongs to the bacterial family Enterobacteriaceae. It grows aerobically on most culture media, including blood agar and MacConkey's agar. It does not ferment lactose and it forms small colonies on MacConkey's agar after 24 h incubation at 35°C. On triple-sugar–iron agar, *Y. pestis* produces an alkaline slant and acid butt, because it ferments glucose. It is non-motile and negative for citrate utilization, urease and indole.

Like the other yersiniae, the plague bacillus produces V and W antigens, which confer a requirement for calcium to grow at 37°C. This property, mediated by a 45 MDa plasmid, is essential for virulence and plays a part in adapting the organism for intracellular survival and growth. Other important virulence factors include the production of lipopolysaccharide endotoxin, a capsular envelope containing the antiphagocytic principal fraction I antigen, the ability to absorb organic iron in the form of a haemin and the presence of the temperature-dependent enzymes coagulase and fibrinolysin.

Clinical symptoms

Although plague infection of humans can assume many and protean clinical forms, the most common presentation is bubonic plague, which has a distinctive clinical picture. The people of plague-endemic regions know the disease and have local names, such as *dich hach* in Vietnamese, that conjure up the horror of recalled fatalities during previous seasons. During an incubation period of 2–8 days following the bite of an infected flea, bacteria proliferate in the regional lymph nodes. Patients are typically affected by the sudden onset of fever, chills, weakness and headache. Usually, at the same time, after a few hours or on the next day, they notice the bubo, which is signalled by intense pain in one anatomical region of the lymph nodes, usually the groin, axilla or neck. A swelling evolves in this area, which is so tender that patients typically avoid any motion that might provoke discomfort. For example, if the bubo is in the femoral area (Fig. 1), the patient will characteristially flex, abduct and externally rotate the hip to relieve pressure on the area and will walk with a limp. When the bubo is in an axilla, the patient will abduct the shoulder or hold the arm in a splint. When a bubo is in the neck, patients will tilt their head to the opposite side.

The buboes are oval swellings that vary from 1 to 10 cm in length and elevate the overlying skin, which may appear stretched or erythematous. They may appear either as a smooth, uniform, ovoid mass or as an irregular cluster of several nodes with intervening and surrounding oedema. Palpation will typically elicit extreme tenderness. There is warmth of the overlying skin and an underlying, firm, non-fluctuant mass. Around the lymph nodes there is usually considerable oedema, which can be either gelatinous or pitting in nature. Occasionally, there is a large area of oedema extending from the bubo into the region drained by the affected lymph nodes. Although infections other than plague can produce acute lymphadenitis, plague is virtually unique for the suddeness of onset of the fever and bubo, the rapid development of intense inflammation in the bubo and the fulminant clinical course, which can produce death as quickly as 2–4 days after the onset of symptoms. The bubo of plague is also distinctive for the usual absence of a detectable skin lesion in the anatomical region where it is located, as well as for the absence of an ascending lymphangitis near it.

In uncomplicated bubonic plague the patients are typically prostrate and lethargic and often exhibit restlessness or agitation. Occasionally, they are delirious with high fever, and seizures are common in children. Temperatures are usually elevated in the range 38.5–40.0°C, and the pulse rates are increased to $110–140 \, min^{-1}$. Blood pressures are characteristically low, in the range of 100/60 mmHg, owing to extreme vasodilatation. Lower pressures, which are unmeasurable, may occur if shock ensues. The liver and spleen are often palpable and tender.

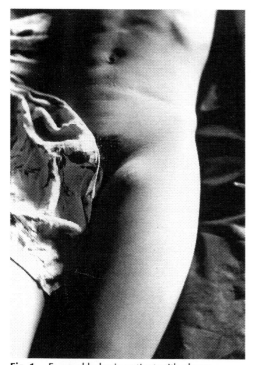

Fig. 1. Femoral bubo in patient with plague.

Most patients with bubonic plague do not have skin lesions; however, about one-quarter of patients in Vietnam did show varied skin findings. The most common were pustules, vesicles, eschars or papules near the bubo or in the anatomical region of skin that is lymphatically drained by the affected lymph nodes, and they presumably represent sites of the flea bites. When these lesions are opened they usually contain white cells and plague bacilli. Rarely, these skin lesions progress to extensive cellulitis or abscesses. Ulceration, however, may lead to a larger plague carbuncle.

Another kind of skin lesion in plague is purpura, which is a result of the systemic disease. The purpuric lesions may become necrotic, resulting in gangrene of distal extremities, the probable basis of the epithet 'Black Death' attributed to plague through the ages. These purpuric lesions contain blood-vessels affected by vasculitis and occlusion by fibrin thrombi, resulting in haemorrhage and necrosis.

A distinctive feature of plague, in addition to the bubo, is the propensity of the disease to overwhelm patients with a massive growth of bacteria in the blood. In the early acute stages of bubonic plague, all patients probably have intermittent bacteraemia. Single blood cultures obtained at the time of hospital admission in Vietnamese patients were positive in 27% of cases. A hallmark of moribund patients with plague is high-density bacteraemia, so that a blood smear revealing characteristic bacilli has been used as a prognostic indicator in this disease. Occasionally in the pathogenesis of plague infection, bacteria are inoculated and proliferate in the body without producing a bubo. Patients may become ill with fever and actually die with bacteraemia but without detectable lymphadenitis. This syndrome has been termed 'septicaemic plague', to denote plague without a bubo. In New Mexico, 25% of plague was septicaemic in 1980–1984 and the case fatality rate of 33% in these instances was three times higher than in bubonic plague, because of delays in diagnosis and treatment.

One of the feared complications of bubonic plague is secondary pneumonia. The infection reaches the lungs by haematogenous spread of bacteria from the bubo. In addition to the high mortality, plague pneumonia is highly contagious by airborne transmission. It presents in the setting of fever and lymphadenopathy as cough, chest pain and often haemoptysis. Radiographically, there is patchy bronchopneumonia, cavities or confluent consolidation. The sputum is usually purulent and contains plague bacilli.

Primary inhalation pneumonia is rare now but is a potential threat following exposure to a patient with plague who has a cough. Plague pneumonia is invariably fatal when antibiotic therapy is delayed more than a day after the onset of illness.

Plague meningitis is a rarer complication and typically occurs more than a week after inadequately treated bubonic plague. It results from a haematogenous spread from a bubo and carries a higher mortality rate than uncomplicated bubonic plague. There appears to be an association between buboes located in the axilla and the development of meningitis. Less commonly, plague meningitis presents as a primary infection of the meninges without antecedent lymphadenitis. Plague meningitis is characterized by fever, headache, meningism and pleocytosis, with a predominance of polymorphonuclear leucocytes. Bacteria are frequently demonstrable with a Gram stain of spinal-fluid sediment, and endotoxin has been demonstrated by the limulus test in spinal fluid.

Plague can produce pharyngitis, which may resemble acute tonsillitis. The anterior cervical lymph nodes are usually inflamed, and *Y. pestis* may be recovered from a throat culture or by aspiration of a cervical bubo. This is a rare clinical form of plague, which is presumed to follow the inhalation or ingestion of plague bacilli.

Plague sometimes presents with prominent gastrointestinal symptoms of nausea, vomiting, diarrhoea and abdominal pain. These symptoms may precede the bubo or, in septicaemic plague, occur without a bubo; they commonly result in diagnostic delay.

Diagnosis

Plague should be suspected in febrile patients who have been exposed to rodents or other mammals in the known endemic areas of the world. A bacteriological diagnosis is readily made in most patients by smear and culture of a bubo aspirate. The aspirate is obtained by inserting a 20-gauge needle on a 10 ml syringe containing 1 ml of sterile saline into the bubo and withdrawing it several times until the saline becomes blood-tinged. Because the bubo does not contain liquid pus, it may be necessary to inject some of the saline and immediately reaspirate it. Drops of the aspirate should be placed on microscope slides and air-dried for both Gram and Wayson's stains. The Gram stain will reveal polymorphonuclear leucocytes and Gram-negative coccobacilli and bacilli ranging from 1 to 2 μm in length. Wayson's stain is prepared by mixing 0.2 g of basic fuchsin (90% dye content) with 0.75 g of methylene blue (90% dye content) in 20 ml of 95% ethyl alcohol. This mixture is then poured slowly into 200 ml of 5% phenol. A smear, after being fixed for 2 min in absolute methanol, is stained for 10–20 s in Wayson's stain, washed with water and dried. *Yersinia pestis* appears as light-blue bacilli with dark-blue polar bodies and the remainder of the slide has a contrasting pink counterstain. Smears of blood, sputum or spinal fluid can be handled similarly.

The aspirate, blood and other appropriate fluids should be inoculated on to blood and MacConkey's agar plates and into infusion broth for bacteriological identification. At some reference laboratories, a serological test, the passive haemagglutination test utilizing fraction I of *Y. pestis*, is available for testing acute- and convalescent-phase serum. In patients with negative cultures, a fourfold or greater increase in titre or a single titre of 1 : 16 or higher is presumptive evidence of plague infection. At reference laboratories, enzyme-linked immunosorbent assay (ELISA) testing for antibodies against fraction I antigen may be available, and rapid diagnosis can be accomplished by applying a fluorescent antibody against fraction I antigen to a bubo aspirate or other body fluids.

Transmission

More than 220 species of rodents can harbour plague bacilli. Rodents are the natural hosts and humans are an accidental host (Fig. 2). Transmission among rodents, such as American red squirrels (e.g. *Tamiasciurus* species), gerbils (e.g. *Gerbillus*, *Meriones* and *Rhombomys* species), marmots (*Marmota* species), ground squirrels (*Spermophilus* (= *Citellus*) species) and voles (e.g. *Microtus* species), is referred to as sylvatic, campestral, rural or endemic plague, with many different species of fleas feeding on these rodents and maintaining transmission among them. When fur trappers and hunters handle these wild rodents, they can be bitten by rodent fleas and develop plague.

Urban plague describes the situation where plague circulating among wild rodents (e.g. *Mastomys* (= *Praomys*) *natalensis* (Multimammate rat), *Gerbillus* and *Meriones* species (gerbils)) has been transmitted to commensal rats, such as *Rattus norvegicus* (Brown or Norwegian rat), *Rattus rattus* (Black rat or House rat), *Rattus*

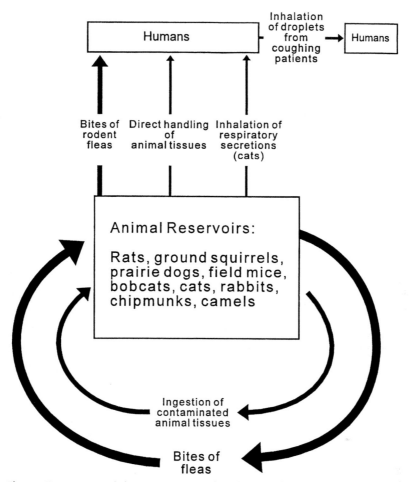

Fig. 2. Transmission of plague among animals and to humans, with thick arrows indicating common, medium arrows occasional and thin arrows rare transmission pathways.

exulans (Polynesian rat) and *Bandicota bengalensis* (Lesser bandicoot rat). The infection is maintained in the rat population by fleas, such as *Xenopsylla cheopis* (Asia, Africa, Europe and the Americas), *Xenopsylla astia* (South-East Asia) and *Xenopsylla brasiliensis* (Africa, India and South America). When rats are living in close association with people, such as in rat-infested slums, fleas normally feeding on rats may jump to humans. This usually happens when the rats are infected with plague and die of the infection. On their death, infected fleas abandon the dead rodents and feed on humans. In this way bubonic plague is spread by rat fleas to the human population. The most important vector is *X. cheopis*, but other fleas, such as *X. astia* and *X. brasiliensis* and, more rarely, *Nosopsyllus fasciatus* and *Leptopsylla aethiopica*, are vectors in some areas. However, as the last two species are reluctant to feed on people, they are not usually involved in transmission of plague to humans.

More rarely, plague is spread directly from person to person by fleas, such as *Xenopsylla* species and the so-called human flea, *Pulex irritans*. This method, however, appears to play a minor role in the transmission of plague.

In the USA plague sometimes infects domestic cats, resulting from their contact with rodents during hunting. Infected cats have developed submandibular lymphadenitis and pneumonia and have caused a few cases of human pneumonic plague after persons had had face-to-face contact with sick cats.

Plague bacilli sucked up with the blood meals of male and female fleas pass to the flea's stomach, where they undergo so great a multiplication that they extend forward to invade the proventriculus (Fig. 3). In some fleas, notably in *Xenopsylla* species, further multiplication of bacilli occurs in the proventriculus and this may become partially or almost completely blocked. This hinders the proventriculus from functioning normally and as a result such blocked fleas regurgitate some of their blood meal during later feeds. In this way bacilli can be injected into a new host during feeding. Because of their inability to feed properly, blocked fleas become starved and repeatedly bite in attempts to take a full blood meal, and are consequently epidemiologically very dangerous. Even if there is no blockage of the alimentary canal, plague transmission can still occur from direct contamination of the flea's mouthparts.

A much less important route of transmission is by the faeces of the flea being rubbed into skin abrasions or coming into contact with mucous membranes. Plague bacilli can remain infective in flea faeces for as long as 3 years. Occasionally the tonsils become infected with plague bacilli due to people crushing fleas between their teeth. In pneumonic plague, where bacilli occur in enormous numbers in the sputum, there is no involvement of fleas in its transmission.

Treatment

Untreated plague has an estimated mortality rate of greater than 50% and can evolve into a fulminant illness complicated by septic shock. Therefore, the early institution of effective antimicrobial therapy is mandatory following appropriate cultures. In 1948, streptomycin was identified as the drug of choice for the treatment of plague, by reducing the mortality rate to less than 5%. No other drug has been demonstrated to be more efficacious or less toxic.

Streptomycin should be given intramuscularly in two divided doses daily, totalling 30 mg kg^{-1} body weight per day for 10 days. Most patients improve rapidly and become afebrile in about 3 days. The 10-day course of streptomycin is recommended to prevent relapses, because viable bacteria have been isolated from buboes of patients with plague during convalescence.

For patients allergic to streptomycin or in whom an oral drug is strongly preferred, tetracycline is a satisfactory alternative. It is given orally in a dose of 2–4 g day^{-1} in four divided doses for 10 days. Tetracycline is contraindicated in children younger than 7 years of age and in pregnant women, because it stains developing teeth.

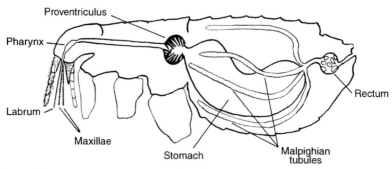

Fig. 3. Diagrammatic representation of the alimentary canal of an adult flea showing the backwardly pointing spines of the proventriculus (from M.W. Service (2000), *Medical Entomology for Students*, Cambridge University Press, Cambridge).

For patients with meningitis, who require a drug with a good penetration into the cerebrospinal fluid, and for patients with profound hypotension, in whom an intramuscular injection may be poorly absorbed, chloramphenicol should be given intravenously, a loading dose of 25 mg kg^{-1} of body weight, followed by 60 mg kg^{-1} of body weight per day in four divided doses. After clinical improvement, chloramphenicol should be continued orally to complete a total course of 10 days.

Other antimicrobial drugs have been used in plague or in experimental animal infections with varying success. These include sulfonamides, trimethoprim-sulfamethoxazole, kanamycin, gentamicin, ampicillin, cephalosporins and fluoroquinolones. These drugs, however, are either less effective than streptomycin or have not been subjected to adequate clinical studies and therefore should not be chosen. An isolate from a 16-year-old boy in Madagascar in 1995 was resistant to streptomycin, tetracycline, chloramphenicol and sulfonamide but was susceptible to trimethoprim-sulfamethoxazole. He recovered after receiving trimethoprim-sulfamethoxazole. Other than this case, antibiotic resistance in *Y. pestis* from humans has never been reported, nor has resistance emerged during antibiotic therapy. The antibiotics streptomycin, tetracycline and chloramphenicol given alone are clinically effective, and relapses are exceedingly rare. Therefore, there is no rationale for using multiple antibiotics to treat plague.

Most patients are febrile, with constitutional symptoms including nausea and vomiting. Hypotension and dehydration are common. Therefore, intravenous 0.9% saline solution should be given to most patients for the first few days of the illness or until improvement occurs. Patients in shock will require additional quantities of fluid, with haemodynamic monitoring and the judicious use of adrenaline or dopamine.

The buboes usually recede without local therapy. Occasionally, however, they may enlarge or become fluctuant during the first week of treatment, requiring incision and drainage. The aspirated fluid should be cultured for evidence of superinfection with other bacteria, but this material is usually sterile.

Control

Prevention

Plague is an internationally quarantinable disease. Accordingly, all patients with suspected plague should be reported to the appropriate health department and to the World Health Organization. Patients with uncomplicated infections who are promptly treated present no health hazards to other people. Those with coughs or other signs of pneumonia must be placed in strict respiratory isolation for at least 48 h after starting antimicrobial therapy or until the sputum culture is negative. The bubo aspirate and blood must be handled with gloves and with care to avoid aerosolization of these infected fluids. Laboratory workers who process the cultures should be alerted to take precautions; however, standard bacteriological techniques that safegaurd against skin contact with and aerosolization of cultures should be adequate.

Vaccines have been developed and used but are not currently available. People living in endemic areas should provide themselves with as much personal protection against rodents and fleas as possible, including living in rat-proof houses, wearing shoes and garments to cover the legs and dusting houses with insecticide. For persons who report close contact with a coughing patient suspected of having pneumonic plague, prophylaxis with oral doxycycline or trimethoprim-sulfamethoxazole is advised.

Flea control

Control of plague should start with killing the vector fleas, not with destroying the reservoir hosts, such as rats and other rodents. During plague outbreaks there should be extensive and well-organized operations. Because of widespread resistance to DDT in *X. cheopis* and, to a lesser extent, in *X. astia* and *X. brasiliensis* this insecticide is not usually used. Instead, insecticides such as the organophosphates, e.g. malathion, fenitrothion or pirimiphos-methyl, carbamates, e.g. carbaryl or bendiocarb, or pyrethroids, e.g. permethrin, deltamethrin or lambdacyhalothrin, are used. Powders of these can be liberally applied to the floors of houses and other buildings where there are known or suspected to be rat fleas and to runways of commensal rodents and blown into their burrows. Insecticidal fogs or aerosols have sometimes been used to fumigate premises harbouring fleas. Alternatively, food baits can be placed into 7–10 cm diameter tubes (plastic, bamboo) and insecticidal powders placed at both openings.

Fleas of wild rodents are not easy to control because of difficulties in locating their runways or burrows. Sometimes aerial insecticidal applications have been made and baits in tubes employed, but usually there is little attempt to control these fleas.

Rodent control

Rodents should not be destroyed before their fleas are killed, because fleas from dead rodents will bite other mammals, including people, and this may result in increased transmission. Rodenticides are usually incorporated into either solid or liquid baits. Basically there are two types of rodenticides: the fast-acting one-dose ones, such as zinc phosphide and calciferol, which are very toxic and are now not commonly used, and the slow-acting multidose ones, most of which are the anticoagulants. The best known is warfarin and other so-called first-generation anticoagulants, include fumarin, coumatetralyl and pindone. Second-generation anticoagulants include difenacoum, bromadiolone and flocoumafen. Anticoagulants are readily ingested by rodents when incorporated into baits and accidental poisoning to humans and to other animals does not occur, but rats developing resistance can be a problem. The fast-acting one-dose rodenticides are very to moderately toxic to humans and can kill a broad spectrum of non-target animals, and rodents often refuse poisoned baits, but they can be useful where there is resistance to the anticoagulants.

Selected bibliography

Buckle, A.P. and Smith, R.H. (eds) (1994) *Rodent Pests and their Control.* CAB International, Wallingford, UK, 405 pp.

Butler, T. (1994) *Yersinia* infections: centennial of the discovery of the plague bacillus. *Clinical Infectious Disease* 19, 655–663.

Galimand, M., Guiyoule, A., Gerbaud, G., Rasoamanana, B., Chanteau, S., Carniel, E. and Courvalin, P. (1997) Multidrug resistance in *Yersinia pestis* mediated by a transferable plasmid. *New England Journal of Medicine* 337, 677–680.

Ratsitorahina, M., Chanteau, S., Rahalison, L., Ratsifasomanana, L. and Boisier, P. (2000) Epidemiological and diagnostic aspects of the outbreak of pneumonic plague in Madagascar. *The Lancet* 355, 111–113.

Russell, P., Eley, S.M., Bell, D.L., Manchee, R.J. and Titball, R.W. (1996) Doxycycline or ciprofloxacin prophylaxis and therapy against experimental *Yersinia pestis* infection in mice. *Journal of Antimicrobial Chemotherapy* 37, 769–774.

World Health Organization (1999) *Plague Manual. Epidemiology, Distribution, Surveillance and Control.* WHO/CDS/CSR/EDC/99.2, WHO, Geneva, 172 pp.

Plasmodium species *see* **Malaria.**

Pongola viruses *see* **Bwamba and Pongola viruses.**

Powassan encephalitis

Donald M. McLean

Encephalitis induced in humans by the tick-borne arbovirus, Powassan (POW) virus (family Flaviviridae) in the genus *Flavivirus*.

Since the initial isolation of POW virus from the brain of a child resident of Powassan, Ontario, Canada (46°N, 79° 30'W), who died with acute encephalitis in September 1958, a total of 27 cases of Powassan encephalitis have been reported in North America through 1998, of whom seven died and 11 of 20 survivors developed severe sequelae.

Distribution

All symptomatic infections with POW virus have arisen in eastern North America. Reported cases have contracted their infections while residing in or visiting forested terrain, interspersed with areas cleared for agricultural pursuits, throughout the south-eastern mixed forest vegetation zone (Fig. 1). This extends from Sault St Marie along the north shore of Lake Huron, eastwards across the Canadian Province of Ontario along the Ottawa River Valley, which joins the St Lawrence River Valley near Montreal (Province of Quebec), and extends further across the Provinces of New Brunswick and Nova Scotia to the Atlantic seaboard. Comparable forested terrain interspersed with farms extends south and east of Lake Ontario and the St Lawrence Valley in the USA, especially across upstate New York from the adjacent state of Pennsylvania eastwards to the adjoining state of Massachusetts.

Although POW virus has been isolated in western USA from *Dermacentor andersoni* ticks collected in the state of Colorado and from *Ixodes spinipalpus* collected in South Dakota, no human cases have been identified in those states, or along the Pacific coast of Canada and USA, where *Ixodes pacificus* is prevalent. Furthermore, during 1972, POW virus was isolated from *Haemaphysalis neumanni* ticks collected in the

Primor'ye region of Siberia, but in the absence of human cases.

In Canada, seven human cases contracted infection in Ontario and four additional cases became infected in Quebec, New Brunswick and Nova Scotia. Neutralizing antibodies to POW virus have been detected in three of 71 (4%) human residents of localities within a 50 km radius of the index case's home in northern Ontario, indicating subclinical infection in that region, but in only 11 of 1008 (1%) residents throughout Ontario, New Brunswick and Nova Scotia, thus demonstrating the focal distribution of POW virus infection.

In the USA, ten humans became infected in upstate New York, and six additional cases arose in adjacent states of Massachusetts and New Jersey. The low incidence of Powassan encephalitis (average 0.4 cases year^{-1}) contrasts with the average of 109 laboratory-confirmed cases of arbovirus encephalitis per year from 1996 through 1999, 80% of which were due to the California serogroup viruses, principally La Crosse serotype (see entry).

Powassan infections occur typically during warmer months, mainly between May and October, when ticks are active. Incubation periods range from 8 to 34 days. Due to the small size of ticks, bites are often overlooked; only seven cases reported tick bites.

Virus

Powassan virus is a tick-borne member of the arbovirus serogroup B, family Flaviviridae. Virions are enveloped icosahedra containing single-stranded positive-sense RNA, molecular weight $4.2-4.4 \times 10^6$, with an average diameter of 45 nm (Fig. 2). Powassan virus multiplies readily after intracerebral injection of suckling mice aged 1–3 days and weaned mice aged 3–4 weeks, inducing fatal encephalitis after 5–7 days' incubation. Although hamsters develop viraemia 1–4 days after subcutaneous

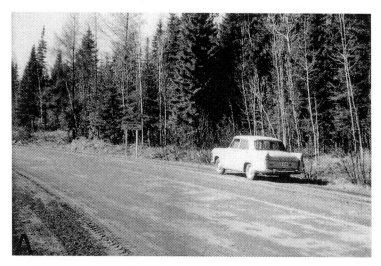

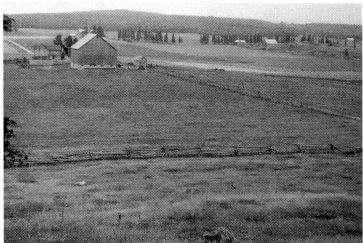

Fig. 1. Natural foci of Powassan virus infection near Powassan, Ontario, Canada (46°N, 79° 30'W). Upper: virus isolation from *Ixodes marxi* ticks and squirrel blood. Lower: farm of index case. (From McLean, D.M. (1989) *Virological Infections*. Courtesy of Charles C. Thomas, Springfield, Illinois.)

injection and subsequently antibodies are detected by haemagglutination inhibition (HI) and neutralization tests (NT), they show no signs of illness. Rabbits and guinea-pigs develop antibodies without overt illness. Woodchuck (*Marmota monax*) also develop viraemia, followed by antibody, after subcutaneous injection, without detectable illness. Propagation of POW virus has been demonstrated in primary monolayer tissue cultures of pig kidney cells, inducing cytopathic effects after 5 days' incubation and also in continuous cultures of dolphin kidney cells.

Haemagglutination of erythrocytes of geese and newly hatched chicks by POW virus occurs optimally at pH 6.4 and 22°C. Haemagglutinin is prepared by extraction of POW virus-infected suckling mouse brains with sucrose and acetone. This preparation also serves as antigen in complement fixation (CF) and enzyme-linked immunosorbent assay (ELISA) tests for POW antibodies in human and animal sera. Before conducting HI tests, it is important to remove non-specific inhibitors of haemagglutination from human and animal sera by extraction with acetone.

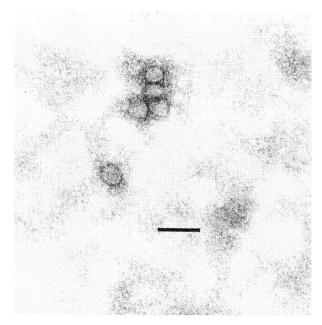

Fig. 2. Powassan virus, prototype LB strain (magnification × 120, 120). Negatively stained preparation after three passages in suckling mouse brain. (Reproduced with permission from McLean, D.M. and Wong, K.K. (1984) *Same-Day Diagnosis of Human Virus Infections.* Courtesy of CRC Press, Boca Raton, Florida.)

Within the Flaviviridae, POW virus shows closer antigenic relationships with the following serotypes within the tick-borne complex of serogroup B, louping ill (see entry) from Scotland, Czech topotype HYPR and other Central European tick-borne viruses, Russian spring–summer encephalitis virus (Sofjin) from Siberia, Langat (see entries) from Malaysia and Kyasanur Forest disease (see entry) from India, than with mosquito-borne serotypes, such as yellow fever and St Louis encephalitis viruses (see entries on both). Recent genotypic analyses have amply confirmed these earlier results of antigenic analyses.

Clinical symptoms

After 1–3 days of fever, headache and drowsiness, sometimes accompanied by slurred speech or possibly limb tremors, signs of encephalitis develop. These include increased temperature, ataxia, spastic hemiplegia, neck stiffness, convulsions and progressive loss of consciousness. Cerebrospinal fluid (CSF) typically shows leucocytosis, with total cell count exceeding 100×10^6 cells l^{-1}, with >60% lymphocytes, and normal levels of glucose and protein. Electroencephalograms show moderate to severe diffuse abnormalities, such as slowing and disorganization. Computerized tomography (CT) and magnetic resonance imaging (MRI) scans reveal no abnormalities. Clinical deterioration may continue for several days, terminating in death in 25% of patients, or slow recovery may occur over many weeks, with severe sequelae, such as hemiplegia, memory deficit or muscle weakness of upper or lower limbs, affecting over 50% of non-fatal cases.

Diagnosis

Encephalitis afflicting a patient who has resided in or visited forested areas of eastern North America during May through October, when ticks are active, raises the possibility of POW virus infection, for which the following tests should be performed.

Serology

Serum collected within 1 week after onset may contain immunoglobulin M (IgM) antibodies to POW virus by the IgM capture ELISA test. Serum collected during subsequent weeks will reveal POW antibodies by HI, NT and IgG ELISA tests; CF antibodies appear 3–4 weeks after onset and become undetectable after 6–12 months. Antibodies should be detected in CSF by IgM ELISA tests within a few days after onset.

Virus identification

In fatal cases, histological examination of brain stained by haematoxylin and eosin reveals features typical of acute encephalitis: perivascular cuffing of cerebral blood-vessels with lymphocytes; and foci of necrotic neurons surrounded by mono-nuclear cells (Fig. 3).

Inoculation of suckling mice intra-cerebrally with brain suspended in saline containing bovalbumin or bovine serum induces fatal encephalitis 5–7 days later, and POW virus is identified by NT in mice, following presumptive identification of POW antigen in brain by HI tests. Recent isolates of POW virus from *Ixodes dammini* (now named *Ixodes scapularis*) ticks in suckling mouse brains have also been identified rapidly by reverse transcriptase–polymerase chain reaction (RT-PCR) and direct sequencing of RNA.

Following identification of the flavivirus West Nile (WN) virus (see entry) in brains of six fatal human cases during an outbreak of encephalitis in New York City and adjacent counties during August and September 1999, by amplification of WN virus-specific gene sequences by RT-PCR or RNA extracted from autopsy specimens within 2–3 days after receipt of specimens, this technique has now become the procedure of choice for prompt diagnosis of fatal cases of Powassan encephalitis, to be followed up with isolation of virus using suckling mice.

Transmission

Powassan virus is maintained in nature by a cycle involving ixodid (hard) ticks (primarily *Ixodes cookei* but also *Ixodes marxi* and *I. scapularis*) as vectors, forest mammals (especially Groundhogs (*M. monax*) but also American red squirrels (*Tamiasciurus hudsonicus*) and White-footed mice (*Peromyscus leucopus*) as reservoir hosts, with humans and other mammals becoming infected tangentially to this cycle as illustrated on the facing page.

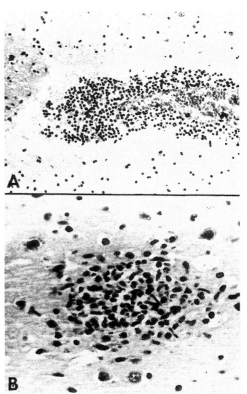

Fig. 3. Powassan virus: sections through cerebral tissue of the index case to show: A, perivascular cuffing of blood-vessels; B, foci of inflammatory cells. H+E stain (× 100). (From Powassan virus: isolation of virus from a fatal case of encephalitis, *Canadian Medical Association Journal* (1959) 80, pp. 708–711. Reprinted with permission of the publisher and of Lippincott Williams & Wilkins, Pennsylvania.)

The principal tick vector species in Ontario is *I. cookei*. The virus isolation rate was 6.6% among 273 pools of ticks removed from groundhogs between May and August in each of the summers of 1964, 1965 and 1966. Tick pools, containing one to 15 ticks each (average 2.5), comprised all the ticks removed from one mammal. Virus titre per pool ranged from 2.5 to 6.0 $\log_{10}$ tissue culture infective dose $(TCID_{50})$ ml^{-1} when tested in pig kidney tissue cultures.

Isolation of POW virus from 12% of eight pools of *I. marxi* ticks collected from Red squirrels during August to October 1962 demonstrated the vector role of this tick species. In Massachusetts, POW virus has been isolated from two pools of *I. scapularis* ticks. Virus transmission to mammals has been demonstrated in the laboratory by all stages of *I. scapularis*, which were infected by feeding on viraemic hamsters. Virus was transferred trans-stadially from larva to nymph and from nymph to adult, plus transovarially to the next tick generation. Although not associated with human POW virus infections to date, *D. andersoni* ticks have become infected as larvae and nymphs by feeding on viraemic rabbits or hamsters, virus has been transferred trans-stadially through each tick stage and both nymphs and adults have transmitted POW virus infection by biting hamsters and rabbits.

The main reservoir species in Ontario is the Groundhog (*Marmota monax*), as shown by the isolation of POW virus from the blood of two Groundhogs collected in May 1964, at titres of 1.7–2.2 $\log_{10}$ $TCID_{50}$ ml^{-1}, and detection of NT antibody in sera from 44% of 993 Groundhogs collected during the summers of 1964, 1965 and 1966, with antibody prevalence increasing from 22% of 225 born in the current year through 30% of 190 juveniles to 57% of 578 adults. This clearly demonstrates their important role as reservoir hosts. *Ixodes cookei* were found feeding on 273 (27%) of these Groundhogs.

Groundhogs are distributed widely throughout New York State and adjoining states. High POW antibody rates signifies their importance as reservoir hosts. They are among 17 mammalian species, including White-footed mice (*Peromyscus leucopus*), in which POW antibodies have been detected. Following subcutaneous injection of juvenile Groundhogs, viraemia was detected 4 days later at titres

sufficient to infect *I. scapularis* ticks, and POW antibodies were detected subsequently.

In Ontario, the Red squirrel (*Tamiasciurus hudsonicus*) serves as an additional reservoir host. During October 1962, POW virus was isolated from the blood of one squirrel among 23 (4%) collected during summer and NT antibodies were detected in three sera from other squirrels.

In Massachusetts, the White-footed mouse has been infected by subcutaneous injection with POW virus, which suggests that it may serve as a reservoir host for *I. scapularis* ticks, whose immature stages feed readily on it.

Treatment
Good supportive nursing care is required to maintain vital functions, including anticonvulsant medication and mechanical ventilation of lungs, where necessary. However, no antiviral medication is currently available.

Preventive measures
Preventive measures should be followed routinely by all visitors and residents within rural forests of eastern Canada and the USA throughout the months of tick activity, May through October. These include clothing that fully covers the trunk and limbs, placing trousers inside socks and always wearing shoes, together with daily or more frequent examination of all skin surfaces. Ticks should be removed promptly, before embedding of their hypostomes. Great care is needed to detect and remove *I. scapularis*, due to their small size; regretfully these are often overlooked until skin swelling and erythema around the

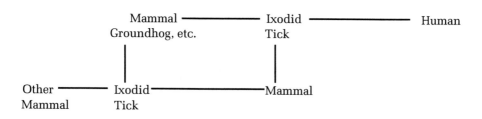

embedded hypostomes becomes obvious. Repellents, such as diethyltoluamide (DEET), are usually ineffective and are not recommended.

Selected bibliography

Chernesky, M.A. and McLean, D.M. (1969) Localization of Powassan virus in *Dermacentor andersoni* ticks by immunofluorescence. *Canadian Journal of Microbiology* 15, 1399–1408.

Costero, A. and Grayson, M.A. (1996) Experimental transmission of Powassan virus (*Flaviviridae*) by *Ixodes scapularis* ticks (Acari: Ixodidae). *American Journal of Tropical Medicine and Hygiene* 53, 536–546.

Deibel, R., Srihongse, S. and Woodall, J.P. (1979) Arboviruses in New York State: an attempt to determine the role of arboviruses in patients with viral encephalitis and meningitis. *American Journal of Tropical Medicine and Hygiene* 28, 577–582.

Gholam, B.I.A., Puska, S. and Provias, J.P. (1999) Powassan encephalitis: a case report with neuropathology and literature review. *Canadian Medical Association Journal* 161, 1419–1422.

McLean, D.M. and Donohue, W.L. (1959) Powassan virus: isolation of virus from a fatal case of encephalitis. *Canadian Medical Association Journal* 80, 708–711.

McLean, D.M. and Larke, R.P.B. (1963) Powassan and Silverwater viruses: ecology of two Ontario arboviruses. *Canadian Medical Association Journal* 88, 182–185.

McLean, D.M., Cobb, C., Gooderham, S.E., Smart, C.A., Wilson, A.G. and Wilson, W.E. (1967) Powassan virus: persistence of virus activity during 1966. *Canadian Medical Association Journal* 96, 660–664.

Telford, S.R., Armstrong, P.M., Katavalos, P. and Foppa, I. (1996) Isolation of a Powassan-like virus from the deer tick *Ixodes dammini*. *American Journal of Tropical Medicine and Hygiene* 55, 139 (abstract no. 122).

US Public Health Service (1999) Update: West Nile virus encephalitis – New York 1999. *Morbidity and Mortality Weekly Report* 48, 944–946.

Protozoa

M.W. Service

The Protozoa comprise more than 200,000 described species of which about 10,000 are parasitic. Some parasitologists use the term Protista, not Protozoa, but this seems to be declining in popularity. They are now usually treated as a kingdom in zoological classification, with the major taxonomic divisions comprising phyla, classes and orders, but their precise classification remains contentious. Protozoa can be regarded as unicellular organisms, rarely containing chlorophyll, consisting basically of a mass of cytoplasm, mitochondria, Golgi bodies and peroxisome. They have one or more nuclei, there is a distinct nuclear membrane and chromosomes are present. Inside the nucleus, usually in a central position, is either a conspicuous or minute mass, known as the karyosome. Protozoa are very small (mostly 1–150 µm), and are possibly the most primitive organisms.

All protozoans reproduce asexually by simple or multiple division, or by budding, and most also reproduce sexually. Some species, such as those of the genus *Plasmodium*, exhibit both asexual and sexual reproduction.

As eukaryotes, Protozoa differ from bacteria in having distinct membrane-bound nuclei and often having complicated life cycles, such as with malarial parasites.

The infections discussed in this encyclopedia are restricted to the so-called parasitic protozoa, of which there are many diverse forms. For example, some species (the flagellates) have flagella to aid their motion, whereas others lack flagella – for example, the amoebae use pseudopodia, while in others, such as sporozoans, locomotion is by 'gliding'.

The hierarchical classification of the Protozoa is complicated and in a state of flux, and therefore remains somewhat unsatisfactory. Phylogenic relationships are based on structure, physiology, biochemistry and molecular biology. Unfortunately, there is no universally recognized taxonomic classification of the Protozoa. The abbreviated scheme adopted here is somewhat of a compromise between differing systems, and places the parasitic protozoans that are vector-borne in the following taxonomic hierarchies.

Phylum: Euglenozoa (The taxa below were previously placed in the Mastigophora, although this is not synonomous with the Euglenozoa).
Class: Kinetoplastidea.
Order: Trypanosomatida. Species in this order have one or two flagella and a single large mitochondrion, with the mitochondrial DNA concentrated in a relatively small body, called the kinetoplast, close to the base of the flagellum.
Genera: Species of two genera, *Leishmania* and *Trypanosoma*, are of economic importance.

1. *Leishmania* species are characterized by intracellular amastigotes in mammalian hosts and extracellular promastigotes in the gut of phlebotomine sand-flies.
2. *Trypanosoma* species are found in a wide variety of vertebrate species, including fish. Nearly all species have trypanomastigote and epimastigote stages in their life cycle.

(See entries on Leishmaniasis, Chagas disease and Human and Animal trypanosomiasis.)

Phylum: Apicomplexa (or Sporozoa).
Class: Haematozoea.
Order: Haemosporida. Members of this order undergo asexual reproduction (schizogony) in vertebrate erythrocytes and sexual reproduction in the blood-sucking insect vectors.

1. *Plasmodium*: schizogony occurs in the host's blood, with the gametocytes developing in the erythrocytes; the end-product of the digestion of haemoglobin is the dark pigment haemozoin. (See entries on Malaria, human and Malaria, avian.)
2. *Leucocytozoon*: schizogony occurs in the tissues; only the gametocytes are found in the peripheral circulation, in both leucocytes and erythrocytes, but no haemozoin is produced. (See entry on Leucocytozonosis.)
3. *Haemoproteus*: schizogony occurs in the tissues, gametocytes develop in mature erythrocytes and haemozoin is produced. (See entry on Haemoproteosis.)

Order: Piroplasmida.
Genera: Species in both the genera *Babesia* and *Theileria* have an intracellular stage in the erythrocytes that is pear-shaped, which is called a piroplasm.

1. *Babesia* species invade the erythrocytes and the haemoglobin is digested without the production of haemozoin. Schizogony occurs in the erythrocytes or lymphocytes, depending on the *Babesia* species. (See entry on Babesiosis.)
2. *Theileria* species have large schizonts called macroschizonts or 'Koch's blue bodies' are produced in the lymphocytes of the host and cause them to divide and produce infected daughter cells. (See entry on Theilerioses.)

Selected bibliography
Baker, J.R. (1982) *The Biology of Parasitic Protozoa*. Studies in Biology No. 136, Edward Arnold, London, 60 pp.
Cavalier-Smith, T. (1993) Kingdom protozoa and its 18 phyla. *Microbiological Reviews* 57, 953–994.
Corliss, J.O. (1994) An interim utilitarian ('user-friendly') hierarchical classification and characterization of the protists. *Acta Protozoologica* 33, 1–51.
Cox, F.E.G. (1998) Classification of the parasitic protozoa. In: Cox, F.E.G., Kreier, J.P. and Wakefield, D. (eds) *Topley and Wilson's Microbiology and Microbial Infections*, Vol. 5, *Parasitology*, 9th edn. Arnold, London, pp. 141–155.
Gilles, H.M. (ed.) (1999) *Protozoal Diseases*. Arnold, London, 707 pp.

Kreier, J.P. and Baker, J.R. (eds) (1991–1993) *Parasitic Protozoa*, 2nd edn. Vol. 1 (1991), 277 pp.; Vol. 2 (1992), 323 pp.; Vol. 3 (1993), 333 pp.; Kreier, J.P. (ed.) (1993–1995), Vol. 4 (1993), 323 pp.; Vol. 5 (1993), 343 pp.; Vol. 6 (1993), 385 pp.; Vol. 7 (1994), 314 pp.; Vol. 8 (1994), 328 pp.; Vol. 9 (1994), 216 pp.; Vol. 10 (1995), 430 pp. Academic Press, New York.

Levine, N.D. (1973) *Protozoan Parasites of Domestic Animals and of Man*, 2nd edn. Burgess, Minneapolis, Minnesota, 406 pp.

Q fever

Todd Hatchette and Thomas J. Marrie

Distribution

Q fever (query fever) is a zoonosis with worldwide distribution. New Zealand is the only country free of the disease. Due to its non-specific presentation, it often goes unrecognized, so the true prevalence of disease in unknown. E.H. Derrick first described Q fever in 1937 while investigating a febrile illness in abattoir workers in Australia. When he was unable to isolate a causative organism, he named the illness Q or 'query' fever. F.M. Burnet and M. Freeman subsequently isolated the causal agent, *Rickettsia burneti*, from guinea-pigs inoculated with blood and urine from Derrick's patients. At the same time G.E. Davis and H.R. Cox isolated the agent from ticks (*Dermacentor andersoni*) in the USA. The organism was renamed *Coxiella burnetii* in honour of Cox and Burnet.

Microorganism

Coxiella burnetii was initially considered to be related to *Rickettsia*. However, current phylogenetic studies suggest that it is most closely related to *Legionella*. *Coxiella burnetii* is an obligate intracellular organism that resides in acidic phagolysosomes in eukaryotic cells. The lipopolysaccharide coat has two distinct antigenic presentations or 'phases'. In nature the microorganism exists in the phase I antigenic state and is highly infectious; as little as one microorganism can induce infection in experimental systems. After numerous passages in cell or animal culture the surface of the organism undergoes a 'phase variation', where it will express a second antigenic form, called phase II, which is its less virulent form. Animals and humans generate antibody responses to both phases, although the predominant antibody response in acute infection is to phase II, whereas the predominant antibody response during chronic infections is to phase I antigen.

Clinical symptoms

Although *C. burnetii* infection can cause abortions and stillbirths, most animals have a persistent, relatively asymptomatic subclinical infection. Infection in humans is often non-specific and can be asymptomatic or manifest as a self-limiting febrile illness, pneumonia, hepatitis or overlapping clinical syndromes. The most common symptoms of acute Q fever are non-specific and include fever, fatigue, chills, myalgias, sweats and a cough. Patients often present with a severe headache, which is a clinical clue to the diagnosis. Mild elevations of liver transaminases are common. Pneumonia can be rapidly progressive or atypical or present as fever without pulmonary symptoms. Pericarditis, myocarditis and meningoencephalitis are also potential manifestations of acute Q fever. Most patients have an 'uneventful' recovery; however, there is evidence that Q fever can lead to a protracted state of fatigue similar to that seen with chronic fatigue syndrome. Chronic infections, such as osteomyelitis, chronic hepatitis, endocarditis and other endovascular infections, are uncommon but well-documented sequelae of infection, particularly in patients who have underlying immunosuppression or cardiac valvular abnormalities.

Diagnosis

Due to its non-specific presentation, Q fever is often difficult to diagnose. *Coxiella burnetii* is considered a level 3 pathogen, making routine culture difficult for most laboratories. Demonstrating seroconversion to *Coxiella* antigens between acute and convalescent serum samples, in conjunction with an appropriate clinical history (exposure to parturient animals or their newborn), is the usual method of diagnosis. Complement fixation, enzyme-linked immunosorbent assay (ELISA) and immuofluorescence assays are used to make the serological diagnosis; however, the indirect immunofluorescence assay (IFA) is the current method of choice. In acute Q fever the antibody response is predominantly to phase II antigen. A titre of $\geq 1 : 800$ to phase I antigen reflects chronic disease. Polymerase chain reaction (PCR) has also been used to confirm the presence of *C. burnetii* in serum, tissue and milk samples.

Transmission

This microorganism has been found in many wild and domesticated animals, including dogs, wild hares (*Lepus* species), Moose (*Alces alces*), Raccoons (*Procyon lotor*), birds, foxes (*Vulpes* species) and deer (Cervidae). In addition, it has been isolated from arthropods, including lice, mites, flies and over 40 species of ticks. The most common reservoir hosts for infection in humans are cats and domesticated farm animals, such as cattle, goats and sheep. *Coxiella* localizes in the uterus and mammary glands of infected animals and is shed in the urine, faeces and milk. It is found in particularly high concentrations in the placenta and amniotic fluid (10^9 organisms g^{-1} of placental tissue), which have consistently been shown to be risk factors for human disease. In Nova Scotia, Canada, many cases of Q fever pneumonia are acquired through exposure to infected parturient cats. The organism is highly resistant to desiccation and can survive in soil for up to 150 days. Inhalation of aerosolized microorganisms is felt to be the most important route of infection. Direct exposure to infected animals, as well as indirect exposures to dusts, manure, hay and clothing contaminated with *C. burnetii*, has been implicated as causing disease in humans. Ingestion of raw milk products has also been suggested as a route of infection and experimental evidence suggests that sexual transmission can occur in mice. Human-to-human transmission can occur but is extremely rare. The only documented cases include direct transmission from a parturient woman to her obstetrician (at the time of delivery) and from a cadaver to the pathologist during autopsy. Infection

can also occur from transfusion of infected blood. Although the microorganism has been isolated from many species of ticks, tick-borne transmission is not a common route of infection in humans. However, there have been a few instances where crushing infected ticks between the fingers resulted in infection. Arthropod-borne disease seems to be more important in maintaining *C. burnetii* infection in wild animals and transmitting the disease to the domestic animal population.

Treatment
Acute Q fever

In the majority of cases, Q fever will resolve spontaneously in approximately 15 days. Patients who present with severe symptoms suspicious for Q fever should be treated empirically, as serological diagnosis is delayed. Tetracycline, doxycycline or quinolone compounds have all been used to treat acute Q fever. At present, doxycycline (100 mg twice daily) for 15–21 days is the treatment of choice. Quinolones can penetrate the blood–brain barrier and should be considered for Q fever meningoencephalitis.

Chronic Q fever

While there is some variation, depending on technique, an IFA titre of $\geq 1/800$ to phase I antigen would signify chronic Q fever. Chronic Q fever endocarditis is a serious complication, with mortality rates of up to 65%. Although doxycycline is the mainstay of therapy in acute Q fever, it does not appear to cure chronic disease. Combination therapy with rifampicin (rifampin) and doxycycline has been used with varying results. Currently the antibiotic regime of choice is a combination of rifampicin (rifampin) and ciprofloxacin. In patients with haemodynamic compromise, valve replacement is often necessary; however, concurrent antibiotic treatment is required to prevent reoccurrence of disease. Response to therapy can be followed by monitoring the antibody titre to the phase I antigen every 3 months, with a phase I titre of <1/200 indicating cure. The duration of treatment is unknown as *C. burnetii* is very difficult to eradicate and can be isolated in patients despite more than 1 year of antibiotic therapy. Patients often require 3 years of therapy to achieve cure. Some authorities recommend continuing therapy indefinitely.

Control

Once an animal infected with *C. burnetii* is introduced into a herd of livestock, the infection quickly spreads throughout the remaining seronegative animals. Outbreaks of Q fever in research institutions have led to a series of recommendations to control and prevent *C. burnetii* infection in the research setting, including using only *C. burnetii* seronegative animals in research, restricting access to animals, vaccination of seronegative animals, using protective clothing and masks while working with the animals, especially pregnant animals, proper decontamination of contaminated surfaces with formalin or bleach solutions and proper disposal of waste by incineration. Recommendations for the control of *C. burnetii* among dairy animals (cows and goats) are necessary but have not been enacted in any country to date. A formalin-inactivated vaccine is available and is used by abattoir workers in Australia with success.

Selected bibliography

Marrie, T.J. and Raoult, D. (1997) Q fever – a review and issues for the next century. *International Journal of Antimicrobial Agents* 8, 145–161.

Raoult, D. (1993) Treatment of Q fever. *Antimicrobial Agents and Chemotherapy* 37, 1733–1736.

Raoult, D. and Marrie, T. (1995) Q fever. *Clinical and Infectious Diseases* 20, 489–496.

Queensland tick typhus *see* **Tick-borne typhuses.**

Rabbit fever *see* **Theilerioses,** *and* **Tularaemia.**

Rabbit haemorrhagic disease

Brian D. Cooke

Distribution

Rabbit haemorrhagic disease is an acute and often fatal disease of the European rabbit, *Oryctolagus cuniculus*. First described in domestic rabbits in China in 1984, it subsequently spread, mainly through trade in rabbit products, to over 40 countries throughout the world. Mortality in excess of 80% was commonly recorded among domestic rabbits until vaccines were developed.

Organism and symptoms

The causative agent, rabbit haemorrhagic disease (RHD) virus, is a calicivirus, which, along with European brown hare syndrome (EBHS) virus, belongs to the genus *Lagovirus* within the family Caliciviridae. Rabbit haemorrhagic disease virus targets the liver, causing fulminating hepatitis, associated with massive cell death. Rabbits usually die 48–72 h after infection. Just before death, the liver, spleen and blood contain large amounts of virus.

Clinical signs and diagnosis

No significant clinical signs are seen in peracute cases of rabbit haemorrhagic disease, but in acute cases rabbits appear quiet; wild rabbits may not move even when approached. Body temperature and respiration rate show increases above normal. Death usually follows within 12 h of the onset of clinical signs. Blood and foamy discharge are occasionally seen from the nostrils of infected animals.

Virus-capture enzyme-linked immunosorbent assays (ELISAs) have been developed to detect RHD virus in tissue samples. Usually tissues such as liver or spleen are used for these analyses because they contain the greatest concentrations of virus.

Transmission and epidemiology

Because its spread was associated with the trade of rabbit meat and fur and the exchange of live rabbits between rabbitries, RHD virus was thought to be transmitted mainly by rabbit-to-rabbit contact and fomites. However, flies of the genus *Phormia* also transmitted in laboratory experiments. Consequently, in assessing RHD virus for use as a biological control for wild European rabbits in Australia, mechanical transmission by insects was considered in some detail. Mosquitoes, *Culex annulirostris*, rabbit fleas, *Spilopsyllus cuniculi* and *Xenopsylla cunicularis*, and bush-flies, *Musca vetustissima*, were shown to be capable of transmitting the virus. In these laboratory trials, insects were first allowed to feed on rabbits that had been infected with RHD virus 16–22 h earlier and then transferred immediately to susceptible rabbits. Viraemia was clearly sufficiently high for biting insects to transmit RHD virus and sufficient virus was present in secretions around the eyes, nose and mouth of rabbits for bush-flies to become infective.

Subsequently, in March 1995, when trials to assess the efficacy of RHD virus were begun on Wardang Island, 4 km off the coast of South Australia, elaborate precautions were taken to minimize the risk of spread of the virus by insects. These included the control of mosquito larvae in swamps using *Bacillus thuringensis* subsp. *israelensis*, the spraying of rabbit burrows in experimental sites with a pyrethroid insecticide (deltamethrin) and the trapping of flies. Nevertheless, in mid-October 1995, the virus escaped to the Australian mainland under circumstances that further implicated insects as vectors. Warm weather followed by an intense low-pressure system apparently allowed the first spring migrations of flying insects from inland Australia to reach Wardang Island and then dispersed them over parts of mainland South Australia. Rabbit haemorrhagic disease was initially seen where rabbits were most abundant but was later confirmed over wider areas (Fig. 1).

Insect vectors were also implicated in the subsequent spread of virus across southern Australia. The progressive appearance of new rabbit haemorrhagic disease outbreaks showed that the virus spread at over 400 km month[-1]. Such high rates are consistent with insect transmission; they cannot be explained in terms of rabbit-to-rabbit spread, given that the disease takes 2 days to incubate and that rabbits have home ranges limited to a few hectares. Furthermore, RHD virus survives best at low temperature and is rapidly destroyed at high temperature. On this basis, virus persistence and spread should occur most rapidly in the Australian winter. Nevertheless, relatively high rates of disease spread in autumn and spring may mean that high insect activity offsets lower virus survival. The low rate of spread of

RHD virus in summer probably reflects lower abundance and limited movements of insects during hot weather, as well as poor virus survival.

Trapping of insects as the virus first spread across Australia quickly revealed that many insects readily became contaminated with RHD virus. Reverse-transcription polymerase chain reaction (RT-PCR) showed that over ten species of flies, including bush-flies (*M. vetustissima*) and blow-flies (Calliphoridae), were involved. Additionally, viable virus was confirmed in wild-caught rabbit fleas, *S. cuniculi*, by both RT-PCR and by allowing them to feed on susceptible rabbits. Likewise, homogenates of RT-PCR-positive mosquitoes, *Ochlerotatus[1] postspiraculosus*, inoculated into rabbits contained viable virus.

Most investigations of insect transmission concentrated on large blow-flies. These flies are closely associated with rabbits, often entering and sheltering in rabbit burrows. Rabbits that die from RHD virus are prime sites for flies to deposit eggs. Virus has not been detected in fly puparia, despite

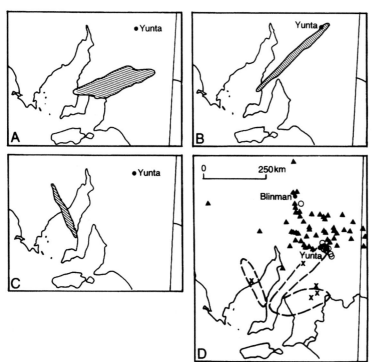

Fig. 1. Maps of part of South Australia showing the surface wind pattern from Wardang Island on (A) 12 October 1995, (B) 13 October 1995 and (C) 14 October 1995, during periods when temperatures were suitable for the flight of bush-flies. Map D shows where RHD virus-infected rabbits were found in October (open circles), November (triangles) and December (crosses) 1995. (From Fenner and Fantini (1999) *Biological Control of Vertebrate Pests. The History of Myxomatosis – an Experiment in Evolution.* CAB International, Wallingford, UK, with permission.)

virus having been ingested by the larvae, so vertical transfer of virus to adult flies is unlikely. Rather, adult flies become contaminated as a result of depositing eggs on or feeding on cadavers. In flies experimentally fed on liver from infected rabbits, virus is detectable within the gut for up to 9 days. However, virus on the feet of the flies persists for less than 12 h. Most importantly, the regurgitated food and faeces of flies contain viable virus. Faeces from a single fly contain an estimated 2–3 lethal dose (LD_{50}) of RHD virus and cause infection when fed to susceptible rabbits. Presumably, blow-flies transmit virus in the field by feeding on cadavers and then defecating on pasture vegetation that is subsequently eaten by rabbits. Pasture harvested from rabbit haemorrhagic disease outbreak sites in Australia contains sufficient RHD virus to infect susceptible domestic rabbits. Outbreaks of rabbit haemorrhagic disease in domestic rabbits in Europe are also linked to the practice of harvesting forage from fields.

Despite good evidence that insects are involved in the transmission and rapid spread of RHD virus, this may not be the most common means of spread. Within social groups of rabbits, contact transmission of virus in urine and faeces (used as social signals for marking territory) or direct contact with cadavers is also very important. Antibody responses of rabbits to infection and reinfection in the field usually involve a strong immunoglobulin A (IgA) component, typical of a mucosal immune response. This implies infection by the oral route and involvement of gut-associated lymphoid tissues. Although this does not rule out flies as common vectors, it indicates that the intradermal route of infection, e.g. by mosquito- or flea-bite, may be relatively unimportant.

Insect transmission of RHD virus is clearly important in the long-distance movement of the virus in natural rabbit populations in Australia. Its importance in other countries has not been confirmed, although this may depend on the suitability of the climate and the range of insects present. However, insect transmission should be regarded as a risk factor in the potential transfer of RHD virus from wild rabbit populations to domestic rabbits.

Treatment
There is no known treatment for rabbits infected with RHD virus.

Control and prevention
Killed-virus vaccines are available for immunizing pet rabbits and commercial herds against RHD virus. Revaccination every 12 months is recommended. Eradication of the disease has usually been achieved by killing stock in infected rabbitries, carefully decontaminating cages and the walls of buildings with sodium hypochlorite and reintroducing uninfected stock from a reliable source after several weeks.

Note
[1] *Ochlerotatus* was formerly a subgenus of *Aedes*.

Selected bibliography

Asgari, S., Hardy, J.R.E., Sinclair, R.G. and Cooke, B.D. (1999) Field evidence of mechanical transmission of rabbit haemorrhagic disease virus (RHDV) by flies (Diptera: Calliphoridae) among wild rabbits in Australia. *Virus Research* 54, 123–132.

Fenner, F. and Fantini, B. (1999) *Biological Control of Vertebrate Pests. The History of Myxomatosis – an Experiment in Evolution.* CAB International, Wallingford, UK, 399 pp.

Kovaliski, J. (1998) Monitoring the spread of rabbit haemorrhagic disease virus as a new biological agent for the control of European rabbits in Australia. *Journal of Wildlife Diseases* 34, 421–428.

Red bugs *see* **Mites.**

Red-eye *see* **Eye-flies.**

Redwater fever *see* **Babesiosis.**

Rickettsiae

C.A. Hart

Rickettsiae are small (0.8 μm × 0.4 μm) Gram-negative coccobacilli that are obligate intracellular bacterial pathogens. They are members of the family *Rickettsiaceae* in the order *Rickettsiales* (see entry). There is a large number of species, but they are usually grouped into those causing typhus and those causing spotted fevers. *Rickettsia prowazekii* causes epidemic typhus (see entry), also called louse-borne typhus, but chronic carriage following a primary infection can recrudesce (Brill–Zinsser disease). *Rickettsia typhi* causes endemic typhus (see entry), sometimes called murine or 'shop' typhus, which is transmitted by the rat flea (*Xenopsylla cheopis*). Most of the spotted fevers are transmitted by ticks, the major exception being rickettsialpox (*R. akari*) (see entry), which is transmitted by a mite (*Allodermanyssus sanguineus*). The spotted fevers tend to be geographically limited (see Tick-borne typhuses). *Rickettsia rickettsii*, which causes Rocky Mountain spotted fever (see entry) or Brazilian fever, is found in North and South America, Mediterranean spotted fever (*R. conorii*) or fièvre boutonneuse, is found around the Mediterranean region, Siberian tick typhus (*R. siberica*) is found in northern Asia and Japan, Japanese spotted fever (*R. japonica*) in Japan and Queensland tick typhus (*R. australis*) in Australia. Some are rare causes of human infection; these include *R. helvetica*, *R. mongolotimonae*, *R. slovaca*, *R. honei* (Flinder's Island spotted fever), *R. africae* (African tick-bite fever) and *R. felis* (California flea typhus). Others have been isolated from ticks or animals and are of unknown pathogenicity for humans. These include *R. rhipicephali*, *R. mossiliae*, *R. montana*, *R. parkeri*, *R. heilongjanji* and *R. belli*.

Selected bibliography

Cowan, G.O. (1996) Rickettsial infections. In: Cook, G.O. (ed.) *Manson's Tropical Diseases*, 20th edn. W.B. Saunders, London, pp. 798–814.

Fournier, P.-E., Gunnenberger, F., Jaulhace, B., Gastinger, G. and Raoult, D. (2000) Evidence of *Rickettsia helvetica* infections in humans, eastern France. *Emerging Infectious Diseases* 6, 389–392.

Olsen, J.G. and Anderson, B.E. (1997) Rickettsia. In: Emerson, A.M., Hawkey, P.M. and Gillespie, S.H. (eds) *Principles and Practice of Clinical Bacteriology*. John Wiley & Sons, Chichester, UK, pp. 745–763.

Walker, D.H. (ed.) (1988) *Biology of Rickettsial Diseases*, Vol. 1, 146 pp., Vol. 2, 164 pp. CRC Press, Boca Raton, Florida.

Rickettsia africae see **Tick-borne typhuses.**

Rickettsia akari see **Rickettsialpox.**

Rickettsia australis see **Tick-borne typhuses.**

Rickettsia conorii see **Tick-borne typhuses.**

Rickettsia helvetica see **Tick-borne typhuses.**

Rickettsia honei see **Tick-borne typhuses.**

Rickettsia japonica see **Tick-borne typhuses.**

Rickettsia mongolotimonae see **Tick-borne typhuses.**

Rickettsia prowazekii see **Epidemic typhus.**

Rickettsia rickettsii see **Rocky Mountain spotted fever.**

Rickettsia sibirica see **Tick-borne typhuses.**

Rickettsia slovaca see **Tick-borne typhuses.**

Rickettsia typhi see **Endemic typhus.**

Rickettsiales

C.A. Hart

The order *Rickettsiales* contains a large variety of small Gram-negative bacteria, most of which are obligate intracellular parasites. Currently there are three families (*Rickettsiaceae, Bartonellaceae* and *Anaplasmataceae*) within the order. The family *Rickettsiaceae* comprises the genera *Orientia, Rickettsia, Coxiella, Ehrlichia, Neorickettsia, Wolbachia, Cowdria* and *Rickettsiella*, although some authors include *Cowdria* species in the genus *Ehrlichia*. The family *Bartonellaceae* includes the genera *Bartonella* and *Grahamella*, and the *Anaplasmataceae* the genera *Anaplasma,* *Aegyptianella, Haemobartonella* and *Eperythrozoon*. Insect transmission occurs for *Rickettsia* and *Ehrlichia*, for some *Bartonella* and *Anaplasmataceae* and for *Orientia tsutsugamushi*.

Selected bibliography

Walker, D.H. (ed.) (1988) *Biology of Rickettsial Diseases*, Vol. 1, 146 pp., Vol. 2, 164 pp. CRC Press, Boca Raton, Florida.
Walker, D.H. and Fishbein, D.B. (1991) Epidemiology of rickettsial diseases: 4th international symposium on rickettsiae and rickettsial diseases. *European Journal of Epidemiology* 7, 237–245.

Rickettsialpox

Alan S. Boyd

Rickettsia, Coxiella and *Ehrlichia* (and formerly *Rochalimaea*) comprise the Rickettsiaceae family. One of the disease groups caused by these organisms is termed spotted fever and is probably responsible for the most morbidity worldwide of all Rickettsiaceae. Rickettsialpox is one of the spotted fevers and the only one not initiated by a tick. The disease is caused by infection with *Rickettsia akari* and is transmitted by the bite of an infected house mite, *Liponyssoides sanguineus*. Fevers, sweats, headaches and myalgia are present initially, followed in a few days by a mildly papular rash, initially, appearing centrally and then spreading acrally. An eschar is often present at the mite bite.

Distribution

Rickettsialpox was initially described in the Kew Gardens section of Queens, New York, and is most often seen in the eastern half of the USA. Other countries reporting cases include South Africa, Russia and Korea, but not Europe. Urban areas with crowding seem particularly prone to outbreaks. There is some evidence that this disease is greatly under-reported.

Parasite

Rickettsia akari is a Gram-negative, prokaryotic coccobacillus. It is morphologically indistinguishable from *Rickettsia rickettsii*. These organisms measure up to 600 nm in length and are obligate intracellular parasites. They prefer to invade endothelial cells and propagate within the nucleus. *Rickettsia akari* may be visualized with Giemsa's and Machiavello's stains.

Clinical symptoms

Men and women are equally affected, there being no sex or age preference. Twenty-four hours to 48 h after being bitten by an infected mite, an eschar begins to develop. Patients are frequently unaware of the bite or eschar. Initially the skin becomes red and is occasionally itchy. Blistering and suppuration may ensue, followed by the production of a dark, hardened eschar. Swelling and discomfort of regional lymph nodes are common.

After an incubation period of 7–14 days, the patient becomes febrile. Temperatures typically remain under 39.9°C but may reach 41.1°C. Headache, myalgias, neck stiffness and drenching sweats with chills are common. Mild photophobia may be noted. Upper respiratory symptoms may also occur, but less frequently.

The rash of rickettsialpox begins 2–3 days after the onset of systemic symptoms. Papules measuring 2–10 mm erupt on the trunk and face and spread to the extremities. These lesions are asymptomatic, are slightly red and can develop a small vesicle or pustule in the centre. More than 40 such lesions is uncommon. An enanthem of the oral mucous membranes has been described. The palms and soles are not affected. Post-inflammatory hyperpigmentation may result, but scarring does not.

Initially patients demonstrate a lymphocytosis, which is later replaced by mild leucopenia. Cerebrospinal fluid is normal and blood cultures are negative.

Symptoms resolve in 6–10 days without therapy. Reinfections and relapses have not been described, meaning that human immunity appears complete. Infection with *R. akari* does not confer immunity to infection with other rickettsial organisms.

Diagnosis

Previously, infected blood leucocytes were injected into the peritoneal cavities of mice to confirm the presence of *R. akari*; however, serological studies have replaced this method. The Weil–Felix test evaluates for the presence of antibodies capable of agglutinating cell wall antigens from *Proteus* species (OX-19, OX-K, OX-2). Among the spotted fever group, rickettsialpox is the only Weil–Felix-negative organism.

Complement fixation evaluation is the most prevalent means of diagnosing this infection. Paired sera antibody titres are compared and a fourfold increase or more than 1 : 64 dilution is considered diagnostic. Antibodies may be detected 10 days after the onset of symptoms, but less than 20% of patients will have a positive titre during the acute stage. Titres peak after 3–4 weeks if therapy has not begun or 6–8 weeks if patients have been treated. Anti-rickettsial fluorescent antibodies have been found on formalin-fixed eschar tissue but rarely from biopsies of the cutaneous eruption. More specific antibody tests are being developed.

Transmission

The typical vector for *R. akari* is the mouse mite *Liponyssoides sanguineus* (previously named *Allodermanyssus sanguineus*). This mite parasitizes the common House mouse (*Mus musculus*) but has also been found on rats, Mongolian gerbils (*Meriones unguiculatus*), the Korean vole (*Eothenomys regulus*) and Egyptian gerbils (*Gerbillus pyramidum*). A substantial portion of the mite's life cycle is spent away from the mouse. Following a blood meal, the mite abandons its host and may be found in mouse-infested housing and mouse bedding. The infectious organisms are passed transovarially among mice and to other hosts by biting. Human infection may occur when the mite finds the murine host less attractive and seeks nourishment elsewhere.

Treatment

Rickettsialpox is a comparatively benign infection and typically runs its course in 7–10 days if untreated. Antibiotics, however, are recommended in patients who are known to be infected. Since *R. akari* is an intracellular organism, antimicrobials which inhibit cell wall synthesis, such as beta-lactams, are ineffective. Antibiotics, such as tetracycline, which arrest protein assimilation are efficacious. One gram per day given in four divided doses is recommended. Fever and systemic symptoms begin to subside within 48 h of beginning treatment. This drug is typically withheld in paediatric cases, since tooth and bone deposition have been described; however, in particularly sick children, dosing at 25 mg kg^{-1} 24 h^{-1} in divided doses for 2 days is acceptable. Chloramphenicol is also effective when given at 250 mg four times day^{-1}. However, idiosyncratic reactions may ensue and this drug is not recommended for mild illness. Successful use of erythromcyin in an 11-month-old child has been reported. Sulfonamides are unhelpful in this disease.

Control

Prevention of this condition is directed at removing the vector by controlling the mouse population. Removal of conditions favourable to rodent proliferation will usually suffice and this revolves around improved living conditions. Rodent traps and poison baits are also useful.

Selected bibliography

Barker, L.P. (1949) Rickettsialpox: clinical and laboratory study of twelve hospitalized cases. *Journal of the American Medical Association* 141, 119–125.

Boyd, A.S. (1997) Rickettsialpox. *Dermatologic Clinics of North America* 15, 313–318.

Boyd, A.S. and Neldner, K.H. (1992) Typhus disease group. *International Journal of Dermatology* 31, 823–832.

Burnett, J.W. (1980) Rickettsioses: a review for the dermatologist. *Journal of the American Academy of Dermatology* 2, 359–373.

Kass, E.M., Szaniawski, W.K., Levy, H., Leach, J., Srinivasan, K. and Rives, C. (1994) Rickettsialpox in a New York city hospital, 1980 to 1989. *New England Journal of Medicine* 331, 1612–1617.

Myers, S.A. and Sexton, D.J. (1994) Dermatologic manifestations of arthropod-borne diseases. *Infectious Diseases Clinics of North America* 8, 689–712.

Sussman L.N. (1946) Kew Gardens' spotted fever. *New York Medicine* 2, 27–28.

Walker, D.H. and Dumler, J.S. (1994) Emerging and reemerging rickettsial diseases. *New England Journal of Medicine* 331, 1651–1652.

Rift Valley fever virus

Michèle Bouloy

In 1931, R. Daubney and colleagues described a disease called Rift Valley fever, which affected sheep and lambs on the northern shores of Lake Naivasha in the Rift Valley of Kenya. Retrospectively, it is likely that the disease described by R.E. Montgomery and R.J. Stordy in the same region, in 1912, was a Rift Valley fever outbreak. However, identification of the outbreak became possible in 1931 when the causative viral agent was isolated for the first time, by Daubney and co-workers. In 1973, the virus was classified in the Bunyaviridae family and the genus *Phlebovirus*.

Among viruses of the Bunyaviridae family, only a few are zoonotic. Rift Valley fever (RVF) virus is probably one of most important in Africa: it is transmitted by mosquitoes, infects livestock and is a serious public health problem, as it is highly pathogenic for humans and causes fatal haemorrhagic fevers.

Human infections

Before 1975, Rift Valley fever was known as a disease essentially affecting domestic animals, such as sheep, cattle and goats, and producing high mortality rates in newborn animals and abortions in pregnant animals. A few human cases, due only to laboratory accidents, were reported. In 1975, human infections occurred during a major epizootic in South Africa. Among 17 diagnosed cases, 12 suffered from encephalitis and four died from haemorrhagic fever. The severity of the disease and the haemorrhagic forms were recognized later in 1977 with the Egyptian outbreak.

Distribution

Although phleboviruses related to RVF virus have been isolated worldwide, Rift Valley fever has until recently been described only on the African continent, namely in Egypt and in sub-Saharan countries; but in 2000 it was found in Saudi Arabia and Yemen.

Major outbreaks have been recorded since 1931: in Kenya in 1931, 1968, 1978–1979 and recently in 1997–1998; in South Africa in 1950–1951, 1969 and 1974–1976; in Zimbabwe in 1957–1958, 1969–1970 and 1978; in Sudan in 1973; and in Zambia in 1973–1974 and 1978 (Fig. 1). In 1997–1998 in Kenya, Tanzania and Somalia, outbreaks occurred in flooded areas after a period of very abundant rainfall. The RVF virus was isolated in 1974 for the first time in West Africa, from *Aedes* mosquitoes. Later, it was detected in Mauritania, Mali and Guinea. In 1987, in Mauritania, a major outbreak occurred in association with implementation of the Diama dam. Circulation of the virus was monitored in Senegal and recently in 1998 in Mauritania, where human cases were reported.

Rift Valley fever virus had not been reported as circulating outside the sub-Saharan countries until 1977, when it provoked a sudden and dramatic outbreak in Egypt in the Nile Valley and re-emerged in the same region in 1993–1997. Manifestations of the virus were observed in 1990–1991 in Madagascar during an epizootic. A recent study indicated that the viruses circulating in Madagascar in 1990 and in Kenya in 1997 were closely related. Interestingly, RVF virus was isolated for the first time in Madagascar in 1979 but serological and phylogenetic analyses of the strain showed that it was closely related to the virus circulating in Egypt in 1977. These data suggest that RVF viruses were imported into the island from different sources and emphasize the risk of emergence of this virus outside its established geographical area, via transportation or travelling.

Virus

Rift Valley fever virus is classified in the Bunyaviridae family and the *Phlebovirus* genus. Examination by electron microscopy and biochemical analysis reveals enveloped particles measuring 90–110 nm in diameter,

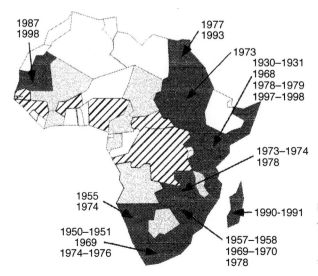

1987
1998

1977
1993

1973
1930–1931
1968
1978–1979
1997–1998

1973–1974
1978

1955
1974

1990-1991

1950–1951
1969
1974–1976

1957–1958
1969–1970
1978

Fig. 1. Circulation of RVF virus in Africa. Dark areas represent epidemics/epizootics; hatched areas, virus isolations; and light grey areas, serological evidence.

composed of four structural proteins and a tripartite single-stranded RNA genome. The protein components consist of two glyco-proteins G1 (60 kDa) and G2 (55 kDa), a nucleoprotein N (27 kDa) and an RNA-dependent RNA polymerase L of approximately 250 kDa (Fig. 2A). Rift Valley fever virus is sensitive to ionic and non-ionic detergents, hypochlorite and common disinfectants.

The three segments of the genome (L, M and S for large, medium and small, respectively), associated with multiple copies of the N nucleoprotein and a few copies of the L protein, form the inner circular and helical ribonucleoproteins. Genomic RNAs possess the 3' terminal sequences UCUCUUUC . . . specific to phleboviruses, which are complementary to the 5' terminal ones AGAGAAAG . . . and form panhandle structures. The sequence of the complete genome of this virus indicates that the L and M segments are of negative polarity and code, respectively, for the L protein and for a polypeptide precursor to the glycoproteins (Fig. 2B). The S segment utilizes an ambisense strategy and expresses the N and NSs proteins from the antigenomic- and genomic-stranded RNA, respectively. It is noteworthy that the NSs protein of RVF virus possesses specific properties, as it is phosphorylated and forms filamentous structures in the nuclei of infected cells (Fig. 3). The nuclear localization of a viral component is surprising since RVF virus, like other members of the family, replicates only in the cytoplasm. The role of NSs has been elucidated. It is an accessory protein for the viral growth in cell culture, since there exists a natural isolate, Clone 13, which possesses an internal deletion in the NSs open-reading frame and replicates in vertebrate and mosquito cells. However, NSs plays a major role in pathogenicity as an antagonist of interferon production.

The virus grows and produces plaques in many continuous line and primary cell cultures, including VERO and BHK-21 cells, the only exceptions being primary macrophages and lymphoblastoid cell lines. The viral cycle occurs in the cytoplasm. During transcription, four subgenomic messenger RNAs (mRNAs) are synthesized, one from each of the L and M segments and two from the S segment, the N and NSs mRNAs, all of them lacking poly-A at their 3' ends (Fig. 4). The N mRNA is transcribed from the S genomic segment, whereas the NSs mRNA is transcribed from the antigenomic RNA molecule. All the mRNAs are subgenomic,

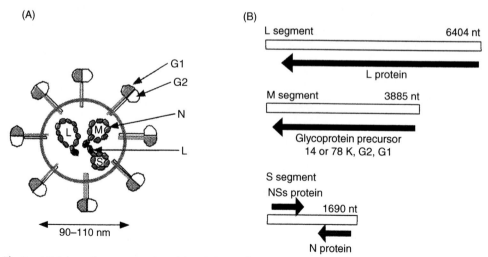

Fig. 2. (A) Schematic representation of the viral particle. (B) Rift Valley fever virus genomic organization; the rectangles and the black arrows represent the genomic strand and the ORFs, respectively. Orientation from right to left: ORF present in the antigenomic strand; and from left to right: ORF present in the genomic strand. ORF, open-reading frame.

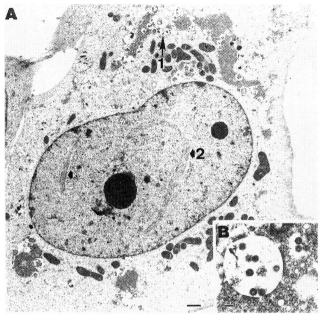

Fig. 3. Electron microscopic examination of: (A) a VERO cell infected with RVF virus MP12 strain showing the presence of particles in the Golgi vesicles (arrow number 1) and (B) the presence of fibrous structures in the nucleus (arrow number 2). The bar represents 100 nm. (Kindly provided by P. Gounon.)

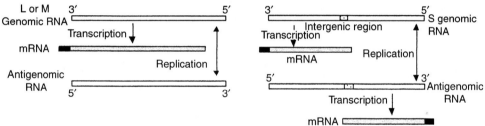

Fig. 4. Transcription and replication of the negative-stranded L and M segments, and the ambisense S segment. The black area represents the additional oligonucleotides derived from cellular RNAs and used as primers for transcription of mRNAs.

resulting from transcription that terminates in the intergenic region for the S segment or before the end of the templates for the L and M segments. Moreover, mRNAs possess a 5′ methylated cap and 10–18 additional non-viral nucleotides derived from cellular RNAs, which are used to initiate the mRNA synthesis with a cap-snatching mechanism, like influenza virus. Full-length antigenomic RNAs, representing the complete copies of the genome and terminating with a 5′ triphosphate, serve as templates for replication. Full-length S antigenomic RNA is also the template for the synthesis of NSs mRNA (Fig. 4).

Translation of the mRNAs leads to the expression of the four structural (N, L, G1 and G2) and three non-structural proteins, NSs, which form filaments in the nuclei and two proteins, 14K and 78K, coded by the M segment, the role of which is not known. The M segment mRNA synthesizes a polypeptide precursor, which is cleaved co-translationally and generates, in this order, the 14K non-structural protein, followed by G2 and G1. Expression of the 78K protein results from translation initiation at the first (instead of the second) in-frame AUG codon (the translation initiation codon), which leads to a polypeptide, uncleaved at the site usually recognized between 14K and G2. Like all the viruses of this family, the viral particles maturate by budding through the membranes of the Golgi apparatus.

Exceptions to this rule were reported: the plasma membranes of infected rat hepatocytes and epithelial cells of the mid-gut of infected mosquitoes were found to be the site for particle maturation.

No significant antigenic differences were detected among RVF virus isolates. However, phylogenetic analysis of strains of various geographical origins and isolated from different hosts (humans, animals, mosquitoes) during epidemics/epizootics or endemic/enzootic periods indicated the existence of three lineages: Egyptian, West African and East–Central African. Extended analyses performed by sequencing regions in the three genomic segments strongly suggested that some of the strains were generated by genomic reassortment between phylogenetically different viruses, indicating that RVF viruses from different origins were present at the same time and place and coinfected mosquito or vertebrate hosts.

Clinical symptoms

In 1977, some 18,000–200,000 human cases were estimated in Egypt, with 600 recorded deaths from encephalitis and haemorrhagic fevers. In 1987, 224 human patients died from RVF virus infection in Mauritania. Although it was difficult to estimate the number of cases in 1997–1998 in East Africa, because of the circulation of numerous pathogens, probably more than 89,000 humans were infected with RVF virus.

Infections in humans occur from contact with infected animals or with viraemic blood or from mosquito bites. Contaminated aerosols may also be implicated. The disease leads to a wide variety of clinical manifestations. Usually Rift Valley fever begins as an influenza-like illness, with fever, headache and myalgia, followed by a complete recovery. However, in some cases, infection progresses to severe and sometimes fatal complications, such as retinitis, encephalitis or haemorrhagic fever, with acute hepatitis. In Egypt, approximately 800 patients had ocular disease appearing after the febrile illness, between 7 and 20 days after the onset of the symptoms, and had a diminution in visual acuity and sometimes a permanent loss of central vision.

Meningoencephalitis was frequent in Egypt. The timing of encephalitic and ocular diseases is similar; the febrile phase is followed in 5–10 days by hallucination, disorientation and vertigo. Immunoglobulin G (IgG) and IgM antibodies were found in the cerebrospinal fluids of patients with central nervous system (CNS) involvement. Fatalities were not frequent but neurological complications were reported.

Most of the haemorrhagic forms are fatal. Usually, the acute febrile phase is followed in 2–4 days by jaundice and haemorrhages. Death usually occurs 3–6 days later.

Diagnosis

Major Rift Valley fever epizootics/epidemics have been preceded by heavy rains, a high density of mosquitoes and frequent abortions in sheep and cattle. These criteria should be considered as a suspicious indication of the circulation of the virus. However, during an outbreak, the clear demonstration of the presence of the RVF virus must be obtained by virological and serological methods. Isolation of the virus after inoculation of suckling mice or VERO cells is considered to be the method of choice. Virus has been isolated from the blood of patients up to 10 days after the onset of the symptoms, and from many organs at autopsy.

Diagnosis can also be performed by detection of RVF virus-specific IgM or IgG antibodies in animal or human sera, IgM being the signature of a recent infection. Enzyme-linked immunosorbent assays (ELISAs), widely used in reference laboratories, are preferred to the previously established methods of complement fixation, inhibition haemagglutination and plaque-reduction neutralization.

The N protein appears as the major antigen during infection. The envelope glycoproteins G1 and G2 carry epitopes inducing neutralizing antibodies, which were shown to play an important protective role against infection. The presence of serum antibodies to RVF virus seems to be the major immunological defence mechanism in recovery. Very little is known about the cellular immune response.

Liver lesions found by histopathological examinations also provide a good indication of RVF virus infection. Immunostaining or *in situ* hybridization to detect RVF virus antigens or its genome is useful to confirm diagnosis. When liver sections were observed under an electron microscope, many hepatic cells were found to be disorganized, with nuclei containing rod- or fibre-like structures composed of the NSs protein.

More recently, detection of the viral genome by reverse transcription–polymerase chain reaction (RT-PCR) amplification has been developed and found to be very useful for rapid diagnosis. This provides material for sequencing and further characterization of the strains.

Transmission

Except for contamination by contact with infected tissues, the virus is generally transmitted by mosquito bites. Numerous strains of RVF virus have been isolated from various mosquito species, especially from species of *Aedes*, *Ochlerotatus*,[1] *Culex* and *Mansonia* (Table 1). Virus isolations have also been reported from *Culicoides*, *Simulium* and ticks, but their role in transmission is as yet unproved.

The occurrence of epidemics/epizootics following periods of heavy rains or in association with dam implementation, e.g. the Aswan dam in 1977 or Diama dam on the Senegal River in 1987, appears to be related to a dense population of mosquitoes. Analysis of records of rainfall, Pacific and Indian Ocean sea-surface temperature anomalies and vegetation index data, coupled with satellite observations, has shown that outbreaks could be predicted up to 5 months in advance in East Africa.

During inter-epidemic periods, the virus is maintained in nature via transovarial transmission in mosquitoes, as was shown in *Aedes lineatopennis* in Kenya and in *Aedes vexans* in Senegal. Recently, it has been reported that RVF virus could infect rodents, such as Namaqua Rock mice (*Aethomys namaquensis*), which were able to propagate the virus and might be involved in a vertebrate–mosquito cycle,

constituting a possible reservoir host in South Africa.

Animal infections

Depending on the animal species, up to 30% of adults could die and 80–100% of pregnant animals abort. During a notable epizootic of Rift Valley fever in South Africa in 1950–1951, 100,000 sheep died and 500,000 aborted. In less developed countries, these outbreaks produce substantial economic losses and sometimes reduce the animal protein available for humans. Restriction of animal exportation from countries where the virus is endemic contributes to the economic losses.

The disease affects sheep and cattle, the most susceptible animals of veterinary interest being lambs, calves and kids. Pigs, horses, domestic Buffaloes (*Syncerus caffer*) and camels (*Camelus* species) do not become ill, but abortion due to RVF virus has been observed in camels and buffaloes. A recent serosurvey of RVF virus infections in wildlife in Zimbabwe showed that RVF virus antibodies were most prevalent in the Black rhinoceros (*Diceros bicornis*), the White rhinoceros (*Ceratotherium simum*), Buffalo (*S. caffer*) and the Waterbuck (*Kobus ellipsiprymnus*).

In newborn lambs, the mortality rate is 90–100% for less than 1-week-old animals. The incubation period may be as short as 12 h but usually lasts 24–36 h, after which the animal develops a high fever, exhibits abdominal pain and dies within 24–36 h after the onset of the first clinical symptoms. Older animals exhibit various clinical signs, from inapparent to peracute or acute infection, the latter form being frequent under field conditions. Sick animals exhibit fever, anorexia, nasal discharge, bloody or fetid diarrhoea and, in some cases, a severe icterus. For pregnant animals, abortion may occur at any stage of pregnancy. Abortion rates are usually very high, ranging from 40 to 100% in southern Africa and 80 to 100% in Egypt in 1977. Adult cattle and sheep may suffer mortality rates of 10–30% or higher, depending on the nutritional state of the animal. The disease primarily affects the liver, with rapid hepatocellular changes

Table 1.   Arthropods naturally infected with RVF virus. Subgenera in parentheses.

Species	Country
Aedes	
(*Aedimorphus*)	
cumminsii	Burkina Faso 1983
dalzieli	Kenya 1982, Senegal 1975, 1983
dentatus	Zimbabwe 1969
durbanensis	Kenya 1937
ochraceus	Senegal 1993
tarsalis	Uganda 1955
vexans	Senegal 1933
(*Neomelaniconion*)	
circumluteolus	Uganda 1955, South Africa 1955, 1981
lineatopennis	Zimbabwe 1969, South Africa 1975, Kenya 1982, 1984
palpalis	Central African Republic 1969
(*Stegomyia*)	
africanus	Uganda 1956
dendrophilus	Uganda 1948
(*Diceromyia*)	
furcifer	Burkina Faso 1983
Ochlerotatus*	
caballus	South Africa 1953
juppi	South Africa 1978
Culex	
(*Culex*)	
antennatus	Kenya 1982, Nigeria 1967, 1970
antennatus, annulioris grp., simpsoni, vansomereni	Madagascar 1979
antennatus, simpsoni, vansomereni	Kenya 1982, Madagascar 1979
theileri	Kenya 1982, South Africa 1953, 1970, 1975, Zimbabwe 1969,
zombaensis	Kenya 1982
(*Eumelanomyia*)	
rubinotus	Kenya 1982
Eretmapodites	
quinquevittatus species	South Africa 1971, Uganda 1948
Coquillettidia	
fuscopennata	Uganda 1960
grandidieri	Madagascar 1979
Mansonia	
africana	Uganda 1959, 1968, Central African Republic 1969
uniformis	Madagascar 1979, Uganda 1960
Anopheles	
(*Anopheles*)	
coustani	Zimbabwe 1969
coustani, fusicolor	Madagascar 1979
(*Cellia*)	
pauliani, squamosus	Madagascar 1979
christyi	Kenya 1982
pharoensis	Kenya 1982
Ticks	
Amblyomma variegatum	Central African Republic 1983
Rhipicephalus appendiculatus	Kenya 1933

Continued

Table 1. *Continued*

Species	Country
Other arthropods	
Culicoides	Nigeria 1967
Simulium	South Africa 1953

*Ochlerotatus was formerly a subgenus of Aedes.

progressing to massive necrosis. In some animals, haemorrhages are observed in the liver.

Experimental infections of susceptible animals have helped towards a better understanding of Rift Valley fever pathogenesis. Infections of mice, hamsters and some strains of rats, by peripheral routes, with virulent strains lead to a transient viraemia, followed by an acute hepatitis and death. In other strains of rats, RVF virus infection provokes encephalitis. Some other strains are completely resistant, with asymptomatic infection. Resistance was shown to be governed by a dominant Mendelian gene. Rhesus monkeys (*Macaca mulatta*) represent an excellent model for human infection, exhibiting a variety of clinical symptoms, including haemorrhagic forms with disseminated intravascular coagulation.

Prevention and treatment

Because of the economic importance of the disease in sheep and cattle, efforts have been to produce a veterinary vaccine. To this end, the Smithburn neurotropic strain was obtained by intracerebral passages of the virulent strain Entebbe in suckling mice and embryonated chicken's eggs. However, the strain was not completely attenuated, being neurotropic, and provoked a range of anomalies of the central nervous system in fetuses. Vaccination of ewes may also result in abortion and stillbirth. Teratogenic effects associated with vaccination have been reported in up to 15% of pregnant ewes. For this reason, other attenuated strains have been produced or isolated. One of them, the mutagenized strain MP12, which derived from a virulent strain isolated in Egypt in 1977, appeared to be a

good candidate because of the presence of attenuating mutations in each of the three segments of the genome. However, although it was an efficient immunogen in adult and young animals, deleterious effects were observed after vaccination of pregnant ewes in the first trimester (B. Erasmus and D.H.L. Bishop, personal communication). Recently, a naturally attenuated strain, Clone 13, isolated from a benign human case was found to be highly immunogenic for mice. Interestingly, this RVF virus possesses a large deletion in the gene coding for the non-structural NSs, which seems to be an important determinant for attenuation.

An inactivated RVF virus vaccine, produced in 1967 and improved in 1978, is used to protect at-risk personnel, but it is too expensive for veterinary use. Administration of immune plasma or serum, interferon, interferon inducer or ribavirin in experimentally RVF virus-infected mice, rats or monkeys has proved efficient in protecting against the disease.

Control

Recent epidemics in East and West Africa have emphasized the importance of irrigation and rainfall in the re-emergence of the virus, as well as a risk of exportation from Africa. Since mosquitoes play an important role for viral transmission and propagation, vector control measures are often appropriate. In emergency situations, such as dealing with epidemics, the most appropriate measures are space-spraying, particularly using ultra-low-volume (ULV) techniques, with insecticides such as malathion, propoxur or the pyrethroids to kill the adult mosquitoes, including infected ones. Aerial applications are the method of choice for covering large areas. In the 1977–1978 epidemic in Egypt the number of cases was reduced following aerial spraying of malathion. Preventive control measures include spraying houses or animal quarters with residual insecticides, if the vectors are known to be, or are suspected of being, endophilic. Because of the often extensive mosquito larval habitats, larviciding is unlikely to be very effective.

During epizootics, relocation of animals where mosquitoes are absent has been suggested. Of utmost importance is the control of the circulation of the virus during serological surveys or virus isolation from captured mosquitoes or a sentinel herd. To this end, methods for the rapid detection of the virus by immunocapture ELISA or RT-PCR amplification are extremely useful.

Note

[1] *Ochlerotatus* was formerly a subgenus of *Aedes*.

Selected bibliography

Caplen, H., Peters, C.J. and Bishop, D.H.L. (1985) Mutagen-directed attenuation of Rift Valley fever virus as a method for vaccine development. *Journal of General Virology* 66, 123–133.

Meegan, J.M. and Bailey, C.L. (1986) Rift Valley fever. In: Monath, T.P. (ed.) *The Arboviruses: Epidemiology and Ecology*, Vol. IV. CRC Press, Boca Raton, Florida, pp. 51–76.

Peters, C.J. and Linthicum, K.J. (1994) Rift Valley fever. In: Beran, G.W. (ed.) *Handbook of Zoonoses, Section B: Viral*, 2nd edn. CRC Press, Boca Raton, Florida, pp. 125–148.

Pretorius A., Oelofsen, M.J., Smith, M.S. and van der Ryst, E. (1997) Rift Valley fever virus: a seroepidemiologic study of small terrestrial vertebrates in South Africa. *American Journal of Tropical Medicine and Hygiene* 57, 693–698.

Sall, A.A., Zanotto, P. M. de A., Sene, O.K., Zeller, H.G., Digoutte, J.P., Thiongane, Y. and Bouloy, M. (1999) Genetic reassortment of Rift Valley fever virus in nature. *Journal of Virology* 73, 8196–8200.

Schmaljohn, C. (1996) Bunyaviridae: the viruses and their replication. In: Fields, B.N., Knipe, D. and Howley, P.M. (eds) *Fields Virology*, Vol. 1, 3rd edn. Lippincott, Williams & Wilkins, Philadelphia, pp. 1447–1471.

Swanepoel R. and Coetzer, J.A.W. (1994) Rift Valley fever. In: Coetzer, J.A.W., Thompson, G.R. and Tustin, R.C. (eds). *Infectious Disease of Livestock with Special Reference to Southern Africa*, Vol. 1. Oxford University Press, Cape Town, pp. 688–717.

Vialat, P., Billecocq, A., Kohl, A. and Bouloy, M. (2000) The S segment of Rift Valley phlebovirus (Bunyaviridae) carries determinants for attenuation and virulence in mice. *Journal of Virology* 74, 1538–1543.

River blindness *see* **Onchocerciasis, human.**

Roaches *see* **Cockroaches.**

Rochalimaea quintana *see* ***Bartonella quintana*** **and** ***Bartonella henselae.***

Rocio encephalitis

Carl J. Mitchell

Distribution

Rocio (ROC) virus was responsible for epidemics of meningoencephalitis in coastal communities in southern São Paulo State, Brazil, during 1975–1977. Epidemics were confined to 20 counties in the Santista Lowlands and the Ribeira Valley; 1021 cases were diagnosed. Outside the epidemic area, five cases were diagnosed in Parana State across the border to the south from the Ribeira Valley. Subsequently, no further outbreaks have occurred and ROC virus activity has decreased markedly.

Aetiological agent

The prototype strain of ROC virus (SP H 34675) was isolated in 1975 from cerebellum and spinal cord tissues of a fatal encephalitis case, who previously resided in the small village of Rocio. Rocio virus belongs to the genus *Flavivirus* (family Flaviviridae) and is closely related serologically to Ilheus, St Louis encephalitis, Japanese encephalitis and Murray Valley encephalitis viruses (see entries). Rocio virus particles are typical of flaviviruses, spherical in shape and about 43 nm in diameter. The virus causes encephalitis and death in suckling and weaned mice and suckling hamsters, after intracerebral inoculation. Rocio virus replicates in a variety of vertebrate and insect cell lines.

Clinical symptoms

The incubation period is estimated to be between 7 and 14 days, with an average of 12 days. The main symptoms and signs among 234 patients with encephalitis included headache (94%), fever (91%), vomiting (51%), weakness (45%), anorexia (24%), abdominal distension (21%), nausea (19%) and hyperaemia of the oropharynx (19%) and conjunctivae (16%). Signs of central nervous system involvement included meningeal irritation (57%), alteration of consciousness (51%), motor abnormalities (50%), alteration of deep tendon reflexes (25%), alteration of muscle tone (25%), presence of pathological reflexes (14%), abnormalities of the cranial nerves (12%), dyslalia (10%), sensory disturbance (2%) and convulsions (2%). Death followed fulminating or prolonged coma. Serious neurological sequelae were observed in about 20% of patients.

Diagnosis

Infections with ROC virus cannot be diagnosed on the basis of clinical symptoms, which may be the same or similar to those caused by a variety of aetiological agents. Laboratory procedures for diagnosis are based on isolation of ROC virus or specific serological tests. Rocio virus can usually be isolated from the central nervous tissues of patients who die within 5 days of the onset of illness. Serological tests, including haemagglutination inhibition (HI), complement fixation (CF) and neutralization tests (NT), can be used. Serological diagnosis is based on a significant rise between paired acute and convalescent sera collected with at least a 10-day interval between samples. The HI test is less reliable because of cross-reactivity between ROC virus and related flaviviruses. An immunoglobulin M (IgM) antibody-capture enzyme-linked immunosorbent assay (MAC-ELISA) is also useful, especially when only a single serum is available, which results in inconclusive results by HI and CF tests.

Epidemiology

The affected area is bordered to the north and north-west by the Serra do Mar Mountains and the Atlantic Ocean to the south. The Ribeira Valley has the lowest population density in São Paulo State; two-thirds of the population is rural. It is extensively forested, and humid tropical forests often extend up to the edges of urban and rural centres. Basic sanitation services are frequently lacking and unpaved streets are common. The Santista Lowlands lie to the north-east in a long, narrow corridor along the coastal plain. Tourism, industry, banana plantations and fishing contribute to a well-developed economy.

The initial outbreak involved primarily adult males who worked close to or inside forests, suggesting an arbovirus aetiology even before the virus was isolated. Subsequently, fishermen and agricultural workers were at greatest risk, especially males in the 15–30-year age bracket. In 1975, the incidence in males in this age group was 82/1000, whereas for males in general it was 49/1000, and for females 15–30 years of age it was 24/1000. The coastal counties were most affected, with attack rates ranging from 718 to 1915 per 100,000 population. From 1978 to 1983, annual encephalitis attack rates in the Ribeira Valley decreased gradually from 19.6/100,000 to 0.9/100,000. The overall case–fatality rate was 10%, with the highest rates in children under 1 year of age (31%) and in people over 60 years of age (28%). Most cases in the Santista

Lowlands occurred from March through May, whereas peak incidence in the Ribeira Valley was during the summer and early autumn.

Transmission cycles

Neither the epidemic nor the epizootic cycles of ROC virus have been defined; however, field and laboratory studies have provided information about the probable involvement of birds and mosquitoes. During the 1975 outbreak, 14,490 mosquitoes, representing at least eight species belonging to three tribes, were collected in the epidemic zone and tested for the presence of virus by inoculating triturated suspensions of mosquito pools into suckling mice. The results were negative. Subsequently, an additional 38,896 mosquitoes collected in the epidemic zone later in 1975, and during 1976, were tested in VERO and primary duck embryo cell cultures. A single isolate of ROC virus was recorded from a pool of *Psorophora ferox* collected in a Shannon trap in Cananeia, along the south-east coast of the Ribeira Valley, on 26 February 1976. The positive pool included 16 unfed, one gravid and two blood-engorged specimens. The abdomen of one of the two engorged mosquitoes was saved for precipitin testing and was found to contain canine blood. Only 283 *P. ferox* (0.7% of the total mosquitoes) were present in the collections. Among the mosquitoes tested, species of *Culex* (*Melanoconion*) were most commonly represented (36%), followed in decreasing abundance by *Coquillettidia chrysonotum*, *Mansonia indubitans*, *Ochlerotatus*[1] *scapularis*, *Ochlerotatus serratus*, other Culicini, Anophelini and Sabethini.

Experimental studies showed that ROC virus produced high-level viraemias in young chicks following subcutaneous inoculation of virus or the bite of a single infected mosquito. Use of a mosquito–chick model permitted an evaluation of the susceptibility of a variety of mosquito species and strains to infection *per os*, measurement of virus infection and transmission rates, determination of the virus content of infected mosquitoes and growth patterns of ROC virus

in infected mosquitoes. Initially, because of the availability of mosquitoes, such studies were carried out with colony strains of mosquitoes from the USA and one from Argentina. Based on the results of these studies, the vector competence of various species and strains was classified as high (*Culex tarsalis* from Colorado and Arizona, and *Culex pipiens* sensu stricto from Illinois), moderate (*C. pipiens* group from Tennessee, and *Culex quinquefasciatus* from Argentina), or low (*P. ferox* from Louisiana, and *Culex opisthopus* and *Culex nigripalpus* from Florida).

Subsequent studies with *P. ferox*, *O. scapularis* and *O. serratus* from the epidemic zone showed that the first two species could be classified as potential vectors, but *O. serratus* was relatively insusceptible to *per os* infection, even following ingestion of high-titre blood meals. Field investigations during the late 1970s and 1980s showed that *O. scapularis*, *O. serratus* and species of *Culex* (*Melanoconion*) were the predominant mosquitoes in the epidemic zone, and that *O. scapularis* was the most common and abundant mosquito in human settlements and human-made environments.

Haemagglutination inhibition antibody to flaviviruses was found in approximately 25% of wild birds in the epidemic zone during the time of the outbreaks, and ROC virus was the most reactive antigen. In addition, strains of ROC virus were isolated from the blood of a Rufous collared sparrow, *Zonotrichia capensis*, and from sentinel mice. The latter were exposed in a suspended cage, indicating that a flying arthropod was the probable vector. Experimental studies with House sparrows, *Passer domesticus*, from Colorado indicated that the population tested was not a good amplification host for Rocio virus.

Treatment

There is no specific treatment for patients infected with ROC virus. Hospitalization with good supportive therapy and general nursing care currently offer the best hope for reducing the risk of complications leading to more severe or fatal cases.

Prevention and control

A formalin-treated extract of infected suckling mouse brains was used to prepare an inactivated vaccine against ROC virus in 1977. Employees of an industry located in the epidemic area were given three doses of the vaccine 1 month apart and another dose 15 months later. Seroconversion rates were low and induced antibodies were short-lived; therefore, the vaccine was not used extensively.

Mosquito control activities undertaken during the epidemic included the use of larvicides in ditches and flooded areas, perifocal application of adulticides around residences with encephalitis cases, and area-wide ultra-low-volume (ULV) applications of malathion from vehicles and aircraft. Also, some areas with stagnant water were drained. It is impossible to determine what impact these control efforts had on ROC virus transmission. Personal protection by the use of bed nets, especially pyrethroid-impregnated ones, and mosquito repellents may be useful for protecting people living in or near the epidemic area, especially when there is evidence of ROC virus activity.

Future perspective

The ecological variables that accounted for the sudden appearance and disappearance of intense Rocio virus transmission in the affected area are unknown. It seems likely that low-level enzootic transmission continues to occur. With increasing deforestation and population expansion in south-eastern São Paulo State and other areas of Brazil, it is highly probable that epidemics caused by ROC virus will occur in the future. The apparent importance of birds, perhaps involving migratory species, in the virus transmission cycle and the ease with which Rocio virus can be transmitted experimentally by a wide variety of mosquito species both suggest that the virus may become more widely distributed in the future. The encephalitis outbreak caused by West Nile virus (see entry), a related flavivirus, in the north-eastern USA in 1999 illustrates the potential for arboviruses to cause severe problems far from previously recognized enzootic foci.

Note

[1] *Ochlerotatus* was formerly a subgenus of *Aedes*.

Selected bibliography

Forattini, O.P., Gomes, A. de C., Galati, E.A.B., Rabello, E.X. and Iversson, L.B. (1978) Estudos ecólogicos sobre mosquitos Culicidae no Sistema da Serra do Mar, Brasil. Parts 1 and 2. Observações no ambiente extra-domiciliar. *Revista de Saúde Pública* 12, 297–325 and 476–496.

Iversson, L.B. (1989) Rocio encephalitis. In: Monath, T.P. (ed.) *The Arboviruses: Epidemiology and Ecology*, Vol. IV. CRC Press, Boca Raton, Florida, pp. 77–92.

Mitchell, C.J., Forattini, O.P. and Miller, B.R. (1986) Vector competence experiments with Rocio virus and three mosquito species from the epidemic zone in Brazil. *Revista de Saúde Pública* 20, 171–177.

Mitchell, C.J., Monath, T.P. and Cropp, C.B. (1981) Experimental transmission of Rocio virus by mosquitoes. *American Journal of Tropical Medicine and Hygiene*, 30, 465–472.

Vasconcelos, P.F.C., Travassos da Rosa, A.P.A., Pinheiro, F.P., Shope, R.E., Travassos da Rosa, J.F.S., Rodrigues, S.G., Degallier, N. and Travassos da Rosa, E.S. (1998) Arboviruses pathogenic for man in Brazil. In: Travassos da Rosa, A.P.A., Vasconcelos, P.F.C. and Travassos da Rosa, J.F.S. (eds) *An Overview of Arbovirology in Brazil and Neighbouring Countries*. Evandro Chagas Institute, Bélem, Brazil, pp. 72–99.

Rocky Mountain spotted fever

Daniel J. Sexton

Rocky Mountain spotted fever, human

Rocky Mountain spotted fever (RMSF) was first recognized as a distinct clinical entity in settlers of the Bitterroot Valley of western Montana over 100 years ago. During the first decade of the 20th century Howard Ricketts discovered that ticks were vectors of RMSF and further discovered that the causative organism (which he isolated from guinea-pigs) circulated in nature between ticks and mammals, and that infected ticks transmitted the causative organism to their progeny. These discoveries paved the way for later investigators, who discovered the causative organisms of other rickettsial diseases and deduced their basic epidemiological features.

Distribution

Rocky Mountain spotted fever is an endemic but highly seasonal disease throughout most of the continental USA, south-western Canada, Mexico, Central America, Colombia and Brazil. In the USA, RMSF is most prevalent in the south-eastern and south central states. In addition, there are several well-known 'hot spots' of spotted fever activity, including Cape Cod (Massachusetts) and Long Island (New York State). Although it is primarily a disease of rural and suburban locations, occasionally RMSF occurs in urban locations, such as Central Park in New York City. Currently available surveillance data probably under-estimate the true incidence of the disease, as proof of diagnosis usually requires collection of paired serological samples and because many cases are treated presumptively without subsequent serological testing.

Aetiological agent

Rickettsia rickettsii is a Gram-negative coccobacillus measuring 0.3–0.7 μm by 0.8–2.0 μm. It is an obligate intracellular parasite that stains weakly with Gram's stain but can be visualized with Giemsa, Machiavello and Gimenez stains, or by fluorescent antibody conjugates. *Rickettsia rickettsii* has ribosomes and indistinct strands of DNA in an amorphous cytosol, surrounded by a plasma membrane. An indistinct microcapsular layer is present on the outer surface of the cell wall. An electron-lucent zone, which is thought to be a slime layer important in pathogenicity, separates the microcapsular layer from the host cytosol. *Rickettsia rickettsii* cannot

be propagated on agar or in broth but the organism grows readily in the yolk sac of chicken embryos and in several tissue culture monolayers, such as chicken embryo fibroblasts, mouse L cells and golden hamster cells. *Rickettsia rickettsii* also grows readily in male guinea-pigs after intraperitoneal inoculation. *In vivo*, *R. rickettsii* has a striking tropism for endothelial cells, where it grows in both the nucleus and the cytosol of infected cells. Cell-to-cell spread of *R. rickettsii* infection occurs *in vivo* and in tissue culture systems without lysis of infected cells. *Rickettsia rickettsii* infection in humans produces a widespread lymphocytic vasculitis, which may secondarily result in dysfunction of virtually any tissue or organ. Severe infections in humans may result in cerebritis, myocarditis, retinitis, cutaneous necrosis or even gangrene, as well as focal necrosis of peripheral nerves and intra-abdominal organs, and diffuse pulmonary infiltrates.

Clinical symptoms

Infected patients become symptomatic 2–14 days after being bitten by an infected tick, with most cases occurring between 5 and 7 days after exposure. In the early phases of illness, most patients have non-specific signs and symptoms, such as fever, headache, malaise, myalgia and nausea, with or without vomiting. Children and occasionally adults may have abdominal pain in the early phases of illness. In fact, gastrointestinal involvement may be severe and lead to erroneous diagnoses, such as acute appendicitis, cholecystitis and even bowel obstruction. A small number of patients in the early phases of RMSF have been admitted to surgical services and some have undergone laparotomy.

Most patients with RMSF develop a rash between the third and fifth days of illness. However, a skin rash is often absent when the patient first contacts a physician. Approximately 15% of patients have a rash on the first day of illness, and less than one-half of all patients develop a rash in the first 72 h of illness. In a small percentage of patients, the rash may be delayed in onset past 5 days and/or is atypical (e.g. confined to one body region). Furthermore, a rash never occurs in up to 10% of patients. These cases of 'spotless' RMSF may be severe and end fatally. The typical rash of RMSF begins on the ankles and wrists and spreads both centrally and to the palms and soles. It often begins as a macular or maculopapular eruption and then usually becomes petechial. The evolution of a skin rash can vary greatly from one patient to another. For example, in some patients the rash may suddenly appear as a petechial eruption, whereas in other patients, especially dark-skinned individuals, the rash may be faint or difficult to see.

In addition to a rash, most patients with RMSF complain of intense headache, myalgias and arthralgias. Cough, abdominal pain, bleeding, confusion, focal neurological signs and seizures may occur together or singly in severe cases. Gangrene of the digits, ears and scrotum can also occur in severe cases, as can widespread organ dysfunction, resulting in renal failure, heart failure or diffuse lung injury. Children with RMSF may develop striking oedema of the hands, feet and periorbital tissues.

The prognosis in RMSF is dependent upon both host factors and as yet poorly characterized virulence factors of the infecting organism. Depending upon the geographical location, 20–80% of patients with Rocky Mountain spotted fever who do not receive anti-rickettsial therapy will die of their illness. The disease is more severe in adults, males and individuals with glucose-6-phosphate dehydrogenase deficiency. However, fulminant disease may occur in patients of both sexes and all ages and races. Delay in the institution of anti-rickettsial therapy is an additional prognostic factor. Patients treated with effective therapy within the first 5 days of onset have significantly better outcomes than those treated later. Long-term sequelae, such as mononeuropathy, neurogenic bladder and paralysis, may occur in patients with severe disease.

Diagnosis

The diagnosis of RMSF is based upon the probability that individual clinical features represent RMSF in the appropriate epidemiological setting. There is no completely reliable diagnostic test in the early phases of illness when therapy should begin. The initial clinical features of Rocky Mountain spotted fever are so non-specific that, even in areas where the disease is endemic, the majority of patients with this disease are not correctly diagnosed at their first physician visit. During the early phases of illness RMSF is frequently mistaken for a wide array of other febrile illnesses, including common viral exanthems and other viral illnesses without skin rash. Individuals with RMSF are often empirically treated with beta-lactam antibiotics in the early phases of illness, and then mistakenly thought to have a drug eruption when a skin rash appears a few days later. Gastrointestinal manifestations are often dominant symptoms in the early phases of illness; indeed, some children and adults with RMSF have undergone appendectomies because of an erroneous initial diagnosis of appendicitis.

Occasionally patients with RMSF present with unusual focal or generalized neurological symptoms that mimic viral meningoencephalitis or bacterial meningitis. Rarely, bizarre neurological symptoms, such as hallucinations, dominate the early presentation of illness, leading to misdiagnosis as psychiatric disease or an intoxication. Severe cases of RMSF fever may mimic meningococcaemia to a point that even experienced clinicians cannot distinguish between the two diseases. In addition, RMSF has been confused with thrombotic thrombocytopenic purpura, streptococcal bacteraemia and measles. Occasionally, more than one person in a household will acquire RMSF nearly simultaneously, leading to the logical, but mistaken, assumption that the cause of illness is a common viral pathogen.

Later in the course of illness, the diagnosis of RMSF can be made by skin biopsy and confirmed serologically. Rickettsial blood cultures are highly sensitive and specific but are only available in research centres with specialized laboratories.

Most patients with RMSF have a normal white blood cell count at presentation. However, the white blood cell count may be low, normal or elevated in individual patients and is therefore not diagnostically helpful.

As the illness progresses, thrombocytopenia becomes more prevalent and may be severe. Hyponatraemia, elevated plasma levels of aminotransferases (transaminases) and bilirubin, azotaemia, and prolongation of the partial thromboplastin and prothrombin times are often present in severe cases of RMSF.

Biopsy of a skin lesion obtained with a 3 mm punch biopsy can establish the diagnosis of RMSF. Fresh or formaldehyde-fixed tissue can be examined for rickettsiae using direct immunofluorescence or immunoenzyme methods. Direct immunofluorescent staining can provide an answer in a few hours if the necessary conjugates are available locally. If local facilities are not able to do direct immunofluorescence, reference laboratories can perform immunoperoxidase stains on fixed tissue specimens. However, any delay in obtaining results makes this technique of little or no use for initial patient management.

The diagnosis of RMSF can be confirmed serologically using the indirect fluorescent antibody (IFA) test. The minimum diagnostic titre in most laboratories is 1 : 64. Antibodies typically appear 7–10 days after the onset of the illness. The optimal time to obtain a convalescent antibody titre is at 14–21 days after the onset of symptoms. Thus, serological testing is usually not helpful during the first 5 days of symptoms, when therapy should be initiated. Patients who are treated within the first 48 h after symptoms have appeared may not develop convalescent IFAs. The Weil–Felix test, which detects cross-reacting antibodies against *Proteus vulgaris* antigens (OX2 and OX19), lacks sensitivity and specificity and its use is no longer recommended.

Transmission

Rickettsia rickettsii circulates in nature between ixodid (hard) ticks and small rodents, such as Ground squirrels (e.g. *Spermophilus lateralis tescorum*), Yellow-pine chipmunks (*Tamias amoenus*), White-footed mice (*Peromyscus leucopus*) and voles (Muridae, Microtinae). A number of different tick species have been implicated in this tick–rodent sylvan cycle of infection. Horizontal transmission of *R. rickettsii* can occur during feeding of ticks on small mammals that are rickettsaemic. Subsequently, infected ticks can in turn infect further animals. Also ticks can be infected trans-stadially and by transovarial transmission of infection. Finally transmission of rickettsial infection may also occur when an infected male mates with an uninfected female tick – that is, venereal transmission.

Humans are only an accidental host for *R. rickettsii*. The principal vectors of human *R. rickettsii* infection in the USA and Canada are *Dermacentor andersoni* (in the Rocky Mountain region) and *Dermacentor variabilis* (in the eastern and south-western USA). In Mexico and Central America, *Rhipicephalus sanguineus* is the primary vector for human infections. In Brazil and Colombia the principal tick vector is *Amblyomma cajennense*. However, *A. cajennense* has also been described as a vector of spotted fever group (SFG) rickettsiae in Mexico and in Central America.

Rickettsia rickettsii has also been isolated from rabbit ticks (*Haemaphysalis leporispalustris*) and from the lone star tick (*Amblyomma americanum*). The latter tick is probably an insignificant or minor vector of RMSF. The rabbit tick is not thought to be a vector for human infection, even though it may be partially responsible for maintaining *R. rickettsii* in rodent populations. Moreover, although rickettsiae recovered from *H. leporispalustris* are antigentically similar to *R. rickettsii*, they do not cause disease in laboratory animals.

Treatment

The only two drugs effective against *R. rickettsii* are tetracyclines and chloramphenicol. The latter drug is generally reserved for the treatment of pregnant women and for empirical treatment of severe cases in which meningococcaemia is thought to be a possible alternative diagnosis. Tetracycline (usually in the form of doxycycline) is the preferred treatment for most cases – both in adults and in children. Although repeated doses of tetracycline can cause dental staining in children, a short course of doxycycline therapy has little chance of dental damage and doxycline is considered to be the drug of choice even in children. The recommended dose of doxycyline for children is 200 mg day^{-1} in two divided doses for children heavier than 45 kg in weight; children weighing less than 45 kg should receive 4.4 mg kg^{-1} body weight day^{-1}. The recommended dose of chloramphenicol for children is 25 mg kg^{-1} day^{-1} in four divided doses, up to a maximum dose of 2 g day^{-1}. Fluoroquinolones have been shown to have *in vitro* activity against spotted fever group (SFG) rickettsiae, including *R. rickettsii*, but they have not been adequately tested in humans with RMSF. Duration of treatment of SFG rickettsial infections has not been systematically studied in a large cohort of humans. Most authorities recommend that tetracycline or chloramphenical be continued for at least 5–7 days or until the patient has been afebrile for at least 48 h and is clinically improving.

Prevention and control

As the tick vectors of SFG rickettsia are widespread and as control of tick populations is not practical or even feasible in most regions, the cornerstone of public health control of all tick-borne rickettsial diseases is prompt empirical treatment of suspected cases. Vaccines developed in the 1930s and 1940s to control RMSF are no longer available because they lacked efficacy, and also because the low frequency of illness even in highly endemic regions made vaccination strategies impractical and prohibitively expensive. Because infected ticks need to feed on hosts for several hours before rickettsial transmission occurs, prompt identification and removal of attached ticks may prevent disease transmission to humans.

Rocky Mountain spotted fever, animal

Although cats and other domestic animals in endemic areas can be shown to have antibodies that react with *R. rickettsii* antigens, the only domestic animal that is known to acquire clinical illness due to *R. rickettsii* is the dog.

Clinical symptoms

Dogs experimentally infected with *R. rickettsii* via inoculation or by the bite of an infected tick may have fulminant clinical illness or subclinical infection. A similar range of severity from asymptomatic infection to fulminant illness has been described after naturally occurring canine infection. Dogs with symptomatic *R. rickettsii* infection usually have fever, anorexia, mental depression, cough and a stiff gait. Examination may reveal subcutaneous oedema, petechiae of the mucosa and skin and epistaxis. Neurological abnormalities, including seizures, may be present.

Some infected dogs make a complete recovery without specific anti-rickettsial treatment; others may die during the second week of illness or recover with significant sequelae. Severely affected dogs may develop necrosis of the extremities, shock with cardiovascular collapse or manifest signs of severe meningoencephalitis.

As in infected humans, canines infected with *R. rickettsii* may have thrombocytopenia, abnormal hepatic serum enzyme levels, hyperbilirubinaemia and abnormal renal function tests.

Necropsy findings in canines with severe *R. rickettsii* infection show histopathological abnormalities almost identical to those of humans with fatal RMSF. These abnormalities include intense vasculitis, with perivascular lymphocytic infiltrates and secondary damage of tissues and organs. Focal myocardial and hepatic necrosis is characteristically present in fatal cases, along with intense vasculitis of the skin, testicles, meninges, retina and skeletal muscle.

Diagnosis

Diagnosis in canines is similar to diagnosis in infected humans. The mainstay of diagnosis is serological testing. Microimmunofluorescent, enzyme-linked immunosorbent assay (ELISA) and latex agglutination tests can be used to demonstrate antibodies to *R. rickettsii*. Paired sera should always be tested to prove infection. In endemic areas 5–25% of asymptomatic dogs have serological evidence of prior infection with

SFG rickettsial antigens; thus a fourfold rise along with a compatible clinical illness is required before acute infection with *R. rickettsii* is considered to be present. None of these serological tests is useful in the acute phases of illness; thus, in virtually all cases of acute infection, diagnosis must be based on the epidemiological setting (time of year, likelihood of exposure to ticks and geographical location) and the presence of compatible clinical features. In virtually all clinical situations, initial therapy must be empirical, as proof of diagnosis requires skin biopsy, a technique that is not readily available or practical for most veterinarians. As infected dogs may have a rather high-grade rickettsaemia, veterinarians and their staff should use caution and care when obtaining blood samples and when performing necropsies on dogs with fatal infection; otherwise they may become infected.

Treatment

The best treatment for *R. rickettsii* infection in dogs is tetracycline or oxytetracycline at a dose of 22 mg kg^{-1} three times daily. Doxycycline, minocycline or chloramphenicol can also be used in treatment. Enrofloxacin has also been shown to be an effective treatment in dogs.

Control

Pet dogs living in areas endemic for RMSF can be restricted from potentially tick-infested brushy areas or locales with long grass, but such measures are generally impractical and ineffective in completely preventing tick exposures. Periodic immersion of dogs in acaricidal baths is also of limited long-term efficacy in preventing tick-to-dog transmission of *R. rickettsii* infection. As in humans, prompt empirical treatment with tetracycline is the best way to prevent canine mortality due to *R. rickettsii* infection.

Selected bibliography

Badger, L.F. (1933) Rocky Mountain spotted fever: susceptibility of the dog and sheep to the virus. *Public Health Reports* 48, 791–795.

Cale, D.F. and McCarthy, M.W. (1997) Treatment of Rocky Mountain spotted fever in children. *Annals of Pharmacotherapy* 31, 492–494.

Conlon, P.J., Procop, G.W., Fowler, V., Eloubeidi, M.A. and Sexton, D.J. (1996) Predictors of prognosis and risk of acute renal failure in patients with Rocky Mountain spotted fever. *American Journal of Medicine* 101, 621–626.

Dumler, J.S. and Walker, D.H. (1994) Diagnostic tests for Rocky Mountain spotted fever and other rickettsial diseases. [Review.] *Dermatology Clinics* 12, 25–36.

Greene, C.E. and Breitschwerdt, E.B. (1993) Rocky Mountain spotted fever in dogs. In: Woldehiwet, Z. and Ristic, M. (eds) *Rickettsial and Chlamydial Diseases of Domestic Animals.* Pergamon Press, Oxford, pp. 153–167.

Kirkland, K.B., Wilkerson, W.E. and Sexton, D.J. (1995) Therapeutic delay and mortality in cases of Rocky Mountain spotted fever. *Clinical Infectious Diseases* 20, 1118–1121.

Norment, B.R. and Burgdorfer, W. (1984) Susceptibility and reservoir potential of the dog to spotted fever-group rickettsiae. *American Journal of Veterinary Research* 45, 1706–1710.

Quintal, D. (1997) Historical aspects of the rickettsioses. *Clinics in Dermatology* 14, 237–243.

Raoult, D. and Roux, V. (1997) Rickettsioses as paradigms of new or emerging infectious diseases. *Clinical Microbiology Reviews* 10, 694–719.

Rutgers, C., Kowalski, J., Cole, C.R., Sherding, R.G., Chew, D.J., Davenport, D., O'Grady, M. and Murtaugh, R.J. (1985) Severe Rocky Mountain spotted fever in five dogs. *Journal of the American Hospital Association* 21, 361–369.

Sexton, D.J. and Corey, G.R. (1992) Rocky Mountain 'spotless' and 'almost spotless' fever: a wolf in sheep's clothing. *Clinical Infectious Diseases* 15, 439–448.

Thorner, A.R., Walker, D.H. and Petri, W.A.J. (1998) Rocky Mountain spotted fever. *Clinical Infectious Diseases* 27, 1353–1360.

Wolbach, S.B. (1919) Studies on Rocky Mountain spotted fever. *Journal of Medical Research* 41, 1–197.

Ross River virus and Ross River virus disease

John S. Mackenzie

Infection of humans with Ross River virus

Ross River (RR) virus is recognized as the aetiological agent of epidemic polyarthritis, now more commonly known as Ross River virus disease to distinguish it from other viruses causing similar symptoms, and sometimes colloquially but erroneously as Ross River fever. It is the most common arboviral disease in Australia, with between 4000 and 8000 cases reported annually. Epidemic polyarthritis as a disease entity was first described in 1928 following unusual epidemics in New South Wales (NSW). Subsequent epidemics occurred in troops stationed in the Northern Territory and Queensland during the Second World War (1939–1945). Serological studies carried out during an epidemic in south-eastern Australia, using Bebaru virus as antigen (Bebaru virus is a Group A arbovirus, later classified as an alphavirus), strongly indicated that the causative agent was an arbovirus. Shortly afterwards the virus was isolated from *Ochlerotatus*[1] *vigilax* mosquitoes trapped in 1959 at the Ross River near Townsville in Queensland.

Distribution

The virus occurs in all states of Australia including Tasmania. A number of cases have been diagnosed in Papua New Guinea, and one isolate has been obtained from mosquitoes there. The virus has not been isolated from the Solomon Islands, although seroepidemiological studies have suggested that it is present. A single large disease outbreak occurred in 1979–1980 in a number of Pacific islands, including Fiji, Samoa, Cook Islands, French Polynesia, New Caledonia and Wallis and Futuna, but the virus did not become established and disappeared in 1981 shortly after the epidemic subsided. Virus was isolated from mosquitoes and from viraemic human cases during the outbreak.

Virus

Ross River virus is an alphavirus with a positive single-stranded RNA genome of about 11,650–11,875 nucleotides. In common with other alphaviruses, the 5′ two-thirds of the genome encodes the four non-structural proteins (nsP1, nsP2, nsP3 and nsP4), whereas the 3′ one-third of the genome encodes the structural proteins (C-E1–6K-E2). Ross River virus is closely related antigenically to chikungunya and Getah viruses in the Semliki Forest serological complex (see entries). The complete sequence has been elucidated for several strains of RR virus, and an infectious clone has been constructed to investigate aspects of replication and immunogenicity and for gene function studies.

Clinical symptoms and pathogenesis

The clinical disease occurs most commonly in adults from 20 to 50 years of age, with the highest incidence in the 30–40-year age group. Clinically apparent infections are rare in children. The incubation period may vary from 5 to 21 days but is usually 7–9 days. Onset is relatively sudden and the first symptom is usually joint pain. The disease is characterized by marked arthralgia and myalgia, with an arthritis in over 40% of patients. Anorexia, headache, photophobia, lymphadenopathy and sore throat may occur. Lethargy is common, and a fever is observed in up to about 50% of cases and a maculopapular rash in about 50% of the cases. The joints of the extremities are most commonly affected, but back involvement is also relatively frequent. Most patients report joint pain, with between 60 and 85% having stiff and swollen joints. Knees, wrists, ankles and the metacarpophalangeal and interphalangeal joints of the fingers are most commonly involved. The next most frequently involved joints are elbows, toes, tarsal joints, vertebral joints, shoulders and hips. Signs of joint involvement can vary from restricted joint movement to prominent swelling and tenderness. A rash can appear from about 11 days before to 15 days after the arthritis as pale, erythematous macules and papules, but may be vesicular. The rash is usually found on the limbs and trunk, but can occur less frequently on the face, palms of the hands or soles of the feet. Purpura can also be found, mainly on the limbs.

In some studies, about 50% of patients were sufficiently well to return to work within a month of the onset of symptoms, although a significant number still suffered residual arthralgia, with a few experiencing relapses for a year or more. However, other studies have suggested that symptoms may persist for much longer, with nearly 50% of patients still experiencing symptoms such as joint pains and stiffness after a year, sometimes with joint swelling. Symptoms and signs generally diminish over time, but may follow a relapsing course, and it is known that symptoms can persist for at least 6 years in a few patients. The persistent joint pain and tenderness is often accompanied by fatigue and myalgia, which may contribute significantly to the morbidity.

Most studies have shown that the rate of disease is about the same for men and for women. Subclinical infections may be common, particularly in endemic areas where infection occurs throughout the year.

The pathogenesis of acute and persistent RR virus infection has been investigated by studying aspirated synovial fluid. Cells in the aspirates were found to be largely mononuclear, with macrophages predominating in the early stages and small lymphocytes becoming the major cell type in later effusions. The persistence of virus-specific immunoglobulin M (IgM) antibodies for months after acute infection raises the question of whether there is ongoing antigenic challenge. Viral antigen can be detected by immunofluorescence in the cytoplasm of leucocytes aspirated from joint effusions during the first few days of clinical infection, and viral genomic sequences have been detected by reverse transcriptase–polymerase chain reaction (RT-PCR) in biopsy material

from cells of the synovial lining in two patients 5 weeks after onset of symptoms. However, RR virus has never been isolated from infected joints, and there is no evidence of immune complexes or complement activation in synovial fluid. Thus it has been believed that synovial tissue damage was caused by non-specific cytotoxic effector cells rather than cytotoxic T cells directed at RR virus. However, recent studies have indicated that RR virus is able to persist within macrophages, and thus may play a role in ongoing joint symptoms. Indeed, in a murine model system, treatment of mice with macrophage-toxic agents (e.g. silica) prior to RR virus infection completely abrogated disease symptoms without significantly affecting titres of virus in organs.

The rash in Ross River virus disease is a cell-mediated immune response to viral antigen in epidermal cells.

Diagnosis

Serological tests are the mainstay of laboratory diagnosis. Most cases are diagnosed by detection of specific IgM antibodies, usually by a capture enzyme-linked immunosorbent assay (ELISA). Diagnoses are frequently made on a single serum specimen, and thus can only be regarded as presumptive, as IgM antibodies can often persist for months and may represent past infection. To confirm a case of RR virus infection, a second serum specimen is needed to demonstrate seroconversion or a greater than fourfold rise in IgG antibodies. False-positive IgM responses have been reported with some commercially available tests, and a false positive should be considered when specific IgG antibody is absent. Immunoglobulin G antibodies nearly always appear within 10 days of the onset of symptoms, although occasionally their appearance can be delayed by a month or more. Virus isolation is rarely attempted, as the period of viraemia is relatively short and, in most cases, viraemia is over by the time a patient presents at the surgery. Viral genomic sequences can be detected and identified by RT-PCR from serum specimens, but is not usually employed in diagnostic laboratories because of the cost and labour involved.

Transmission

The natural wildlife transmission cycles of RR virus are believed to be between macropods and various mosquito species, depending on the season and the geographical location. The major vertebrate hosts of RR virus are believed to be macropods, especially Eastern grey kangaroos (*Macropus giganteus*) and Western grey kangaroos (*Macropus fuliginosus*), but a number of other domestic and wild animals have been implicated on serological and/or epidemiological grounds, including horses, Rabbits (*Oryctolagus cuniculus*) and Flying foxes (Fruit bats) (*Pteropus* species). Two virus isolations have been made from Wallabies (*Macropus* species), a single virus from a horse and three isolations from birds. Despite these latter avian isolates, there has been no subsequent evidence to suggest that birds are involved in RR virus transmission cycles in nature. There is also evidence that humans may act as vertebrate hosts in urban transmission cycles to a limited extent, but transmission cannot be maintained.

Ross River virus has been isolated from over 30 species of mosquitoes, although only a few have been shown to be involved in natural transmission cycles. The most important mosquito species involved in RR virus transmission cycles are the two salt-marsh-breeding species *Ochlerotatus vigilax* and *Ochlerotatus camptorhynchus*, particularly in coastal areas, and the freshwater-breeding species *Culex annulirostris* in inland areas, especially in semi-permanent water. *Ochlerotatus vigilax* is found from southern NSW northwards around the north of the continent, and down the Western Australia (WA) coast to south of Perth, whereas *O. camptorhynchus* occurs along the southern coastline from Gippsland in Victoria to just north of Perth. Other species may be important in specific localities or conditions. Thus *Ochlerotatus notoscriptus* and *Coquillettidia linealis* are important vectors in urban areas, while *Ochlerotatus normanensis*, the *Ochlerotatus sagax* group, *Ochlerotatus pseudonormanensis*, and *Ochlerotatus*

bancroftianus and other temporary ground-pool-breeding species are important for initiating outbreaks following heavy rainfall events and flooding. Indeed, RR virus is transmitted seasonally by different mosquito species in different ecological and climatic situations. In coastal areas of northern and north-eastern Australia, Ross River virus disease exhibits an endemic pattern of disease, with virus activity and human cases occurring all year, but, elsewhere in Australia and particularly in southern areas, virus activity tends to be seasonal and epidemic, although low levels of virus transmission can be detected in some areas all year round.

Epidemiology and ecology

Epidemics and outbreaks are driven by environmental conditions, especially heavy rainfall events and flooding, and by tidal inundation of salt-marshes. Epidemic activity is also dependent on the recruitment of sufficient numbers of non-immune vertebrate hosts, and this may be a limiting factor in the genesis of epidemics in successive years, even when environmental conditions favour mosquito breeding. However, modelling to account for the effects of climate change have proved difficult, because of the importance of local rather than regional climatic conditions. There is strong evidence to indicate that virus can persist in the environment during adverse conditions by vertical transmission in desiccation-resistant mosquito aedine eggs.

There was a significant increase in the number of cases of Ross River virus disease reported throughout Australia in the 1980s, due largely to a combination of increased general medical practitioner awareness and of improvements and availability of diagnostic reagents. Ross River virus disease is a notifiable disease in Australia. However, the number of reported cases is probably a significant underestimate because of under-presentation and under-reporting. In the 8-year period between 1991 and 1998, over 38,000 cases of Ross River virus disease were reported, at an annual average of about 4800. The highest number of cases was 7800 in 1996, and the lowest 2700 in 1995. The national annual notification rate of reported cases varied between 14.4 and 50.3 per 100,000 population. However, at a state or regional level incidence rates are much higher, particularly following epidemic activity. Thus, in an outbreak in South Australia, the regional rate was 670 per 100,000. In endemic areas with year-round transmission, annual incidence rates can exceed 350 per 100,000.

Minor variations among RR virus strains have been found with comparisons of biological properties, such as mouse pathogenicity, antigenicity (kinetic haemagglutination inhibition (HI)) and genetic variation (restriction enzyme maps of complementary DNA (cDNA), sequence variation), but none of these properties has been related to differences of medical significance. Nevertheless, a number of medical practitioners have noted that signs and symptoms varied in different outbreaks, suggesting that strains differing in pathogenicity occurred naturally. The best example of this was in the 1979–1980 outbreak in the Pacific, where, for the first time, virus could be readily isolated from sera collected from patients. This may have been because of a delayed antibody response to the Pacific virus strains, or because the course of disease was biphasic in the acute stage in some patients. These patients developed a second clinical phase after a short period of remission, which might coincide with the appearance of detectable HI antibody. Thus virus could be isolated because of the earlier presentation during the first acute phase. This differs from the disease in Australian patients, who have a clinically silent first phase, and, by the time they present, a detectable antibody response would normally have occurred. Although sequencing parts of the genomes of Pacific island RR virus strains revealed amino acid substitutions, there was no evidence to link specific substitutions with any changes in the disease. Genetic variants (or topotypes) have been described in different areas, which have been useful in molecular epidemiological investigations, such as outbreak origins. Thus two major topotypes have been found in western and eastern Australia, respectively, with the eastern topotype being

associated with the major outbreak in the Pacific in 1979–1980. Thus it is believed that the virus was introduced into the Pacific through a viraemic tourist from eastern Australia. A third topotype, found only in north-eastern Australia and including the prototype strain of RR virus, has not been detected since the mid-1970s.

Treatment

No treatment is available for Ross River virus disease, but aspirin or non-steroidal anti-inflammatory drugs can be used for relief of joint pains.

Prevention and control

Prevention has been largely directed at behavioural changes, with local warnings disseminated when epidemic activity is predicted. These warnings suggest the use of insect repellents and wearing long sleeves and long trousers at dusk and dawn. Adult mosquito control measures using insecticides are rarely used because of the difficulty in applying such agents effectively in most settings and because of environmental concerns. Larvicides have been employed successfully in certain habitats close to human habitation. Runnelling and improved drainage have been important in decreasing mosquito breeding in salt-marsh habitats.

A killed vaccine has been suggested but too many difficulties remain unresolved before a vaccine can be contemplated. These include the reports of immune enhancement, improved understanding of the pathogenesis of the disease, recent studies of the persistence of the virus in macrophages and synovial cells and the choice of virus strain for vaccine development.

Infections of animals with Ross River virus

Ross River virus only causes disease naturally in humans and possibly horses, although some strains of laboratory mice and hamsters are susceptible to lethal infections. The evidence for disease in horses requires further investigation, but, as RR virus is very closely related to the alphavirus Getah virus (see entry), a known equine pathogen, it may not be altogether surprising that disease may occur in horses. There was a suggestion from serological studies that RR virus infection of horses may lead to muscle and joint stiffness, reluctance to move, leg swelling, ataxia and nervous disease. Subsequent studies in Victoria and Tasmania demonstrated a rising ELISA IgG antibody titre in horses presenting with reluctance to move, pyrexia, swollen legs, abdominal discomfort or mild colic, inappetence and shifting lameness. Ross River virus was also isolated from a horse exhibiting ataxia with muscle rigidity and twitching. This animal was also hypersensitive to sound and had a rapid heart rate, with occasional arrhythmia. Inoculation of horses with RR virus has given equivocal results, with the animals exhibiting a vague inappetence, mild transient pyrexia and a reluctance to move. It is interesting to note that RR virus was also isolated more frequently from traps, such as carbon dioxide-baited light-traps, set in locations close to horses than in traps placed elsewhere during surveillance studies in WA.

Note

[1] *Ochlerotatus* was formerly a subgenus of *Aedes*.

Selected bibliography

Burness, A.T.H., Pardoe, I., Faragher, S,G., Vrati, S. and Dalgarno, L. (1988) Genetic stability of Ross River virus during epidemic spread in non-immune humans. *Virology* 167, 639–643.

Flexman, J.P., Smith, D.W., Mackenzie, J.S., Fraser, R.E., Bass, S., Hueston, L., Lindsay, M.D.A. and Cunningham, A.L. (1998) A comparison of the diseases caused by Ross River virus and Barmah Forest virus. *Medical Journal of Australia* 169, 159–163.

Fraser, J.R.E. (1986) Epidemic polyarthritis and Ross River virus. *Clinics in Rheumatic Diseases* 12, 369–388.

Kay, B.H. and Aaskov, J.G. (1989) Ross River virus (epidemic polyarthritis). In: Monath, T.P. (ed.) *The Arboviruses: Epidemiology and Ecology*, Vol. IV. CRC Press, Boca Raton, Florida, pp. 93–112.

Lindsay, M.D., Broom, A.K., Wright, A.E., Johansen, C.A. and Mackenzie, J.S. (1993) Ross River virus isolations from mosquitoes in arid regions of Western Australia: implication of vertical transmission as a means of persistence of the virus. *American Journal of Tropical Medicine and Hygiene* 49, 686–696.

Mackenzie J.S. and Smith, D.W. (1996) Mosquitoborne viruses and epidemic polyarthritis. *Medical Journal of Australia* 164, 90–93.

Mackenzie, J.S., Lindsay, M.D., Coelen, R.J., Broom, A.K., Hall, R.A. and Smith, D.W. (1994) Arboviruses causing human disease in the Australasian region. *Archives of Virology* 136, 447–467.

Marshall, I.D. and Miles, J.A.R. (1984) Ross River virus and epidemic polyarthritis. *Current Topics in Vector Research* 2, 31–56.

Russell, R.C. (1994) Ross River virus: disease trends and vector ecology in Australia. *Bulletin of the Society for Vector Ecology* 19, 73–81.

Russell, R.C. (1995) Arboviruses and their vectors in Australia: an update on the ecology and epidemiology of some mosquito-borne arboviruses. *Reviews of Medical and Veterinary Entomology* 83, 141–158.

Sammels, L. Coelen, R.J., Lindsay, M.D. and Mackenzie, J.S. (1995) Geographic distribution and evolution of Ross River virus in Australia and the Pacific Islands. *Virology* 212, 20–29.

Russian spring–summer encephalitis *see* **Tick-borne encephalitis.**

St Louis encephalitis

Laura D. Kramer

St Louis encephalitis (SLE) virus was first recognized as the cause of central nervous system disease in the USA, when it was isolated from brain tissue of deceased humans during an epidemic in St Louis, Missouri, in 1933. Over 1000 cases were reported in people resident in the area. Extensive breeding of two domestic mosquitoes, *Culex pipiens* and *Culex quinquefasciatus*, was noted in the urban and suburban environs of Missouri, Kentucky, Ohio and Illinois, where the disease occurred. The causative agent was first isolated from field-collected *Culex tarsalis* mosquitoes in Yakima Valley, Washington State, in 1941 by W.McD. Hammon and W.C. Reeves. Subsequent intermittent epidemic transmission was followed by a relative lull from 1969 to 1973, after which the largest and most widespread outbreak occurred in the Ohio River Valley from 1974 to 1975. There were 1815 documented cases from 30 states and the District of Columbia, but the most intensive activity occurred in the east north central and east south central states. This trend continued through 1998, as is evident from an analysis of the distribution of 4478 St Louis encephalitis cases by state from 1964 to 1998 (Fig. 1). Large outbreaks have occurred approximately every 10 years.

Distribution

St Louis encephalitis virus is widely distributed throughout the Americas, having been isolated in Canada, the USA, Mexico, Central and South America and the Caribbean islands. In the continental USA, St Louis encephalitis has occurred, in both endemic and epidemic forms, in all but five states. A small number of human cases of St Louis encephalitis have been reported in Central and South America, but no large outbreaks in the region have been attributed to this virus. St Louis encephalitis virus strains isolated from different sections of the USA have phenotypic variations in their virulence for mice and monkeys, and they differ in their ability to produce viraemia in House sparrows (*Passer domesticus*) and chickens and in their vector competence in *C. quinquefasciatus*.

Phylogenetic analyses indicate that SLE virus isolates from tropical and temperate America, including the USA, Mexico, the

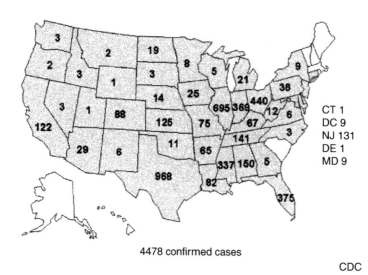

CT 1
DC 9
NJ 131
DE 1
MD 9

4478 confirmed cases

CDC

Fig. 1. Human St Louis encephalitis cases by state, in the USA, 1964–1998. CT, Connecticut; DC, District of Columbia; NJ, New Jersey; DE, Delaware; MD, Maryland.

Caribbean and Central and South America, form a monophyletic group, indicating a common ancestor. Isolates generally tend to cluster according to geographical origin: isolates from Panama and South America predominantly form two large groupings, whereas isolates from the USA form two additional major groups. Several South and Central American strains are more closely related to strains isolated in the USA than to other South American strains; e.g. one isolate each from Mexico and Panama are closely related to two Tampa Bay, Florida, isolates, and an isolate from Brazil is closely related to three isolates from Texas. The USA isolates were also not strictly grouped according to geographical source. For example, some California isolates were closely related to Texas or midwestern isolates, and a Florida isolate was closely related to three isolates from Maryland. The results of these phylogenetic analyses indicated that SLE virus is predominantly maintained locally, but has occasionally been transported between areas, both within and outside the USA.

Virus

St Louis encephalitis virus is a mosquito-borne virus and a member of the genus *Flavivirus* in the family Flaviviridae. Along with other important human pathogens, such as Murray Valley encephalitis (MVE), West Nile (WN) and Japanese encephalitis (JE) viruses (see entries), SLE virus is a member of the JE serocomplex, and is the only member of this serocomplex that is endemic in the Nearctic north of Mexico, with the possible exception of WN virus, introduced into New York City in 1999. The members of the JE serocomplex are related mostly through broad serological inter-relationships and cross-react extensively with each other.

The genome of the flaviviruses is single-stranded, linear, positive-sense infectious RNA, approximately 10,800 nucleotides long and composed of one open-reading frame. The 5′ terminus has a methylated nucleotide cap, and the 3′ terminus has no poly-(A) tract. Structural proteins are located at the 5′ end of the genome and the non-structural genes, involved in viral replication, at the 3′ end of the genome in the order 5′ C-PrM-E-NS1-NS2A-NS2B-NS3-NS4A-NS4B-NS5 3′. The non-structural proteins include a protease, a helicase and a polymerase. The virion structural proteins are glycosylated. The virus particles are uniform in shape, spherical, enveloped and 40–60 nm in diameter, with glycoprotein surface projections. Antigenic determinants on the envelope are type-specific and group-specific and are involved in antibody-mediated neutralization. The virion contains an icosahedral nucleocapsid, 25–30 nm in diameter.

Clinical symptoms

Humans

Multiple environmental, biological and social factors contribute to disease occurrence. In naïve populations in the eastern USA the incidence of disease in persons >60 years old is 5–40 times higher than in the 0–9-year-old age group. As many as 30% of the elderly die following infection. However, the majority of infections in other age groups are subclinical or result in mild illness. Having an outdoor occupation which increases exposure represents another risk factor. The incubation period between infection and the onset of clinical symptoms is usually 5–15 days. Most people who are infected with SLE virus have no symptoms or only a mild non-specific flu-like illness. However, in some individuals, especially the elderly, SLE virus can cause serious illness that affects the central nervous system. Symptoms often include a rapid onset of headache, high fever, stiff neck, disorientation and tremor. Coma, convulsions and paralysis may also occur. Clinical syndromes, besides febrile headache, include encephalitis and aseptic meningitis. Convalescence can take as long as 3 years in 30–50% of the cases, with long-term sequelae in approximately 20% of these patients, particularly old and acutely ill people.

Other vertebrates

Domestic animals and horses do not usually develop clinical symptoms.

Diagnosis

In fatal cases, virus may be recovered from suspensions of brain tissue by intracerebral inoculation of suckling mice; however, isolation from serum or cerebral spinal fluid (CSF) is unusual. Diagnosis is usually accomplished by demonstration of immunoglobulin M (IgM) antibodies in CSF or by a fourfold rise in IgG antibody titre between acute and convalescent sera. Serological diagnosis may be confounded by cross-reaction with other flaviviruses. Sera can be initially screened by the broadly reacting haemagglutination inhibition (HI) assay or enzyme-linked immunosorbent assay (ELISA) tests, which detect group-reactive antigens. The most specific assay is the neutralization test; neutralizing antibody titres following the first infection with SLE virus rise rapidly the week after onset and persist over the lifetime of the person. A diagnosis can be made by demonstrating a fourfold rise in neutralizing antibody titre between acute and convalescent sera. Complement-fixing (CF) antibodies develop in the second week, peak after 3–4 weeks and then decrease to low levels by 9–12 months. Evidence of CF antibody in a single serum sample indicates recent infection. The presence of IgM antibodies, which appear in the serum by 4 days after onset, also suggests recent infection. However, approximately one-quarter of all patients demonstrate IgM antibodies even 1 year after infection.

SLE Transmission Cycle

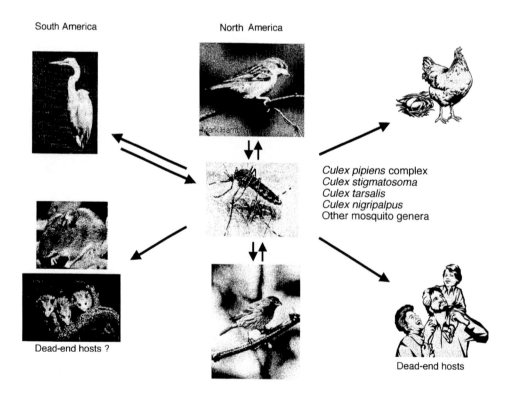

South America   North America

Culex pipiens complex
Culex stigmatosoma
Culex tarsalis
Culex nigripalpus
Other mosquito genera

Dead-end hosts ?   Dead-end hosts

Fig. 2. St Louis encephalitis transmission cycles.

Transmission
Virus cycle
In the USA, SLE virus is maintained and amplified by horizontal transmission in an enzootic cycle involving wild birds, primarily passeriformes and columbiformes, and *Culex* mosquitoes (Fig. 2). Specific mosquito vectors vary regionally. Humans may acquire the infection tangentially, but are dead-end hosts. On the Gulf Coast and in the Ohio and Mississippi River Valleys, two *C. pipiens* complex mosquitoes, *C. pipiens* and *C. quinquefasciatus*, are the primary vectors. In these regions, SLE virus occurs in both urban and suburban areas. In contrast, in the western USA, SLE virus occurs more frequently in rural settings, especially in heavily irrigated areas, where *C. tarsalis* is the primary vector. Urban transmission has been recognized in the west since the 1984 outbreak in Los Angeles, and *C. quinquefasciatus* and *Culex stigmatosoma* may play a secondary role in these environments. A third distinct SLE virus cycle occurs in Florida, where *Culex nigripalpus* is the primary vector.

Less is known of the natural transmission cycle in Mexico, the Caribbean and Central and South America, where SLE virus has been isolated from *Culex* species, including *C. quinquefasciatus*, *Culex* species of the subgenus *Melaniconion*, and *C. nigripalpus*, as well as species in other genera, such as *Mansonia*, *Haemagogus* and *Sabethes*. Birds are presumed to be the primary vertebrate host in the cycle, but conclusive studies have not been conducted. In South America, there are a number of isolates from mammals other than humans, including *Calomys musculinus* (Vesper mouse), *Mus musculus* (House mouse), *Akodon* species (field mice) and other rodents, and *Didelphis marsupialis* (Opossum), but it is not known whether these are dead-end or amplification hosts.

Factors that affect the transmission cycle include mosquito population genetics and densities, virus strain and environmental factors, such as temperature. The duration of the transmission season is delineated by temperatures that permit viral replication in the mosquito host and by photoperiods conducive to vector host-feeding activity. The length of extrinsic incubation in the mosquito host decreases as the temperature of extrinsic incubation increases above the thermal minimum of 17°C.

Infection in the arthropod host
The replication and dissemination of SLE virus has been characterized in *Culex* mosquitoes. The genetics of both the virus and the mosquito influence the transmission of virus. Interspecies variation in susceptibility to peroral infection with SLE virus has been demonstrated. *Culex stigmatosoma* was found to be more susceptible to infection with SLE virus than were most populations of *C. tarsalis*, followed by *C. quinquefasciatus*; *Culex erythrothorax* was refractory to infection. The extrinsic incubation period before which 50% of the infected mosquitoes were able to transmit virus was delayed for *C. quinquefasciatus*, from 14 to 21 days as compared with *C. tarsalis*. It is thought that the delay in ability to transmit is associated with a delay in dissemination of virus from the infected mesenteron into the haemocoel. The number of infected cells in the mesenteron of *C. pipiens* infected with SLE virus increased progressively from day 6 to day 12, reaching a maximum of one infected cell in five cells examined. Salivary glands were initially infected 8 days after infection, with increasing numbers of virus particles through day 32, the end of the experiment. This explains the observation that transmission rates increase with increasing length of extrinsic incubation; it has been observed that once a *Culex* mosquito becomes infected after ingestion of SLE virus, it will probably transmit virus if allowed to incubate for a sufficient period of time. None the less, there were never more than one in 20 epithelial cells infected in a particular site of the salivary gland.

A homoeostatic situation is established in the mosquito which causes viral replication to plateau and not increase without limit. Comparative vector competence studies with different geographical strains of SLE virus and geographical strains of *Culex* mosquitoes demonstrated little evidence of variation in infectivity for females of the same mosquito population, but did reveal differences in transmission between different virus strains. These differences were most probably a result of differences in replication of virus, because significant differences were noted in virus titres of transmitting versus non-transmitting females.

Infection in the vertebrate host

St Louis encephalitis virus produces a cytopathic effect in various continuous and primary vertebrate cell lines, such as baby hamster kidney cells (BHK-21), monkey kidney cells (VERO and LLC-MK2), porcine kidney, Pekin duck kidney and chick embryo. In vertebrate cell culture, the virus replicates at a slower rate than do alphaviruses. There is a latent phase of approximately 11 h, followed 12 h later by the production of maximal titres of virus. Infectious viral RNA is produced as early as 6 h after infection and continues at low levels until the formation of virions begins. Replication in arthropod cells is usually long-term and inapparent. A wide variety of mammals and birds can be infected experimentally with SLE virus. Infections range from asymptomatic to lethal, with the outcome dependent on age of host, route of infection, virulence of isolate and dose on infection. St Louis encephalitis viraemia usually occurs in birds within 18–48 h after the mosquito bite and usually lasts no longer than 3–4 days. Persistence of SLE virus for 1–5 months in brains of mice has been reported.

St Louis encephalitis virus strains from different hosts and geographical locations differ in biological characteristics, such as virulence and the ability to replicate in mosquito vectors. In general, virus strains isolated from birds were highly virulent and disseminated from the mesenteron of the mosquito vector, whereas SLE virus isolates from rodents and carnivores were attenuated (as determined by mouse inoculation), indicating that these vertebrates might be dead-end hosts.

Epidemiology

St Louis encephalitis usually appears in the summer, with peak incidence in August–September. Several studies of both urban and rural forms of St Louis encephalitis have shown recurrence of transmission of the virus in a single geographical area, e.g. in Texas and California, suggesting that the virus is maintained locally from year to year. Phylogenetic analysis of isolates from the San Joaquin Valley of California over a period of more than 34 years also indicated local persistence of virus, although the mechanism(s) by which the virus cycle is maintained during periods when active transmission is not detected is not known. The most likely hypotheses proposed to explain the maintenance of SLE virus over adverse seasons and years include: (i) local maintenance in arthropod vectors, either through vertical transmission or persistence in diapausing adults; (ii) reactivation of virus in chronically infected vertebrate hosts; and/or (iii) annual reintroduction of the virus from tropical and subtropical areas by migratory birds.

Vertical transmission in mosquitoes

In the laboratory, SLE virus was transmitted vertically to <1% of the progeny of perorally and parenterally infected female *Culex* and *Ochlerotatus*[1] mosquitoes, including natural vectors. The low rate of filial infection observed with SLE virus may be related to the mechanism by which eggs become infected – i.e. virus enters through the micropyle of the fully formed egg rather than through infected ovarian tissues. In addition, a temperature-dependent barrier to trans-stadial transmission has been observed in some *Ochlerotatus* species, in that higher vertical transmission rates of SLE virus have been observed in larvae reared at 18°C rather than 27°C. The low rate of vertical transmission would allow for short-term persistence of SLE virus, but probably not long-term persistence without significant recruitment from horizontally infected females.

Persistence in diapausing adult Culex *species*

Field studies conducted over a 5-year period (1950–1955) in Kern County, California, yielded isolates of SLE virus from *C. tarsalis* collected in June to September, with one isolate being made in March. In the laboratory, infection persisted in and was transmitted by experimentally infected *C. tarsalis* maintained outdoors in Kern County, for 3–8 months after peroral infection. However, the mosquitoes infected by feeding on viraemic chicks were not in reproductive diapause. In the field, SLE virus was isolated from overwintering *C. pipiens* in Maryland; however, the method of infection of these adult mosquitoes was not known. Related experiments indicated that this species may undergo gonotrophic dissociation and possibly become infected through feeding on viraemic birds during the autumn.

Chronic infection in birds

No infectious SLE virus was isolated from more than 3000 wild birds of 84 species collected from October through February over a 5-year period in Kern County, California, or recovered from more than 350 experimentally infected birds. Recent experiments have detected possible chronic infections in experimentally infected House finches (*Carpodacus mexicanus*), using a reverse transcriptase–polymerase chain reaction (RT-PCR), but recrudescence of infectious virus has not been detected.

Alternative vectors

There is no evidence that alternative arthropods, such as ticks or mites, contribute to the maintenance of SLE virus in nature. These arthropods become incidentally infected when feeding on viraemic nestlings, but they are incompetent vectors.

Alternative vertebrate hosts

Precipitin tests on more than 2000 blood-engorged *C. tarsalis* collected in November through April from an area with enzootic SLE virus activity identified 98% of the blood meals as avian in origin. Therefore, it is unlikely that other vertebrates are involved in the virus cycle.

Reintroduction – bird flyways

Although spring bird migrations are generally completed before amplification of SLE virus is detected in the USA, avian transport of SLE virus may nevertheless be important in viral dispersal. The majority of birds observed to move between the Mississippi and Pacific flyways, or between California and Texas, are species of Anseriformes (especially Northern pintails (*Anas acuta*), Mallards (*Anas platyrhynchos*), Green-winged teal (*Anas crecca*) and Redheads (*Aythya americana*)), largely because they are captured during hunts, but species of Columbiformes (especially Mourning doves (*Zenaidura macroura*)) have also been banded and recaptured in the three flyways.

Mourning doves provide an excellent potential means of viral transport, because these birds have been observed to travel, at least occasionally, between the Mississippi and Pacific flyways, as well as between the Rocky Mountain and Pacific flyways, and to migrate to the Gulf states and Mexico for the winter. Approximately equal numbers of birds appear to travel to and from California, except for the Northern pintail, which was predominantly banded in California and recaptured either in the Mississippi flyway or in Texas. There has also been considerable movement of birds noted between Texas and the Mississippi flyway. Therefore, migratory birds may provide a means of viral movement and reintroduction.

Treatment

There is no vaccine which protects against SLE virus infection. Treatment of the illness is supportive.

Control

Changes in human behaviour, such as the use of air-conditioning and television watching at dusk, which keeps people indoors, may have led to decreased infection and immunity in areas where the virus is being transmitted enzootically. None the less, surveillance activities must be vigilant because of the unpredictable and intermittent occurrences of outbreaks.

Prevention and control of the disease is accomplished through proactive surveillance of virus amplification within the enzootic cycle and timely vector control. Active surveillance is a collaboration between state and local health departments and mosquito control districts. National expenditures for mosquito control activities approach US$150 million, with SLE virus surveillance and control activities 0–70% of the total, but this figure varies by state. Deterioration of inner cities and global warming may increase vector abundance and transmission.

Note

[1]   *Ochlerotatus* was formerly a subgenus of *Aedes*.

Selected bibliography

Kramer, L.D. and Chandler, L.J. (2001) Phylogenetic analysis of the envelope gene of St. Louis encephalitis virus. *Archives of Virology* (in press).

Monath, T.P. (1980) *St. Louis Encephalitis*. American Public Health Association, Washington, DC, 680 pp.

Monath, T.P. and Heinz, F.X. (1996) Flaviviruses. In: Fields B.N., Knipe, D.M. and Howley, P.M. (eds) *Fields Virology*, Vol. 1, 3rd edn. Lippincott-Raven, Philadelphia, pp. 961–1034.

Reeves, W.C. (ed.) (1990) *Epidemiology and Control of Mosquito-borne Arboviruses in California,1943–1987*. Californian Mosquito and Vector Control Association, Sacramento, California, 508 pp.

Schlesinger, S. and Schlesinger, M. J. (1986) *The Togaviridae and Flaviviridae*. Plenum Press, New York, 687 pp.

Tsai, T. F. and Mitchell, C.J. (1989) St. Louis encephalitis. In: Monath, T.P. (ed.) *The Arboviruses: Epidemiology and Ecology*, Vol IV. CRC Press, Boca Raton, Florida, pp. 113–144.

***Salmonella* infections** *see* **Flies** *and* **Cockroaches.**

San Angelo virus

Bruce F. Eldridge

San Angelo (SA) virus is a mosquito-borne arbovirus transmitted to medium- to large-sized mammals in the south-western USA. The virus has been used extensively as a model for transovarial transmission of arboviruses in mosquitoes; however, it is of no known public health importance, although, in one instance, neutralizing antibodies were detected in humans. Although well studied in the laboratory, there have been few studies of the natural ecology of this virus.

Distribution

Virus isolations from mosquitoes have been made from Arizona, Colorado, New Mexico and Texas, USA (Fig. 1).

Virus

San Angelo virus is a member of the genus *Bunyavirus* and the California serogroup. Along with California encephalitis, Tahyna and La Crosse viruses (see entries), it is classified as a subtype of the California encephalitis virus division of the serogroup. San Angelo virus was first isolated in 1958 from a pool of *Anopheles pseudopunctipennis* mosquitoes collected near San Angelo, Tom Green County, Texas. Viral cultures injected into mice or baby chicks cause central nervous system impairment and death. San Angelo virus has been used as a model pathogen to study transovarial transmission in various species of mosquito. It has been shown to produce stable infections in germ cells in *Aedes albopictus*. The genomic sequence of the small segment of the SA viral genome has been determined.

Clinical symptoms

No symptomatic infections have been reported in humans. A rise in antibody titre

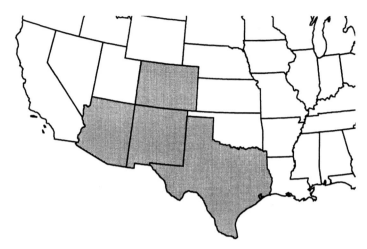

Fig. 1. Known distribution of San Angelo virus in the south-western USA.

to La Crosse viral antigen by complement fixation test was detected in a 3-year-old child from Texas. The antibodies were later shown to be specific for SA virus by the neutralization test.

Diagnosis

Confirmation of arboviral disease requires isolation of virus from an infected patient or a fourfold or greater increase in antibody titre between acute and convalescent human serum samples. Isolation of fully typed virus from mosquitoes or detection of antibodies in sentinel mammals may demonstrate enzootic viral activity.

Transmission

The natural vertebrate hosts of SA virus are unknown. Neutralizing antibody has been detected in Coyotes (*Canis latrans*), Raccoons (*Procyon lotor*), Opossums (*Didelphis marsupialis*) and White-tailed deer (*Odoileus virginianus*). In one study, neutralizing antibody was detected in one of 255 human serum samples tested.

San Angelo virus has been isolated from only a few species of mosquitoes. The original isolate was from *A. pseudopunctipennis*; other isolates have been made from *Ochlerotatus*[1] *atlanticus* (or *Ochlerotatus infirmatus*), *Psorophora columbiae*, *Psorophora signipennis* and *Psorophora ferox*. There are insufficient numbers of reports of virus isolation from wild-caught mosquitoes to permit an analysis of the relative importance of these species as vectors.

The relative importance of horizontal transmission between mosquitoes and mammals in SA virus ecology is unknown.

Control

Usually none.

Note

[1]   *Ochlerotatus* was formerly a subgenus of *Aedes*.

Selected bibliography

Calisher, C.H. and Thompson, W.H. (eds) (1983) *California Serogroup Viruses*. Progress in Clinical and Biological Research, Vol. 123. Alan R. Liss, New York, 399 pp.

Karabatsos, N. (ed.) (1985) *International Catalogue of Arboviruses Including Certain Other Viruses of Vertebrates*, 3rd edn. American Society of Tropical Medicine and Hygiene, San Antonio, Texas, 1147 pp.

Parkin, W.E., Hammon, W.McD. and Sather, G.D. (1972) Review of current epidemiological literature on viruses of the California arbovirus group. *American Journal of Tropical Medicine and Hygiene* 21, 964–978.

Sand-flies *see* **Phlebotomine sand-flies.**

Sandfly fever *see* **Phlebotomus fevers.**

Scrub typhus

Daniel Strickman

Scrub typhus remains the most common English designation for symptomatic infection with the bacteria, *Orientia tsutsugamushi* (formerly *Rickettsia tsutsugamushi*, but raised to a separate genus in 1995 based on major differences in the genome, cell wall characteristics and antigenicity). Various authors have attempted to popularize other names for the disease (e.g. chigger-borne rickettsiosis, tsutsugamushi disease, Japanese river fever, mite-borne typhus), because transmission is not restricted to 'scrub' habitats (i.e. non-forested secondary vegetation), nor is the aetiological agent closely related to the organisms causing epidemic typhus (*Rickettsia prowazekii*) and endemic typhus (*Rickettsia typhi*) (see entries).

    Good estimates of prevalence are unavailable over most of the range of scrub typhus because of the disease's protean symptomatology, formerly difficult laboratory diagnosis and tendency to affect rural populations that are distant from sophisticated medical care. The best indications of the potential burden of human suffering from this disease come from frightening accounts of mortality in Japan and New Guinea during the pre-antibiotic era, the documented high incidence in Allied soldiers during the Second World War (1939–1945) in certain locations (Myanmar, Australasian islands and Pacific islands) and organized studies in Thailand and Malaysia showing that up to 20% of all fevers in some areas was caused by scrub typhus.

Distribution

The disease affects people in a large geographical area sometimes called the 'scrub typhus triangle', with apices in Pakistan, Primorye (south-eastern Siberia) and New Zealand. Reports from Africa remain unconfirmed and uncertain (Fig. 1). This geographical range corresponds to the distribution of the major vector species of chigger (leptotrombiculid) mites. Biogeographically, *O. tsutsugamushi* appears

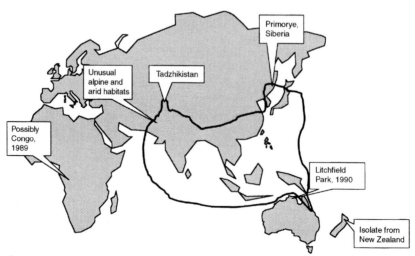

Fig. 1. Distribution of scrub typhus, showing the major transmission areas within the so-called 'scrub typhus triangle'.

to be centred in South-East Asia, which is also the area of greatest diversity of *Leptotrombidium* mites and their principal rodent hosts in the genus *Rattus*.

Pathogen

Orientia are obligate intracellular bacteria in the order *Rickettsiales*, family *Rickettsiaceae*. They are Gram-negative, short rods 0.5–0.8 μm in diameter and 1.2–3.0 μm long. *Orientia tsutsugamushi* is characterized by a soft cell wall, which, unlike members of the genus *Rickettsia*, lacks peptidoglycan and lipopolysaccharide and has the outer leaflet of the cell wall thicker than the inner leaflet. The bacteria grow by binary fission (doubling time 9–18 h) in the cytoplasm of host cells without the formation of a distinct vacuole. In at least some host membranes, however, naked bacterial particles are observed in tissue culture. The major outer membrane protein antigens are 50–62 kDa, with the major human antigenic protein usually designated as the 56 kDa protein.

Orientia tsutsugamushi has almost always been characterized from mammalian cells, but can appear as a very different elongated (up to 4.0 μm long) form, with unique microtubular structures in the cells of chigger mites. Isolates of the rickettsia have been classified into eight basic serotypes (including the well-known Karp, Kato and Gilliam types) for many years, together with several more serotypes recently described from Japan and Korea. Recent work with genetic methods, however, has failed to show any correlation between genotypes and serotypes, raising much doubt about the value of phylogenetic interpretation of serotyping.

Clinical symptoms

Illness begins suddenly, an average of 12 days after an infective bite of a chigger mite, beginning with fever, headache and myalgia. The disease often progresses to include lymphadenopathy and conjunctival suffusion. Other common signs are a cough, rash and diarrhoea. The formation of an eschar (small, painless area of necrosis surrounded by reddened induration) at the site or sites of infective chigger bites is a much more specific sign, but the eschar is present in only about half of the cases and may be missed during medical examination. Approximately a week after the illness begins, a macular rash often appears on the trunk and progresses to a papular state also involving the extremities. Clinically, scrub typhus could be easily confused with Korean haemorrhagic fever (see Haemorrhagic fever with renal syndrome), malaria, dengue, Japanese encephalitis (see entries) or leptospirosis. Untreated, scrub typhus can progress to any of a number of serious and potentially mortal problems, including pulmonary oedema, pneumonitis, myocarditis, splenomegaly, hepatomegaly, renal dysfunction and impairment of the central nervous system (including deafness). If fatal, death usually occurs within 30 days; otherwise, untreated patients may experience a prolonged convalescence. Even with appropriate antibiotic treatment, patients may require 2 weeks of hospitalization. All infection-related pathology is completely reversible in patients who survive. Apparently, patients do not completely clear the infection, since isolations of the pathogen have been made from lymph glands up to a year after cessation of symptoms. The severity of illness depends greatly on the strain of *O. tsutsugamushi* and the immune status of the patient (heterologous protection for a few months after infection, homologous protection for 2–3 years after infection). Before the advent of effective antibiotics, mortality ranged as high as 50% in some outbreaks. In contrast, some strains in Japan produce either mild illness or asymptomatic infection.

Diagnosis

Clinical presentation

Despite the protean character of the disease, scrub typhus is often suspected based on initial presentation. The presence of an eschar on a febrile patient in an endemic area is highly suggestive. Even in the absence of an eschar, fever with a cough and lymphadenopathy should raise suspicion of the disease. Unfortunately, scrub typhus is sometimes only suspected following exclusion of similar diseases, such as dengue (when fever persists longer than 4–5 days), malaria (when antimalarials fail to reduce fever) and salmonellosis/shigellosis (when fluoroquinolones or sulfa drugs fail to stop diarrhoea and fever).

Serology

Although immunoglobulin M (IgM) antibodies may not be present until 5 days after the beginning of fever, serology is still useful for three reasons: first, many patients suffer with fever for at least several days before seeking medical care, thus presenting with positive serological tests; secondly, physicians need tools to continue to find a diagnosis after initiation of the wrong presumptive treatment; and, thirdly, retrospective proof of diagnosis builds statistics that raise the index of suspicion so that presumptive treatment is more likely to be successful in subsequent patients. The old serological test, called Weil–Felix, used *Proteus* antigens, which cross-react with IgM antibody from some rickettsial infections. Historically, the Weil–Felix test produced the first evidence that certain South-East Asian fevers were a form of rickettsial disease. Although this test is cheap and commercially available, it is not ideally sensitive for detection of scrub typhus. The modern standard, indirect immunofluorescence assay (IFA), is more accurate, but it depends on the availability of non-commercial reagents (the rickettsial antigens), a fluorescence microscope and highly trained technicians. A very similar test that has been used extensively in South-East Asia is the indirect immunoperoxidase (IIP) assay. This test avoids the complications of handling and detecting fluorogens, but the results can be somewhat more difficult to interpret than with IFA. A dot–blot assay is commercially available and registered in the USA, but involves the use of a heat-block or water-bath and requires about 2 h. This test is based on exposure of a nitrocellulose strip with spots of antigen to solutions of test serum, alkaline phosphatase-linked anti-human antibodies and a developing agent. A positive result is a colour change at the location of the antigen.

A newer assay, based on a medium in which all reagents are embedded in an absorbent material (commonly called a wicking assay), is also commercially available, but not yet registered in the USA. The test consists of a card with a shallow well, which receives a small sample of the test serum. This liquid moves by capillary action over conditioning reagents and a band of *Orientia* antigen, which is fixed in place. If specific antibodies are present in the serum, they bind to the antigen; other antibodies are carried past the antigen band. Another part of the card is folded against the antigen band, placing gold-labelled anti-human detection antibody against it. Human antibodies bound to the antigen then bind to the labelled detection antibodies, producing a colour reaction. It is almost as accurate as IFA, produces results in 15 min and does not require specialized equipment other than that necessary to produce a serum sample. Other serological tests include complement fixation, serum neutralization, Western blot and enzyme-linked immunosorbent assay (ELISA), but these assays have only been used for research purposes.

Genetic methods

Numerous investigators have used genetic methods to detect and analyse *O. tsutsugamushi*. Methods have ranged from sequencing of antigenic operons, comparison of sequences of 16s ribosomal DNA (rDNA), extensive restriction fragment length polymorphism (RFLP) analysis of antigenic and heat-shock protein operons and refinements to achieve practical detection in mammalian tissues and chigger mites. The DNA of this pathogen is easily lost during handling, so that either huge quantities of the organism are necessary for analysis or extraordinary care must be exercised during extraction. Surprisingly, one of the best ways of preserving *Orientia* DNA is to dry the sample on filter paper. Amplification of *Orientia* DNA by polymerase chain reaction (PCR) has been used for detection of human infection in dried blood specimens. This technique may eventually provide better practical diagnosis than the serological techniques.

Isolation and culture

Isolation of a live culture of *O. tsutsugamushi* is a long, specialized procedure requiring the use of biosafety level 3 facilities. The procedure usually involves injection and passage in mice, followed by adaptation of the culture to tissue culture. All stages of the procedure are usually conducted in the absence of antibiotics, increasing the challenge of maintaining sterility in tissue culture. Fertile chicken eggs have also been used for culture of *Orientia*, producing large quantities of very useful IFA reagent.

Transmission

Vectors

Orientia tsutsugamushi is transmitted to mammals during feeding by the larval stage of some species of chigger mites in the genus *Leptotrombidium* (Table 1). Other genera of chiggers (e.g. *Ascoschoengastia*, *Blankaartia*, *Gahrliepia*, *Eutrombicula*, *Microtrombicula* and *Odontocarus*) commonly contain the pathogen and have been suspected of having a role in transmission. The life cycles of these mites follow the same general pattern, with a long-lived adult form that deposits on the ground as many as 15 eggs per day, which hatch into the six-legged larvae, or chiggers. The chigger mite seeks reptiles, birds or mammals as hosts, cementing itself to the outer layers of the skin for about 4 days and engorging on fluids extracted from cells. The chiggers drop off to become eight-legged nymphs, which feed on arthropod eggs in the soil for about 2 weeks before developing into adults. The adults also feed on arthropod eggs. As a result of the life cycle, in which an individual feeds on a host only once per generation, maintenance of *Orientia* is totally dependent on vertical (trans-stadial and transovarial) transmission. Surprisingly, uninfected larvae that feed on an infected host may pass the infection transstadially, but never transovarially. As a result, vertebrates are always 'dead-end' hosts for *O. tsutsugamushi* and the pathogen is only maintained within infected maternal lines of chigger mites. This situation seems unlikely from an evolutionary standpoint, but direct experimentation and the recent discovery of dozens of genetically distinct strains of the species lend support to this widely held hypothesis.

Transmission foci

Vector chigger mites are consistently associated with habitats that experience ecological disruption, favouring small mammals (especially rodents in the genera *Rattus* and *Apodemus*, shrews in the genus *Suncus* and other tree-shrews in the genus *Tupaia*), which serve as maintenance hosts. Disruption results in secondary vegetation associated with the designation 'scrub'; hence the common name of the disease. Disruption is often the result of human activity, such as clearing vegetation for cultivation, gathering agricultural waste together (most notably, piles of palm fronds in Malaysian oil-palm estates), flooding rice-fields and various construction activities. Natural disruption, caused by erosion, large animal activity and tree falls, can also create foci. Despite their small size (approximately 100 µm), chigger mites are capable of crawling to favourable microhabitats, sometimes resulting in concentrations of larvae in so-called 'mite islands'. People who linger at these mite islands may acquire scrub typhus, while those only a few metres away remain uninfected. The distribution of mites can sometimes, however, be much

Table 1. Major chigger mite vectors of scrub typhus.

Leptotrombidium species	Areas where recorded as vector
L. akamushi	Japan
L. arenicola	Malaysia
L. chiangraiensis	Northern Thailand (suspected)
L. deliense	Pakistan, South-East Asia, Indonesia, Australia
L. fletcheri	Malaysia
L. pallidum	Japan, Korea, Primorye
L. palpale	Suspected in Japan, Korea, Primorye
L. pavlovskyi	Primorye
L. scutellare	Japan, Korea, Thailand (suspected)
L. tosa	Japan (suspected)
L. umbricola	Malaysia

more widely dispersed, so that the mite island phenomenon is not observed.

Occupational associations

Most people infected with *O. tsutsugamushi* pursue various rural occupations in endemic areas. Those who become re-infected regularly by the same strain from their local surroundings may remain perfectly healthy, but maintain high titres of antibodies. Symptomatic cases occur when people enter new areas, for such activities as construction, seasonal agriculture, fishing and military operations, and are bitten by infected mites. Infection of tourists visiting rural areas of endemic regions occurs regularly, sometimes with tragic mortality due to misdiagnosis and subsequent inappropriate treatment. Although not typical, urban foci of scrub typhus can result in disease in people who have never visited a rural area. Urban foci could include vacant land, abandoned construction sites, drainage embankments and any other sites where secondary vegetation encourages proliferation of rodents and chigger mites. The difficulty of diagnosing scrub typhus and the rural distribution of the disease result in gross under-reporting by public health authorities. Specific studies of prevalence rates showed that 20% of all fever cases in endemic areas of Malaysia and Thailand and 44% of undiagnosed fevers in Korea were due to infection with *Orientia*. The recent discovery that *O. tsutsugamushi* survives blood-banking procedures in an infective state raises the possibility that some scrub typhus is caused by transfusions.

Treatment

Scrub typhus was a frightening disease prior to the development of effective antibiotics. Despite attempts to use supportive therapy and para-aminobenzoic acid, patients essentially suffered the full extent of morbidity and mortality regardless of treatment. The first effective antibiotic for scrub typhus was chloramphenicol (its use being first published in 1948), which is still commonly used in some endemic areas because of the drug's low cost. Tetracycline antibiotics came into use during the 1950s and are now the treatment of choice, because of their greater effectiveness and lower toxicity. Although all tetracycline drugs are effective, doxycycline is used most often and generally results in elimination of fever within 36 h. There is some concern over finding alternative drugs because neither chloramphenicol nor tetracyclines can be recommended for use by pregnant women. Recent evidence for doxycycline resistance in northern Thailand also justifies the search for alternative antibiotics. Rifampicin (rifampin), ciprofloxacin and azithromycin have been used successfully in preliminary studies.

Prevention and control

Chemoprophylaxis

Although chemoprophylaxis with weekly doses of doxycycline was shown to be effective in a single study, it has never been added as a registered use of the drug. Weekly rather than daily administration of doxycycline is important for successful prophylaxis. Those bitten by an infected chigger mite build their immune responses between doses of antibiotic while suffering minimal or no signs of infection. The antibiotic prevents further multiplication but does not kill the pathogen (i.e. it is bacteriostatic), so that the immune response can successfully and permanently control the infection before the appearance of symptoms. Daily administration of doxycycline only delays symptomatic illness until prophylaxis ends.

Personal protection from chigger bites

TOPICAL REPELLENTS Diethyltoluamide (DEET) is a very effective repellent of chiggers. If a person is wearing short trousers when travelling through an infested area, a DEET-based repellent can be applied to the tops of shoes, socks and at least to the lower legs. If long trousers are worn, it is best to tuck their bottoms into the tops of boots or socks so that the mites are forced to walk on the outside of the trousers, which, together with the socks, can be treated with DEET. This should prevent mites from attaching to the lower parts of the body, their favoured sites. Direct application of DEET to the skin will provide further protection. The duration of protection depends greatly on both the concentration and the formulation of the DEET product. Generally, increases in concentration up to 30–50% will result in an increase in the duration of effectiveness; concentrations above 50% result in, at best, marginal improvement in performance when applied directly to the skin. Rain, washing or sweating and abrasion (e.g. from rubbing against objects or tools) will decrease the effectiveness of repellents.

CLOTHING REPELLENTS Another method for preventing bites from chigger mites is application of a product containing permethrin (a pyrethroid insecticide) to clothing. The common commercial products are sprayed directly on outer clothing (not underwear or hats). Depending on the thoroughness of the application, such treatments may last through several launderings. Products are available for military clothing which result in longer-lasting protection. These treatments would be particularly effective when wearing long trousers tucked into boots.

AVOIDANCE OF CHIGGERS Finally, avoiding contact with microhabitats favouring chigger mites can prevent bites. Although difficult to quantitate the effectiveness of these measures, common sense would suggest that travellers should avoid areas with obviously high populations of rodents, avoid areas where tall vegetation brushes directly against them and avoid sitting or lying directly on the ground. Local populations sometimes claim to know particular areas or particular kinds of plants associated with chigger mites. Although such local knowledge may be accurate, it is usually difficult for the traveller to put this to practical application.

Community vector control

The presence of chigger mites can be detected by several survey methods, including using black plates (shiny black squares of plastic briefly placed on the ground and then examined for chigger mites), Tullgren funnels (a technique for extracting organisms from soil), examination of captive or wild rodents, or a black cloth combined with carbon dioxide as an additional attractant. Infection rates of the chigger mites can be determined either by the direct fluorescence antibody assay or by PCR.

Killing chiggers over a large area is difficult. Many texts have recommended the use of organochlorine insecticides (e.g. lindane, dieldrin), which are now known to be unacceptable legally, environmentally and toxicologically. The organophosphate insecticide chlorpyrifos was also once registered for mite control, but is now also considered unacceptable. Probably the most practical recommendation is to spray suspected or known mite-infested areas with insecticides such as fenthion, propoxur or permethrin, but their effectiveness for chigger control is largely unknown. In the absence of insecticidal measures, burning vegetation or applying herbicides (with caution for the applicator's safety from toxic compounds) can temporarily eliminate chigger mites from infested areas, though populations return quickly as the area is re-vegetated. Rodent control can reduce mite populations over the long term, though the immediate effect could be increased biting of humans, due to lack of suitable rodent hosts. Current methods for community vector control of chigger mites are entirely inadequate, justifying further research in this area.

Selected bibliography

Dasch, G.A., Strickman, D., Watt, G. and Eamsila, C. (1996) Measuring genetic variability in *Orientia tsutsugamushi* by PCR/RFLP analysis: a new approach to questions about its epidemiology, evolution, and ecology. In: Kazan, J. and Toman, R. (eds) *Rickettsiae and Rickettsial Diseases, Proceedings of the Vth Symposium.* Slovak Academy of Science, Bratislava, pp. 79–84.

Frances, S.P. and Khlaimanee, N. (1996) Laboratory tests of arthropod repellents against *Leptotrombidium deliense* – noninfected and infected with *Rickettsia tsutsugamushi* – and noninfected *L. fletcheri* (Acari: Trombiculidae). *Journal of Medical Entomology* 33, 232–235.

Philip, C.B. (1948) Tsutsugamushi disease (scrub typhus) in World War II. *Journal of Parasitology* 34, 169–191.

Raoult, D. and Drancourt, M. (1991) Antimicrobial therapy of rickettsial diseases. *Antimicrobial Agents and Chemotherapy* 35, 2457–2462.

Ree, H.-I., Cho, M.-K., Lee, I.-Y. and Jeon, S.-H. (1995) Comparative epidemiological studies on vector/reservoir animals of tsutsugamushi disease between high and low endemic areas in Korea. *Korean Journal of Parasitology* 33, 27–36.

Smadel, J.E., Woodward, T.E. Ley, H.L., Philip, C.B., Traub, R., Lewthwaite, R. and Savoor, S.R. (1948) Chloromycetin in the treatment of scrub typhus. *Science* 108, 160–161.

Tamura, A., Ohashi, N., Urakami, H. and Miyamura, S. (1995) Classification of *Rickettsia tsutsugamushi* in a new genus, *Orientia* gen. nov., as *Orientia tsutsugamushi* comb. nov. *International Journal of Systematic Bacteriology* 45, 589–591.

Traub, R. and Wisseman, C.L. (1974) The ecology of chigger-borne rickettsiosis (scrub typhus). *Journal of Medical Entomology* 11, 237–303.

Twartz, J.C., Shirai, A., Selvaraju, G., Saunders, J.P., Huxsoll, D.L. and Groves, M.G. (1982) Doxycycline prophylaxis for human scrub typhus. *Journal of Infectious Diseases* 146, 811–818.

Uchikawa, K., Kawamore, F., Kawai, S. and Kumada, N. (1993) Suzuki's method (MITORI-HO), a recommended method for the visual sampling of questing *Leptotrombidium scutellare* larvae in the field (Trombidiformes, Trombiculidae). *Journal of the Acarological Society of Japan* 2, 91–98.

Watt, G., Chouriyagune, C., Ruangweerayud, R., Watcharapichat, P., Phulsuksombati, D., Jongsakul, K., Teja-Isavadharm, P., Bhodhidatta, D., Corcoran, K.D., Dasch, G.A. and Strickman, D. (1996) Scrub typhus infections poorly responsive to antibiotics in northern Thailand. *The Lancet* 348, 86–91.

Wright, J.D., Hastriter, M.W. and Robinson, D.M. (1984) Observations on the ultrastructure and distribution of *Rickettsia tsutsugamushi* in naturally infected *Leptotrombidium* (*Leptotrombidium*) *arenicola* (Acari: Trombiculidae). *Journal of Medical Entomology* 21, 17–27.

Scrub typhus mites *see* **Mites.**

Semliki Forest virus

Martin Pfeffer

Semliki Forest (SF) virus was first isolated in 1942 from a pool of *Aedes abnormalis* mosquitoes trapped in the Semliki Forest, Bwamba, Uganda.

Distribution

Isolations of this virus have been reported from much of sub-Saharan Africa, from Senegal in the west eastwards to Kenya, from central Africa to as far south as Mozambique. In Asia, the virus has been isolated from mosquitoes in far eastern Russia and Vietnam.

Virus

Semliki Forest virus belongs to the genus *Alphavirus* (family Togaviridae) and is the group representative of an antigenic complex within the genus, including closely related human pathogens. Zingilamo (iso-

lated from wild birds in the Central African Republic) and Me Tri viruses (Vietnam) are considered to be strains of SF virus, based on nucleotide sequence similarities, although classical typing may justify a distinct virus species for the latter. The entire genomic nucleotide sequences of mouse neurovirulent and avirulent strains of SF virus have been determined and infectious complementary DNA (cDNA) clones have been constructed. Semliki Forest virus is one of the most intensively studied viruses and was used to analyse the molecular basis of age-dependent neurovirulence (see Sindbis virus) and teratogenesis in rodent models. *In vitro* experiments with SF virus added much to our knowledge of the cascade leading to programmed cell death (apoptosis) and the intracellular processes involved in virus replication, protein biosynthesis and maturation within the infected host cell.

Clinical symptoms

Studies in various parts of Africa in the 1950s to 1980s demonstrated that up to half of the human population had antibodies to SF virus. Consequently, SF virus was not considered to be a human pathogen until a fatal case of human encephalitis in a German virologist was traced to the handling of SF virus, strain Osterrieth, as the causative agent. Neurological signs included convulsions, generalized as well as focal epileptic seizures and hemiplegia. Subsequent integration of SF virus into surveillance programmes in central Africa confirmed that SF virus produces illness in humans. The clinical picture always included fever, headache, arthralgia and myalgia. Sometimes abdominal pain, with or without diarrhoea, was seen, and there is one report of conjunctivitis as part of the clinical picture. The headache is described as very severe and long-lasting (up to 2 weeks). Serosurveys in Vietnam indicate that Me Tri virus may be responsible for aseptic meningitis and viral encephalitis in children.

Diagnosis

Virus isolation from diluted serum samples of viraemic patients in tissue cultures (e.g. VERO cells) or baby mice, with subsequent identification using monovalent polyclonal or monoclonal antibodies in an indirect immunofluorescence assay is the 'gold standard'. Sensitive alphavirus genus-specific antigen-capture enzyme-linked immunosorbent assay (ELISA) and reverse transcription–polymerase chain reaction (RT-PCR) techniques have been described. Subsequent virus identification can be achieved with an SF virus-specific monoclonal antibody or sequence determination of the amplicon. Although group-reactive immunoglobulin M (IgM) antibody-capture (MAC-) and IgG ELISAs are available for alphaviruses, the use of SF virus antigen has never been described. Semliki Forest virus agglutinates goose and chicken erythrocytes at a pH of 6.0–7.2 (optimum: 6.4–6.8) over a broad temperature range (4–37°C). The haemagglutination inhibition (HI) test has been widely used because of its low cost, but HI antibodies are cross-reactive to other members of the SF virus antigenic complex, mainly chikungunya and o'nyong-nyong viruses (see entries). Thus, there is need for caution in the interpretation of HI test results. Cross-neutralization assays, mostly performed as plaque-reduction neutralization test using the respective hyperimmune antisera, allow a precise species identification within the genus.

Transmission

Known vectors in Africa are mainly *Aedes* mosquitoes, such as *A. vittatus*, *A. jamoti*, *A. palpalis*, *A. aegypti*, *A. africanus*, *A. opok*, *A. abnormalis* and *A. argenteopunctatus*. There is one SF virus isolate each from *Culex quinquefasciatus* and *Eretmapodites chrysogaster* from the Central African Republic and from *Eretmapodites grahami* from Cameroon, and one from a pool of *Rhipicephalus guilhoni* ticks from Senegal.

The Russian SF virus isolates are mostly from *Aedes vexans* and the *Culex pipiens* complex. (Me Tri viruses were isolated from *Culex tritaeniorhynchus* in northern Vietnam.) Literally nothing is known about the maintainence of SF virus in nature. Considering the numerous mosquito species and ticks from which SF virus has been isolated and the broad spectrum of antibody-positive domesticated animals (e.g. cattle, pigs, horses), it would appear that a transmission cycle involving only a few vector species and a few specific vertebrate hosts, as is known for other alphaviruses, is unlikely. However, based on a comprehensive study from the Central African Republic, it was suggested that *A. africanus* transmitted SF virus in the Vervet (= Green) monkey (*Chlorocebus aethiops*[1]) population, with a spillover into human populations living in proximity to the monkeys. The magnitude of the involvement of *A. aegypti* in both this spillover and/or a subsequent human-to-human transmission is unknown.

Treatment

Since there is no specific treatment known to combat the virus infection, medication has to concentrate on the patient's symptoms. Pain relief of the severe headache (e.g. paracetamol, oral dose of up to 4 g adult^{-1} day^{-1}, or ibuprofen, with up to 2.5 g adult^{-1} day^{-1}) and prevention of dehydration are of most importance. Depending on the severity of both the arthralgia and the myalgia, anti-inflammatory and antirheumatic medication may be indicated (e.g. diclofenac-sodium, oral dose of up to 150 mg adult^{-1} day^{-1}).

Control

Efficient use of insecticides in endemic areas is hampered by the lack of detailed knowledge of the behaviour of the vectors involved. However, repellents such as *N,N*-diethyl-*m*-toluamide (DEET) can give protection against mosquitoes for up to 6 h. New long-acting formulations of DEET seem to protect for up to 72 h (LIPODEET, morpel 220). Synthetic pyrethroids (e.g. permethrin, deltamethrin and lambdacyhalothrin) and organophosphates (e.g. malathion, fenitrothion, pirimiphos methyl) can be applied as ultra-low-volume (ULV) sprays from ground-based equipment or aircraft, to kill adult mosquitoes, especially infected ones in outbreak situations. Organophosphate larvicides (e.g. malathion, pirimiphos methyl, temephos), microbial insecticides, such as *Bacillus thuringiensis* subsp. *israelensis* and *Bacillus sphaericus*, and insect growth regulators (IGRs) can be used if the larval habitats are known and sufficiently localized for operational logistics. Since SF virus has been repeatedly isolated from *A. aegypti*, control measures should be aimed at eradicating, or at least reducing, container-type breeding places, such as domestic water-storage pots, and unused and discarded containers.

Note

1   This monkey was formerly in the genus *Cercopithecus*.

Selected bibliography

Atkins, G.J., Sheahan, B.J. and Liljeström, P. (1999) The molecular pathogenesis of Semliki Forest virus: a model virus made useful? *Journal of General Virology* 80, 2287–2297.

Ha, D.Q., Calisher, C.H., Tien, P.H., Karabatsos, N. and Gubler, D.J. (1995) Isolation of a newly recognized alphavirus from mosquitoes in Vietnam and evidence for human infection and disease. *American Journal of Tropical Medicine and Hygiene* 53, 100–104.

Mathiot, C.C., Grimaud, G., Garry, P., Bouquety, J.C., Mada, A., Daguisy, A.M. and Georges, A.J. (1990) An outbreak of human Semliki Forest virus infections in Central African Republic. *American Journal of Tropical Medicine and Hygiene* 42, 386–393.

Roehrig, J.T., Brown, T.M., Johnson, A.J., Karabatsos, N., Martin, D.A., Mitchell, C.J. and Nasci, R.S. (1998) Alphaviruses. In: Stephenson, J.R. and Warnes, A. (eds) *Diagnostic Virology Protocols*. Humana Press, Totowa, New Jersey, pp. 7–18.

Willems, W.R., Kaluza, G., Boschek, C.B., Bauer, H., Hager, H., Schütz, H.-J. and Feistner, H. (1979) Semliki Forest virus: cause of a fatal case of human encephalitis. *Science* 203, 1127–1129.

Sepik virus

John S. Mackenzie

Sepik (SEP) virus has been implicated as a possible aetiological agent of febrile disease in humans in Papua New Guinea.

Distribution

Sepik virus was first isolated in the mid-1960s from mosquitoes collected near Maprik in the East Sepik Province of Papua New Guinea. A subsequent isolation was made from mosquitoes trapped near Balimo in Western Province of Papua New Guinea in 1998. Seroepidemiological investigations have suggested that SEP virus may infect domestic animals on Lombok and possibly on other islands of the eastern Indonesian archipelago. A related virus, identified initially as Wesselsbron virus (see entry), was isolated in Thailand, but whether it actually represents another strain of SEP virus remains to be determined.

Virus

Sepik virus is in the family Flaviviridae, genus *Flavivirus*, and is closely related to Wesselsbron virus (see entry). Sepik virus has recently been classified in the yellow fever (see entry) complex. The possible infection of domestic animals with SEP virus may not be unexpected, given the host range and pathogenicity of Wesselsbron virus.

Clinical symptoms and pathogenicity

Little is known of the clinical features and pathogenicity of SEP virus. It was implicated as a possible aetiological agent of human disease on the basis of high neutralizing antibodies in serum taken from a New Guinea patient hospitalized with a febrile illness.

Transmission

Four isolates of SEP virus were obtained from mosquitoes collected near Maprik in the East Sepik Province in the late 1960s. The isolates came from a pool of *Mansonia septempunctata*, a mixed pool of *Ficalbia flavens* and other *Ficalbia* species, a pool of *Armigeres* species and a pool of mixed mosquito species. A further isolate was obtained from *Culex palpalis* trapped in 1998 at Balimo in Western Province. The roles of these different mosquito species in transmission cycles and the identity of vertebrate host(s) for SEP virus are unknown.

Selected bibliography

Johansen, C.A., Van den Hurk, A.F., Ritchie, S.A., Zborowski, P., Nisbet, D., Paru, R., Bockarie, M.J., Macdonald, J., Drew, A.C., Khromykh, T.I. and Mackenzie, J.S. (2000) Isolation of Japanese encephalitis virus from mosquitoes (Diptera: Culicidae) collected in the Western Province of Papua New Guinea. *American Journal of Tropical Medicine and Hygiene.* 62, 631–638.

Karabatsos, N. (ed.) (1985) *International Catalogue of Arboviruses Including Certain Other Viruses of Vertebrates.* American Society of Tropical Medicine and Hygiene, San Antonio, Texas, 1147 pp.

Woodroofe, G.M. and Marshall, I.D. (1971) Arboviruses from the Sepik district of New Guinea. In: *John Curtin School of Medical Research Annual Report.* Australian National University, Canberra, pp. 90–91.

Setaria species *see* **Setariosis**

Setariosis

W.S.S. Wijesundera

Setariosis is an infection of ungulates with the filarial worms of the genus *Setaria*. In the natural hosts (e.g. bovids), these parasites are considered to be non-pathogenic. However, the transmission of the infective-stage larvae to abnormal hosts (e.g. sheep) causes serious neuropathological disorders.

Infections in goats, sheep and horses (abnormal hosts)

The neurological disorders in goats and horses caused by *Setaria digitata* were earlier referred to as 'lumbar paralysis' and 'weak back', or 'kumri', respectively, by farmers for many years. The disease occurs seasonally during late summer and autumn or in the tropics, during the rainy season or soon after, when the mosquito vectors are active. The infection, often referred to as cerebrospinal nematodiasis (epizootic cerebrospinal nematodiasis), causes locomotor defects, including paralysis, leading to secondary infections. These defects can also severely affect the breeding and production capability of the animal, leading to substantial economic losses in animal husbandry.

Distribution

The disease occurs mainly in Asian countries and in the Far East, such as in Japan, Korea, China, India, Myanmar and Sri Lanka. For example, in China, as many as 30–40% of goats and sheep are affected by the disease.

Parasite

The parasite found in sheep, goats and horses is the immature form of *S. digitata*. The adults are commonly found in the peritoneal cavity of cattle and Buffalo (*Bubalus bubalis*), which are its natural hosts.

The adult male worm is about 4–6 cm in length and the female approximately double the size of the male (6–12 cm). The female worm produces sheathed microfilariae, about 190 μm in length. The microfilariae occur in the blood and do not show periodicity. Further development of the microfilariae into the infective larval stage takes place within 10–14 days (depending on the temperature) in the insect vector. The life cycle of the parasite is completed once the infective larvae find their way into a host via a mosquito bite and develop to the adult stage in the appropriate parasite location, such as the peritoneal cavity. It takes 8–10 months for the larvae to reach sexual maturity. The parasite lives for about 1.5 years in the natural host (bovids). However, if the infective-stage larvae enter an abnormal host, such as sheep, goats or horses, it is unable to complete the life cycle. The immature worms are, however, attracted to and migrate erratically to the central nervous system of these abnormal hosts, causing cerebrospinal nematodiasis. Although goats and horses are considered to be abnormal hosts, there are a few instances where *S. digitata* adult worms have been reported in the peritoneal cavity of these animals.

Clinical symptoms

Both young and adult animals are affected, but there are no reports of the disease in newborn lambs, kids or foals. The latent period varies from 14 to 33 days for goats and 15 to 66 days for horses, this being followed by the appearance of neurological signs. The onset of disease may be dramatically acute in some, while at other times it may develop gradually. The disease is generally non-febrile; typically, animals develop motor weakness and ataxia in the hind or all four limbs leading to swaying, tumbling and paralysis. Affected animals also show visual impairment, dullness and incoordination. Some animals die while others recover but suffer from residual neurological signs, such as weakness in the limbs, impaired gait and head tilt. The variation observed in the degree of severity of the clinical signs is related to the neuroanatomical location of the migrating worm and the lesion it produces. A small lesion located in the lower lumbar part of the spinal cord is less serious than a lesion at a higher level, such as in the brain stem.

Diagnosis

Diagnosis is based on the clinical manifestations. There is no diagnostic method to confirm the disease in live animals. Serological assays based on the enzyme-linked immunosorbent assay (ELISA) technique to detect antibodies against the parasite are still at the laboratory stage. Pathological examination for the identification of the disease is often laborious, as the focal process may attack any part of the nervous system in a haphazard manner and the microscopic lesion itself can take a meandering path. In certain instances, the entire nervous system is processed to obtain sections for microscopic examination. Deoxyribonucleic acid (DNA)-based polymerase chain reaction (PCR) assay may be useful in overcoming this strenuous procedure of examination.

Transmission

Transmission is through a number of mosquitoes, the species depending on geographical area. Known vectors of *S. digitata* include *Aedes togoi* (Japan), *Aedes vitattus* (India), *Anopheles sinensis* (Japan) and *Armigeres subalbatus*[1] (India, Sri Lanka). Certain *Culex* species, such as *C. tritaeniorhynchus* and the *C. pipiens* complex, have also been reported as vectors in Japan.

Once ingested by the mosquito, the microfilariae shed their sheaths and penetrate the stomach wall to enter the thoracic muscles, where they develop into sausage-shaped larvae. The sausage-shaped larvae moult twice before developing into elongate (1.9–2.5 mm) third-stage infective larvae. The infective stage larvae find their way to the proboscis of the mosquito. When the infected mosquito feeds, the infective larvae actively pass down the proboscis to be deposited on the host's skin, and then enter the host through the puncture caused by the mosquito bite.

Experiments have shown that a large number of infective-stage larvae are necessary at a given time to produce an infection in abnormal hosts. However, in nature this type of infection may be produced due to prolonged exposure of animals to large numbers of bites from *Setaria*-infected mosquitoes.

Treatment

Diethylcarbamazine citrate (Hetrazan) (20 mg kg^{-1} body weight) and ivermectin (200 µg kg^{-1} body weight) are the most common drugs administered. When given at the onset of the disease, these drugs can prevent further damage to the central nervous system. Broad-spectrum antibiotics can be administered to treat secondary infections.

Control

During the high-risk period susceptible animals are given Hetrazan once or twice a month as a prophylactic measure. Experiments using vaccines produced from the infective stage larvae have been shown to be effective in preventing the disease. The success of control measures will also depend on the reduction of *Setaria* parasites in cattle and buffaloes, which act as reservoir hosts in harbouring the parasite. Treatment of infected cattle and buffaloes with anti-filarial drugs, especially during the rainy season, when microfilarial production increases, can be effective in controlling the disease. The disease can also be controlled by separating goats and sheep from cattle and buffaloes, with respect to both breeding and grazing.

Setariosis – natural hosts

There are around 43 *Setaria* species and certain members have a worldwide distribution, especially in cattle and horses. Species allocation of *Setaria* has been somewhat confusing in the past. However, scanning electron-microscopic studies, together with other studies, have made specific distinctions among species and hence allocation of specific names is now possible. Species commonly found in domesticated animals are listed in Table 1.

Setaria species are mainly found in the peritoneal cavity and, on rare occasions, some parasites have been located in the urinary bladder, eye, pleural cavity, scrotum and heart of these natural hosts. Prenatal infection of *Setaria* species (especially *S. marshalli*) in cattle has been reported, where adult worms were detected in the peritoneal cavity of neonatal calves.

In endemic areas, the infection rate may be more than 90% in cattle. However, the infection is asymptomatic and not considered pathogenic, but sometimes it may cause mild fibrinous peritonitis. *Setaria digitata* has been found to cause eosinophilic granulotomatus lesions in the urinary bladder of cattle. In some instances the young *S. digitata* and *Setaria equina* worms

Table 1. *Setaria* species in domesticated animals.

Livestock host	Setaria species	Distribution
Cattle (*Bos taurus,* *Bos indicus*)	S. digitata	Asia, Far East
	S. labiatopapillosa	Cosmopolitan
	S. cervi	Asia, Eastern Europe
Newborn calves	S. marshalli	Far East
Water buffalo (*Bubalus bubalis*)	S. digitata	Asia, Far East
	S. labiatopapillosa	Cosmopolitan
	S. leichungwingi	Asia
Horse (*Equus caballus*)	S. equina	Cosmopolitan
Pig (*Suis scrofa domesticus*)	S. congolensis	Afrotropical
	S. thomasi	Asia
	S. bernardi	Asia
Reindeer (*Rangifer tarandus*)	S. tundrae	Northern Eurasia

are found in the anterior chamber of the eye of cattle and horses, causing inflammation leading to eye opacity and blindness.

Transmission

The development of the microfilariae into the infective-stage larvae has been studied in only a few species of *Setaria*. The intermediate hosts for *S. equina*, in western parts of the Commonwealth of Independent States (CIS) are *Ochlerotatus*[2] *communis* and *Ochlerotatus rusticus*.[3] In Japan the vectors of *Setaria labiatopapillosa* are *Ochlerotatus togoi*, *Anopheles hyrcanus* and *Armigeres subalbatus*. In East Africa *Aedes aegypti* and *Aedes pembaensis* have been found infected after feeding on an infected donkey; *Mansonia* species are also considered likely vectors. In western CIS vectors are *Ochlerotatus caspius*, *Ochlerotatus flavescens*, *Aedes cinereus*, *Aedes vexans* and *Anopheles claviger*[4]. The vector of *Setaria cervi* in the western CIS appears to be the stable-fly (*Stomoxys calcitrans*).[5]

Treatment

Hetrazan (20 mg kg^{-1} body weight) reduces the microfilariae burden, but mass-scale treatment is not usually carried out.

Control

No large-scale control programmes are undertaken.

Notes

[1]   In some publications the vector is given as *Armigeres obturbans*, but this is usually based on misidentification.

[2]   *Ochlerotatus* was formerly a subgenus of *Aedes*.

[3]   In some previous publications the junior synonym, *Aedes maculatus*, is given.

[4]   In some previous publications the junior synonym, *Anopheles bifurcatus*, is given.

[5]   In some previous publications stable-flies are incorrectly named as *Haematobia stimulans*.

Selected bibliography

Anderson, R.C. (2000) *Nematode Parasites of Vertebrates. Development and Transmission.* CAB International, Wallingford, UK, pp. 479–482.

Hagiwara, S., Suzuki, M., Shirasaka, S. and Kurihara, F. (1992) A survey of the vector mosquitoes of *Setaria digitata* in Ibaraki Prefecture, central Japan. *Japanese Journal of Sanitary Zoology* 43 291–295.

Innes, J.R.M. and Saunders, L.Z. (1962) *Comparative Neurology.* Academic Press, New York, 839 pp.

Innes, J.R.M. and Shoho, C. (1952) Nematodes, nervous disease, and neurotropic virus infection. *British Medical Journal* 2, 366–368.

Radostis, O.M., Gay, C.C., Blood, D.C. and Hinchcliff, K.W. (1999) *Veterinary Medicine. A Textbook of the Diseases of Cattle, Sheep, Pigs and Horses,* 9th edn. Baillière-Tindall, London, 1881 pp.

Shoho, C. and Uni, S. (1977) Scanning electron microscopy (SEM) of some *Setaria* species (Filariodea Nematoda). *Zeitschrift für Parasitenkunde* 53, 93–104.

Sonin, M.D. (1977) *Filariata of Animals and Man and the Diseases Caused by Them. Fundamentals of Nematology,* Vol. 28, Part IV. *Onchocercidae.* (In Russian, translated into English by Amerind Publishing, New Delhi, India, 1985.)

Soulsby, E.J.L. (1982) *Helminths, Arthropods and Protozoa of Domesticated Animals,* 7th edn. Baillière-Tindall, London, 809 pp.

Sheep keds *see* **Hippoboscids.**

***Shigella* infections** *see* **Flies** *and* **Cockroaches.**

Siberian tick typhus *see* **Tick-borne typhuses.**

***Simulium* species** *see* **Black-flies.**

Sindbis virus

Diane E. Griffin

A mosquito-transmitted arbovirus belonging to the *Alphavirus* genus of the family Togaviridae.

Fever, rash and arthritis caused by Sindbis (SIN) virus are known in different regions by the local names Ockelbo disease (Sweden), Karelian fever (western Russia) and Pogosta disease (Finland), as well as Sindbis. Sindbis virus infection of humans is widespread, but clinically apparent disease occurs primarily in northern Europe and South Africa. A mild form of the illness has been recognized in Australia.

Distribution

Sindbis virus is the most widespread of the alphaviruses that cause fever, rash and arthritis (Fig. 1). It was originally isolated in 1952 from a pool of *Culex univittatus* mosquitoes collected near Sindbis, Egypt.

Seroprevalence in humans in this region at the time was 27%, but SIN virus was not recognized to cause human disease. The virus has now been isolated throughout much of Africa, Europe, the Middle East, India, Asia, the Philippines and Australia from a variety of mosquito and vertebrate species.

Virus

Sindbis virus is an Old World alphavirus within the western equine encephalitis (WEE) (see entry) antigenic complex. Like other alphaviruses, it has an enveloped icosahedral virion and a genome composed of a single strand of message-sense RNA containing 11,700 nucleotides. The genome is capped, polyadenylated and infectious. There are three main structural proteins: the E1 and E2 surface glycoproteins and a

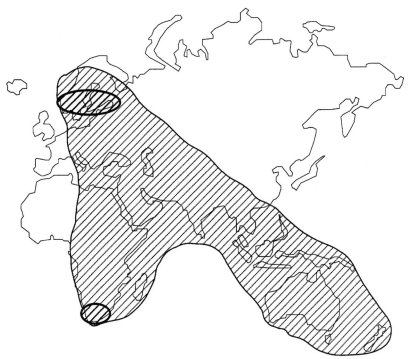

Fig. 1. Distribution of Sindbis virus. Darker encircled areas are regions where clinical disease occurs most often.

capsid protein. There are four genes for non-structural proteins (nsPs) that encode the components of the viral replicase.

The structural proteins and nsPs are translated as polyproteins, which are processed by viral and host proteases to the individual proteins. Viral protease function is found in nsP2 for the nsPs and in the capsid protein for the structural proteins. The nsPs function as polyprotein P123 and nsP4 to synthesize a minus-strand copy of the genomic RNA (Fig. 2). The papain-like protease nsP2 cleaves first in *cis* to produce P123 and nsP4 and later in *trans* to produce the fully processed nsP1, nsP2, nsP3 and nsP4, which synthesize plus-strand genomic and subgenomic RNAs (Fig. 2). For this reason, minus-strand synthesis continues for only a few hours after infection, because, as levels of nsP2 increase, the non-structural polyprotein is rapidly processed and the lack of polyprotein P123 leads to cessation of minus-strand synthesis and continuation of plus-strand synthesis with nsP1, nsP2 and nsP3.

The structural polyprotein is translated from a subgenomic RNA. The chymotrypsin-like serine protease in the C-terminal portion of the capsid protein (C) cleaves itself co-translationally from the nascent chain. After cleavage, the C terminus remains in the active site, inactivating the protease. The two transmembrane glycoproteins E1 and E2 are translocated and processed in the endoplasmic reticulum (ER). E2 is synthesized as a precursor PE2, cleaved by signal peptidase and folded with E1 as a heterodimer. The small 6K protein is transported through the Golgi to the cell surface with the PE2–E1 heterodimers; it is important for efficient budding, but only small amounts are incorporated into the virion. PE2 is cleaved in the trans Golgi by the cellular protease furin to E2 and E3. The E1–E2 heterodimers trimerize and form flower-like spikes on the virion surface. C, E2 and E1 are present in the virion in equimolar amounts. E3 is shed from the cell surface. Capsid proteins assemble around genomic RNA, which has a packaging signal within the coding region for nsP2, to form nucleocapsid cores, which are transported to the cell surface for assembly into virions. The cytoplasmic tail of E2 interacts with the capsid to initiate assembly, leading to virion budding from the cell surface.

Sindbis virus can infect a wide variety of cells in culture and enters the cell by receptor-mediated endocytosis. The low pH of the endosome triggers a conformational change in the E1–E2 heterodimer, which results in fusion of the viral membrane with the cell membrane and delivery of the virus nucleocapsid to the cytoplasm of the cell. The virus replicates rapidly and infection often induces death of the virus-infected cell. Extensive studies in animal models, primarily mice with encephalitis, have shown that important determinants of virulence are present in the E1 and E2 protein sequences and in the 5′ non-translated region of the genome.

Different genotypes of the virus have been identified and these genotypes correlate with the likelihood that infection will cause clinical illness in humans. Sindbis viruses from Europe and Africa form one major lineage and those from Asia and Australia form another, suggesting that ancestral SIN virus has diverged into at least two distinct groups. A third lineage has recently been identified in south-western Australia. Sindbis virus-like viruses isolated in Azerbaijan (Kyzyagach virus) and western China (XJ-160) are distantly related to the African/European genetic lineage of SIN virus. Strains isolated in northern Europe and South Africa, where most SIN virus-induced disease occurs, are more closely related to each other than to strains isolated in south and central Europe and the Middle East, where recognized clinical disease is rare. Within this region strain divergence is temporal rather than geographical, consistent with migratory birds as the major vertebrate host.

Clinical symptoms

Sindbis virus was first isolated from the blood of febrile humans in Uganda in 1961 and recognized in South Africa as a cause of rash and arthritis in 1963. The primary manifestations of infection are rash, joint pain and mild fever, which usually appear concurrently without a significant prodrome.

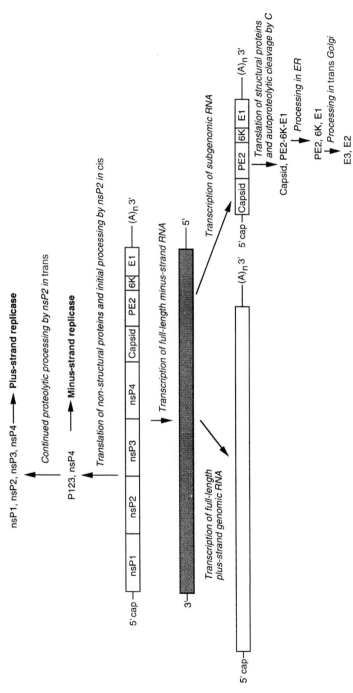

Fig. 2. Schematic diagram of the replication of Sindbis virus showing the processing necessary for the switch from full-length minus-strand to plus-strand synthesis, the production of the subgenomic RNA and the processing pathway of the structural proteins.

The rash is distributed diffusely over the trunk and limbs and often involves the palms and soles. The skin lesions begin as macules, which become papular and progress to central vesicle formation and are occasionally haemorrhagic. The lesions may be irritating, but are not pruritic. Lesions occur in crops, may last up to 10 days, are occasionally recurrent and leave brown stains. An enanthem is not present but the pharynx may become mildly inflamed. Arthralgias occur in large and small joints and may be severe enough to be immobilizing. Extremities may swell. Joint pain usually resolves within 1–2 weeks, but moderate pain and stiffness may persist for months to years. Fever, when present, is generally low-grade and may be accompanied by anorexia and occasionally lymphadenopathy. In Australia, SIN virus-induced arthritis and rash are milder and less frequent than Ross River (see entry) virus-induced arthritis and rash and SIN virus-induced disease in northern Europe and South Africa.

Diagnosis

Although the virus can occasionally be isolated from the skin lesions, and can be detected by reverse transcription–polymerase chain reaction (RT-PCR), SIN virus-induced disease is usually a serological diagnosis. Anti-SIN virus immunoglobulin M (IgM) antibody is usually present at the time of clinical presentation and can be detected using a virus-specific IgM capture enzyme immunoassay. Immunoglobulin M decreases slowly over 3–4 years, independent of persistent symptoms.

The major differential diagnosis is with other causes of rash and arthritis, such as infections with other alphaviruses in the region (e.g. chikungunya, o'nyong-nyong, Barmah Forest and Ross River viruses (see entries)), and with parvovirus B19 and rubella virus.

Transmission

Sindbis virus is maintained in a natural cycle between mosquitoes (*Culex* and *Culiseta* species) and wild birds. In Sweden the enzootic cycle involves *Culex torrentium*, *Culiseta morsitans* and passerine birds. In Australia isolates are primarily from *Culex annulirostris*. Spread of SIN virus from its enzootic cycle between birds and ornithophagic mosquitoes to humans involves introduction of the virus into *Aedes* mosquitoes with less specialized feeding habits and which serve as 'bridge' vectors. In northern Europe the primary bridge vector is *Aedes cinereus*, and the availability of this species may determine the frequency of human infection, which is greatest in zones between the 60th and 64th parallels. Human cases of disease in this region usually begin to appear in late July and continue into the autumn. The mechanism of overwintering in temperate climates is not clear, but evidence of vertical transmission has been obtained.

Treatment

There is no recognized specific treatment for SIN virus-induced disease. Symptomatic treatments may be beneficial.

Control

As with most alphaviruses, prevention of infection relies primarily on efforts to control mosquito populations by insecticidal spraying and reducing breeding sites. The need for mosquito abatement can be assessed by monitoring mosquito population densities and the presence of SIN virus in populations of mosquitoes capable of transmitting the virus to humans. Use by individuals of protective measures, such as applying mosquito repellents and wearing protective clothing, preferably impregnated with insect repellents or pyrethroids, such as permethrin, is important. There is no vaccine.

Selected bibliography

Espmark, Å. and Niklasson, B. (1984) Ockelbo disease in Sweden: epidemiological, clinical and virological data from the 1982 outbreak. *American Journal of Tropical Medicine and Hygiene* 33, 1203–1211.

Francy, D.B., Jaenson, T.G.T., Lundström, J.O., Schildt, E.-B., Espmark, Å., Henrickson, B. and Niklasson, B. (1989) Ecologic studies of mosquitoes and birds as hosts of Ockelbo virus in Sweden and isolation of Inkoo and

Batai viruses from mosquitoes. *American Journal of Tropical Medicine and Hygiene* 46, 355–363.

Jupp, P.G., Blackburn, N.K., Thompson, D.L. and Meenehan, G.M. (1986) Sindbis and West Nile virus in the Witwatersrand–Pretoria region. *South African Medical Journal* 70, 218–220.

Liang, G.D., Li, L., Zhou, G.L., Fu, S.H., Li, Q.P., Li, F.S., He, H.H., Jin, Q., He, Y., Chen, B.Q. and Hou, Y.O. (2000) Isolation and complete nucleotide sequence of a Chinese Sindbis-like virus. *Journal of General Virology* 81, 1347–1351.

Lundström, J.O. (1999) Mosquito-borne viruses in western Europe: a review. *Journal of Vector Ecology* 24, 1–39.

Mackenzie, J.S., Lindsay, M.D., Coelen, R.J., Broom, A.K., Hall, R.A. and Smith, D.W.

(1994) Arboviruses causing human disease in the Australasian zoogeographic region. *Archives of Virology* 136, 447–467.

Niklasson, B., Espmark, Å. and Lundström, J. O. (1988) Occurrence of arthralgia and specific IgM antibodies three to four years after Ockelbo disease. *Journal of Infectious Diseases* 157, 832–835.

Sammels, L.M., Lindsay, M.D., Poidinger, M., Coelen, R.J. and Mackenzie, J.S. (1999) Geographic distribution and evolution of Sindbis virus in Australia. *Journal of General Virology* 80, 739–748.

Turunen, M., Kusesto, P., Uggedahl, P.E. and Toivanen, A. (1998) Pogosta disease: clinical observations during an outbreak in the province of North Karelia, Finland. *British Journal of Rheumatology* 37, 1177–1180.

Sleeping sickness *see* **African trypanosomiasis, human.**

South African tick typhus *see* **Tick-borne typhuses.**

Spirochaetes

C.A. Hart

Spirochaetes (family *Spirochaetaceae*) are slender, winding or helically coiled Gram-negative bacteria. They are from 0.1 to 0.75 µm in diameter and 2 to 250 µm long. Wrapped longitudinally around the surface of the bacteria are endoflagella, by which the bacteria are motile. Within the spirochaetes there are five genera (*Spirochaeta, Christispira, Treponema, Borrelia* and *Leptospira*). Of these only the latter three are pathogenic for humans and only *Borrelia* species are transmitted by arthropods. The important species are those causing Lyme disease (*B. burgdorferi, B. afzelli* and

B. garinii: transmitted by ticks), louse-borne relapsing fever (*B. recurrentis*) and tick-borne relapsing fevers (*B. duttonii, B. hermsii, B. parkeri* and *B. turicatae*).

Selected bibliography

Nordstrand, A., Barbour, A.G. and Bergstrom, S. (2000) *Borrelia* pathogenesis research in the post-genomic and post-vaccine era. *Current Opinion in Microbiology* 3, 86–92.

Dattwyler, R.J. and Luft, B.J. (1997) *Borrelia burgdorferi.* In: Emmerson, A.M., Hawkey, P.M. and Gillespie, S.H. (eds) *Principles and Practice of Clinical Bacteriology.* John Wiley & Sons, Chichester, UK, pp. 691–707.

Splendidofilaria fallisensis *see* **Splendidofilariasis.**

Splendidofilariasis

R.C. Anderson

Infections of birds with filarial worms of the genus *Splendidofilaria*. Vectors are ornithophagic simuliid black-flies or ceratopogonids (i.e. *Culicoides* species), depending on the filarial species.

Distribution

Reported in domestic ducks in eastern North American, where black-fly vectors and wild duck reservoir hosts occur.

Parasite

Splendidofilaria fallisenisis (syn. *Ornithofilaria fallisensis*) are delicate, rather transparent nematodes found in the subcutaneous tissues of wild American black ducks (*Anas rubripes*) and Domestic (Mallard) ducks (*Anas platyrhynchos domesticus*). Males are 9–15 mm and females 24–40 mm in length. Microfilariae occur in the blood, are 90–121 mm in length, are without obvious sheaths and have blunt tails.

Clinical signs

None reported, probably absent.

Diagnosis

Microscopic examination of fresh blood or films of blood stained with Giemsa's stain.

Transmission

Vectors are nettaphagic (duck-loving) and chenophagic (goose-loving) simuliids, which attack birds in the spring. In Ontario, Canada, adults of *Simulium anatinum* emerge during the early part of May and persist for about 2 weeks. *Simulium rugglesi* emerges at the end of May and adults persists to the middle of July in diminishing numbers. Both species feed only during the day and will range widely in search of ducks, being attracted by secretions of their preen gland (uropygial gland) and carbon dioxide. Flies invade the feathers of the birds at the water-line and then crawl to various places on the body to feed; they do not attack birds that are on land or are elevated above the water level.

In the vector, microfilariae develop in the haemocoel (unique among filarial parasites transmitted by black-flies), and attain the infective stage in 7–14 days, depending on ambient temperatures (about 8 days at 17.1°C). Infective larvae from the mouthparts of flies are 389–486 μm in length. The tail of the infective larva has two prominent lateroterminal swellings and the oesophagus is short, narrow and undivided.

In ducklings the pre-patent period is 30–36 days and microfilariae persist for perhaps 2 years. In experiments birds could not be reinfected by later exposure to black-flies or by the subcutaneous inoculation of infective larvae.

Control

Avoid raising ducks and geese in enzootic areas or keep birds in fly-proof pens during May, June and the first 2 weeks of July (applicable to conditions in Ontario, Canada).

Selected bibliography

Anderson, R.C. (1954) *Ornithofilaria fallisensis* n. sp. (Nematoda, Filarioidea) from domestic ducks with descriptions of microfilariae in waterfowl. *Canadian Journal of Zoology* 32, 125–137.

Anderson, R.C. (1956) The life cycle and seasonal transmission of *Ornithofilaria fallisensis*, a parasite of domestic and wild ducks. *Canadian Journal of Zoology* 34, 485–525.

Anderson, R.C. (2000) *Nematode Parasites of Vertebrates, their Development and Transmission*, 2nd edn. CAB International, Wallingford, UK, 650 pp.

Spondweni virus

Oyewale Tomori

Distribution

Spondweni (SPO) virus, a flavivirus, was first isolated in 1955 from a pool of *Mansonia uniformis* mosquitoes collected at Lake Simbu, in Natal, South Africa. The virus has been subsequently recovered from several species of mosquitoes from Natal. Isolations of the virus have also been made from mosquitoes in Mozambique, Côte d'Ivoire and Cameroon. Spondweni virus has been isolated from cases of natural and laboratory-acquired human infections in various African countries. The virus was isolated from the blood of an anicteric child with fever and headache. Spondweni virus was originally identified as Zika virus (see entry). However, a recent analysis of the isolate using monoclonal antibodies suggests that the virus was a mixture of yellow fever and another flavivirus most closely resembling SPO virus. Two persons acquired SPO virus infections in the laboratory in South Africa. Serological evidence for other natural infections have been found in expatriates who resided in Burkina Faso, Cameroon and Gabon, indicating that the virus might be a cause of acute febrile infections throughout West Africa. Neutralizing antibodies have been found in humans in South Africa, Mozambique, Angola, Botswana, Ethiopia and Namibia and in cattle, sheep and goats in South Africa.

Virus

Spondweni virus is in the genus *Flavivirus* of the Togaviridae family, most closely related to Zika virus.

Clinical symptoms, pathogenesis and pathology

The virus is pathogenic for suckling and weanling baby mice inoculated intracerebrally (i.c.), but not intraperitoneally (i.p.), with the development of high virus titres ($10^{9.4}$ ml^{-1}) in the brain. Only 3–4-week-old mice succumb to intracerebral infection with SPO virus. Histopathology in mice inoculated by the i.c. route show perivascular round-cell infiltration and cerebral nerve cell necrosis. The virus produces plaques (1–3 mm in size) in Vervet monkey (VERO), pig kidney (PS), African green monkey (BS-C-1), human heteroploid (MA 104) and Rhesus monkey (LLC-MK2) cells. Spondweni virus infection of guinea-pigs, rabbits and Vervet (= African green) monkeys (*Chlorocebus aethiops*[1]) by the i.c. route and of day-old chicks by the intravenous (i.v.) route results in the development of antibodies. Wild rodents experimentally infected with SPO virus do not develop viraemia or antibody.

Human clinical disease following SPO virus infections varies from mild febrile illnesses with headache (disease resulting from acquired laboratory infection) to fever, chills, aches and pains, nausea, dizziness and epistaxis.

Other reported symptoms include myalgia, photophobia and maculopapular pruritic rash.

Diagnosis

Diagnosis is by virus isolation from blood or by serology.

Transmission

Spondweni virus has been recovered from *Mansonia africana*, *M. uniformis*, *Aedes circumluteolus*, *Aedes cumminsii*, *Eretmapodites silvestris* and *Culex neavei* from Natal, South Africa, from a pool of *Ochlerotatus*[2] *fryeri* and *Aedes fowleri* collected in Mozambique, from *Aedes abnormalis* group and *Aedes cumminsii* in Côte d'Ivoire and from *Eretpmapodites* species in Cameroon.

Although SPO virus has been successfully transmitted by *A. circumluteolus* and antibodies have been detected in domesticated animals, the vertebrate hosts involved in natural transmission are unknown.

Treatment

Treatment is symptomatic.

Control

There are no specific control measures.

Notes

[1] This monkey was formerly in the genus *Cercopithecus*.

[2] *Ochlerotatus* was formerly a subgenus of *Aedes*.

Selected bibliography

Karabatsos, N. (ed.) (1985) *International Catalogue of Arboviruses Including Certain Other Viruses of Vertebrates*, 3rd edn. American Society of Tropical Medicine and Hygiene, San Antonio, Texas, 1147 pp.

Kokernot, R.H., Smithburn, K.C., Paterson, H.E. and McIntosh, B.M. (1957) Studies on arthropod-borne viruses of Tongaland. VIII. Spondweni virus, an agent previously unknown, isolated from *Taeniorhynchus* (*Mansonioides*) *uniformis* Theo. *South African Journal of Medical Science* 22, 103–112.

McIntosh, B.M., Kokernot, R.H., Paterson, H.E. and de Meillon, B. (1961) Isolation of Spondweni virus from 4 species of culicine mosquitoes and a report of 2 laboratory infections with the virus. *South African Medical Journal* 35, 647–650.

Macnamara, F.M. (1954) A report of 3 cases of human infection during an epidemic of jaundice in Nigeria. *Transactions of the Royal Society of Tropical Medicine and Hygiene* 48, 139–145.

Monath, T.P. and Heinz, F.X. (1996) Flaviviruses. In: Fields, B.N., Knipe, D.M., Howley, P.M., Chanock, R.M., Melnick, J.L., Monath, T.P., Roizman, B. and Straus, S.E. (eds) *Fields Virology*, Vol. 1, 3rd edn. Lippincott-Raven Publishers, Philadelphia, pp. 961–1034.

Wolfe, M.S., Calisher, C.H. and McGuire, K. (1982) Spondweni virus infection in a foreign resident in Upper Volta. *The Lancet* 2, 1306–1308.

Stable-flies (Muscidae)

M.W. Service

Stable-flies (biting house-flies, dog-flies) have a worldwide distribution. They belong, like *Haematobia* species (see Horn-flies), to the subfamily Stomoxyinae. There are four species, all in the genus *Stomoxys*, the most common species being *Stomoxys calcitrans* (Fig. 1).

Biology

Both sexes take blood meals from wild and domesticated animals, especially horses, cattle, dogs and pigs; they also feed on people if their preferred hosts are scarce or absent. Most biting is on the legs and bites can be quite painful. In hot weather flies digest their blood meal within 12–24 h, but in cooler areas digestion can take as long as 2–4 days. Feeding is repeated every 2–10 days, depending on temperature, and is restricted to the daytime. Most biting occurs out of doors, but stable-flies sometimes enter houses to feed. Adult flies are more common in rural areas, being especially common around farms and horse stables.

Eggs are usually laid in horse manure, but also among rotting vegetable material, cut grass, weeds or hay, or in compost pits. They hatch within 1–5 days and the resultant larvae are typically maggot-shaped and closely resemble larvae of house-flies. Larvae are mainly found in wet mixtures of manure and straw and in vegetable matter

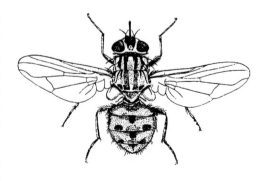

Fig. 1.   An adult stable-fly (*Stomoxys calcitrans*).

in advanced stages of decay. There are three larval instars and development may take only 6–10 days, but under unfavourable conditions can be prolonged to 4–5 weeks or even longer. The puparium is barrel-shaped (like that of house-flies) and in warm areas this stage lasts 5–7 days. The life cycle is basically similar to that depicted in the figure accompanying the biology of house-flies (see entry on Flies). The time from oviposition to adult emergence is 12–42 days, duration depending mostly on temperature.

Diseases

In addition to inflicting painful bites and causing distress to horses and cattle, stable-flies can mechanically transmit sleeping sickness in Africa, although there is no evidence that they play any part in its epidemiology. In contrast, they are probably involved in the transmission of trypanosomes that cause the disease surra in horses and camels. Stable-flies are also intermediate hosts of *Setaria cervi*, a filarial parasite of cattle, and several species of *Habronema* that infect horses (see entries on these infections).

Control

Control measures advocated for house-flies are generally applicable, with some minor modifications, for stable-flies – for example, preventing piles of rotting vegetation and horse manure from accumulating and providing breeding sites. Larval habitats that cannot be removed can be sprayed with insecticides, but large volumes may be needed to penetrate deep into piles of manure, where most larvae are found. Insecticidal spraying of horse stables and other animal shelters, or hanging insecticide- impregnated cords in these shelters, may help reduce the numbers of stable-flies.

Selected bibliography

Greenberg, B. (1973) *Flies and Disease*, Vol. 2, *Biology and Disease Transmission.* Princeton University Press, Princeton, New Jersey, 447 pp.

Skidmore, P. (1985) *The Biology of the Muscidae of the World.* W. Junk Publishers, Dordrecht, 550 pp.

Zumpt, F. (1973) *The Stomoxyine Biting Flies of the World. Diptera: Muscidae. Taxonomy, Biology, Economic Importance and Control Measures.* Gustav Fischer, Stuttgart, 175 pp.

Steam bugs *see* **Cockroaches.**

Stephanofilariasis

R.C. Anderson

Infection of ungulates with nematodes of the genus *Stephanofilaria*, which live in the dermis and create a skin lesion attractive to muscid flies, which serve as intermediate hosts. Microfilariae occur in the dermal papillae.

Parasites

Stephanofilaria assamensis

Small nematodes with a circle of 16–24 cephalic spines (Fig. 1) and 14–18 peribuccal spines. Males are 2.5–6.0 mm and females 7.0–12.7 mm in length. Eggs are thin-shelled and 38–42 μm × 25–36 μm in size. Microfilariae are 93–148 μm in length.

DISTRIBUTION Mainly in cattle in India, Bangladesh, Pakistan and southern Russia. Also reported in Buffaloes (*Bubalus bubalis*; Murrah breed), goats and the Indian elephant (*Elephas maximus*).

CLINICAL SIGNS Early lesions are probably usually raw and bloody or covered with serous exudate, as reported in infections with *Stephanofilaria stilesi* in the USA. Lesions of some duration are described as circumscribed, raised, dry, alopecic–hyperkeratotic or scab-encrusted. In an active state the surface may be raw or cracked, with haemorrhage and serum

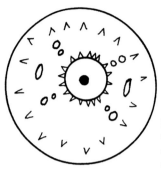

Fig. 1.
Cephalic end of
*Stephanofilaria
assamensis.*

Musca species or in stable-flies (*Stomoxys calcitrans*) collected while feeding on sores.

CONTROL   Control of horn-flies in the environment may be feasible by the proper handling of manure and the use of insecticides.

A single treatment of cattle with ivermectin given subcutaneously at 200 mg kg^{-1} body weight is effective. In endemic areas it is recommended that the treatment is repeated every 28 days. Intramuscular or subcutaneous injection of levamisole at 9.1–12.1 mg kg^{-1} body weight and daily topical application of zinc oxide ointment on lesions has proved to be effective, but topical application of zinc oxide on its own was not effective. Application of 98% trichlorfon (Neguron®) to lesions repeated 24 and 48 h later resulted in wound-healing within 21 days.

exudation. Lesions in cattle are commonly on the hump ('hump-sore') but lesions have been reported in the medial canthus of the eye and on the neck, poll, base of the horns, ears, muzzle, back, base of the tail, abdomen and feet. In buffaloes, lesions are reported on the navel flap and in Indian elephants the lesions may occur on the feet and flanks.

DIAGNOSIS   Scrapings of the lesions soaked in saline should reveal the typical eggs and the coiled microfilariae within them. Eggs and microfilariae occur in the superficial region of the lesions. Biopsy may reveal the adult worms as well.

TRANSMISSION   A suitable intermediate host attracted to the lesions in India was reported to be *Musca conducens*. A pre-existing lesion may be necessary to initiate transmission, since the mouthparts of *Musca* species cannot penetrate the skin (cf. horn-flies, such as *Haematobia* species). In the fly the first moult occurred in 5–6 days and the second 13–14 days post-infection. Third-stage infective larvae appeared after 23–25 days at 25.5°C. Infective larvae were of two sizes, 0.75–0.97 mm and 1.08–1.26 mm; these are presumably sexual differences. Infected *M. conducens* were allowed to feed on two minor surgical lesions on the hump of calves. One lesion became infected and a circular lesion appeared about 6 weeks post-infection. In Uzbekistan the vector of *S. assamensis* is the horn-fly *Haematobia titillans.* Microfilariae reached the infective stages in thoracic muscles in 21–24 days in this fly, in which greatest activity is in June and July. Larvae were not found in

Stephanofilaria stilesi

Small nematodes with only four or five cephalic spines (cf. *S. assamensis*) and 18–19 peribuccal spines (Fig. 2). Males are 2.6–3.7 mm and females 3.7–6.9 mm in length. Thin-shelled eggs are 58–72 µm × 42–55 µm in size. Microfilaria are 45–60 µm in length.

DISTRIBUTION   In cattle in North America, Hawaii, Japan and the Commonwealth of Independent States (CIS).

CLINICAL SIGNS   Lesions are probably initiated by the bites of horn-flies. Active lesions are raw, bloody and covered with serous exudate. In chronic conditions the infected area becomes smooth, dry and thickened, usually in older animals. Lesions are most common along the midventral line between the brisket and the navel, especially in young cattle. Lesions are also reported on the udder, scrotum, flanks and ears. Adult nematodes occur in the dermis 1–2 mm below the epidermis. Microfilariae within shells are found in dermal papillae of lesions and not in adjacent healthy tissue.

DIAGNOSIS   Deep skin scrapings macerated in saline will release microfilariae and adult worms for microscopical study. Biopsy

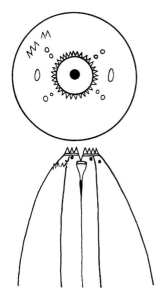

Fig. 2.
Cephalic end of
*Stephanofilaria
stilesi.*

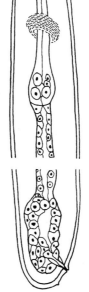

Fig. 3. Infective larva of
Stephanofilaria stilesi.

sections will readily reveal microfilaria and
adults.

TRANSMISSION   Vectors of *S. stilesi* are the
horn-flies, *Haematobia irritans* and *H. titillans*, which develop in cattle manure.
(The genus name *Lyperosia* is a synonym of
Haematobia.) The flies feed predominantly
along the midventral line of the host
and their bites create lesions that permit
infective larvae to invade the skin. Obvious
lesions appear about 2 weeks after flies have
fed on the skin. These mature lesions are
attractive to both species of horn-flies, as
well as to non-biting muscids (e.g. *Musca*
species). Microfilariae ingested by the vector
develop in the abdominal haemocoel.
At room temperature, the first moult occurs
after 8–10 days and the second in
14–16 days. Infective larvae (Fig. 3)
(695–900 µm in length) migrated to the head
and proboscis 2–5 days after the final moult.
The larva is characterized by a peribuccal
elevation with a single spine and a short and
rounded tail.

CONTROL   Much as for *S. assamensis.*

Selected bibliography

Anderson, R.C. (2000) *Nematode Parasites of
Vertebrates, their Development and
Transmission*, 2nd edn. CAB International,
Wallingford, UK, 650 pp.
Dikman, G. (1934) Observations on stephanofila-
riasis in cattle. *Proceedings of the Helmintho-
logical Society of Washington* 1, 42–43.
Hibler, C.P. (1966) Development of *Stephano-
filaria stilesi* in the horn fly. *Journal of
Parasitology* 52, 890–898.
Ivashkin, V.M., Shmitova, G.Y. and Koishibaev,
G.K. (1971) Stephanofilariasis in herbivorous
animals. *Veterinariya* 48, 66–68. (In Russian.)
Johnson, S.J. (1987) Stephanofilariasis – a review.
Helminthological Abstracts 56, 287–299.
Kabilov, T.K. (1980) New data on the biology
of *Stephanofilaria assamensis* (Nematoda,
Filariata). *Helminthologia* 17, 191–196.
Patnaik, B. (1973) Studies on stephanofilariasis in
Orissa. III. Life cycle of *S. assamensis* Pande,
1936. *Zeitschrift für Tropenmedizin und
Parasitologie* 24, 457–466.
Patnaik, B. and Roy, S.P. (1966) On the life cycle
of the filariid *Stephanofilaria assamensis*
Pande, 1936, in the arthropod vector *Musca
conducens* Walker, 1859. *Indian Journal of
Animal Health* 5, 91–101.
Srivastava, H.D. and Dutt, S.C. (1963) Studies
on the life history of *Stephanofilaria*

assamensis. *Indian Journal of Veterinary Science* 33, 173–177.

Sultanova, M.A., Kabilov, T.K. and Siddikov, B.K. (1979) The developmental cycle of the nematode *Stephanofilaria assamensis* Pande, 1936, in Uzbekistan (USSR). *Doklady Akademii Nauk Uzberskoi SSR* 9, 73–74. (In Russian.)

***Stephanofilaria* species** *see* **Stephanofilariasis.**

Stercorarian trypanosomes *see* **Animal trypanosomiasis.**

***Stomoxys* species** *see* **Stable-flies.**

Stratford virus

John S. Mackenzie

Stratford (STR) virus is a mosquito-borne flavivirus enzootic in Australia and possibly in Papua New Guinea. It was first isolated from *Ochlerotatus*[1] *vigilax* mosquitoes collected in Cairns in north Queensland in 1961. Subsequent seroepidemiological studies carried out in New South Wales suggested that occasional human infections occurred, but there has been no reported association with human disease.

Distribution

Stratford virus has been isolated from mosquitoes trapped at various localities in Queensland and New South Wales, ranging from south coastal New South Wales to northern Queensland.

Virus

Stratford virus is in the genus *Flavivirus* and is closely related to Kokobera virus (see entry). Both viruses were classified as members of the Japanese encephalitis (see entry) serological complex of flaviviruses. However, the recent Seventh Report from the International Committee for the Taxonomy of Viruses (in Sydney, 1999) has reclassified Stratford and Kokobera viruses into a separate complex of their own.

Clinical symptoms and pathogenesis

Although seroepidemiological studies carried out in New South Wales suggested that occasional human infections have occurred, there has been no reported association with human disease.

Transmission

Stratford virus has been isolated from several mosquito species, including *O. vigilax* in Queensland and New South Wales, and *Culex annulirostris*, *Ochlerotatus procax* and *Ochlerotatus notoscriptus* in New South Wales. However, the role of each of these in transmission is unknown.

Ecology

The vertebrate hosts of Stratford virus are thought to be marsupials. Birds are not believed to play a role in transmission cycles.

Note

[1] *Ochlerotatus* was formerly a subgenus of *Aedes*.

Selected bibliography

Mackenzie, J.S., Lindsay, M.D., Coelen, R.J., Broom, A.K., Hall, R.A. and Smith, D.W. (1994) Arboviruses causing human disease in the Australasian region. *Archives of Virology* 136, 447–467.

Poidinger, M., Hall, R.A. and Mackenzie, J.S. (1996) Molecular characterisation of the Japanese encephalitis serocomplex of the flavivirus genus. *Virology* 218, 417–421.

Surra *see* **Animal trypanosomiasis.**

Swamp fever *see* **Equine infectious anaemia.**

Tabanids *see* **Horseflies.**

Tahyna virus

Milan Labuda

Distribution

Tahyna (TAH) virus was first isolated from mosquitoes (*Aedes vexans, Ochlerotatus*[1] *caspius*) in Slovakia (Tahyna and Krizany villages, East Slovakia) in 1958. It became one of the first recognized mosquito-borne viruses isolated in Europe. Later isolates were obtained from the Czech Republic, Austria, Hungary, Slovenia, Serbia, Romania, France, Italy, Germany, Norway, Estonia, Moldavia, Ukraine and Russia. Anti-TAH virus antibodies were detected in all the above-mentioned countries and also in most other European countries, as well as in Asia and Africa. In fact the virus occurs throughout Europe, depending on the abundance of local *Aedes* mosquito populations. In Central Europe in flood-plain forest ecosystems, following summer floods, which result in large populations of mosquitoes, there are local periodic outbreaks of TAH virus.

The closely related Inkoo virus is known from Finland, Norway, Sweden, Estonia and Russia. Snowshoe hare (SSH) virus, another closely related virus, has been isolated from *Ochlerotatus communis* mosquitoes in northern Russia. A virus antigenically indistinguishable from TAH virus, Lumbo virus, was isolated from mosquitoes in Mozambique.

Virus

Tahyna virus (family Bunyaviridae, genus *Bunyavirus*) is a member of the California serogroup, the California encephalitis complex, together with Inkoo virus and the North American California encephalitis, La Crosse (see entry), SSH and other viruses.

The spherical TAH virus virions are 90–120 nm in diameter. An envelope composed of a lipid bilayer containing glycoprotein spikes (G1 and G2) surrounds a core consisting of the genome and its associated proteins (nucleocapsid protein, viral polymerase). The genome is single-stranded RNA of negative polarity divided into three segments – large (coding for large polymerase protein), medium (coding for G1 and G2 glycoproteins) and small (coding for nucleocapsid protein). A number of non-structural proteins have also been described and assigned to specific segments. Each viral particle contains three internal nucleocapsids, composed of three genomic segments, many copies of nucleocapsid protein and a few copies of viral polymerase. Each nucleocapsid is arranged in a non-covalently closed circle. Reassortment of genomic segments of closely related viruses can occur when cells are co-infected with two California serogroup viruses.

Clinical symptoms

Many infections with TAH virus are inapparent, but the antibody prevalence among inhabitants of endemic foci can be as high as 60–80%. When symptomatic, the infection produces an acute influenza-like disease, mainly in children, with sudden onset of fever lasting for 3–5 days, with headache, malaise, conjunctivitis, pharyngitis, myalgia, nausea, gastrointestinal disorders, anorexia and occasional arthralgia. Meningitis or other signs of central nervous system (CNS) involvement have been observed. In contrast to La Crosse virus, no fatalities have been attributed to TAH virus. In the endemic region of southern Moravia (Czech Republic), the disease is known as 'Valtice fever'. Several hundred documented Tahyna virus human cases have been recorded.

Diagnosis

Methods used for TAH virus diagnosis are in principle the same as for other arboviruses. Direct virus isolation from mosquitoes or host tissues is still the main proof of TAH virus presence and infection. Further methods of choice are immuno-fluorescence or polymerase chain reaction (PCR); however, the lack of circulating virus for subsequent virological studies is a disadvantage of PCR. A variety of cell cultures can be used for virus isolation. Alternatively, intracranial inoculation of suckling laboratory mice can be used. Several standard methods for determining the presence of antibody to TAH virus, such as virus neutralization, haemagglutination inhibition, complement fixation and enzyme-linked immunosorbent assay, are well established.

Transmission

Transmission in an endemic focus is perpetuated via infected mosquito bites. During the long-term ecological studies of TAH virus in southern Moravia (Czech Republic), 45 TAH virus isolates were obtained from seven mosquito species (*A. vexans*, *Ochlerotatus cantans*, *O. caspius*, *Ochlerotatus sticticus*, *Aedes cinereus*, *Culiseta annulata* and *Culex modestus*). The most important TAH virus vector was shown to be *A. vexans* (58% of all isolates resulted from this species) and these observations are in accord with results obtained elsewhere in Europe. It seems that the presence of *A. vexans* is a prerequisite for the maintainance of TAH virus transmission cycles in an area. Nevertheless, other *Aedes* and *Ochlerotatus* species contribute to transmission and *Culiseta* and *Culex* mosquitoes may be important in the overwintering of TAH virus.

The most important vertebrate hosts of TAH virus in Central Europe appear to be Brown hares (*Lepus europaeus*) and Rabbits (*Oryctolagus cuniculus*). They are highly susceptible to TAH virus, develop sufficiently high and long-lasting viraemias to infect vectors and are also abundant and attractive hosts for mosquitoes. In addition, certain species of rodents and insectivores, as well as several species of domestic animals can serve occasionally and locally as TAH virus hosts. It has been suggested that direct transmission from human to human

may occur during periods when there are very large mosquito populations in urban areas.

Treatment

The disease is self-curable. No specific treatment is known or required.

Control

Because the treatment of TAH virus infections is only symptomatic, control measures in endemic foci of infection are important. Among them the most important is the control of mosquitoes through application of insecticides to and/or drainage of their breeding places. Personal protection against mosquito bites by wearing protective clothes or using insect repellents can give some degree of protection from the vectors. Because of the mild influenza-like clinical picture of most human illnesses caused by TAH virus, vaccine preparation is not a priority.

Note

[1] *Ochlerotatus* was formerly a subgenus of *Aedes*.

Selected bibliography

Bárdos, V. (1974) Recent state of knowledge of Tahyna virus infections. *Folia Parasitologica* 21, 1–10.

Bárdos, V. (1975) The role of mammals in the circulation of Tahyna virus. *Folia Parasitologica* 22, 257–264.

Bárdos, V. and Danielova, V. (1959) The Tahyna virus – a virus isolated from mosquitoes in Czechoslovakia. *Journal of Hygiene, Epidemiology, Microbiology and Immunology* 3, 264–276.

Gonzales-Scarano, F. and Nathanson, N. (1996) Bunyaviridae. In: Fields, B.N., Knipe, D.M. and Howley, P.M. (eds) *Fields Virology*, Vol.1, 3rd edn. Lippincott-Raven Publishers, Philadelphia, pp. 1473–1504.

Hubálek, Z. and Halouzka, J. (1996) Arthropod-borne viruses of vertebrates in Europe. *Acta Scientiarum Naturalium Academiae Scientiarum Bohemicae Brno* 30(4–5), 1–95.

Rosick , B. and Málková, D. (1980) Tahyna virus natural focus in southern Moravia. *Rozpravy Ceskoslovenske Akademie Ved Rada Matematickych a Prirodnich Ved Akademie Prague* 90(7), 1–107.

Tataguine virus

Oyewale Tomori

Distribution

Tataguine (TAT) virus was originally isolated in 1962 from a pool of adult unidentified female *Anopheles* and *Culex* mosquitoes aspirated from dwelling places in M'Betit Gouye, near Tataguine in Senegal. The virus was subsequently isolated from various species of mosquitoes in other countries. Tataguine virus has also been isolated from febrile (human) patients in Nigeria, Senegal, Central African Republic and Cameroon. Serological studies revealed widespread prevalence of neutralizing antibodies to TAT virus in humans in Senegal and Nigeria. None of the domestic animals, monkeys, rodents, bats and birds tested for TAT neutralizing antibody has been positive.

Virus

Tataguine virus is classified as an ungrouped member of the *Bunyavirus* genus in the Bunyaviridae family. It is moderately sensitive to treatment with sodium deoxycholate, with a 2-$\log_{10}$ decrease in virus titre following treatment. Virus-infected suckling mouse brains contain haemagglutinin activity for goose and chick erythrocytes.

Clinical symptoms, pathogenesis and pathogenicity

Tataguine virus is pathogenic for suckling mice only when inoculated intracerebrally, resulting in the development of high virus titres and death within 5 days after inoculation. Adult mice do not succumb to TAT virus infection by either the intracerebral or the intraperitoneal routes. Intracerebral inoculation of suckling hamsters with TAT virus results in 100% mortality; however, by the intraperitoneal route, less than 50% die. Histopathological lesions in mice and hamsters dying from TAT virus infections, irrespective of route of infection, are limited to the brain. These lesions include interstitial and perivascular oedema of the cerebral cortex and the spinal cord and cuffing of the blood-vessels, with small foci of neuronal degeneration and necrosis in the anterior horns, mid-brain and pons. There is evidence of lymphocytic meningitis, but no inclusion bodies are seen. Bunyavirus-like particles are seen within cytoplasmic vacuoles of neurons in thin-section electron microscopy of infected mouse brains. Guinea-pigs are refractory to TAT virus infection. Tataguine virus replicates but does not cause cytopathic effects (CPE) in Vervet monkey (VERO) cells, baby hamster kidney (BHK-21) cells and *Aedes albopictus* monolayers. The virus produces plaques (1–1.5 mm in diameter) in VERO cells and virus antigen can be detected in the cytoplasm of VERO cells by the immunofluorescence test. Rhesus monkey kidney (LLC-MK2) and porcine kidney (PK-15) cells do not support the replication of TAT virus.

The clinical manifestations of TAT virus are mild and characterized by fever and a rash, and are similar to those of malaria and pyrexias of unknown origin in West Africa. However, during the period 1966–1975, when active surveillance for arbovirus infections was in place in West Africa, TAT virus was one of the five viruses most frequently isolated from human blood in Nigeria and Senegal.

Diagnosis

Diagnosis is by virus isolation from blood or by serology. Tataguine virus presents a special diagnostic problem, because serological response to infection, as measured by complement fixation, is generally low or without serological conversion. Therefore detection of neutralizing or immunoglobulin M (IgM) antibodies may prove useful and essential for diagnosis.

Transmission

The virus has been isolated from *Anopheles funestus* in Nigeria and the Central African Republic, from *Anopheles gambiae* in Burkina Faso, the Central African Republic,

Cameroon and Senegal, from *Anopheles nili* in Senegal and from *Mansonia aurites* in Cameroon.

Although TAT virus has been successfully transmitted by *Aedes circumluteolus* mosquitoes and antibodies detected in domesticated animals, the vertebrate hosts involved in the natural cycle of transmission are unknown.

Treatment

Treatment is symptomatic.

Control

No control measures are applicable.

Selected bibliography

Brès, P., Williams, M.C. and Chambon, L. (1966) Isolement au Senegal d'un nouveau prototype d'arbovirus, la souche 'Tataguine' (IPD/A 252). *Annales de l'Institut Pasteur 3*, 585–591.

Fagbami, A.H. and Tomori, O. (1981) Tataguine virus isolations from humans in Nigeria 1971–1975. *Transactions of the Royal Society of Tropical Medicine and Hygiene 75*, 788.

Fagbami, A.H., Monath, T.P., Tomori, O., Lee, V.H. and Fabiyi, A. (1972) Studies on Tataguine virus infection in Nigeria. *Tropical and Geographical Medicine 24*, 298–302.

Gonzalez, J.P. and Georges, A.T. (1988) Bunyaviral fevers: Bunyamwera, Ilesha, Germiston, Bwamba and Tataguine. In: Monath, T.P. (ed.) *The Arboviruses: Epidemiology and Ecology*, Vol. II. CRC Press, Boca Raton, Florida, pp. 87–98.

Institut Pasteur, Dakar (1997) *Annual Report*, 65 pp.

Karabatsos, N. (ed.) (1985) *International Catalogue of Arboviruses Including Certain Other Viruses of Vertebrates*, 3rd edn. American Society of Tropical Medicine and Hygiene, San Antonio, Texas, 1147 pp.

Moore, D.L., Causey, O.R., Causey, D.E., Reddy, S., Cooke A.R., Akinkugbe, F.M., David-West, T.S. and Kemp, G.E. (1975) Arthropod-borne viral infections of man in Nigeria (1964–1970). *Annals of Tropical Medicine and Parasitology 69*, 49–64.

Tensaw virus

Bruce F. Eldridge

Tensaw (TEN) virus is a mosquito-borne arbovirus that occurs in the south-eastern USA. It is transmitted by many species of mosquitoes, especially members of the genus *Anopheles*. It occurs in the south-eastern USA from Texas to Georgia. Its public health importance is unknown, but evidence of infection has been demonstrated by the presence of haemagglutination inhibition (HI) antibodies in human serum samples. A single case of encephalitis associated with TEN virus has been reported from Indiana, but this is outside the known geographical distribution of the virus. Tensaw virus is classified in the genus *Bunyavirus*, Bunyamwera serogroup.

Distribution

Virus isolations from mosquitoes have been made from the states of Alabama, Florida, Georgia, Mississippi, Louisiana and Texas in the USA (Fig. 1).

Virus

Tensaw virus is a member of the family Bunyaviridae, genus *Bunyavirus*, and the Bunyamwera serogroup. The prototype for this genus and serogroup is Bunyamwera virus. Other members of the serogroup include Northway virus and Cache Valley (see entry) viruses. Tensaw virus was first isolated in 1960 from a pool of *Anopheles crucians* collected in Baldwin County, Alabama, at Stream Mill Landing. The collection was made at the edge of a swamp close to the Tensaw River.

Clinical symptoms

Human cases of illness are unknown except for a single case of encephalitis reported from Indiana. Because no isolations of TEN virus have ever been reported from Indiana, this case may represent infection by some other bunyavirus. However, surveys conducted in Alabama have shown that about

9% of the human serum samples tested were seropositive by HI test.

Diagnosis

Confirmation of arboviral disease requires isolation of virus from an infected patient or a fourfold or greater increase in antibody titre between acute and convalescent human serum samples. Isolation of fully typed virus from mosquitoes or detection of antibodies in sentinel mammals may demonstrate enzootic viral activity.

Transmission

Based on the presence of HI antibodies and isolation of virus from blood, the natural vertebrate hosts of TEN virus appear to be a variety of small- to medium-sized mammals. Virus has been isolated from the blood of domestic cats, Hispid cotton rats (*Sigmodon hispidus*), Swamp-rabbits (*Sylvilagus aquaticus*), Cotton mouse (*Peromyscus gossypinus*) and Gray foxes ((*Vulpes* (= *Urocyon*) *cinereoargenteus*)). In addition, HI antibody has been detected in domestic dogs and Raccoons (*Procyon lotor*).

Tensaw virus has been isolated from many species of mosquitoes. The original isolate was from a pool of *Anopheles crucians*, a species common in or near freshwater swamps in the eastern USA. Since then, many isolations have been made from this species (Table 1). A few isolates have been made from *Anopheles punctipennis*, *Anopheles quadrimaculatus* and *Ochlerotatus*[1] *mitchellae*, but at high rates. *Psorophora columbiae*, *Ochlerotatus atlanticus/tormentor*, *Ochlerotatus infirmatus*, *Ochlerotatus taeniorhynchus*, *Coquillettidia perturbans*, *Culex nigripalpus* and *Culex salinarius* have yielded some isolates. Isolations from most of these species have been at very low frequencies, and they are probably relatively unimportant in the ecology of TEN virus. The greatest number of isolates has been from *A. crucians*, with an overall

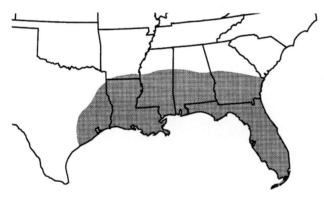

Fig. 1. Distribution of Tensaw virus in the south-eastern USA.

Table 1. Minimum infection rates (MIR) for TEN virus reported in the literature (two or more isolations).

Species	No. tested	No. positive	MIR*
Anopheles punctipennis	874	6	146
Ochlerotatus[†] mitchellae	1,249	3	416
Anopheles crucians	221,314	293	755
Anopheles quadrimaculatus	9,560	5	1,912
Psorophora columbiae	89,459	36	2,485
Ochlerotatus atlanticus/tormentor	48,021	8	6,003
Ochlerotatus infirmatus	105,865	17	6,227
Ochlerotatus taeniorhynchus	34,127	3	11,376
Coquillettidia perturbans	43,594	2	21,797
Culex nigripalpus	754,793	3	251,598

*Number tested positive/total isolations made.
[†]*Ochlerotatus* was formerly in the subgenus *Aedes*.

minimum infection rate (MIR, i.e. the number of mosquitoes tested positive divided by the total number isolations made) of 755. The only other significant species from the standpoint of numbers of isolations are *P. columbiae* (36 isolations) and *O. infirmatus* (17 isolations). However, for both of these species, the MIR is more than threefold higher than for *A. crucians*. This suggests that *A. crucians* is the primary vector of TEN virus, with the other species being of either secondary importance or serving as local vectors. Thus, TEN virus is one of the relatively few *Anopheles*-transmitted arboviruses.

Transmission of TEN virus has been demonstrated in the laboratory in *A. quadrimaculatus* mosquitoes.

Treatment

There are no specific treatments.

Control

Usually none. Mosquito abatement may be indicated in specific situations, such as the close proximity of high-density housing to freshwater swamps and other sources of potential vector mosquitoes. In such cases, control would probably be limited to destruction of adult female mosquitoes by ground application of insecticidal fogs.

Note

1 *Ochlerotatus* was formerly a subgenus of *Aedes*.

Selected bibliography

Calisher, C.H., Francy, D.B., Smith, G.C., Muth, D.J., Lazuick, J.S., Karabatsos, N., Jakob, W.L. and McLean, R.G. (1986) Distribution of Bunyamwera serogroup viruses in North America, 1956–1984. *American Journal of Tropical Medicine and Hygiene* 35, 429–443.

Chamberlain, R.W., Sudia, W.D. and Coleman, P.H. (1969) Isolations of an arbovirus of the Bunyamwera group (Tensaw virus) from mosquitoes in the southeastern United States. *American Journal of Tropical Medicine and Hygiene* 18, 92–97.

Karabatsos, N. (ed.) (1985) *International Catalogue of Arboviruses Including Certain Other Viruses of Vertebrates*, 3rd edn. The American Society of Tropical Medicine and Hygiene, San Antonio, Texas, 1147 pp.

Texas cattle fever *see* **Babesiosis.**

Theileria **species** *see* **Theilerioses.**

Theilerioses

Patricia M. Preston

Infections of ruminants, equids and felids with tick-borne protozoan parasites of the genus *Theileria*.

The malignant theilerioses of cattle and sheep cause morbidity and loss of productivity in indigenous breeds and severe, often lethal, disease in imported animals and cross-bred, high-grade stock throughout Africa and Asia (Tables 1–3). Apathogenic/benign *Theileria* species also cause economically significant infections, especially in imported, immunocompromised or stressed animals. The recent recognition of the parasites formerly known as *Babesia equi* and *Cytauxzoon felis* as species of *Theileria* extended the known host range of the genus *Theileria* and the diseases considered as theilerioses.

Distribution

The distribution and occurrence of the *Theileria* species and the diseases they cause are determined by the distribution and seasonal activity of their particular tick vectors (Tables 1–3). Basically infections occur in Europe, Asia, Africa, North, Central and South America and Australasia.

Table 1.   The family Theileridae. Cosmopolitan species of cattle, buffalo and equids: species, diseases, tick vectors, mammalian hosts and distribution.

Parasites	Diseases	Tick vectors	Mammalian hosts	Distribution
Theileria annulata	Tropical theileriosis, Mediterranean Coast fever (severe disease uncommon in southern Europe)	*Hyalomma* species	Cattle, Asian buffalo (*Bubalus bubalis*)	Southern Europe, northern Africa, Middle East, Russian Federation (Transcaucasian regions), Central Asian republics, China (north of R. Chang Jiang)
Theileria orientalis orientalis (synonym *Theileria sergenti*)	Benign cosmopolitan theileriosis: pathogenic strains Apathogenic strains	*Haemaphysalis* species *Haemaphysalis* species, except N. America: vector unknown	Cattle, Asian buffalo (*Bubalus bubalis*) Cattle	Russian Federation (Far Eastern maritime regions), China, Korea, Japan Europe, Africa, Asia, Australia, New Zealand, North America
Theileria orientalis sergenti (synonym *Theileria sergenti*)	Oriental theileriosis	*Haemaphysalis* species	Cattle	Japan (Ikeda stock)
Theileria new species detected by molecular systematics	Apathogenic	Unknown	Cattle	China, North America, Thailand
Theileria buffeli	Apathogenic	*Haemaphysalis* species	Asian buffalo (*Bubalus bubalis*)	South-East Asia
Theileria equi	Equine biliary fever	*Dermacentor* species *Hyalomma* species *Rhipicephalus* species	Horses, donkeys, mules, Zebra (*Equus burchelli*), humans	Southern Europe, Africa, Asia, Australia, USA (Florida), S. and C. America

Table 2.   The family Theileridae. Parasites of cattle and wild ruminants in sub-Saharan Africa: species, diseases, tick vectors, mammalian hosts and distribution.

Parasites	Diseases	Tick vectors	Mammalian hosts	Distribution
Theileria parva	East Coast fever Corridor (buffalo) disease January disease	*Rhipicephalus appendiculatus** *Rhipicephalus duttoni** *Rhipicephalus zambeziensis**	Cattle, Waterbuck (*Kobus ellipsiprymnus*), African buffalo (*Syncerus caffer*), Asian buffalo (*Bubalus bubalis*)	Eastern, Central and Southern Africa
Theileria mutans	Benign African theileriosis I Usually benign but may be pathogenic	*Amblyomma* species	Cattle, some strains of African buffalo (*S. caffer*)	Sub-Saharan Africa, Madagascar, Islands of Réunion and Mauritius, Lesser Antilles
Theileria taurotragi	Benign African theileriosis II Usually benign, may cause cerebral theileriosis	*Rhipicephalus appendiculatus**	Eland (*Taurotragus oryx*), cattle, sheep, goats and wide range of wild ungulates	Eastern, Central and Southern Africa
Theileria velifera	Apathogenic	*Amblyomma* species	Cattle, African buffalo (*S. caffer*)	Africa

*Main field vectors.

The genus *Theileria*

The distinguishing features of the genus are given in Table 4; its characteristic life cycle is illustrated in Figs 1–3. Current taxonomic research recognizes at least 17 species of *Theileria*, of which six cause important diseases of domestic stock (Tables 1–3). Four of these six species are geographically cosmopolitan parasites: *T. annulata* and *T. orientalis* in cattle, *T. lestoquardi* in sheep and *T. equi* in horses. The fifth, the most pathogenic species in cattle, *T. parva*, is confined to sub-Saharan Africa, along with three apathogenic/benign species (*T. mutans*, *T. taurotragi* and *T. velifera*). The sixth, a newly recognized pathogenic parasite of sheep in China, is still unnamed.

The apathogenic/benign cosmopolitan parasites of domestic and wild ruminants are assigned to five species: *T. buffeli*, *T. cervi*, *T. orientalis*, *T. ovis* and *T. recondita*. Another (unnamed) cosmopolitan apathogenic parasite of cattle has recently been described as occurring in China, North

Table 3. The family Theileridae. Parasites of sheep, goats and cervids : species, disease, tick vectors, mammalian hosts and distribution.

Parasites	Diseases	Tick vectors	Mammalian hosts	Distribution
Theileria lestoquardi (synonym *Theileria hirci*)	Malignant ovine and caprine theileriosis	*Hyalomma* species	Sheep, goats	South-East Europe, North Africa, Middle East, India
Theileria new species?	Pathogenic	*Haemaphysalis quinghaiensis*	Sheep	China
Theileria ovis (possibly several species)	Benign ovine theileriosis	*Rhipicephalus* species	Sheep, goats	South-east Europe, Asia, Africa and Madagascar
Theileria recondita	Apathogenic	*Haemaphysalis* species (UK)	Sheep, goats, deer, Moufflon (i.e. wild sheep)	Western Europe: Germany, UK
Theileria separata	Apathogenic	*Rhipicephalus evertsi*	Sheep, goats	Sub-Saharan Africa
Theileria cervi (possibly several species)	Apathogenic	Unknown	Fallow deer (*Dama dama*), Red deer (*Cervus elaphus*), Sika deer (*Sika nippon*), Canadian Elk (*Cervus elaphus canadiensis*), White-tailed deer (*Odocoileus virginianus*)	Europe, Japan, North America

Table 4. Distinguishing features of the families Theileridae and Babesidae.

Kingdom	Protozoa	Single-celled eukaryotes
Phylum	Apicomplexa	Apical complex present in some stages; syngamy
Class	Haematozea	Sporogonic stages producing sporozoites
Subclass	Piroplasmia	Pyriform, rod-shaped or amoeboid parasites of erythrocytes
Order	Piroplasmida	Asexual and sexual reproduction; transmitted by ticks
Family	Theileridae	
Genus	*Theileria*	Exoerythrocytic schizogony in lymphocytes, macrophages or 'reticuloendothelial' cells
		Parasites of ruminants, equids or wild and domestic North American felids
		Trans-stadial transmission by ticks
Family	Babesidae	
Genus	*Babesia*	No schizogonic stages
		Widespread parasites of warm-blooded vertebrates
		Transovarial transmission by ticks

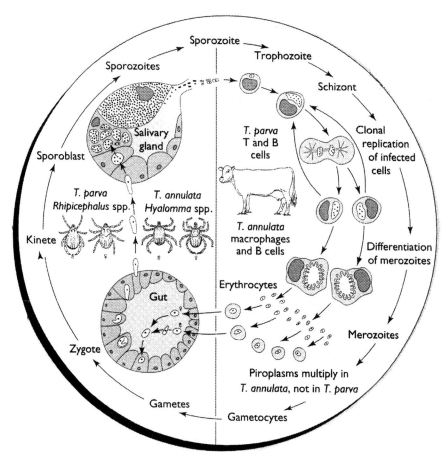

Fig. 1. The life cycle of a typical *Theileria* species, as illustrated by those of *T. annulata* and
T. parva, comprises a cycle of clonal replication of schizonts in mononuclear cells in lymphoid
and reticuloendothelial tissues, followed by the appearance of 'piroplasms' – small (<3 μm) and
pleomorphic organisms – in erythrocytes. *Theileria parva* proliferates as schizonts; its piroplasms
do not multiply. Schizonts are the major proliferating stage of *T. annulata*, *T. lestoquardi* and
T. felis. In infections of *T. annulata*, at least, elevated parasitaemias arise when erythrocytes
are invaded by massive numbers of merozoites produced by large populations of schizonts.
Theileria orientalis, *T. mutans* and *T. equi* proliferate mainly as piroplasms. In every species,
piroplasms include parasites undergoing gametogony and producing the gametocytes which are
infective for ticks. Differentiation into gametes and sexual recombination occurs in the tick gut.
Kinetes developing from zygotes in the gut cells appear to migrate directly to the tick's salivary
gland, where they undergo sporogony and differentiate into sporozoites, which are injected into
the next host by the tick. The different clinical manifestations of the theilerioses are broadly due
to the relative pathogenic effects of schizonts and piroplasms. Both schizonts and piroplasms
of *T. annulata*, *T. lestoquardi* and *T. felis* are pathogenic; the schizonts of *T. parva* cause East
Coast fever; piroplasms cause the diseases induced by *T. equi* and *T. orientalis*. The identity
of the schizont-infected mononuclear cells is only known so far for *T. annulata*, *T. parva* and
T. lestoquardi, the latter living mainly in macrophages. (Figure reprinted from Preston, P.M. and
Jongejan, F. (1999), Protective immune mechanisms in ticks and tick-borne diseases,
Parasitology Today 15, with permission from Elsevier Science.)

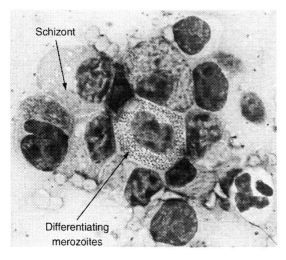

Schizont

Differentiating merozoites

Fig. 2. Schizonts and parasites differentiating into merozoites as seen in an impression smear of the spleen of a calf undergoing tropical theileriosis. (Photograph by L.M.G. Forsyth. Reprinted from Preston, P.M. and Jongejan, F. (1999) Protective immune mechanisms in ticks and tick-borne diseases, *Parasitology Today* 15, with permission from Elsevier Science.)

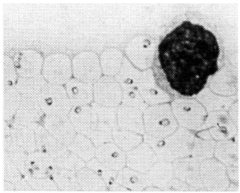

Fig. 3. Intraerythrocytic piroplasms as seen in a smear made from the blood of a calf undergoing tropical theileriosis. (Photograph by L.M.G. Forsyth.)

America and Thailand. Three other species have been linked to disease, namely *Theileria felis* in North American wild and domestic cats; *T. tarandi rangeriferis* in Reindeer, *Rangifer tarandus*; and *T. tachyglossis* in the monotreme, the Short-nosed echidna, *Tachyglossus aculeatus*. So far schizonts have been found in all species except for apathogenic strains of *T. orientalis orientalis*, which occur in Africa, Asia, Europe and North America, *T. buffeli* and *T. cervi*. Molecular systematics indicate that most *Theileria* species form a monophyletic taxon derived from a paraphyletic group that includes *T. equi*, *T. felis* and *Babesia rodhaini*. The genus *Theileria* comprises

two monophyletic clades: one includes *T. annulata*, *T. lestoquardi* and *T. parva;* the other includes *T. orientalis* and the 'new' pathogenic parasite of sheep in China. *Babesia* species sensu stricto are a sister taxon, which diverged from the paraphylectic group before most species of *Theileria* and lost the capacity to inhabit mononuclear cells.

Transmission

Transmission is trans-stadial, depending on gametocytes in the blood of infected animals being ingested by the larvae or nymphs of the particular species of two- or three-host ixodid (hard) ticks, in which a parasite can undergo sexual recombination and sporogony, and the sporozoites being inoculated into an appropriate mammalian host by the next stage of the tick, nymph or adult (Fig. 1). The identity of specific vector ticks helps to distinguish different *Theileria* species and subspecies (Tables 1–3).

Hosts and parasite factors influencing the outcome of infection

Theileria species are generally well adapted to their indigenous ruminant hosts, whether domesticated or wild animals. Disease occurs when potentially pathogenic organisms infect 'susceptible' stock, susceptibility being due to genetic or breed factors, loss of immunocompetence or stress due to lactation, parturition, management changes or concomitant infections. 'Pathogenic' species show strain variation, with virulent and mild strains coexisting in one region and cosmopolitan 'benign' species varying in pathogenicity from region to region. The different clinical manifestations of the theilerioses can be broadly attributed to the relative pathogenic effects of the different parasite stages (Fig. 1) and, in certain cases, to the nature of the schizont-infected mononuclear cells. Parasite dose also influences the outcome of infection – whether subclinical or clinical, self-limiting or lethal; the time to appearance and population size of different parasite stages; and the nature and extent of haematological responses. Cytokine production appears to determine many of the typical clinical features and pathological responses of the theilerioses.

Tropical theileriosis (*T. annulata*)

Although *T. annulata* exhibits extensive strain variation in virulence and molecular diversity in all endemic areas (Table 1), it causes similar disease symptoms across most of its range (from North Africa to China). Infection may cause severe, often lethal, disease in susceptible taurine or cross-bred cattle and significant morbidity and loss of productivity in local stock. Animals may survive disease but recovery and convalescence may be prolonged and incomplete, leading to permanent debilitation, loss of productivity and a prolonged carrier state. The parasite is maintained by cattle-tick transmission. In the Asian buffalo, *Bubalus bubalis*, which is probably its original host, *T. annulata* causes only subclinical or very mild infections. Cattle become infected when at pasture and under conditions of 'zero grazing', because the hyalommid tick vectors of *T. annulata* live in animal housing. *Theileria annulata* differs markedly from *T. parva* in that its schizonts inhabit macrophages, which undergo clonal replication, and it does not induce lymphocytic hyperplasia.

Clinical features of tropical theileriosis

Theileria annulata causes acute, mild, subacute, peracute and chronic disease, according to strain virulence and host susceptibility. The initial stages of disease accompany the metastasis of schizont-infected cells throughout the lymphoid system and reticuloendothelial tissues; later stages accompany the invasion of erythrocytes by merozoites and proliferation of piroplasms. In acute lethal disease, cattle exhibit increasingly pronounced symptoms (Table 5) from 5–7 days after infection, when schizonts become detectable in the lymph node draining the site of infection. Death may occur within 2–3 weeks following the proliferation of schizont-infected cells or the haemolytic anaemia resulting from intraerythrocytic piroplasms. Parasitaemias may reach 60% during the terminal stages of disease. Peracute disease is fairly common: onset is sudden, animals exhibit the symptoms of acute disease but death, preceded by hypothermia, occurs within a few days. Mild strains may cause subclinical infections, mild symptoms lasting a few days or subacute disease, with an irregularly intermittent fever lasting for up to 2 weeks and less marked symptoms than in acute infections. Animals usually recover, but pregnant animals may abort. In chronic disease, intermittent fever, inappetence, marked emaciation, anaemia and icterus may persist for a month or more, with animals taking more than 2 months to return to normal.

Pathology

The major pathological features are listed in Table 6. Damage to lymphoid tissues and reticuloendothelial tissues progresses as schizont-infected cells metastasise, often accompanied by lymphocytic infiltrations. Lymph nodes, including the paracortical areas, are dominated by schizont-infected cells and uninfected macrophages. Haemorrhagic lesions in the paracortex begin with extravasation of erthryocytes and macrophages and loss of integrity of the high endothelial venules. By the late stages of disease, schizonts throughout the body have differentiated into merozoites to form a vast pool of merozoites infective for erythrocytes. Anaemia has been linked to parasitaemia exacerbated by the proliferation of intraerythrocytic stages, autoimmune mechanisms and erythrophagocytosis by macrophages.

Table 5. Clinical features of acute fatal disease.

Tropical theileriosis

Early clinical signs	Pyrexia coinciding with the appearance of schizonts in the lymph node draining the site of inoculation; leucopenia; enlarged superficial lymph nodes; inappetence; drooling; serous nasal discharge; swelling of the eyelids; drooping ears; lowered head; sluggish gait; lacrimation; accelerated pulse; general weakness; decreased milk production; sometimes nervous symptoms
As disease progresses	Cachexia followed by wasting; marked anaemia with bilirubinaemia and bilirubinuria; superficial lymph nodes greatly enlarged; thrombocytopenia; conjunctiva icteric with petechial haemorrhages; diarrhoea
During later stages	Faeces are often mixed with blood and mucus; the skin may bear petechiae and, more rarely, raised nodules containing schizont-infected cells; marked emaciation; recumbency. If erythrocytes do not regenerate, anaemia becomes so severe and dyspnoea so pronounced that death ensues 8–15 days after the onset of the disease

East Coast fever

Early clinical signs	Pyrexia; leucopenia; listlessness; appetite wanes; bodily condition and milk production deteriorate; lymph nodes draining the site of inoculation of the parasite enlarge; other external nodes become palpably enlarged and hot
As disease progresses	Appetite and rumination cease; bodily condition degenerates rapidly; wasting follows cachexia; lethargy, weakness and recumbency increase; animals are reluctant to move, are tucked up and hang their heads; constipation; lacrimation and photophobia; mucous membranes unaffected, slightly hyperaemic or even anaemic; petechial haemorrhages common under the tongue and on the vulva
During later stages	If disease is prolonged, diarrhoea and dysentery may develop, blood may appear in the faeces; anaemia and icterus may occur; nodular skin lesions may develop
In the terminal stages	Severe respiratory distress with a watery cough due to pulmonary oedema; as oedema increases, watery frothy fluid runs from the mouth and nostrils; recumbency; copious quantities of fluid may pour from the nostrils; death is normally due to asphyxiation following pulmonary oedema

The production of cytokines, in particular tumour necrosis factor alpha (TNF-α), by both schizont-infected cells and uninfected host cells appears to underlie many of the symptoms (fever, inappetence, weight loss, emaciation) and pathological reactions (haemorrhagic necrosis). The presence of parasites in the pituitary glands and in badly damaged adrenal glands may underlie the disruption of the endocrine and immune systems.

Immunity

Theileria annulata clearly induces very effective immune responses in the vertebrate host, because recovered cattle are solidly immune to challenge. Isolates from widely separated regions (Morocco/India) are cross-protective, indicating that stocks across the parasite's range share the same protective antigens. Innate and adaptive responses appear to cooperate in protection. During primary infection, schizonts are eliminated by macrophage-derived nitric oxide (NO); schizont-infected cells are lysed by CD8$^+$ T cells and natural killer (NK) cells, piroplasms are killed by antibodies and piroplasm-infected cells are phagocytosed by macrophages. After challenge, antibodies may kill sporozoites and merozoites, but protection appears to be largely due to the rapid onset of innate immune responses and recall of memory CD4$^+$ T cells, which enhance macrophage activity. Nitric oxide and gamma-interferon (IFN-γ) produced by NK cells, CD4$^+$ T and CD8$^+$ T cells kill trophozoite-infected cells; CD8$^+$ T and NK cells lyse schizont-infected cells arising from parasites that evade the initial immune responses.

East Coast fever, Corridor disease and January disease (*T. parva*)

Theileria parva is a parasite of the African buffalo (*Syncerus caffer*); it is highly pathogenic to cattle causing the lymphoproliferative diseases known as East Coast fever, Corridor disease and January disease (Table 2). The parasites isolated from the different

Table 6.   Gross pathology of acute fatal disease.

Tropical theilerosis

Carcasses	Emaciated; anaemic; icteric; yellowish and gelatinous connective tissues
Blood	Watery
Subcutaneous tissues	Numerous petechial or larger haemorrhages
Mucous membranes (pharynx, larynx, trachea, bronchi)	Pale; numerous petechial or larger haemorrhages
Serous membranes	Numerous petechial or larger haemorrhages
Lymph nodes	Markedly enlarged; oedematous; varying degrees of haemorrhage
Thymus	Mildly congested
Heart	Myocardial muscular degeneration; petechial and ecchymotic haemorrhages on the epi- and endocardium
Lungs	Frequently oedematous; congested
Spleen	Splenomegaly due to lymphoid hyperplasia; soft; prominent Malpighian corpuscles
Liver	Hepatomegaly; pale brown or yellow; friable; evident parenchymatous degeneration
Gall-bladder	Often markedly distended; dark green viscid bile
Kidneys	Pale; congested; infarcts
Adrenal glands	Cortical haemorrhages
Abomasum, small and large intestines	Characteristic ulcers surrounded by a haemorrhagic zone
Nervous system	Occasionally cerebral haemorrhages

East Coast fever

Carcasses	Often a frothy exudate around the nostrils; emaciation, dehydration in protracted cases
Lymph nodes	In acute cases, oedematous, hyperaemic, may be greatly enlarged; in protracted cases, shrunken, necrotic
Thymus	Atrophy, necrosis common in young animals
Heart	Petechial and ecchymotic haemorrhages common on the epicardium and endocardium; serous fluid in pericardium
Trachea and bronchi	May be full of white, frothy exudate
Lungs	Interlobular oedema, emphysema and hyperaemia
Pleural cavity	Petechial and ecchymotic haemorrhages on serosal surfaces; serous fluid
Spleen	Mushy or dry, swollen or shrunken; subcapsular ecchymotic haemorrhages common
Liver	Usually normal although may be enlarged and mottled
Gall-bladder	Usually normal
Kidneys	Petechial haemorrhages common on surface; greyish white 'pseudoinfarcts' of lymphoid tissue; cortex may be congested
Bladder	Small haemorrhagic lesions on the mucosal and serosal surface
Peritoneum and viscera	Petechial and ecchymotic haemorrhages common on serosal surfaces
Abomasum	Ecchymotic and larger haemorrhages (up to 1 cm) with ulceration common on mucosa
Small and large intestines	Petechial haemorrhages on mucosal surfaces throughout
Peyer's patches	May be swollen
Nervous system	Changes rarely obvious; some hyperaemia

Malignant ovine and caprine theileriosis

Carcasses	Emaciated; icteric; intramuscular and subcutaneous tissues gelatinous
Blood	Changes characteristic of anaemia, being thin, watery, clear red
Lymph nodes	Markedly and generally enlarged, reddish and oedematous
Heart	Hydropericardium; muscles pale, flabby; no petechial haemorrhages
Lungs	Oedematous, congested
Spleen	Splenomegaly, pulp soft
Liver	Hepatomegaly, brownish-yellow or yellow, very friable
Gall-bladder	Distended, full of viscid bile
Kidneys	Pale due to anaemia, infarcts

Continued

Table 6. *Continued.*

Abomasum	Generally empty; mucous membranes slight to severe congestion; haemorrhages rare, if present, small
Intestines	Congested with petechial haemorrhages; mucous membranes, particularly caecum and colon, severely congested; sometimes haemorrhages and haemorrhagic patches; contents enlarged, reddish

diseases are genetically identical and the variations in morphology, pathogenicity, and incidence seen in *T. parva* in different geographical areas reflect its extreme antigenic diversity, and variations in host and vector relationships. Immunity to one stock of parasites may not protect against another. Distribution of *T. parva* reflects that of its three main vectors (Table 2). Assigning the agents of the three diseases to three subspecies (*T. parva parva*, *T. p. lawrencei*, and *T. p. bovis* respectively) is a controversial issue, as the use of the trinomial system is biologically invalid, but there is no zoological objection to calling them the *parva*-type, *lawrencei*-type and *bovis*-type for the time being. *Theileria parva* differs from *T. annulata* in living mostly in αβ CD4$^+$ T lymphocytes and in producing piroplasms of low pathogenicity.

East Coast fever

The parasites causing East Coast fever are mostly maintained by cattle-tick transmission. Infection is subclinical or mild in the African buffalo (*Syncerus caffer*), which serves as a maintenance host in some areas. In the Asian buffalo (*B. bubalis*), the disease resembles that seen in oxen. East Coast fever is fatal in cattle of European origin (*Bos taurus*). African zebu or Sanga cattle (predominantly *Bos indicus*) respond variably to infection. Mortality among indigenous cattle may be negligible, but the disease significantly reduces growth and productivity. Significant numbers of clinical cases occur in endemic areas only where susceptible cattle, particularly improved dairy or cattle breeds, are introduced and become infested with ticks.

Clinical features

East Coast fever is caused by the invasion of lymphoid and non-lymphoid tissues with schizont-infected lymphoblasts; disease may occur as a mild, peracute, acute or subacute form. In susceptible cattle, acute lethal disease normally lasts about 3 weeks, with a pre-patent period of 5–10 days after infection with sporozoites. Pronounced clinical symptoms (Table 5) develop as the schizont-infected cells rapidly disseminate. Death may follow within a week; more commonly the clinical phase lasts about 2 weeks. In peracute cases, animals may die before marked respiratory symptoms arise. Pregnant animals may abort during the pyrexic stage of recovery. Animals that develop severe respiratory or nervous symptoms rarely recover; those which survive often fail to regain normal levels of productivity. Sublethal acute disease may be followed by complete recovery or may persist for months, leading to chronic, often irreversible, wasting.

Pathology

The most dramatic pathological changes are seen in the respiratory organs (Table 6). The failure of animals undergoing primary infection to mobilize protective cytotoxic CD8$^+$ T cells and to control infection has been attributed to the down-regulation of type 1 T-cell responses by interleukin-10 (IL-10) produced by the schizont-infected lymphocytes. Schizont-infected cells activate autologous lymphocytes non-specifically *in vitro*; if such activation occurs *in vivo*, it could cause a cascade of detrimental cytokine-related effects. The extensive lymphocytolysis and leucopenia seen in the late stages of disease may be caused by the marked non-specific lytic activity observed in the peripheral blood mononuclear cells at this time.

Immunity

Recovery from infection with *T. parva* and protection against challenge appear to be mediated primarily by parasite-specific

CD8[+], major histocompatibility complex class I restricted and cytotoxic T lymphocytes. Gamma-delta (γδ) T-cell responses occur during infection and are linked to the generation of parasite inhibitory cytokines and lytic activity. Strong CD4[+] T-cell responses occur in immune cattle and may directly inhibit infection through cytokine production and cytolysis. Innate immune mechanisms may also protect against infection.

Corridor disease or buffalo disease

Corridor disease is an acute, usually fatal, disease of cattle, which occurs sporadically wherever ticks transmit *T. parva* from infected African buffaloes to cattle. It is a major constraint to accepting the presence of buffaloes in cattle-raising areas. The parasites causing this disease are usually non-pathogenic to African buffaloes, in which both schizonts and piroplasms persist indefinitely. They are not well adapted to cattle; the schizonts are fewer and smaller than in East Coast fever and usually fail to develop into piroplasms. These parasites also cause fatal infections in Asian buffaloes. Corridor disease has the same clinical signs as East Coast fever but its course is shorter – lasting only 3–4 days after the first signs. Emaciation and diarrhoea do not occur, nor do the lymph nodes regress. Severe pulmonary oedema precedes death, which occurs before piroplasms can develop.

January disease, Zimbabwe theileriosis or Fortuna disease

January disease is an acute, frequently fatal, disease of cattle caused by *T. parva* in the high and low veld of Zimbabwe. Its strictly seasonal occurrence (December to May) coincides with the seasonal distribution of adult *Rhipicephalus appendiculatus* ticks. Primary outbreaks are associated with new additions to the herd. January disease has the same clinical features as East Coast fever, but its course is often shorter – lasting for only a few days after first onset of signs – and emaciation and diarrhoea are not seen. Schizonts and piroplasms, when present, are scanty.

Malignant ovine and caprine theileriosis (*T. lestoquardi*)

Theileria lestoquardi causes highly fatal, acute or subacute diseases, with heavy losses, in many tropical and subtropical regions (Table 3). Unusually for a *Theileria* species, it causes high morbidity and mortality in indigenous sheep and goats, as well as exotic (imported) breeds. Animals that recover from the disease are immune to challenge. In some areas, young kids and lambs are more resistant to infection than adult animals.

Clinical features

Tick transmission studies suggest an incubation period of about 12 days, with disease lasting from 5 to 40 days. Acute, subacute and chronic forms occur, the acute form being most usual. Schizont proliferation is accompanied by lymph node enlargement, pyrexia, leucopenia, listlessness, nasal discharge, atony of the rumen and weakness. Piroplasm parasitaemia is accompanied by anaemia, often icterus. In experimental, sporozoite-induced, acute infections in European sheep, fever was first noted around day 12 and lasted for 1–2 weeks. Schizonts were first detected from days 7–9 and piroplasms from days 10–12. Peak parasitaemias in animals that died ranged from 10 to 32% and in those that survived from 5 to 10%.

Pathology

Pathological changes (Table 6) resemble those of *T. annulata* infections and are associated with schizont proliferation and dissemination and piroplasm parasitaemia. Schizonts are most numerous in the liver, present in the petechiae of the intestines and absent from the spleen. While relatively few infected erythrocytes may occur in the circulation, virtually all the erythrocytes in the capillaries of the kidney, liver and heart may be parasitized.

New species of *Theileria* in small ruminants in China

A newly recognized, as yet unnamed, pathogenic *Theileria* parasite of small ruminants from north-western China (Table 3) is distinguished from other species in sheep and goats by its tick vector (*Haemaphysalis quinghaiensis*), the failure to establish schizont-infected cells in culture and its close relationship to *T. orientalis* (see p. 490). The parasite is most pathogenic in lambs and imported animals: morbidity may reach 65% and mortality 76%, according to geographical locality. Infected animals show typical signs of theileriosis: fever, inappetence, cessation of rumination, rapid heartbeat, dyspnoea, weakness, listlessness, swelling of superficial lymph nodes, marked anaemia and icterus.

Benign cosmopolitan bovine theileriosis and oriental theileriosis (*T. orientalis*)

Knowledge of the benign parasites of cattle is scanty but there is sound evidence that many cause disease. Attempts to establish their taxonomic relationships have been hindered by the extensive molecular diversity displayed across their distribution and within stocks isolated from individual hosts and by the occurrence of mixed infections within individual hosts. Molecular systematics indicate that members of the *T. orientalis/buffeli* group represent four different types (Table 1), which resemble previous groupings based on morphological, serological and biochemical features. In the scheme adopted here (Table 1), marked differences between the Japanese Ikeda stock and other benign parasites led to the tentative creation of two separate subspecies of *T. orientalis*. Differences between the benign parasites of the Asian buffalo (*B. bubalis*) and cattle suggest that the name *T. buffeli* should be kept for the parasites of the buffalo. The fourth, as yet unidentified, parasite occurs in Thailand, China and America. An alternative, more recent, scheme designates all four types as *T. buffeli*, on the grounds that they probably all arose from a group of buffalo-derived parasites that adapted to cattle and there is, as yet, insufficient evidence to recognize separate species within the group.

Theileria orientalis orientalis is a very widespread complex of pathogenic and apathogenic strains (Table 1). Pathogenic strains usually occur as subclinical infections in the Far Eastern maritime region of the Russian Federation, northern China, Korea and Japan, but often cause the economically significant disease, benign cosmopolitan theileriosis. Schizonts are readily detected in infections with Korean, Chinese or Russian stocks. Apathogenic strains in Europe, Africa, America and Australia very rarely cause disease, except in stressed animals; schizonts have only been reliably described for Australian strains. A distinct but closely related pathogen in Japan, tentatively named *Theileria orientalis sergenti*, causes oriental theileriosis; it produces schizonts, but they do not appear to contribute to disease.

Overall, outbreaks of disease appear to be related to the behaviour of particular geographical strains of *T. orientalis* and the breed, origin, age and physiological condition of the cattle. Increased levels of stress and decreased immunocompetency appear to convert subclinical infections to overt disease. In China, where almost all cattle are infected with *T. o. orientalis*, the incidence rates and numbers of fatalities vary widely between areas and cattle breeds. The parasite is normally avirulent in indigenous cattle, but dairy, exotic and hybrid cattle are highly susceptible; outbreaks involving 100% of exotic cattle, with 40% mortalities, have occurred. In this context, 'exotic' includes indigenous breeds moved between different regions, as well as animals imported into China. In Korea and Japan, *T. o. orientalis* and *T. o. sergenti* usually cause little harm in healthy and immunocompetent animals, but subclinically infected animals may develop severe anaemia if stressed by pregnancy, parturition or sudden environmental changes. Exotic imported cattle are more prone to infection than indigenous cattle; exotic dairy cattle have died from infection within several weeks of being imported into Korea. Mortality is low, but the cost of controlling and treating the disease is high.

The major clinical symptoms are pyrexia, superficial lymph node enlargement, inappetence, weakness, listlessness, haemorrhages in the visible mucosa, hyperaemic or haemorrhagic conjunctiva, thinning of the blood, haemolytic anaemia and icterus, related to the proliferation of piroplasms. Parasitaemia may reach 30%, accompanied by a 70% reduction in haematocrit, but haemoglobinuria is not seen. Pathological changes, as described for Chinese and Russian stocks, include: pale mucosa; lymph node enlargement; haemorrhages in subcutaneous tissues, serosa, abomasal and intestinal mucosa and mesenteric lymph nodes; hepatomegaly; tawny-coloured bile; splenomegaly; and enlarged heart, with haemorrhagic foci in the auricle.

Benign African theilerioses (*T. mutans, T. taurotragi, T. velifera*)

Theileria mutans is a parasite of the African buffalo (*S. caffer*) that is infective for cattle and may cause latent infection in sheep (Table 2). It is widespread throughout the range of its vectors; almost 100% of calves may be infected by the age of 6 months. Schizonts are scanty and transient; parasites mainly multiply as piroplasms. Severity of infection is proportional to intensity of piroplasm parasitaemia. Infection usually results in a mild febrile reaction lasting for 2–5 days, but pathogenic strains in East Africa cause anaemia, icterus and sometimes death. *Theileria taurotragi* is widely distributed throughout eastern and southern Africa (Table 2). It is infective to Eland (*Taurotragus oryx*), ox, sheep and goats. In cattle, subclinical or mild febrile infections last 1–14 days; the superficial lymph nodes draining the site of inoculation of sporozoites are slightly enlarged, but there are no other signs of clinical disturbance. *Theileria taurotragi* is benign in sheep, but sometimes causes severe or fatal disease in Eland. Turning sickness of cattle is an aberrant form of infection, characterized by the sudden onset of nervous signs, caused by an accumulation of parasitized lymphoblasts in the cerebral blood-vessels, leading to thrombosis and infarction. In East Africa it is usually caused by *T. parva* and in South Africa by *T. taurotragi*. *Theileria velifera* is apathogenic and of no practical significance, except for differential diagnosis.

Benign ovine, caprine and cervine theilerioses (*T. ovis, T. separata, T. recondita, T. cervi*)

The interrelationships of the four apathogenic/benign species of *Theileria* described in sheep, goats and cervids (Table 3) are unclear. Morphological, serological and biological features suggest that the parasites found in sheep in the Mediterranean basin and Asia may be *T. ovis*, a species first described in Central Africa. In *T. ovis* infections, schizonts and piroplasms are relatively scarce and distinct clinical signs are rare. The second benign parasite of sheep, *T. separata*, is confined to sub-Saharan Africa; its piroplasms have a distinctive morphology (Fig. 4). The morphology, distribution and tick vectors of the parasite known as *T. recondita* distinguish it from *T. ovis*, but it could be the parasite first described in Fallow deer (*Dama dama*) as *T. cervi* by A. Bettencourt, C. Franca and I. Borges in 1907. Clinical signs following *T. recondita* infection in normal sheep last only a few days in the field; many infections are subclinical and recovered animals are carriers. Experimentally infected sheep underwent a transient, low parasitaemia accompanied by slight fever, depression, anorexia, listlessness, loss of condition, transient macrocytic hypochromic anaemia, neutrophilia and lymphocytopenia. The parasites identified as *T. cervi* are very widely distributed. Their infectivity for ovids and caprids make it difficult to know whether parasites in sheep and goats are parasites of domesticated stock or of wild ruminants. Both *T. cervi* and *T. ovis* may prove to be more than one species.

Equine piroplasmosis/equine biliary fever (*T. equi*)

Although schizonts have rarely been recorded in natural field infections, experimental sporozoite-induced infections showed that the causative agent of equine biliary fever undergoes exoerythrocytic schizogony and merogony in mononuclear cells. The parasite is therefore now generally accepted as *T. equi* (Table 1), a very widely distributed species with different geographical strains varying in virulence. In endemic

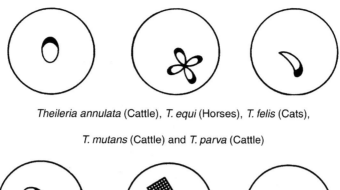

Theileria annulata (Cattle), T. equi (Horses), T. felis (Cats),

T. mutans (Cattle) and T. parva (Cattle)

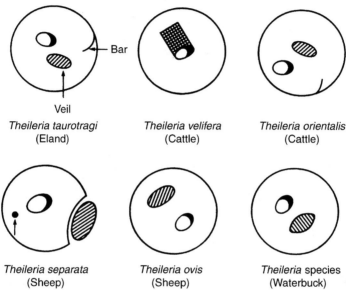

Fig. 4. Diagrammatic representation of the intraerythrocytic stages of members of the genus *Theileria*. Some forms of piroplasms predominate in certain species: round and oval forms in *T. annulata, T. felis, T. lestoquardi, T. ovis, T. recondita, T. separata, T. taurotragi* and the new species in Chinese sheep; rods in *T. parva*; rods and elongate forms in *T. orientalis*; and round forms and typical tetrads (Maltese crosses) in *T. equi*. Piroplasm morphology cannot be used to identify *Theileria* species reliably as piroplasms are polymorphic and vary in size and shape during infection, but the presence or absence of a rectangular veil-like body and a bar-like structure in the cytoplasm of infected erythrocytes is useful. Veils consist of a haemoglobin-derived crystalline substance; bars are connected with the parasite and the outside of the cell. Both structures are thought to be of parasite origin. *Theileria parva* only produces a veil in *Syncerus caffer*. Bars occur in all strains of *T. orientalis*; veils are absent in North American strains and not yet recorded for Chinese and African strains. The arrow points to reduced bar structure of *T. separata*. *Theileria recondita* resembles *T. ovis* in lacking a bar, and its veil protrudes from the surface of the erythrocyte. To date, it is not known whether *T. buffeli, T. cervi, T. equi, T. felis, T. lestoquardi*, and the new Chinese parasite of sheep produce bars and/or veils. (Figure reprinted from, Norval, R.A.I., Perry, B.D. and Young, A.S. (eds) (1992) *The Epidemiology of Theileriosis in Africa*, 1st edn, p. 90, with permission from Academic Press Ltd.)

areas, most horses are symptomless carriers; overt infection only occurs if host immunity wanes or is reduced by stress due to racing, transportation or pregnancy or if susceptible animals are imported. The clinical signs and pathological changes resemble those attributed to piroplasms in bovine and ovine theilerioses. Neonatal infections have serious consequences. *Theileria equi* sporozoites infect and transform equine lymphocytes into lymphoblastoid cell lines *in vitro*. *Theileria equi* is unique in that it is not just the only *Theileria* species known to infect equids but also the only *Theileria* species known to have infected humans.

Clinical features

Acute disease lasts 8–10 days and is characterized by pyrexia, coinciding with the first piroplasms in the blood, icterus and anaemia. Fever is often accompanied by sweating, congestion of mucous membranes, tachycardia and palpitating cardiac sounds. Faecal balls are yellowish-green, small and dry. Parasitaemia may be low in adult animals that die. Peracute disease, in which animals die 1–2 days after the onset of signs, is rare. Subacute infections develop slowly and are prolonged; recovery may take many weeks. Such cases undergo anorexia, malaise, weight loss, fever and increased pulse and respiratory rates. Mucous membranes vary from pale pink to pale yellow to bright yellow, with petechial or ecchymotic haemorrhages. Anaemia is accompanied by thrombocytopenia, hypophosphataemia, hypoferronaemia, and bilirubinaemia. Normal bowel movements may be slightly depressed: animals may show signs of colic pawing, looking at the flank or lying down. Faecal balls are small and may be covered in mucus. Constipation may be followed by diarrhoea. Urine is often dark yellow, orange or even brown, and sometimes reddish-brown, due to haemoglobin and bile pigments. Moderate supraorbital oedema is common; peripheral and dependent oedema of the limbs and ventral abdomen occurs during terminal stages. Untreated or neglected horses may become severely anaemic and show signs of general weakness. Chronic cases show non-specific clinical signs, including mild inappetence, poor performance, a drop in body mass, pale pink mucous membranes, mild tachycardia and splenomegaly. Animals that recover become carriers and are immune.

Gross pathological changes

Changes include: emaciation; anaemia; icterus; oedema of subcutaneous and subserosal tissues; enlarged lymph nodes; pale, flabby heart; epi- and endocardial haemorrhages; pulmonary congestion and oedema; splenomegaly; hepatomegaly; enlarged pale or, in haemoglobinuric cases, red-brown kidneys with subcapsular and cortical haemorrhages; and ascites, hydrothorax and hydropericardium.

Abortions and neonatal infections

Mares may abort at any stage of gestation, due to systemic disease and pyrexia, but most commonly in the last 3 months after intrauterine infection. Fetal foals may be infected and born with overwhelming parasitaemia. Neonatal infections are characterized by weakness, pyrexia, listlessness, anaemia, icterus and malaise; mucous membranes may exhibit petechial haemorrhages. Foals are progressively lethargic and finally unable to stand or suck. Some appear normal at birth but rapidly develop clinical signs. Mortality is particularly high. Aborted fetuses are usually moderately autolysed, anaemic and icteric. Fetuses and neonatal foals show hydrothorax, congestion and oedema of the lungs, splenomegaly, hepatomegaly and parasitaemias higher than 50%.

Feline theileriosis (*T. felis*)

Theileria felis causes a relatively common acute disease in cats that roam in wooded areas in the southern states of North America (south-western Missouri, Georgia, Arkansas, Texas). The Lynx (Bobcat), *Lynx rufus*, is presumed to be the primary host, with ticks acting as vectors. In fatally ill cats, massive accumulations of schizonts occur in cells in lymph nodes and in 'reticuloendothelial' cells attached to or close to the endothelial lining of blood-vessels in a number of organs; the exact identity of these cells is unknown. Round piroplasms occur in erythrocytes. The clinical signs – fever, anorexia, listlessness, anaemia, icterus, dehydration and death – are reminiscent of other theilerioses. Schizonts partially or completely occlude the major venous channels of the lungs, liver and spleen, appearing to cause severe circulatory impairment; haemolytic anaemia may be linked to the piroplasms. Pathological changes resemble those caused by other *Theileria* species: marked dehydration; paleness; icterus; numerous petechial and ecchymotic haemorrhages of the epicardium, beneath the visceral pleura of the lungs, in the serosal membranes of the abdominal organs and in the mucosa of the urinary bladder; icteric fluid in pericardial sacs; enlarged, congested or haemorrhagic, oedematous lymph nodes; splenomegaly; orange-brown livers; and swollen and congested parenchymatous organs.

Diagnosis of *Theileria* infections

Diagnosis is based on characteristic haematological, clinical and post-mortem findings (Tables 5 and 6), the detection of intraerythrocytic stages (Fig. 3) in thin blood films and the presence of vector ticks (Tables 1–3). Where suspected parasites are known to produce detectable levels of schizont-infected cells (e.g. *T. annulata*, *T. parva* and *T. lestoquardi*), these should be looked for in thin smears prepared from biopsy material of lymph nodes or the liver (Fig. 2). In fatal cases, schizonts and merozoites can be detected in impression smears of affected organs – notably, liver, spleen and lymph nodes. *Theileria* species cannot be identified reliably from the structure of their schizonts or piroplasms, although some may be distinguished by 'bars' and 'veils' in infected erythrocytes (Fig. 4). The indirect fluorescent antibody (IFA) and enzyme-linked immunosorbent assay (ELISA) tests are useful for identifying infected animals and herds that contain carriers of infection and, more recently, polymerase chain reaction (PCR)-based tests are being used for species-specific identification.

Treatment

Tetracyclines have prophylactic and therapeutic activity against *T. annulata* and *T. parva*. The naphthoquinone, parvaquone, has high therapeutic activity against *T. annulata* and *T. parva*; buparvaquone has been shown to cure clinical infections of *T. annulata*, *T. lawrencei*, *T. parva* and *T. orientalis*.

Control of *Theileria* infections

Control of theilerioses depends upon an integrated approach against the parasite and its vectors; the exact methods depend upon the *Theileria* species involved, the epidemiology of the disease and the behaviour of the vectors.

Vector control

Tick control is based on the treatment of animals with acaricides. Livestock animals can be periodically sprayed or dipped in solutions or emulsions of acaricides such as the organophosphates, carbamates or pyrethroids. The problem is that ticks are notorious for rapidly becoming resistant to a broad spectrum of chemicals, resistance to different classes of acaricides is often developed in a single species. Another constraint is the increasing sensitivity to the possible contamination of meat with chemical residues.

The development of methods for stimulating immunity to ticks, to be used in conjunction with acaricides, is considered to be a rational approach for improving methods for controlling ticks.

Parasite control

Control of the parasite depends upon immunization and therapeutic compounds. Attenuated schizont-infected cell line vaccines are used very effectively against *T. annulata* and *T. lestoquardi* in endemic areas; these vaccines succeed because the schizonts of the two species can establish and multiply sufficiently in the recipients' macrophages to induce protection against challenge. *Theileria parva* schizont-infected cell lines cannot be used as vaccines because only the administration of extremely high numbers of cells will result in sufficient schizonts transferring to the recipients' lymphocytes to induce protection. The most successful form of immunization for East Coast fever so far is the 'infection and treatment' method, which involves injection of virulent cryopreserved sporozoites and concurrent treatment with a long-acting oxytetracycline. Strategies for vaccine development are aimed at multicomponent subunit vaccines capable of targeting more than one stage of the parasite.

Selected bibliography

Boulter, N. and Hall, R. (2000) Immunity and vaccine development in the bovine theilerioses. *Advances in Parasitology* 44, 41–97.

De Waal, D.T. and van Heerden, J. (1994) Equine babesiosis. In: Coetzer, J.A.W., Thomson, G.R. and Tustin, R.C. (eds) *Infectious Disease of Livestock with Special Reference to Southern Africa*, Vol. 1. Oxford University Press, Cape Town, pp. 295–304.

Gubbels, M.-J., Hong, Y., van der Weide, M., Qi, B., Nijman, I.J., Guangyuan, L. and Jongejan, F. (2000) Molecular characterisation of the *Theileria buffeli/orientalis* group. *International Journal for Parasitology* 30, 943–952.

Irvin, A.D. and Mwamachi, D.M. (1983) Clinical and diagnostic features of East Coast fever (*Theileria parva*) infection of cattle. *Veterinary Record* 113, 192–198.

Kawazu, S., Kamio, T., Kakuda, T. Terada, Y., Sugimoto, C. and Fujisaki, K. (1999) Phylogenetic relationships of the benign *Theileria* species in cattle and Asian buffalo based on the major piroplasm surface protein (p33/34) gene sequences. *International Journal for Parasitology* 29, 613–618.

Lawrence, J.A., de Vos, A.J. and Irvin, A.D. (1994) Theilerioses. In: Coetzer, J.A.W., Thomson, G.R. and Tustin, R.C. (eds) *Infectious Disease of Livestock with Special Reference to Southern Africa*, Vol. 1. Oxford University Press, Cape Town, pp. 307–340.

McKeever, D.J., Taracha, E.L.N., Morrison, W.I., Musoke, A.J. and Morzaria, S.P. (1999) Protective immune mechanisms against *Theileria parva*: evolution of vaccine development strategies. *Parasitology Today* 15, 263–267.

Mehlhorn, H., Schein, E. and Ahmed, J.S. (1994) Theileria. In: Kreier, J.P. (ed.) *Parasitic Protozoa*, Vol. 7, 2nd edn. Academic Press, San Diego, pp. 217–304.

Neitz, W.O. (1957) Theileriosis, gonderiosis and cytauxzoonosis. A review. *Onderstepoort Journal of Veterinary Research* 27, 275–318.

Norval, R.A.I., Perry, B.D. and Young, A.S. (eds) (1992) *The Epidemiology of Theileriosis in Africa*, 1st edn. Academic Press, London, 481 pp.

Pipano, E. (1994) *Theileria annulata* theileriosis In: Coetzer, J.A.W., Thomson, G.R. and Tustin, R.C. (eds) *Infectious Disease of Livestock with Special Reference to Southern Africa*, Vol. 1. Oxford University Press, Cape Town, pp. 341–348.

Preston, P.M. and Yin Hong (eds) (1997) Proceedings of the European Union International Symposium on Ticks and Tick-borne diseases, Xi'an, China, 1996. *Tropical Animal Health and Production* 29 (suppl.), 1S–144S.

Preston, P.M., Hall, F.R., Glass, E.J., Campbell, J.D.M., Darghouth, M.A., Ahmed, J.S., Shiels, B.R., Spooner, R.L., Jongejan, F. and Brown, C.G.D. (1999) Innate and adaptive immune responses cooperate to protect cattle against *Theileria annulata*. *Parasitology Today* 15, 268–274.

Schnittger, L., Yin, H., Jianxun, L., Ludwig, W., Shayan, P., Rahbari, S., Voss-Holtmann, A. and Ahmed, J.S. (2000) Ribosomal small-subunit RNA gene-sequence analysis of *Theileria lestoquardi* and a *Theileria* species highly pathogenic for small ruminants in China. *Parasitology Research* 86, 352–358.

Sergent E., Donatien, A.L., Parrot, L.M. and Lestoquard, F. (1945) *Etudes sur les Piroplasmoses Bovines*. Institut Pasteur d'Algérie, Alger, 816 pp.

Uilenberg G. (1981) Theilerial species of domestic livestock. In: Irvin, A.D., Cunningham, M.P. and Young, A.S. (eds) *Advances in the Control of Theileriosis*. Martinus Nijhoff Publishers, The Hague, pp. 4–37.

Thelaziasis

E.T. Lyons

Thelazia species are spirurid nematodes of the orbital, nasal and oral cavities of birds and mammals. Some of their features, such as parenteral location and life cycle requiring an intermediate host, are similar to those of filariids. Typically, infections are benign, but these parasites may cause varying degrees of eye problems, including impairment of vision. Thelazids associated with the eyes of mammals, especially cattle and horses, will be stressed here.

Distribution

Thelazids are found worldwide. Geographical distribution is related to the presence of appropriate intermediate hosts for successful completion of the life cycle.

Parasite

Over a dozen species of *Thelazia* have been described from mammals. In domestic animals, some of the species are *T. gulosa*, *T. rhodesii* and *T. skrjabini* in cattle and *T. lacrymalis* in horses. *Thelazia californiensis* is unusual in being found in several different types of hosts, such as the Black bear (*Ursus americanus*), Black-tailed deer[1] (*Odocoileus hemionus*), Californian or Black-tailed jack rabbit (*Lepus californicus*), cat, Coyote (*Canis latrans*), dog, sheep and humans. *Thelazia callipaeda* is a parasite of canids, humans and other mammals.

Adult worms are small – lengths vary with species and sex of the worms. Measurements for the type species, *T. rhodesii*, are 8–12 mm for males and 12–18 mm for females. Location of *Thelazia* species in the eye orbit varies somewhat with species. They do not invade the eyeball but are associated with its adnexa, including the lachrymal gland and its ducts, nictitating membrane gland and its ducts, conjunctival sac and nasolachrymal ducts and under the eyelids. Eye-worms are not usually visible in live animals. They do move around more during general anaesthesia and also after the death of the host. In these situations, they may be seen on the cornea or conjunctiva and on the eyelashes and hair of the periorbital area.

Clinical symptoms

The most pathogenic species of eye-worms (*T. rhodesii* in cattle) is found in many countries but not in North America. *Thelazia rhodesii* have a pronounced serrated cuticle, which may irritate conjunctiva and cornea, resulting in inflammation. Clinical signs of thelaziasis, especially in cattle, are most evident in summer months during the fly season. There is some indication that the condition is an immunological response to immature stages, including first-instar larvae (L_1). Pathological conditions, especially with *T. rhodesii*, consist initially of slight conjunctivitis and lachrymation. With progressive severity, there is keratitis, blockage, irritation of lachrymal and nictitating membrane ducts, with collections of pus and cellular debris, and ulceration, with perforation and/or permanent fibrosis of the cornea. Except for *T. rhodesii*, thelaziasis is usually devoid of clinical signs. The eye-worm of horses, *T. lacrymalis*, generally causes only slight irritation and inflammation.

Diagnosis

Ante-mortem diagnosis of thelaziasis is difficult. Two possibilities are: (i) detection of adult or larval stages during inspection of the eye; and (ii) clinical signs. Gross examination may reveal adult worms, especially *T. rhodesii*, which are more commonly present in the conjunctival sac than some of the other species, e.g. *T. lacrymalis*. Administration of a local anaesthetic may be a diagnostic aid. It causes the adults to become active initially and move across the eyeball, where they are visible; later, they become inactive. Flushing the eyes with saline and a collection of washings may reveal immature stages, such as L_1 by microscopic examination. Clinical signs may be an aid in diagnosis of thelaziasis, because this disease is characterized by chronic conjunctivitis.

Transmission

Species of *Thelazia*, where the life cycle is known, utilize an insect (dipteran) as an intermediate host. Female eye-worms are viviparous and release numerous embryos into the lachrymal fluid. The larvae (L_1) gravitate to the eye secretions around and under the lower eyelids. These L_1 are in a thin, tight-fitting eggshell, with a slight knob-like swelling at the anterior end of at least some species. Research with one species (*T. callipaeda*) revealed that placing L_1 in a container of saline resulted in the swelling of the eggshell, producing a ballooning effect and the flotation of the L_1. This led to a theory that flotation of the L_1 in the secretions in the lower eyelid of the host would favour chances of ingestion by the intermediate host.

Intermediate hosts are flies, such as *Musca autumnalis* (face-fly) for *T. lacrymalis* and several other *Thelazia* species; they ingest L_1 as they feed, usually around the medial canthus of the eye. Development of the L_1 to the infective third stage (L_3) occurs in the haemocoel and head of the fly in about 2–4 weeks. The L_3 are mechanically transferred to the definitive host through the proboscis of the fly as it feeds around the eyes. Prepatent periods (time for development of the L_3 to the mature adult worm) are approximately 2–4 weeks for *T. rhodesii*, 6 weeks for *T. gulosa* and 10–11 weeks for *T. lacrymalis*. Infections are present throughout the year; these parasites can overwinter in the eyes of the host. With *T. lacrymalis* and at least some other species, young animals present a higher infection prevalence than older ones.

Treatment and control

Adult eye-worms can be removed with forceps following instillation of a local anaesthetic. Irrigation of the eyes with various solutions, including 50–75 ml aqueous solution of 0.5% iodine and 0.75% potassium iodide, has been recommended for *T. gulosa* and *T. skrjabini* and might be useful in infections of *T. lacrymalis*. Topical application of 0.03% echothiophate iodide or 0.02% isofluorophate has been recommended for controlling *T. lacrymalis*. Systemically, certain antiparasitic compounds (e.g. levamisole and ivermectin) have been reported as effective against *T. gulosa*, *T. rhodesii* and *T. skrjabini*. Ivermectin and probably other macrocyclic lactones are not effective on *T. lacrymalis*; this may be the result of the horse metabolizing this group of compounds differently from some other mammalian species.

Control of the intermediate hosts, such as *M. autumnalis*, aids in controlling thelaziasis in cattle and horses. This can be by chemical usage, usually insecticides, against adult flies and larvae in cattle faeces, which is the breeding material for the face-fly and other fly species.

Note

[1] Black-tailed deer and Mule deer are usually considered to be the same species.

Selected bibliography

Anderson, R.C. (2000) *Nematode Parasites of Vertebrates: Their Development and Transmission*, 2nd edn. CAB International, Wallingford, UK, 650 pp.

Levine, N.E. (1968) *Nematode Parasites of Domestic Animals and of Man*. Burgess Publishing, Minneapolis, 600 pp.

Skrjabin, K.I., Sobolev, A.A. and Ivashkin, V.M. (1971) Spirurata of animals and man and the diseases caused by them. Part 4, Thelazioidea. In: *Nematodology*, Vol. XVI. Israeli Program for Scientific Translations, Jerusalem, 610 pp.

Soulsby, E.J.L. (1965) *Textbook of Veterinary Clinical Parasitology*, Vol. 1, *Helminths*. F.A. Davis, Philadelphia, 1120 pp.

Thogoto virus

Jack Woodall

This causes a viral infection of humans and other mammals.

Thogoto virus infection, human

Viral disease of livestock, occasionally transmitted to humans. Thogoto (THO) virus was first isolated from two pools of ticks, one being of mixed ixodid species, the other of *Boophilus decoloratus*, collected in September 1960 from cattle set out as disease sentinels in the Thogoto forest near Nairobi, Kenya. It was subsequently found to be the cause of abortion storms in sheep and of a fatal human case of meningitis in Nigeria. Although the virus belongs to the same family as the influenza viruses, it is transmitted by ticks, not by aerosol.

Distribution

Africa north of the equator, Portugal, Italy (Sicily) and Iran. Virus isolates from Kenya, Portugal, Italy, Iran, Nigeria, the Central African Republic and Cameroon were cross-tested by haemagglutination inhibition and serum dilution plaque reduction neutralization tests, and shown to differ only slightly. This suggests that the virus is repeatedly introduced into those countries from a common source, possibly tick-infected domesticated animals and/or migrating birds. Human cases are rare, with only two recorded, from Nigeria. Two humans with plaque-reduction neutralizing antibody were found in southern Portugal.

Virus

Family Orthomyxoviridae, enveloped, negative-sense RNA virus budding from the outer plasma membranes of infected cells, with six size classes of single-stranded RNA, sensitive to actinomycin D and alpha-amanitin. The genome is transcribed and replicated in the cell nucleus by a unique cap-stealing mechanism involving the cleavage of only the m(7)GpppAm structure from cellular heterogeneous nuclear RNAs (hnRNAs). The envelope glycoprotein has a highly significant homology with the gp64 glycoprotein of two DNA-containing insect baculoviruses, but not with the envelope glycoproteins of the influenza viruses. Thogoto virus is thus sufficiently different from the other orthomyxoviruses to be placed in a separate genus, *Thogotovirus*, as the prototype, along with Batken and Dhori viruses. Reassortment, just as with influenza viruses, has been shown to occur between temperature-sensitive mutants of THO virus and wild-type virus, in both hamsters and ticks.

Clinical symptoms

Only two cases are recorded in the literature, both from Ibadan, Nigeria, in July 1966. Case 1, an adult male, had an onset of generalized tension, joint cramps, bilateral optic neuritis and papilloedema, followed by pyramidal signs in the limbs. He made a complete recovery without sequelae. Case 2 was a 14-year-old male, with fever and possible neck stiffness, followed by anorexia, dysphagia, hepatosplenomegaly and lymphadenitis. He died on the sixth day in sickle-cell crisis. Post-mortem findings were leptomeningitis, hepatic haemorrhage and extensive necrosis, splenic haemorrhage with sickled erythrocytes, lung haemorrhage and congestion, gross renal congestion and necrosis.

Diagnosis

By virus isolation. Case 1 had virus in the cebrospinal fluid (CSF) but not in the blood; case 2 had the reverse.

Transmission

This is by ticks of numerous species in the genera *Amblyomma*, *Boophilus*, *Hyalomma*, and *Rhipicephalus*. Ticks can become infected and transmit at any stage of their life cycle, and they carry the virus trans-stadially. Laboratory transmission between infected and uninfected hamsters by feeding ticks has been demonstrated for *Rhipicephalus appendiculatus* and *Amblyomma variegatum*. Direct transmission between virus-positive and virus-negative ticks feeding on uninfected guinea-pigs has been demonstrated, but this was markedly reduced if the guinea-pigs were allowed to develop resistance to tick infestation. The virus is suspected of being transported between Africa and Eurasia by ticks on migrating birds. The virus has been isolated from a Banded mongoose (*Mongos mungo*) (Herpestidae) in Uganda, where 2/7 other mongooses were found to be seropositive, suggesting that they could be possible reservoir hosts. Transmission to humans is infrequent; 48 sera from humans living in the Rift Valley of Kenya in close contact with immune livestock were negative for neutralizing antibodies to THO virus. In Africa, transmission takes place mainly in the dry season, which is when ticks are most abundant.

Treatment

There is no specific treatment. The case which survived was treated with steroids and vitamin B complex.

Control

No specific measures except avoidance of tick bites.

Thogoto virus, animal

Bovine, ovine, caprine, camelid

Thogoto virus has been responsible for abortion storms in sheep, without the maternal mortality associated with Nairobi sheep disease (see entry). It also infects cattle and goats, and has been isolated from a Camel (*Camelus dromedarius*) in northern Nigeria. In one flock of 600 ewes in Kenya in 1983, more than 500 aborted over a 2-month period. *Rhipicephalus* and *Hyalomma* ticks, species from which THO virus has been isolated elsewhere, were found on the sheep, but the rapid spread led to suspicions that the virus was not entirely tick-transmitted. Experimental inoculation of sheep produces a fever of 1–3 days' duration, a raised respiratory rate and slight malaise.

Treatment

There is no specific treatment for infected animals.

Control

There are no specific control measures, except trying to prevent tick infestations of animals.

Selected bibliography

Calisher, C.H., Karabatsos, N. and Filipe, A.R. (1987) Antigenic uniformity of topotype strains of Thogoto virus from Africa, Europe, and Asia. *American Journal of Tropical Medicine and Hygiene* 37, 670–673.

Darwish, M.A., Hoogstraal, H. and Omar, F.M. (1979) A serological survey for Thogoto virus in humans, domestic mammals, and rats in Egypt. *Journal of the Egyptian Public Health Association* 54, 1–8.

Davies, F.G., Soi, R.K. and Wariru, B.N. (1984) Abortion in sheep caused by Thogoto virus. *Veterinary Record* 115, 654.

Degallier, N., Cornet, J.-P., Saluzzo, J.-F., Germain, M., Hervé, J.-P., Camicas, J.-L. and Sureau, P. (1985) Ecologie des arbovirus à tiques en République Centrafricaine. *Bulletin de la Société de Pathologie exotique* 78, 296–310. (In French, English summary.)

Filipe, A.R. and Calisher, C.H. (1984) Isolation of Thogoto virus from ticks in Portugal. *Acta Virologica* 28, 152–155.

Filipe, A.R., Calisher, C.H. and Lazuick, J. (1985) Antibodies to Congo–Crimean haemorrhagic fever, Dhori, Thogoto and Bhanja viruses in southern Portugal. *Acta Virologica* 29, 324–328.

Haig, D.A., Woodall, J.P. and Danskin, D. (1965) Thogoto virus: a hitherto undescribed agent isolated from ticks in Kenya. *Journal of General Microbiology* 38, 389–394.

Johnson, B.K., Chanas, A.C., Squires, E.J., Shockley, P., Simpson, D.I., Parsons, J., Smith, D.H. and Casals, J. (1980) Arbovirus isolations from ixodid ticks infesting livestock, Kano Plain, Kenya. *Transactions of the Royal Society of Tropical Medicine and Hygiene* 74, 732–737.

Jones, L.D., Davies, C.R., Steel, G.M. and Nuttall, P.A. (1989) Vector capacity of *Rhipicephalus appendiculatus* and *Amblyomma variegatum* for Thogoto and Dhori viruses. *Medical and Veterinary Entomology* 3, 195–202.

Leahy, M.B., Dessens, J.T., Weber, F., Kochs, G. and Nuttall, P.A. (1997) The fourth genus in the Orthomyxoviridae: sequence analyses of two Thogoto virus polymerase proteins and comparison with influenza viruses. *Virus Research* 50, 215–224.

Moore, D.L., Causey, O.R., Carey, D.E., Reddy, S., Cooke, A.R., Akinkugbe, F.M., David-West, T.S. and Kemp, G.E. (1975) Arthropod-borne viral infections of man in Nigeria, 1964–1970. *Annals of Tropical Medicine and Parasitology* 69, 49–64.

Ogen-Odoi, A., Miller, B.R., Happ, C.M., Maupin, G.O. and Burkot, T.R. (1999) Isolation of Thogoto virus (Orthomyxoviridae) from the banded mongoose, *Mongos mungo* (Herpestidae), in Uganda. *American Journal of Tropical Medicine and Hygiene* 60, 439–440.

Sureau, P. and Klein, J.-M. (1980) Arbovirus en Iran. *Médecine Tropicale* 40, 549–554. (In French, English summary.)

Williams, R.E., Hoogstraal, H., Casals, J., Kaiser, M.N. and Moussa, M.I. (1973) Isolation of Wanowrie, Thogoto, and Dhori viruses from *Hyalomma* ticks infesting camels in Egypt. *Journal of Medical Entomology* 10, 143–146.

Wood, O.L., Lee, V.H., Ash, J.S. and Casals, J. (1978) Crimean–Congo hemorrhagic fever, Thogoto, Dugbe, and Jos viruses isolated from ixodid ticks in Ethiopia. *American Journal of Tropical Medicine and Hygiene* 27, 600–604.

Three-day fever *see* **Phlebotomus fevers.**

Tick-borne encephalitis

Franz X. Heinz and Heidemarie Holzmann

Disease caused by tick-borne encephalitis (TBE) virus, a member of the genus *Flavivirus* within the family Flaviviridae. Other closely related important human-pathogenic flaviviruses are yellow fever virus, Japanese encephalitis virus, the dengue viruses and West Nile virus (see entries). More distantly related are the hepatitis C viruses and the animal-pathogenic pestiviruses, which form independent genera in the family Flaviviridae.

Tick-borne encephalitis virus is the most important tick-transmitted human-pathogenic flavivirus. It is endemic in many European countries as well as in Asia, and about 10,000 hospitalized tick-borne encephalitis cases are officially registered each year. However, due to under-reporting in certain countries, the actual number of cases is higher. A number of synonyms for tick-borne encephalitis can be found in the literature, e.g. Central European encephalitis, Kumlinge disease, Russian spring–summer encephalitis and biphasic milk fever, which are related to its geographical occurrence, seasonal distribution or potential transmissibility by raw milk (see below).

Distribution and molecular epidemiology

Tick-borne encephalitis virus is endemic in natural foci (see below) that exist in all European countries, with the exception of Great Britain, the Benelux countries and the Iberian Peninsula (Fig. 1). It also occurs in large areas of the former Soviet Union, as well as in northern China and northern Japan (Hokkaido). Based on nucleotide and amino acid sequence homologies, at least three different TBE virus subtypes can be distinguished. They are designated European, Central Siberian and Far Eastern subtypes, corresponding to their principal region of distribution. However, the extent of the differences between the subtypes is relatively low and does not exceed the differences between different isolates of mosquito-borne flaviviruses, such as yellow fever or the dengue viruses. Infection or immunization with one TBE virus subtype therefore confers immunity against the other subtypes. No cross-protection, however, exists between TBE virus and the mosquito-borne flaviviruses. Under natural ecological conditions the virus is genetically quite stable within the subtypes and does not exhibit a significant degree of antigenic variation.

Virus

Like all flaviviruses, TBE virus is a lipid-enveloped RNA virus, with a diameter of approximately 50 nm, consisting of only three structural proteins, designated C (capsid), E (envelope) and M (membrane) (Fig. 2). Virus assembly occurs in the endoplasmic reticulum and first leads to the formation of immature particles, which contain a precursor form of the M protein (prM). During exocytosis the prM protein is cleaved by a cellular protease (presumably furin) and mature and fully infectious virions are released from infected cells. The E protein is the viral haemagglutinin and mediates important viral functions during early virus–cell interactions, such as receptor binding and fusion of the viral membrane with the membrane of the endosome after uptake by receptor-mediated endocytosis. The E protein is also the major viral antigen, which induces a protective immunity by eliciting neutralizing antibodies. The isometric nucleocapsid encloses the genomic RNA, which is single-stranded and has a positive orientation and a length of about 11,000 nucleotides. In addition to the structural proteins, the genomic RNA encodes a series of non-structural proteins (NS1, NS2A, NS2B, NS3, NS4A, NS4B,

NS5), which are essential for viral replication. They include the viral protease (NS3 + NS2B) and the helicase (also NS3), as well as the RNA-dependent RNA polymerase (NS5).

Clinical symptoms

A significant proportion of infections are clinically inapparent, and a clinically manifest disease of the central nervous system (CNS) occurs in only about 10–30% of those infected. In these cases, tick-borne encephalitis normally takes a biphasic course, but in some cases one of the two phases may be missing. In typical cases, the first phase (viraemic state) starts after an incubation period of about 1 week (3–14 days) as an uncharacteristic flu-like illness,

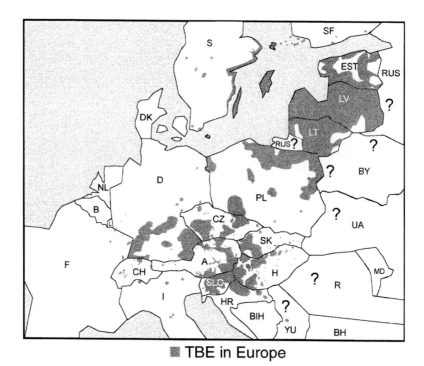

TBE in Europe

Fig. 1. Distribution of tick-borne encephalitis in Europe. The map shows areas with tick-borne encephalitis cases according to data from the individual countries and the World Health Organization (WHO). ?, no data available. (Modified from a map published by Baxter, Vienna, Austria, issued January 1999.)

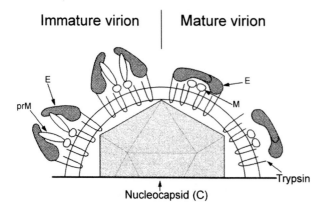

Fig. 2. Model of a TBE virus particle showing the immature (intracellular) and mature form of a virus particle. Mature virions consist of the structural proteins C (capsid), E (envelope) and M (membrane), whereas immature particles contain a precursor of the M protein (prM).

with fever (rarely exceeding 38°C) and non-specific symptoms, such as malaise, headache, myalgia, catarrhal or sometimes gastrointestinal symptoms. This stage lasts for only a few days and is followed by an asymptomatic interval of about 1 week (6–10 days). Ten to thirty per cent of cases (less frequent in children) develop a second phase of the disease with the recurrence of fever (>38°C), a strong feeling of illness and the occurrence of neurological symptoms.

The infection of the CNS may become manifest as aseptic meningitis (~50%), meningoencephalitis (~40%), meningo-encephalomyelitis or -radiculitis (~10%). In rare cases an accompanying hepatitis or myocarditis is observed. The case-fatality rate of the encephalitic course of the disease is 0.5–2% in Europe, whereas 20–30% has been reported in the Far East. It is not clear at present whether this reflects a higher virulence of Far Eastern virus strains or differences in the hospitalization of milder forms and/or the treatment of acute cases. The acute meningitis lasts for about 3–5 days and usually resolves completely. The more severe encephalitic forms may be accompanied by the following symptoms: disturbances of speech and consciousness, ataxia, convulsions, failure of the cranial nerves, breathing insufficiency and hemi- and tetraparesis. Paralysis most often affects the neck, the shoulder girdle and the upper extremities, because the cells of the frontal spinal cord are especially susceptible to the infection. Ten to twenty per cent of the patients have long-lasting or permanent neuropsychiatric sequelae, such as headache, reduced physical capability and depression, but also flaccid paralyses may persist. To a certain degree, the severity of the disease is also affected by the age of the patient. Whereas the majority of children develop meningitis only, the encephalitic forms predominate in individuals >40 years of age. Natural infection results in a lifelong immunity, regardless of whether the course of the infection was clinically manifest or inapparent. Chronic infections have not been reported in Europe.

Diagnosis

Because of the uncharacteristic clinical picture of a TBE virus infection, the actual diagnosis must be established in the laboratory. In principle, it is possible to isolate the virus from the blood or to detect the viral nucleic acid using reverse transcription–polymerase chain reaction (RT-PCR) during the first viraemic phase. However, in practice this is of minor importance, since admission to the hospital usually takes place in the second phase of the disease, when the neurological symptoms become manifest. At this time point, the virus has already been cleared from the blood (and the cerebrospinal fluid), and specific immunoglobulin M (IgM) and IgG antibodies are formed, which rapidly rise to high titres (Fig. 3). Since these antibodies are detectable in practically every case at the time of hospitalization, the demonstration of specific IgM and IgG serum antibodies by enzyme-linked immunosorbent assay (ELISA) is the method of choice for the specific diagnosis of tick-borne encephalitis. Immunoglobulin M (IgM) antibodies may be detectable for several months after infection, whereas IgG antibodies persist for life and mediate an immunity that prevents reinfection. In the cerebrospinal fluid, shortly after onset of the disease, specific antibodies can be found in only 50% of the patients, but by the tenth day of illness they almost invariably become detectable. If an infection occurs after and despite the post-exposure administration of a specific immunoglobulin, the seroconversion can be delayed and may cause diagnostic problems. In cases with fatal outcome, the virus can be isolated or detected by RT-PCR from the brain and other organs.

Transmission

Tick-borne encephalitis virus occurs in foci characterized by ecological habitats favourable for ticks, especially in wooded areas within the 7°C isotherm. The main vectors of the European virus subtype are ticks of the species *Ixodes ricinus*, whereas the Central Siberian and Far Eastern subtypes are primarily transmitted by *Ixodes*

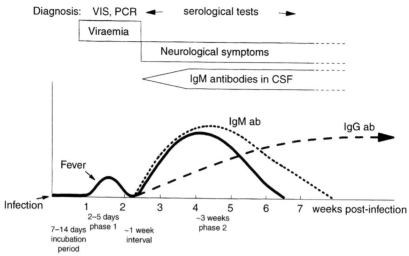

Fig. 3. Biphasic course of a TBE virus infection: detection of the virus or viral nucleic acids and development of specific antibodies (ab) in serum and cerebrospinal fluid. VIS, virus isolation; PCR, polymerase chain reaction.

persulcatus. In its natural foci TBE virus circulates between ticks and small mammals. The latter support virus replication but are asymptomatic (Fig. 4). In particular, small rodents and insectivores, such as Shrews (*Sorex* species), European moles (*Talpa europaea*) and European hedgehogs (*Erinaceus europaeus*), serve as amplifying hosts and act as important virus reservoir hosts. Ixodid (hard) ticks undergo three developmental stages (larva, nymph, adult), which need to engorge blood at each stage for further development. The virus multiplies in several organs, including the salivary glands, and is transmitted via saliva. In ticks the virus can replicate persistently in all developmental stages and also overwinter. Additionally, transovarial virus transmission within the tick population is known to occur. Large domestic animals, such as goats, sheep and cattle, are important hosts for adult ixodid ticks, but have only low viraemias and therefore are not considered to be important sources of tick infection. However, the virus is excreted in the milk of infected animals and can cause local epidemics of milk-borne tick-borne encephalitis (see below). The virus is apathogenic for its natural hosts but in rare cases clinically apparent infections of dogs,

horses or Chamois (*Rupicapra rupicapra*) have been observed.

Humans do not form part of the natural virus transmission cycle and are only accidentally infected by tick bites when they enter a natural focus. It is important to note that about half of the tick bites go unnoticed. Infection of humans, however, can also occur by the consumption of unpasteurized milk from infected animals (especially goats) and milk products, such as cheese. This route of transmission regularly causes small epidemics in the Baltic countries and in Eastern Europe, but does not seem to be an important source of infection in the rest of Europe. Some decades ago most of the cases occurred in people with an occupational risk of infection, such as farmers and forest workers. Today more than 90% of the infections are acquired during leisure activities.

Treatment

Currently no specific antiviral therapy is available and patients can therefore only be treated symptomatically.

Control and prevention

Immunization

The method of choice for the control and prevention of tick-borne encephalitis is

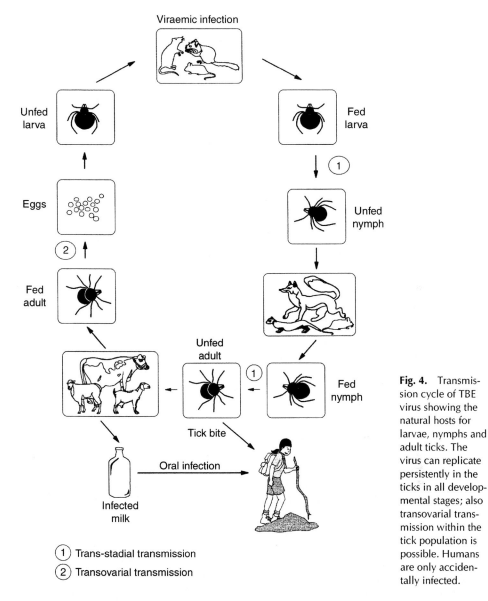

Viraemic infection

Unfed larva

Fed larva

Eggs

Unfed nymph

Fed adult

Unfed adult

Fed nymph

Tick bite

Infected milk

Oral infection

(1) Trans-stadial transmission

(2) Transovarial transmission

Fig. 4. Transmission cycle of TBE virus showing the natural hosts for larvae, nymphs and adult ticks. The virus can replicate persistently in the ticks in all developmental stages; also transovarial transmission within the tick population is possible. Humans are only accidentally infected.

vaccination. Highly purified inactivated whole virus vaccines are available that are well tolerated and mediate a high degree of protection. The immunization schedule consists of two immunizations 1–3 months apart, followed by a third vaccination after 1 year. For maintaining long-term immunity, booster immunizations should be given every 3 years. After the series of three vaccinations seroconversion rates are 98–99% and in children almost 100%. Austria has the highest vaccination coverage of all countries where tick-borne encep- halitis is endemic. About 85% of the total population (in some endemic areas more than 90%) has been protected by vaccination and this has resulted in a dramatic decline of the number of hospitalized cases to about 10% of those recorded in the pre-vaccination era (several hundred per year). The protection rate of the vaccine has been calculated as being approximately 98%. Vaccination is recommended for persons living in or going to endemic arreas – for instance, during holidays or for leisure activities.

In some European countries a TBE hyperimmunoglobulin is available for post-exposure prophylaxis by passive immunization. It should be given as early as possible, but not later than 4 days (96 h) after exposure. The dose depends on the patient's body weight and the length of time elapsed (0.1 ml kg^{-1} body weight within the first 2 days, 0.2 ml kg^{-1} body weight on the third and fourth days). This procedure does not, however, reliably prevent the disease. The extent of the protective efficacy of immuno-globulin has not been definitely clarified. There is a certain concern that the late application of a specific immunoglobulin not only may not prevent the disease but may even lead to an aggravated course of the disease. Therefore passive immuniza-tion after the fifth day post-exposure is con-traindicated. Based on isolated observations of unusually severe courses of tick-borne encephalitis in children after post-expo-sure prophylaxis by immunoglobulin, the approval of this procedure has been sus-pended for children under the age of 14 years in Germany and Austria.

Vector control

The control of the disease by the eradication of tick vectors has sometimes been attemp-ted locally but cannot be successfully app-lied to all endemic areas. Also the wearing of protective clothing and the use of chemi-cal repellents are not nearly as effective in preventing disease as is vaccination.

Determination of immunity after vaccination

Successful vaccination can easily be monitored by the demonstration of IgG antibodies in the serum by ELISA. How-ever, there is a potential for misleading results, because all flaviviruses are serologi-cally related and infections or vaccinations with one flavivirus will give rise to anti-bodies that also react with all other flavi-viruses in IgG ELISAs. Vaccinations against yellow fever or Japanese encephalitis or infections with dengue viruses will thus result in cross-reactive but non-neutralizing antibodies, yielding a positive result in TBE ELISAs. In such cases specific immunity against TBE virus can only be assessed in a virus neutralization assay.

Selected bibliography

Barrett, P.N., Dorner, F. and Plotkin, S.A. (1999) Tick-borne encephalitis vaccine. In: Plotkin, S.A. and Orenstein, W.A. (eds) *Vaccines*, 3rd edn. W.B. Saunders, Philadelphia, pp. 767–780

Ecker, M., Allison, S.L., Meixner, T. and Heinz, F.X. (1999) Sequence analysis and genetic classification of tick-borne encephalitis viruses from Europe and Asia. *Journal of General Virology* 80, 179–185.

Harabacz, I., Bock, H., Jüngst, Ch., Klockmann, U., Praus, M. and Weber, R. (1992) A randomized phase II study of a new tick-borne encephali-tis vaccine using three different doses and two immunization regimens. *Vaccine* 10, 145–150.

Holzmann, H., Kundi, M., Stiasny, K., Clement, J., McKenna, P., Kunz, C. and Heinz, F.X. (1996) Correlation between ELISA, hemag-glutination inhibition and neutralization test after vaccination against tick-borne encep-halitis. *Journal of Medical Virology* 48, 102–107.

Monath, T.P. and Heinz, F.X. (1996) Flaviviruses. In: Fields, B.N., Knipe, D.M. and Howley, P.M. (eds) *Fields Virology*, Vol. 1, 3rd edn. Lippincott-Raven, Philadelphia, pp. 961–1034.

Tick-borne fever *see* **Ehrlichiosis.**

Tick-borne relapsing fever

Philip J. McCall

Tick-borne relapsing fever (TBRF) is a human disease caused by infection with spirochaetes of *Borrelia* and contracted from the bite or coxal fluid of soft ticks (Argasidae) of the genus *Ornithodoros*. The disease is characterized by episodes of febrile illness, separated by afebrile periods, giving rise to its name.

Distribution

Tick-borne relapsing fever has a wide distribution in both the Old and New Worlds, occurring in Africa, Asia and the Americas, with different *Borrelia*–tick vector complexes in each area. It is absent from Australia and New Zealand. With the exception of *Borrelia duttonii* in Africa, TBRF is a zoonosis and can be pathogenic for both human and rodent hosts. Lyme disease (see entry) is also caused by tick-borne borreliae, but does not cause a relapsing fever.

Parasite

Bacteria of the genus *Borrelia* are spirochaetes within the order Spirochaetales, which also includes the genera *Treponema* and *Leptospira*. Borreliae are motile spirochaetes (5–25 μm long and 0.2–0.5 μm wide), with up to ten loose regular waves in shape and periplasmic flagella enclosed within an outer membrane. Spirochaetes enter the skin and subcutaneous tissues without causing a lesion and invade both the systemic and lymphatic circulation, where they multiply by transverse fission. During fever, spirochaetes appear in the peripheral blood.

Historically, borreliae were identified taxonomically (and named) according to their geographical distribution and their tick vectors; however, this specificity may not be exact and the taxonomy of the group is likely to be more complex. Nevertheless, 11 different *Borrelia* species are recognized as being responsible for TBRF in humans, and they have been classified with their tick vectors, as shown in Table 1.

The most important of these is *B. duttonii*, which occurs throughout east, central and southern Africa, from Somalia to South Africa and from Tanzania to Angola, where it is transmitted by ticks of the *Ornithodoros moubata* complex. The other African species, *Borrelia crocidurae*, is found in a range of small mammals in West Africa, occasionally infecting humans.

Immunology

Relapsing fever borreliae undergo antigenic variation within the host, similar to that seen in African trypanosomes. Antigenic variation enables the population of

Table 1. Geographical distribution of the main species of *Borrelia* associated with relapsing fever in humans and their respective *Ornithodoros* vectors.

Species of *Borrelia*	*Ornithodoros* vectors	Distribution
B. duttonii	*O. moubata complex*	East, Central and southern Africa
B. crocidurae	*O. sonrai* (= *O. erraticus* small form)	North Africa, Senegal, Kenya, Turkey, Iran
B. hispanica	*O. erraticus*	North Africa, Iberian Peninsula
B. caucasica	*O. verrucosus*	Caucasus to Iraq
B. latyschewii	*O. tartakowski*	Iran, Central Asia
B. persica	*O. tholozani* (= *O. papillipes*)	Middle East, Iran to Kashmir, former USSR and western China
B. hermsi	*O. hermsi*	Central and western USA, Mexico
B. parkerii	*O. parkeri*	Central and western USA, Mexico
B. turicata	*O. turicata*	Central and western USA, Mexico
B. mazzotti	*O. talaje*	Southern USA, Mexico, Central and South America
B. venezuelensis	*O. rudis* (= *O. venezuelensis*)	Central and South America, southwards to northern Argentina

parasites to overcome the host's specific humoral response, and gives rise to a succession of antigenic types, which are in turn responsible for the series of relapses. On entering the host's bloodstream, those borreliae that are not killed via immunoglobulin M (IgM) antibody mechanisms are antigenically unstable and generate new outer membrane antigen types, called variable membrane proteins (Vmps), and continue to proliferate. Fresh specific antibodies produced in response will eventually remove these types, leading to successive waves of Vmps, each resulting in a fever relapse.

Tick-borne relapsing fever is more serious in newcomers to an endemic area than in the indigenous people, indicating that some level of immunity exists in persons under continuous challenge. Neurological complications are also far more common in visitors than in the local population.

Clinical symptoms

The incubation period of TBRF varies from 2 to 18 days, with a sudden onset of rapidly rising fever, headache, chills and muscle and joint pain, accompanied by nausea, dizziness and vomiting. The fever is caused by the large number of borreliae, which do not produce a toxin but whose outer envelope stimulates the expression of leucocyte pyrogens by host mononuclear phagocytes. Approximately ten times more organisms are found in the peripheral blood during the initial attack than in the subsequent relapses. Untreated, the symptoms intensify over a 4–6 day period ending in a characteristic pathophysiologic crisis, during which spirochaetes rapidly disappear from the circulating blood. Tick-borne relapsing fever may range from a subclinical mild infection to a severe disease with a mortality of 1–8%. Pregnant women and children are most susceptible. Locally the infection can be very important, with TBRF incidences of up to 38% recorded in 1-year-olds and 16% in 1–5-year-olds. *Borrelia duttonii* prevalence rates of 7.5% in pregnant women and 3% in under-5-year-olds have been recorded in Tanzania. Risk of pregnancy interruption can be as high as 30%.

Tick-borne relapsing fever borreliae are neurotropic and can be detected in cerebrospinal fluid. Neurological complications are not uncommon, particularly the involvement of the seventh cranial nerve. Neurological syndromes can appear at the end of the first bout of fever or during relapses. Involvement of other cranial nerves can result in ophthalmoplegia or deafness. Acute adult complications include jaundice, hepatomegaly, pneumonia and mental confusion.

Diagnosis

Relapsing fever can be difficult to distinguish from many other fevers before a remission-relapse cycle has occurred. It can easily be confused with malaria, typhus fevers, typhoid, leptospirosis and arboviral fevers.

Spirochaetes can be visualized in blood films between the red blood cells, although they are usually less numerous than in louse-borne relapsing fever (see entry) caused by *Borrelia recurrentis*. The spirochaetes can be observed by dark-field microscopy and with Giemsa-, Wright-, acridine orange- or Leishman-stained preparations of thin or dehaemoglobinized thick smears of peripheral blood, or in stained buffy-coat preparations. Spirochaetes in mild infections may be more readily detected by microhaematocrit concentration than by microscopy. Detection during afebrile periods can be difficult. Borreliae can be cultured *in vitro*, by inoculation of blood into Barbour–Stoenner–Kelly II (BSK II) medium, or *in vivo*, by intraperitoneal inoculation into immature laboratory mice.

The variety of borreliae causing relapsing fever and the existence of antigenic variation limit the use of serological tests. Immunoblotting can indicate a negative result with some degree of safety, but positive diagnoses are not reliable, as cross-reactions with other spirochaetes can occur. A detection method based upon the polymerase chain reaction has not yet been developed.

Transmission

The tick vectors of *Borrelia* species are all members of the *Ornithodoros* genus

(Table 1). Although the spirochaetes can survive in lice (*Pediculus* species) and bed bugs (*Cimex* species), these insects are not involved in transmission.

Ticks feed rapidly, engorge in 10–45 min and spend the remainder of the life cycle off the host. Larval *Ornithodoros* is unusual in being inactive and not feeding. Ingested spirochaetes multiply in the midgut of the tick, penetrate the gut wall and enter the haemocoel within 24 h of ingestion. They then disperse to the tick's organs and can be found in the salivary glands, ovaries and coxal organs after about 3 days. Spirochaetes are not found in tick faeces. On subsequent feeds, the host can be infected by inoculation with spirochaetes from the infected saliva, or through infected coxal fluid contaminating the relatively large bite wound. Typically, transmission occurs primarily through the saliva, since most tick species leave the host before excreting coxal fluid. However, *O. moubata* excretes coxal fluid while still on the host and this can be an important route of transmission by adult ticks of this species complex.

There is a high rate of transovarial and trans-stadial transmission of borreliae in ticks, permitting maintenance of the parasite in the tick population for generations, without the need for an individual tick to feed on an infected vertebrate at any stage in its life. In combination with the ability of ticks to starve for long periods, this permits natural foci to survive in the absence of any vertebrate hosts.

Epidemiology

Tick-borne relapsing fever is a zoonotic disease in all cases, with the exception of *B. duttonii* in Africa, where humans are the only known host. The reservoir animals are usually rodents, though certain insectivores can also be reservoir hosts for *B. crocidurae*. The diversity of hosts infected with any one species of relapsing fever borrelia is low compared with *Borrelia burgdorferi*, probably a result of the more host-specific feeding preferences of the tick vectors rather than host specificity of the borreliae. Because *Ornithodoros* life cycles are spent in close

association with the microhabitats where their hosts nest or rest, they are unlikely to come into contact with any species other than their normal host. Humans become infected when they come into contact with ticks, either by camping in wilderness areas, by sleeping in remote rodent-infested houses or caves or if the rodent hosts disappear due an epizootic disease (such as plague) and the ticks are driven to search for new hosts.

Due to the sporadic nature of most TBRFs, reliable estimates for the prevalence or incidence of disease worldwide are rare. Tick-borne relapsing fever cases are typically isolated, often in small family clusters and rarely involving more than a few persons. Most patients are unaware of the tick bite and, if a history of camping or wilderness activity is not suspected, it can easily be misdiagnosed. The disease is sustained in endemic areas by both tick and rodent reservoir hosts, but ticks appear to be the main reservoirs.

Where there is no animal reservoir host, *B. duttonii* persists as a low-prevalence disease in humans in communities within endemic areas Transmission occurs in traditional houses, where the vectors, ticks species of the *O. moubata* complex, live within the home in cracks and depressions in the loose earth floors and walls. Wide variations in feeding behaviour are seen within the *O. moubata* complex, influencing tick vectorial capacity. Prevalence of TBRF is higher where a human feeding habit predominates and where certain types of local housing promote the proliferation of indoor tick populations. Ticks probably colonize a new house by being carried unknowingly in the possessions of travellers moving between homes. They are nocturnal and emerge a few hours after dark to feed upon the sleeping occupants. House infestation rates can be as high as 88% in some areas, and biting rates can be so high that the occupants are driven to sleeping outdoors. Ticks may then be found outside the house beneath these sleeping places. In poor rural communities TBRF remains undiagnosed or is often misdiagnosed as malaria or another non-specific fever. It is likely that prevalences of

B. duttonii are much higher than has been recorded.

Treatment

Relapsing fever spirochaetes can be treated effectively with antibiotics. Some TBRF cases can be treated with a single dose of tetracycline (500 mg) or procaine penicillin (300 mg), but in certain areas relapses are common and a 5–10 day treatment with 500 mg at 6-hourly intervals is needed. The Jarisch–Herxheimer reaction, which commonly follows treatment of louse-borne relapsing fever, is less likely to occur in the treatment of TBRF.

Control

Some degree of personal protection against tick bites may be achieved by applying chemical repellents to the skin or clothing, but the effects are short-lived; more lasting protection is achieved by wearing repellent- or insecticide-impregnated clothes.

Where the dwelling is the source of infection, prevention of tick infestation will reduce exposure. In the zoonotic relapsing fevers, prevention of rodent access to house foundations and attics will prevent tick infestation. In houses infested with *B. duttonii*, construction of solid floors and walls with concrete or mortar will obviate tick breeding and resting sites and eliminate infestations. Sleeping on a bed raised from the floor instead of a sleeping mat can greatly reduce or even prevent biting.

Spraying the interior surfaces of walls, ceilings/roofs with a range of residual insecticides, including pyrethroids, carbamates and organophosphates, is the most effective method of controlling indoor tick populations. Such treatments will reduce tick infestation and can eliminate borrelia transmission. Bed nets impregnated with insecticides, such as permethrin or other pyrethroids, may reduce transmission of TBRF by reducing biting rates and killing ticks, but their effect upon domestic tick populations remains to be determined.

Selected bibliography

Cook, G.C. (1996) In: *Manson's Tropical Diseases*, 20th edn. W.B. Saunders, London, pp. 952–955.

Dennis, D.T. (1998) Borreliosis (relapsing fever). In: Palmer, S.R., Soulsby, E.J.L. and Simpson, D.I.H. (eds) *Zoonoses: Biology, Clinical Practice and Public Health Control.* Oxford University Press, Oxford, pp. 17–21.

Goubau, P.F. (1984) Relapsing fevers. A review. *Annales de la Société de Médecine Tropicale* 64, 335–364.

Schwan, T.G., Burgdorfer, W. and Rosa, P.A. (1995) Borrelia. In: Murray, P.R., Baron, E.J., Pfaller, M.A., Tenover, F.C. and Yolke, R.H. (eds) *Manual of Clinical Microbiology.* American Society for Microbiology, Washington, DC, pp. 626–635.

Talbert, A., Nyange, A. and Molteni, F. (1998) Spraying tick-infested houses with lambdacyhalothrin reduces the incidence of tick-borne relapsing fever in children under five years old. *Transactions of the Royal Society of Tropical Medicine and Hygiene* 92, 251-253.

Walton, G.A. (1962) The *Ornithodorus moubata* superspecies problem in relation to human relapsing fever epidemiology. In: Arthur, D.R. (ed.) *Aspects of Disease Transmission by Ticks.* The Zoological Society of London Symposium 6, pp. 83–153.

Tick-borne typhuses

Philippe Parola and Didier Raoult

Tick-borne typhuses are caused by obligate intracellular bacteria belonging to the genus *Rickettsia* and are among the oldest known arthropod-borne diseases. At the beginning of the 20th century, H.T. Ricketts demonstrated the role of the Rocky Mountain wood tick, *Dermacentor andersoni*, in the transmission of *Rickettsia rickettsii*, the agent of Rocky Mountain spotted fever (see entry). In 1910, A. Conor and A. Bruch reported the first case of Mediterranean spotted fever ('boutonneuse fever'). In the

1930s, the role of the brown dog tick, *Rhipicephalus sanguineus*, and the causative agent (*Rickettsia conorii*) were described. However, tick-borne typhuses have to be considered as emerging diseases. Prior to 1974, four tick-borne rickettsioses were recognized: *R. rickettsii* in the Americas, *R. conorii* in Eurasia and Africa, *Rickettsia sibirica* in Siberia and Russia and *Rickettsia australis* in Australia. In subsequent years, a further nine pathogenic rickettsiae have been described throughout the world, seven since 1991 (Table 1). These newly described diseases were discovered not only in countries with poor laboratory facilities (e.g. *Rickettsia africae* in sub-Saharan Africa), but also in well-developed countries (e.g. Japanese spotted fever due to *Rickettsia japonica* in Japan). Some emerging tick-borne typhuses were found in areas where rickettsiae were not previously known to occur (Japan, Tasmania and Astrakhan in Russia), or where *R. conorii* was thought to be the only pathogenic rickettsia, such as the mainly African tick-bite fever, due to

R. africae, and infection with *Rickettsia slovaca* and *Rickettsia mongolotimonae* in southern France.

Distribution

The tick-borne typhuses have an almost worldwide distribution, occurring in many European countries, in Asia, Africa, Australia and the Americas. The distribution and species of rickettsia depends much on the distribution of different tick species, (for more details see under named rickettsiae).

Bacteria

Bacteria of the genus *Rickettsia* are intracellular, short (0.8–2 µm long and 0.3–0.5 µm in diameter), Gram-negative rods, which retain basic fuchsin when stained by the method of Gimenez. The agents of the tick-borne typhuses belong to the spotted fever group of rickettsiae. Their growth in the laboratory requires living organisms (animals, embryonated eggs) or cell cultures such as African green monkey kidney (VERO), mouse fibroblasts (L929),

Table 1. The tick-borne rickettsiae pathogenic to humans and their vectors. Bold-typed rickettsiae were recognized as human pathogens in 1974 or later.

Location by continent	Rickettsia (year of the first documented human case)	Principal tick vector(s)
Americas	*Rickettsia rickettsii*	*Dermacentor andersoni, Dermacentor variabilis*
	Rickettsia africae (West Indies) (1998)	*Amblyomma variegatum*
Europe	*Rickettsia conorii*	*Rhipicephalus sanguineus*
	Rickettsia conorii Astrakhan (1991)	*Rhipicephalus pumillio*
	Rickettsia mongolotimonae (1996)	?
	Rickettsia slovaca (1997)	*Dermacentor marginatus, Dermacentor reticulatus*
	Rickettsia helvetica (1999)	*Ixodes ricinus*
	Rickettsia conorii Israel (1999)	*Rhipicephalus sanguineus*
Asia	*Rickettsia conorii*	*Rhipicephalus sanguineus*
	Rickettsia sibirica	*Dermacentor nuttalli, Haemaphysalis concinna*
	Rickettsia conorii Israel (1974)	*Rhipicephalus sanguineus*
	Rickettsia mongolotimonae	*Hyalomma asiaticum*
	Rickettsia japonica (1984)	*Ixodes ovatus, Dermacentor taiwanensis, Haemaphysalis longicornis, Haemaphysalis flava*
Africa	*Rickettsia conorii*	*Rhipicephalus sanguineus*
	Rickettsia africae (1992)	*Amblyomma variegatum, Amblyomma hebraeum*
	Rickettsia mongolotimonae	*Hyalomma truncatum*
Australia	*Rickettsia australis*	*Ixodes holocyclus*
	Rickettsia honei (1992)	?

human embryonic lung (HEL) or human diploid lung (MRC5). In the cytoplasm, rickettsiae are not enclosed by a vacuole and can rarely be observed in the nuclei of the host cells. In the organism, the target cells of the pathogenic rickettsiae are the endothelial cells, and multiplication of the bacteria in these cells results in vasculitis. Among the rickettsial protein antigens, two high-molecular-mass surface proteins (rOmpA and rOmpB) contain species-specific epitopes. They provide the basis for rickettsial serotyping, using comparative micro-immunofluorescence, which remains the reference method for identification of rickettsiae. However, although protein analyses using sodium dodecyl sulphate polyacrylamide gel electrophoresis (SDS-PAGE) or species-specific monoclonal antibodies have also been used to identify rickettsial species, sequence analysis of polymerase chain reaction (PCR) product is currently the most rapid, convenient and sensitive technique for the identification of rickettsiae. Several rickettsial genes have been used for the study of their phylogeny and the identification of new strains, as well as the description of emerging diseases.

Clinical symptoms

Generally tick-borne typhus clinical symptoms begin 6–10 days after a tick bite and typically include fever, headache, muscle pain, rash, local lymphadenopathy and a characteristic inoculation eschar ('tache noire') at the site of the tick bite. However, the main clinical signs vary depending on the rickettsial species involved (Table 2). Unspecific biological findings include thrombocytopenia, leucocyte count abnormalities and elevated hepatic enzyme levels.

A study of atypical cases in endemic areas has also led to the description of new clinical syndromes caused by organisms previously considered as 'rickettsiae of unknown pathogenicity', including *Rickettsia slovaca* and *Rickettsia helvetica* in Europe. Moreover, new rickettsial strains of unknown pathogenicity have been isolated or detected in ticks in recent years. Their role

in human disease has yet to be determined, but, to date, all of them must be considered potential pathogens.

Diagnosis

In recent years, the advent of novel diagnostic tools has improved the specific diagnosis of rickettsioses and allowed the description of new rickettsial species as well as the recognition of emerging tick-borne typhuses.

Serology is the most valuable test to perform. The Weil–Felix test, the oldest serological assay for rickettsioses, was based on the detection of antibodies to various *Proteus* antigens that cross-react with rickettsiae (*P. vulgaris*, OX2 with spotted fever rickettsiae *P. vulgaris* OX19 with typhus-group rickettsiae and *P. mirabilis* OXK with *Orientia tsutsugamushi*). To date, immunofluorescence is the reference method. Acute and convalescent serum testing allows any rise in antibody titres to be detected. A major limitation is cross-reactivity, and frequently it is not possible to differentiate among spotted fever rickettsiae. Western blot immunoassay, particularly when associated with cross-adsorption studies, can be used to determined the rickettsia species involved, but it is time-consuming and expensive to perform.

Rickettsiae are most commonly isolated using cell culture systems and the centrifugation shell-vial technique, using HEL fibroblasts, is the reference method. Numerous rickettsiae have been isolated from blood, skin biopsy samples, tissues and ticks. Immunodetection methods have been widely used to detect rickettsiae in biopsy specimens and arthropods. The advent of molecular methods based on PCR gene amplification has enabled the development of useful, sensitive and rapid methods to detect and identify rickettsiae from blood and skin biopsy specimens (the 'tache noire' being the most useful specimen). Primers obtained from the sequences within the rOmpA and the rOmpB gene, the citrate synthase gene, the 17 kDa protein gene, and the 16 S ribosomal RNA (rRNA) gene of rickettsiae are all used. Sequencing the PCR amplification products is reproducible and any laboratory with facilities for molecular methods and access to sequence databases is able to identify known rickettsiae or even describe new strains.

Transmission

The tick-borne typhuses are transmitted by ixodid (hard) ticks. Rickettsiae infect and multiply in almost all the organs of ticks, in particular the salivary glands, which enables the rickettsiae to be transmitted to vertebrate hosts during feeding. Moreover, rickettsiae are maintained in ticks through trans-stadial (from larva to nymphs to adults) and transovarial (from one generation to another through the ovaries) transmissions. Thus, ticks act as the main reservoirs of the spotted fever group rickettsiae and tick-borne typhuses are geographical diseases determined by the distribution of ticks. Ecological characteristics of the tick vector influence the epidemiology of the transmission of typhus. For example, *Rhipicephalus sanguineus* ticks wait for passing hosts (essentially dogs) and have a low affinity for people. Cases of Mediterranean spotted fever are sporadic in endemic areas. In contrast, *Amblyomma hebraeum* in southern Africa emerge from their habitats and actively attack and run towards their hosts when these animals appear nearby. They also feed readily on humans that enter their biotopes and numerous ticks can attack a host at the same time. Thus, cases of African tick-bite fever often occur as grouped cases among subjects entering the bush and people can suffer several tick bites simultaneously.

Although many animals (mammals and birds) may present rickettsaemia and clinical signs after tick bites, the role of vertebrates as reservoir hosts in maintaining zoonotic foci has yet to be determined. People do not appear to be reservoir hosts for tick-borne rickettsiae, because they are only occasionally parasitized by ticks and are rickettsaemic for only short periods.

Treatment

Empirical treatment is usually started before laboratory confirmation of the diagnosis, with the treatment of choice being 200 mg doxycycline day^{-1} for 1–7 days, depending on the severity of the disease.

Control and prevention

Reducing and controlling tick populations is difficult. Methods include vegetation management, ground or aerial applications of acaricides, regular dipping of wild or domesticated animal hosts in acaricidal baths or spraying them with acaricides, as well as biological control methods. However, in practice there are usually no vector control measures aimed at reducing typhus transmission, and tick-borne typhuses are best prevented by people avoiding tick bites in infested areas. Tick bites may be prevented by wearing long trousers which are tucked into boots. Currently, the best method of avoiding tick bites comprises two components: a topical *N,N*-diethyl-*m*-toluamide (DEET) repellent applied to exposed skin, and treatment of clothing with permethrin (a pyrethroid acaricide killing ticks on contact). These products are commercially available in a wide variety of formulas (e.g. lotions, sprays). Finally, people should check their clothes and their entire body when staying in infested area and after leaving them, and any ticks found should be removed immediately.

The tick-borne typhuses

The following account describes the various tick-borne typhuses throughout the world, with the exception of Rocky Mountain spotted fever (see entry), which is described in a separate encyclopedia entry.

Mediterranean spotted fever

The disease, due to *R. conorii*, was first described in 1909 and thereafter referred to as 'boutonneuse fever', because of a papular rather than macular rash. It is transmitted by the brown dog tick, *R. sanguineus*, which is well adapted to a human urban environment but is relatively host-specific and rarely feeds on people. Although about 5% (up to 12%) of these ticks are infected with *R. conorii* in southern France, the incidence of the disease and the prevalence of seropositive people are relatively low. The disease occurs in late spring and summer, particularly in August, during the activity of immature forms of the ticks (smaller than adults and usually not observed). The onset of signs is abrupt and typical cases have high fever, rash and a unique eschar (the 'tache noire') at the tick bite site (Table 2). Although it produces a less severe disease than *R. rickettsii*, the agent of Rocky Mountain spotted fever in the Americas, the mortality rate may reach 2.5% and malignant forms include neurological, renal and cardiac or vascular complications. The disease is present all around the Mediterranean Sea, in sub-Saharan Africa, in India, around the Black Sea and in eastern Russia. However, no case has been reported to date in the USA, although *R. sanguineus* ticks (which are also a reservoir of *R. conorii*) are prevalent there.

African tick-bite fever

Although African tick-bite fever has been recognized since the beginning of the century, it has been considered for a long time as a milder form of Mediterranean spotted fever. However, it is usually contracted in rural areas following contact with cattle and ticks of wild animals, particularly *Amblyomma* species. In the 1930s, A. Pijper considered African tick-bite fever to be distinct from Mediterranean spotted fever and suggested that the two diseases were caused by different rickettsiae. His work was not confirmed and *R. conorii* became considered to be the aetiological agent of all cases of tick-bite fever in Africa, until the first case that could reliably be attributed to infection with a new rickettsia was reported from Zimbawe in 1992 by P.J. Kelly and colleagues. The strain was demonstrated to be distinct from *R. conorii* and indistinguishable from an isolate obtained from *Amblyomma variegatum* ticks in Ethiopia and *A. hebraeum* in Zimbabwe (Fig. 1). The strain was subsequently characterized as a distinct species of the spotted fever group rickettsiae and named *R. africae*. In sub-Saharan Africa, this rickettsia is highly prevalent in *Amblyomma* species (e.g. 65% in *A. hebraeum* in Zimbabwe), and these ticks frequently bite people. The seroprevalence of the rickettsioses in sub-Saharan African people is as high as 30–80% and correlated with the geographical distribution of *Amblyomma* species. Moreover, these ticks are aggressive and actively seek out hosts, which explains grouped cases of infection and multiple inoculation eschars in patients (Fig. 2). More than 100 cases of African tick-bite fever have been diagnosed in our laboratory in patients returning from Africa (particularly after safari through southern Africa). Specific features of the disease include an incubation period of 6 days, occurrence as grouped cases, multiple inoculation eschars in 53% of the cases (the main difference from other spotted fever rickettsioses), regional lymphadenopathy, an infrequent rash, which may be vesicular, and the absence of severe forms (Table 2). The disease also occurs in the West Indies where *A. variegatum* ticks were introduced during the 18th or 19th century on cattle shipped from Senegal to Guadeloupe.

Infection due to *Rickettsia slovaca*

In 1997, the first documented case of infection due to *R. slovaca* was reported in a woman bitten by *Dermacentor marginatus*. She had presented with a fever, a necrotic eschar at the site of tick attachment on the head surrounded by a large Lyme-like erythema, enlarged cervical lymph nodes and she suffered fatigue. Similar undocumented cases had been previously reported in France and Hungary where this clinical syndrome was known as 'Tibola' – for tickborne lymphadenopathy. *Rickettsia slovaca* was first isolated in 1968 from *Dermacentor marginatus* ticks in Czechoslovakia. Subsequently, it has been detected or isolated from ticks in all European countries where *D. marginatus* was screened for rickettsial infections, including France, Switzerland, Slovakia, Ukraine, Yugoslavia, Armenia and Portugal. Prevalence in ticks varies from 1 to 17%. To date, 25 cases have been documented in patients from France and Hungary presenting with tick bites on the scalp and lymphadenopathy (unpublished data). The median incubation period was 6 days, general symptoms were rare and sequelae included localized alopecia at the bite site and chronic fatigue (Table 2). Two

Table 2. Location and symptoms of the tick-borne typhuses.

Diseases	Rickettsia	Distribution	Clinical symptoms				
			Fever	Diffuse rash	Inoculation eschar	Enlarged local nodes	Fatality rate without treatment
Rocky Mountain spotted fever	*R. rickettsii*	North and South America	99%	90% (45% purpuric)	Very rare	No	10–50%
Mediterranean spotted fever	*R. conorii*	Mediterranean littoral, Africa, Black Sea, eastern Russia, India	100%	97% (10% purpuric)	72%	Rare	1–2.5%
Israeli spotted fever	*R. conorii* Israel	Israel, Portugal, Sicily	Yes	100%	No	No	<%
Astrakhan fever	*R. conorii* Astrakhan	Caspian sea	Yes	100%	23%	No	No
Siberian tick typhus North Asian tick typhus	*R. sibirica*	Northern China, Pakistan, former USSR (Asian republics, Siberia, Armenia)	Yes	100%	77%	Yes	Low
Queensland tick typhus	*R. australis*	Australia (Queensland)	Yes	100% (vesicular)	65%	Yes	Low
Flinders Island spotted fever	*R. honei*	Flinders Island (Tasmania)	Yes	85% (8% purpuric)	28%	Yes	Low
African tick bite fever	*R. africae*	Sub-Saharan Africa, West Indies	92%	49% (50% vesicular)	98% (55% multiple)	43%	Very low
Japanese or Oriental spotted fever	*R. japonica*	Japan	100%	100%	91%	No	Low
Unnamed	*R. mongolotimonae*	France, Inner Mongolia, Niger	Yes	Yes	Yes	No	No
Unnamed	*R. slovaca*	From western Europe to central Asia	24%	Low (8%)	Yes	Cervical (painful 44%)	No
Unnamed	*R. helvetica*	From north-western Europe to central Asia	Yes	?	?	?	Yes

ticks removed from the scalp were identified as *D. marginatus* and one as *Dermacentor reticulatus*. Both species are prevalent throughout Europe to central Asia (except that *D. marginatus* is absent in northern Europe). Adult ticks inhabit forests and pastures and feed on large mammals, including humans. They frequently bite the scalp of young people. They are active during early spring (March and April) and again in

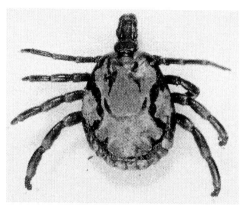

Fig. 1. *Amblyomma hebraeum*, the vector of African tick-bite fever caused by *Rickettsia africae* in southern Africa.

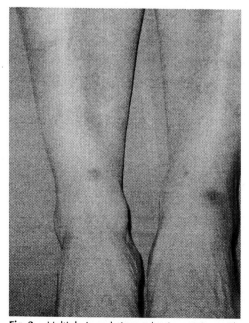

Fig. 2. Multiple inoculation eschar in a patient with African tick-bite fever (courtesy of Dr. G. Caruso).

autumn (September and October). In Spain, bites on humans are frequently reported between December and March.

Japanese or Oriental spotted fever

The first cases of this rickettsiosis were reported in Japan by F. Mahara during the summer of 1984, when three patients presented with high fever and a rash. They lived in the countryside and had collected shoots from bamboo plantations on the same mountain. In two patients an eschar was observed. The Weil–Felix test and immunofluorescence serology suggested a spotted fever group rickettsiosis. In 1986, the causative agent was isolated from patients, characterized and named *R. japonica*. It has been detected in several species of ticks in Japan. Of these, *Haemaphysalis flava*, *Haemaphysalis longicornis* and *Ixodes ovatus* commonly feed on humans and may act as vectors. Since 1984, more than 175 cases have been reported, mainly along the coast of south-western and central Japan, where the climate is warm. The disease occurs from April to October. It has an abrupt onset, with headache, high fever (39–40°C) and chills. A macular rash appears after 2–3 days, all over the body, including the palms and soles. It becomes petechial after 3–4 days and disappears in 2 weeks. An inoculation eschar is frequently observed. No fatal cases have been reported.

Infection due to *Rickettsia mongolotimonae*

In 1991, a spotted fever group rickettsia was isolated from a *Hyalomma asiaticum* tick collected in Inner Mongolia (Nei Monggol), China. It was subsequently characterized and described as a distinct species of the spotted fever group rickettsiae (Ha-91). Its pathogenicity was demonstrated when it was obtained from the blood and skin of a 63-year-old woman from Marseilles in March 1996, who presented with fever, a discrete rash and an eschar in her left groin. She had no previous travel history in Mongolia or contact with individuals from Mongolia. March is not a typical month for Mediterranean spotted fever, which is endemic in southern France. She had collected compost from a garden where migratory birds were resting. Such birds are known to carry ticks, in particular *Hyalomma* species, and to travel from the Arctic to Africa via Mongolia and France. Thus birds were hypothesized as transporting tick vectors that were capable of transmitting diseases.

The name *R. mongolotimonae* was proposed to acknowledge the sites (Mongolia and La Timone Hospital, Marseilles) where the organism has been isolated. A second case was described in May 1998 in a human immunodeficiency virus (HIV) patient living in a rural area 40 km from Marseilles who presented with fever, headache, an eschar, lymphangitis and painful satellite lymphadenopathy. Since then, two other cases have been documented (unpublished data). More recently, we detected *R. mongolotimonae* in *Hyalomma truncatum* collected on cattle in the Republic of Niger, sub-Saharan Africa (unpublished data). Although this discovery does not exclude the possible role of migratory birds in the epidemiology, it may be that *R. mongolotimonae* is associated with *Hyalomma* ticks throughout the world. In southern France, the vector remains to be described, but autochthonous *Hyalomma* species are known to parasitize birds and mammals in the area.

Other tick-borne typhuses
Siberian tick typhus
This has been well described in the former USSR since the 1930s and has been documented in Pakistan and China. This typical spotted fever rickettsiosis is mild and seldom associated with severe complication.

Astrakhan fever
In Astrakhan on the Caspian Sea, this is a summer disease reported since 1983. Dog ticks, *Rhipicephalus pumilio*, are the suspected vectors. The agent is closely related to, but distinct from, *R. conorii*.

Israeli spotted fever
This is also due to a rickettsia closely related to *R. conorii*. The inoculation eschar is lacking. The disease seems to be increasing and may be severe. It has recently been identified in Sicily and Portugal.

Queensland tick typhus
This is due to *R. australis* and has been recognized since 1946, when the first cases were observed among Australian troops training in the bush of northern Queensland. The rash is frequently vesicular. Although the disease is usually mild, a single fatal case has been reported.

Flinders Island spotted fever
This was described in 1991 by R.S. Stewart, the only physician on Flinders Island of Tasmania. He reported 26 cases, over 12 years, of a febrile eruptive disease, which occurred in the summer. The causative agent, *Rickettsia honei*, was isolated in 1992. The vector has yet to be identified.

Rickettsia helvetica
This infection was implicated in fatal perimyocarditis in young patients in Sweden. Furthermore, we recently reported the case of a French patient who seroconverted against *R. helvetica* 4 weeks after the onset of an unexplained febrile illness. The vector is *Ixodes ricinus*, the vector of Lyme borreliosis (see entry) in Europe, which is distributed throughout Europe. People engaged in outdoor activities in forests are particularly exposed to this emerging rickettsiosis.

Conclusions
Numerous factors may explain the increasing number of emerging tick-borne typhuses throughout the world or their increasing incidence. People are undertaking more outdoor activities, which result in increased contact with ticks. Awareness of tick-borne diseases among primary physicians, increased studies on potential pathogenic bacteria found in ticks and the use of new molecular methods have all greatly facilitated studies of the epidemiology of emerging human tick-borne diseases throughout the world. However, some tick-borne disease syndromes remain unexplained and there are a number of *Rickettsia* species that have been found only in ticks. Although their pathogenicity in people is yet to be determined, we anticipate that the number of known tick-borne typhuses will probably increase in the future.

Selected bibliography

Bacellar, F., Beati, L., Franca, A., Pocas, J., Regnery, R. and Filipe, A. (1999) Israeli spotted fever rickettsia (*Rickettsia conorii* complex) associated with human disease in Portugal. *Emerging Infectious Diseases* 5, 835–836.

Fournier, P.E., Tissot-Dupont, H., Gallais, H. and Raoult, D. (2000) *Rickettsia mongolotimonae*: a rare pathogen in France. *Emerging Infectious Diseases* 6, 290–292.

Lascola, B. and Raoult, D. (1997) Laboratory diagnosis of rickettsioses: current approaches to diagnosis of old and new rickettsial diseases. *Journal of Clinical Microbiology* 35, 2715–2727.

Mahara, F. (1997) Japanese spotted fever: report of 31 cases and review of the literature. *Emerging Infectious Diseases* 3, 105–111.

Nilsson, K., Lindquist, O. and Pahlson, C. (1999) Association of *Rickettsia helvetica* with chronic perimyocarditis in sudden cardiac death. *The Lancet* 354, 169–173.

Parola, P. and Raoult, D. (2001) Ticks and tickborne bacterial disease in humans: an emerging infectious threat. *Clinical Infectious Diseases* 32, 897–928.

Parola, P., Jourdan, J. and Raoult, D. (1998) Tick-borne infection caused by *Rickettsia africae* in West Indies. *New England Journal of Medicine* 338, 1391.

Parola, P., Vestris, G., Martinez, D., Brochier, B., Roux, V. and Raoult, D. (1999) Tick-borne rickettsiosis in Guadeloupe, the French West Indies: isolation of *Rickettsia africae* from *Amblyomma variegatum* ticks and serosurvey in humans, cattle and goats. *American Journal of Tropical Medicine and Hygiene* 60, 883–887.

Raoult, D. and Roux, V. (1997) Rickettsioses as paradigms of new and emerging infectious diseases. *Clinical Microbiology Reviews* 10, 694–719.

Raoult, D., Brouqui, P. and Roux, V. (1996) A new spotted-fever-group Rickettsiosis. *The Lancet* 348, 412.

Raoult, D., Berbis, P., Roux, V., Xu, W. and Maurin, M. (1997) A new tick-transmitted disease due to *Ricketssia slovaca*. *The Lancet* 350, 112–113.

Raoult, D., Fournier, P.E., Fenollar, F., Jensenius, M., Prioe, T., de Pina, J.J., Caruso, G., Jones, N., Laferl, H., Rosenblatt, J.E. and Marrie, T.J. (2001) *Rickettsia africae*, a tick-borne pathogen in travelers to sub-Saharan Africa. *New England Journal of Medicine* 344, 1504–1510.

Rolain, J.M., Maurin, M., Vestris, G. and Raoult, D. (1998) *In vitro* susceptibilities of 27 rickettsiae to 13 antimicrobials. *Antimicrobial Agents and Chemotherapy* 42, 1537–1541.

Sekeyova, Z., Roux, V., Xu, W., Rehacek, J. and Raoult, D. (1998) *Rickettsia slovaca* sp. nov., a member of the spotted fever group rickettsiae. *International Journal of Systematic Bacteriology* 48, 1455–1462.

Ticks (Ixodida)

M.W. Service

There are almost 900 species of ticks in 31 genera in the order Ixodida. They have a worldwide distribution. Based on their morphology and life cycle they are placed in two main families, namely the Argasidae (soft ticks) and the Ixodidae (hard ticks). Ticks are the most important vectors of infections to animals and are almost as important as mosquitoes in transmitting infections to humans.

Identification

The two principal families of ticks can be distinguished as follows.

Argasidae

Adults are more or less oval or roundish in outline and have a leathery and wrinkled integument, which is usually covered in fine tubercles. They lack a scutum (dorsal shield). Their mouthparts (capitulum, gnathosoma or 'false head') are not visible when viewed dorsally. (In the larval stage the capitulum projects in front of the body.)

Ixodidae

Adults are usually oval in shape and have a relatively smooth integument. All hard ticks have a dorsal plate (scutum, shield) on the body; often this has so-called enamelled coloured patterns and such species are described as ornate. In the females the scutum is relatively small, being confined to the anterior part of the body, but in males it is very large, covering almost the entire body. (In all immature stages the scutum is small.) The capitulum visibly projects from the front of the body in both sexes and all stages of the life cycle.

Biology

All ticks have a life cycle consisting of the egg, larva and nymphal stages. However, there are considerable differences in the biology of argasid and ixodid ticks and their biologies are best described separately.

Argasidae (soft ticks)

There are about 180 species belonging to 11 genera. The most important species involved in transmission of infections belong to the genera *Ornithodoros* and *Argas*.

Female ticks ingest about 12 times their weight in blood and consequently enlarge considerably in size. After each blood meal the tick generally lays four to six batches of eggs, amounting to several hundred eggs, and, as females can live for many years, thousands of eggs are. laid in her lifetime. Eggs are deposited in cracks and crevices of the ground, the walls and floors of houses or rodent burrows and hatch within 1–3 weeks. The resultant larva superficially resembles the adult but has only three pairs of legs. (The capitulum projects forward and is visible from above.) It climbs on to a suitable host, feeds for 10–20 min and drops to the ground. After a few days it changes into an eight-legged nymph, which seeks out a blood meal, feeds for 20–30 min and then drops off the host. Argasid ticks usually have four or five nymphal instars (Fig. 1). The same or different species of hosts may be fed upon by the different stages in the tick's development. These ticks are often called 'multi-host' or 'many-host' ticks.

Larvae of the tick *Ornithodoros moubata* differ from most other argasid ticks in remaining in the eggshells after hatching and not taking a blood meal, but moulting to produce a first-instar nymph, which crawls from the eggshell and blood feeds.

The life cycle from egg laying to adult typically lasts 6–12 months. Adult ticks can live for 12–20 years, and can survive for many years without feeding. Argasid ticks are usually found in or near the homes, nests or resting places of their hosts, such as live-stock shelters, chicken sheds and animal burrows. Species that commonly feed on people, such as *O. moubata* in Africa, are often found in houses. These ticks do not disperse very far from their breeding places.

Ixodidae (hard ticks)

There are some 690 species in 20 genera. Species of major veterinary and medical importance are found in the genera *Ixodes*, *Hyalomma*, *Rhipicephalus*, *Dermacentor*, *Amblyomma*, *Haemaphysalis* and *Boophilus*.

Adult ticks remain on their hosts blood-feeding for 1–4 weeks. The enormously engorged female tick, sometimes increasing 200 times her size, drops to the ground and after about 3–6 days starts laying eggs. Sometimes, however, several weeks or even occasionally months elapse before the blood meal is digested and oviposition starts. Thousands of eggs are laid in a gelatinous mass that covers part of the tick (Fig. 2). Oviposition can extend over 10 days into 5 weeks, after which the female tick dies. Thus only a single large batch of eggs is laid during her lifetime. After 10–20 days, or sometimes several months, six-legged larvae emerge from the eggs and climb up vegetation and attach themselves to passing hosts, on which they remain blood-feeding for 3–7 days. This process of climbing up vegetation in preparation to attaching to a host is called questing. After feeding, the larvae drop to the ground and about 3–6 days later moult to the eight-legged nymphal stage (Fig. 2), which then ascends vegetation and attaches to a host. After 5–10 days, the engorged nymph drops to the ground and, after a further 3–4 weeks, becomes an adult tick. There is only one nymphal stage in the life cycle of hard ticks. Adult ticks can withstand starvation for 1–2 years and can occasionally live for up to 7 years.

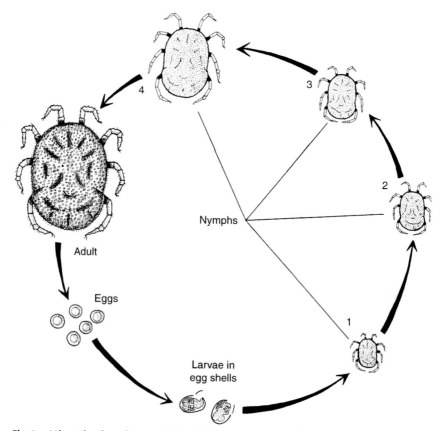

Fig. 1. Life cycle of a soft (argasid) tick (*Ornithodoros* species) showing many nymphal stages (from M.W. Service (2000) *Medical Entomology for Students,* Cambridge University Press, Cambridge).

The larva, nymph and adult of most ticks feed on a different host, which can be of the same species or a different species, and the tick is referred to as a three-host species. With two-host ticks, such as some species of *Rhipicephalus* and *Hyalomma*, the larva and nymph remain attached to and feed on the same individual host, but the adult feeds on a different individual. In a few ticks, such as *Boophilus* species, all three life stages feed on the same individual host, with the female dropping off to lay her eggs. Because all stages remain attached to hosts for several days, ixodid ticks tend to get dispersed long distances.

Diseases

Ticks are very important vectors of disease pathogens to both humans and domesticated animals. For example, ticks transmit spirochaetes causing tick-borne relapsing fever and Lyme disease and rickettsiae causing tick-borne typhuses, as well as a variety of arboviruses, such as Colorado tick fever and Crimean–Congo haemorrhagic fever. Ticks are even more important as vectors of infections to animals, such as avian borelliosis, babesiosis, theileriosis and numerous arboviruses, including those responsible for African swine fever, bluetongue and Nairobi sheep disease. (See entries on these infections.)

Control

Personal protection against tick bites can be obtained by applying chemical repellents to the skin or wearing repellent- or insecticide-impregnated clothing. Houses

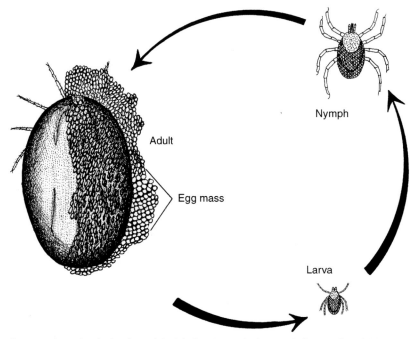

Fig. 2. Life cycle of a hard (ixodid) tick showing a single nymphal stage (from M.W. Service (2000) *Medical Entomology for Students,* Cambridge University Press, Cambridge).

infested with ticks, such as *O. moubata,* can be sprayed with residual insecticides. Ixodid ticks can be controlled to a limited extent by spraying gardens, yards, nearby vegetation or even pastures with residual insecticides, using either ground-based equipment or aircraft applying ultra-low-volume (ULV) techniques. Regular dipping of cattle, sheep and other livestock is practised in many parts of the world. Alternatively livestock can be sprayed or supplied with insecticide-impregnated ear tags or collars. Unfortunately, however, in many areas ticks have developed resistance to some of the more commonly used insecticides.

For the control of *Boophilus* species infecting cattle, 'pasture spelling' is sometimes practised. This involves leaving pastures free of cattle for several months, which results in newly hatched tick larvae dying of starvation. Occasionally habitats can be modified, such as by drainage or scrub clearance, to make them unfavourable for tick survival. Selecting and breeding cattle for resistance to tick infections is also sometimes practised.

Selected bibliography

Baker, A.S. (1999) *Mites and Ticks of Domestic Animals. An Identification Guide and Information Source.* The Stationery Office, London, 240 pp.

Camicas, J.-L., Hervy, J.-P., Adam, F. and Morel, P.-C. (1998) *The Ticks of the World (Acarida, Ixodida). Nomenclature, Described Stages, Hosts, Distribution.* Editions de l'ORSTOM, Paris, 233 pp.

Evans, G.O. (1992) *Principles of Acarology.* CAB International, Wallingford, UK, 563 pp.

Hoogstraal, H. (1981) Changing patterns of tick-borne diseases in modern society. *Annual Review of Entomology* 26, 75–99.

Maroli, M., Uilenberg, G. and Caracappa, S. (1999) Proceedings of the workshop on tick-borne diseases of livestock in the Mediterranean area. Palermo, 3–6 March 1999. *Parassitologia* 41 (suppl. 1), 1–118 (actual publication date 2000).

Oliver, J.H. (1989) Biology and systematics of ticks (Acari: Ixodoidea). *Annual Review of Ecology and Systematics* 20, 397–430.

Sonenshine, D.E. (1991) *Biology of Ticks.* Vol. 1. Oxford University Press, Oxford, 447 pp.

Sonenshine, D.E. (1993) *Biology of Ticks,* Vol. 2, Oxford University Press, Oxford, 465 pp.

Toxoplasma gondii *see* **Cockroaches.**

Trachoma *see* **Flies.**

Trench fever *see **Bartonella quintana*** **and *Bartonella henselae*.**

Triatomine bugs (Triatominae)

C.J. Schofield

There are 130 species of triatomine bugs in 17 genera, ranging from the tiny *Alberprosenia*, with adults just 5 mm long, to the giant *Dipetalogaster*, whose adults can reach 5 cm in length. They occur throughout the Americas, approximately from the Great Lakes of North America (about 42°N) to southern Argentina (about 46°S), where they are important vectors of *Trypanosoma cruzi* (see Chagas disease). Exceptions are the genus *Linshcosteus* of the Indian subcontinent and *Triatoma rubrofasciata*, which appears to have been exported from the Americas (probably on sailing-ships) and is recorded from port areas throughout the tropics and subtropics. Seven closely related species derived from *T. rubrofasciata* are recorded from various parts of South-East Asia, north-eastern Australia and southern China, although these species are generally rare and without epidemiological significance.

In the Americas, triatomine bugs have many local names, including kissing-bugs (USA), pitos (Colombia), chipos (Venezuela), chinchorros (Ecuador), chirimachas (Peru), barbeiros (Brazil), chichá guazu (Paraguay) and vinchuca (Southern Cone countries).

Biology

Eggs may be laid loose or attached to the substrate. They usually hatch within 10–25 days, and the first-instar nymph emerges. After feeding, the nymph moults to the next instar. There are five nymphal stages, followed by adult males and females (Fig. 1). The nymphal stages differ from the adults by being smaller and without wings or external genitalia, but adults and nymphs have similar habits and behaviour. Both sexes and all nymphal stages feed on vertebrate blood (although some sylvatic species may also feed from invertebrates). Their bites can cause severe allergic reactions, although those species that have adapted to living in human dwellings generally have almost imperceptible bites, which rarely provoke a reaction by the hosts.

Most species are active at night, feeding from sleeping hosts. The life cycle from egg to adult is typically about 6 months, although this can extend to 12 months in cool conditions (such as southern Argentina). Some species of *Rhodnius* can complete their life cycle in 3–4 months, but several of the larger species of *Triatoma* may require more than 12 months for their development. Females of most species are able to lay around 200 eggs during their adult life, although the number of eggs depends largely on the amount of blood ingested.

Most species of Triatominae are of sylvatic habit, generally associated with nests or refuges of certain birds and small mammals – especially opossums (*Didelphis* species), armadillos (*Dasypus* species) and small rodents. Species of *Rhodnius* are frequently found in palm-tree crowns, while species of *Triatoma* are more usually associated with terrestrial habitats. Several species have adapted to living in rural houses in Latin America, being found in the cracks and crevices of walls, roofs and floors, and frequently colonizing peridomestic habitats, such as chicken coops and goat corrals. Many sylvatic species seem to be adapting to domestic or peridomestic habitats; they may be brought to houses by being carried by small mammals, or adult bugs may fly to houses at night. Adaptation to domestic

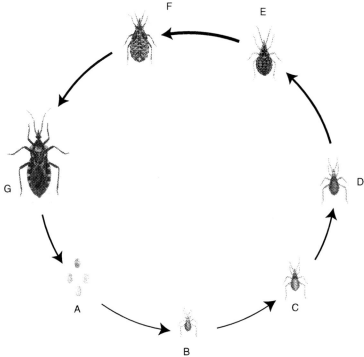

Fig. 1. *Panstrongylus megistus.* A, eggs; B–F, first to fifth nymphal stages; G, adult bug.

habitats seems to be a function of changing land use causing loss of the original sylvatic habitats of the bugs.

Diseases

All species of Triatominae are probably capable of transmitting *T. cruzi*, causative agent of Chagas disease (see entry). Important vectors are those that have adapted to living in human dwellings and can transmit *T. cruzi* to humans and domestic animals – especially *Triatoma infestans* in the Southern Cone countries, *Triatoma brasiliensis* and *Panstrongylus megistus* in northeastern Brazil and *Rhodnius prolixus* and *Triatoma dimidiata* in parts of the Andean Pact countries and Central America. *Triatoma pallidipennis* and other members of the *Triatoma phyllosoma* complex and *Triatoma barberi* are important vectors in Mexico. The domestic species of Triatominae are also important for the nuisance that they can cause, and for the chronic blood loss associated with their feeding. Adults of some species can take up to 300–400 mg of

blood at each feed and may feed every 4–9 days. Heavy domestic infestations numbering several thousand bugs are not uncommon in some rural areas of Latin America, and chronic blood loss due to these bugs is typically around 2 ml person^{-1} day^{-1} (sometimes considerably higher).

Species of *Rhodnius* are also vectors of *Trypanosoma rangeli* (see entry), although this parasite does not seem to be pathogenic to humans. Triatomine bugs can be infected with viruses, including those causing hepatitis, equine encephalitis and human immunodeficiency virus (HIV), but there is no evidence to suggest that they can transmit them.

Control

Domestic bugs are controlled by spraying infested premises with residual formulations of pyrethroid insecticides (mainly deltamethrin, cyfluthrin, lambdacyhalothrin or cypermethrin). A single application covering all internal wall and roof surfaces and furniture is usually sufficient to eliminate the domestic bug population. However, vigilance must be maintained to report any reinfestations so that these can also be sprayed. Reinfestation is generally due to bugs being carried in from untreated foci, for example, among the clothes or baggage of visitors.

Large-scale control programmes are currently in progress against the main domestic vectors of Chagas disease in the Southern Cone countries (Argentina, Bolivia, Brazil, Chile, Paraguay, Peru and Uruguay) and in the Andean Pact (Colombia, Venezuela and Ecuador) and Central American regions (Guatemala, El Salvador, Honduras and Nicaragua) (see Chagas disease).

Selected bibliography

Dujardin, J.P., Schofield, C.J. and Panzera, F. (2000) *Les Vecteurs de la Maladie de Chagas.*

Recherches Taxonomiques, Biologiques et Génétiques. Academie Royale des Sciences d'Outre Mer, Brussels, 162 pp.

Lent, H. and Wygodzinsky, P. (1979) Revision of the Triatominae (Hemiptera, Reduviidae), and their significance as vectors of Chagas disease. *Bulletin of the American Museum of Natural History* 163, 123–520.

Schofield, C.J. (1994) *Triatominae – Biology and Control.* Eurocommunica Publications, Bognor Regis, UK, 80 pp.

Schofield, C.J., Diotaiuti, L. and Dujardin, J.P. (1999) The process of domestication in Triatominae. *Memórias do Instituto Oswaldo Cruz* 94 (suppl. 1), 375–378.

Schofield, C.J. and Dolling, W.R. (1993) Bedbugs and kissing-bugs (bloodsucking Hemiptera). In: Lane, R.P. and Crosskey, R.W. (eds) *Medical Insects and Arachnids.* Chapman & Hall, London, pp. 483–516.

Trichomonas infections *see* Cockroaches.

Tropical theileriosis *see* Theilerioses.

Trubanaman virus

John S. Mackenzie

Trubanaman (TRU) virus is a mosquito-borne infection that is an unassigned member of the family Bunyaviridae. It is enzootic in Australia. It was first isolated from *Anopheles annulipes* mosquitoes trapped in Kowanyama (Mitchell River Mission) in 1965.

Distribution

Trubanaman virus has been isolated from mosquitoes collected in Queensland, New South Wales and Western Australia.

Virus

Trubanaman virus has been grouped with three other antigenically related viruses in the Mapputta antigenic group. This group comprises two other Australian viruses, Gan Gan virus (see entry) and Mapputta virus, and a virus from Papua New Guinea, Maprik virus.

Clinical symptoms

Trubanaman virus has not been associated with human disease, but seroepidemiological studies in New South Wales and Queensland have suggested that occasional subclinical human infections may occur.

Transmission

Trubanaman virus has been isolated from *A. annulipes* in Queensland, New South Wales and the south-west of Western Australia and from *Culex annulirostris* mosquitoes in northern Western Australia and New South Wales. The role of these mosquito species in transmission, however, remains to be elucidated.

Ecology

The vertebrate hosts of TRU virus are unknown, but believed to be terrestrial animals.

Selected bibliography

Newton, S.E., Short, N.J., Irving, A.M. and Dalgarno, L. (1983).The Mapputta group of arboviruses: ultrastructural and molecular studies which place the group in the Bunya-virus genus of the family *Bunyaviridae*. *Australian Journal of Experimental Biology and Medical Science* 61, 201–217.

Trypanosoma cruzi see **Chagas disease.**

Trypanosoma evansi (surra) *see* **Animal trypanosomiasis.**

Trypanosoma melophagium see **Animal trypanosomiasis.**

Trypanosoma rangeli

C.J. Schofield

Trypanosoma rangeli is an enigmatic try-panosome parasite related to *Trypanosoma cruzi* (see Chagas disease) which is also transmitted by triatomine bugs in some parts of South America (see Triatomine bugs). It is rarely (if ever) pathological to humans or other mammals, but can cause high mortality in some strains of the insect vectors. Interest in this parasite is mainly due to sympatry with *T. cruzi* and the need for differential diagnosis between the two.

Distribution
Confined to Latin America, from Mexico to Brazil. There are no confirmed reports of *T. rangeli* from Argentina, Chile, Paraguay or Uruguay. The natural distribution of *T. rangeli* closely matches that of species of *Rhodnius*, which are the main insect vectors, and reports of *T. rangeli* from coun-tries where *Rhodnius* species do not occur (such as Chile and Argentina) have been discounted.

Parasite
Trypanosoma rangeli is a large flagellated protozoan, typically up to 30 µm long, with a small subterminal kinetoplast. Although genetically related to *T. cruzi*, its biology is quite different. There is no conclusive evi-dence for a tissue phase in the vertebrate hosts, and it may be that the parasite only rarely multiplies in vertebrates – generally only during the first few days after entering the bloodstream. In the insect vectors, how-ever, the parasites frequently invade and multiply in the insect haemocoel and sali-vary glands.

Clinical symptoms
Although early observations suggested that *T. rangeli* could produce clinical symp-toms, it is now generally agreed that it is non-pathogenic to humans and other mammals. Infection in humans seems to be self-limiting, generally lasting only 2–3 weeks but sometimes persisting for up to 18 months. Parasitaemia is usually low and rarely reaches patent levels. Cases of tran-sient muscle ache and fatigue have been reported in some infections (but these may not necessarily be due to the parasite).

Diagnosis
Demonstration of bloodstream trypoma-stigotes in thin or thick blood smears, stained with Giemsa, has been widely used, although bloodstream parasites are gener-ally sparse. They can generally be distin-guished from *T. cruzi* by their larger size and smaller kinetoplast. Xenodiagnosis using laboratory-reared species of *Rhodnius* can also be used, examining the bug's haemolymph and/or salivary glands as well as its rectal contents. Some serological tests for *T. cruzi* may cross-react with

T. rangeli, although specific non-cross-reactive enzyme-linked immunosorbent assay (ELISA) tests have recently been developed. Polymerase chain reaction (PCR) of mini-exon gene and kinetoplast DNA targets has also been used for differential diagnosis.

Transmission

Bloodstream forms ingested by a triatomine bug transform and multiply in the mid-gut and rectum, with subsequent discharge of distinct flagellate forms in the bug's faeces. Unlike the case with *T. cruzi*, however, it is generally held that transmission of *T. rangeli* in the bug faeces is of minor importance. Some parasites may escape from the mid-gut into the haemocoel, where multiple division as well as binary fission may occur. In addition, some of the haemolymph parasites may enter and divide in haemocytes. Parasites in the haemolymph can migrate to form a layer around the salivary glands, with some penetrating the glands to be inoculated with the insect's saliva when it next feeds. This is the main route of transmission. A wide variety of mammalian species has been reported naturally infected with *T. rangeli*, including several primate species.

Although a wide variety of triatomine bugs can be experimentally infected with *T. rangeli* (as can some species of *Cimex* – bed bugs), natural infections have almost invariably been reported only from species of *Rhodnius*. The tribe Rhodniini (including *Rhodnius* and *Psammolestes*) are unusual in having salivary nitrophorins, which give a characteristic red colour to their salivary glands, and it has been observed that this red colour is depleted in bugs with heavy infections of *T. rangeli*. It may be that the parasite makes use of the nitrophorins, which could account for its relative specificity for *Rhodnius* species as vectors, as well as the high mortality often caused in infected *Rhodnius*.

Treatment

There is no evidence that specific treatment is required, since the infection is non-pathogenic and probably self-limiting.

Control

There is no case for control directed specifically against *T. rangeli*, although some of its insect vectors are targeted for control of Chagas disease.

Selected bibliography

D'Alessandro, A. and Saravia, N.G. (1992) *Trypanosoma rangeli*. In: Kreier, J.P. and Baker, J.R. (eds) *Parasitic Protozoa*, Vol. 2, 2nd edn. Academic Press, London, pp. 1–54.

Grisard, E.C., Campbell, D.A. and Romanha, A.J. (1999) Mini-exon gene sequence polymorphism among *Trypanosoma rangeli* isolated from distinct geographical regions. *Parasitology* 118, 375–382.

Grisard, E.C., Steindel, M., Guarneri, A.A., Eger-Mangrich, I., Campbell, D.A. and Romanha, A.J. (1999) Characterization of *Trypanosoma rangeli* strains isolated in Central and South America: an overview. *Memórias do Instituto Oswaldo Cruz* 94, 203–209.

Murthy, V.K., Dibbern, K.M. and Campbell, D.A. (1992) PCR amplification of mini-exon genes differentiates *Trypanosoma cruzi* from *Trypanosoma rangeli*. *Molecular Cell Probes* 6, 237–247.

Vallejo, G.A., Guhl, F., Chiari, E. and Macedo, A.M. (1998) Species-specific detection of *Trypanosoma cruzi* and *Trypanosoma rangeli* in vector and mammalian hosts by polymerase chain reaction amplification of kinetoplast minicircle DNA. *Acta Tropica* 72, 203–212.

Trypanosoma theileri see **Animal trypanosomiasis.**

Trypanosomiasis *see* **African trypanosomiasis, human, Animal trypanosomiasis, Chagas disease** *and* ***Trypanosoma* species.**

Tsetse-flies (Glossinidae)

M.W. Service

There are just 21 species of tsetse-flies, all belonging to the genus *Glossina*. Apart from two localities in the Arabian peninsula, tsetse-flies are found only in sub-Saharan Africa, between about 10°N and 20°S, but extending to 30°S on the coastal side of eastern Africa.

Biology

Tsetse-flies are unusual insects in that the female does not lay eggs. Instead an egg hatches within the fly and the resultant larva grows within her 'uterus'. After about 9 days the mature larva is deposited by the female on sandy soil or humus, often underneath bushes, trees or logs, but also in sandy, dried-up river-beds or in animal burrows. As soon as the larva is deposited, it buries itself under a few centimetres of soil and, within 15 min the whitish larva darkens to a reddish-brown and becomes a barrel-shaped puparium (Fig. 1). The puparium remains hidden under the soil for usually about 4–5 weeks before an adult tsetse-fly wriggles out and breaks through the surface of the soil.

Adults of both sexes take blood meals. Hosts range from humans to wild and domesticated mammals, including cattle, pigs and horses, and some species feed on reptiles and birds. Biting takes place out of doors and during the daytime. Tsetse-flies are attracted to dark colours and movements; on Caucasians, they often prefer to bite through dark clothing than exposed white skin. They often follow vehicles moving slowly through scrub vegetation, frequently settling on the dark tyres before finding a suitable host on which to feed. A blood meal is taken about every 2–3 days, and several are required for the complete development of a larva, one of which is deposited by the female about every 9–12 days. Breeding usually continues throughout the year, but largest populations occur at the end of the rainy season. When not host-seeking, adult flies rest on tree trunks or the undersurface of leaves or branches and twigs; at night they

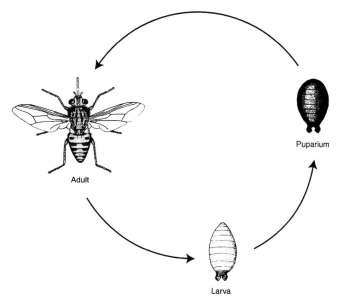

Adult

Puparium

Larva

Fig. 1. Life cycle of a tsetse-fly (*Glossina* species) (modified from M.W. Service (2000) *Medical Entomology for Students,* Cambridge University Press, Cambridge).

may prefer to rest on the upper surfaces of vegetation. Knowledge of the precise resting sites helps determine the type of vegetation needing to be sprayed with insecticides to kill the flies.

Based on their morphology, ecology and behaviour, tsetse-flies can be separated into three main groups of species. The *Glossina fusca* group, or forest flies, comprises 15 species, such as *G. fusca*. Flies in this group are restricted to equatorial forests. They contain a few species that transmit nagana (animal trypanosomiasis) to livestock, but no important vectors of sleeping sickness (human trypanosomiasis). The *Glossina morsitans* group, or savannah flies, contains about seven species and, as the name suggests are mainly found in thicket or scrub vegetation in semi-arid areas or in wooded vegetation at the edges of forests. This group contains important vectors of both sleeping sickness and nagana, such as *G. morsitans* and *Glossina pallidipes*. Finally, the *Glossina palpalis* group, or riverine and forest flies, contains about nine species. Essentially these flies inhabit wetter types of habitats, such as luxuriant scrub and vegetation growing along river-banks and lake shores, and sometimes forests. Important vectors of sleeping sickness and nagana include *G. palpalis* and *Glossina tachinoides*.

Diseases

Tsetse-flies are important in sub-Saharan Africa as vectors of the trypanosome parasites causing both human trypanosomiasis (sleeping sickness) and animal trypanosomiasis (nagana) (see African trypanosomiasis, human, and Animal trypanosomiasis).

Control

Because the immature stages are well protected by the soil, all control measures are directed against the adults. Most control involves using insecticides – for example, the use of strategically placed dark blue and/or black cloth screens (targets) impregnated with residual insecticides, such as the pyrethroids, to kill flies attracted to and resting on them. Visually attractive biconical or monoconical traps made of dark blue material are also used to attract and trap flies; sometimes they are treated with insecticide to kill flies settling on the traps, but probably not entering them (see Fig. 3, p. 22). Such screens and traps need only be retreated with insecticides every 3–4 months. Alternatively vegetation on which the tsetse-flies rest can be sprayed, either from the ground or from fixed-wing aircraft and helicopters, with insecticides such as endosulfan, permethrin, deltamethrin, lambdacyhalothin or cypermethrin. Spraying is often done in the dry season, so that residual deposits are not washed from vegetation by rainfall. Fortunately there are no recorded cases of tsetse flies developing insecticide resistance.

Selected bibliography

Buxton, P.A. (1955) *The Natural History of Tsetse-flies. An Account of the Biology of the Genus* Glossina *(Diptera)*. London School of Hygiene & Tropical Medicine Memoirs, 10, H.K. Lewis, London, 816 pp.

Dransfield, R.D., Williams, B.G. and Brightwell, R. (1991) Control of tsetse flies and trypanosomiasis: myth or reality? *Parasitology Today* 7, 287–291.

Jordan, A.M. (1986) *Trypanosomiasis Control and African Rural Development*. Longman, London, 357 pp.

Leak, S.G.A. (1999) *Tsetse Biology and Ecology: their Role in the Epidemiology and Control of Trypanosomiasis*. CAB International, Wallingford, UK, 568 pp.

Nash, T.A.M. (1969) *Africa's Bane. The Tsetse Fly*. Collins, London, 224 pp.

Tsutsugamushi disease *see* **Scrub typhus.**

Tularaemia

Karim E. Hechemy

Tularaemia is a zoonotic bacterial infection associated with both animals and humans and is transmitted by insect vectors, such as ixodid (hard) ticks and deer-flies (*Chrysops* species). It is caused by the bacterium *Francisella tularensis*. The genus *Francisella* was named for Edward Francis, who extensively studied the aetiological agent and its pathogenesis. The infection's name, tularemia (American spelling) or tularaemia (British spelling) is derived from Tulare County in South Central California. Tularaemia has been referred to in the popular literature as rabbit fever and deer-fly fever.

Two species of the genus *Francisella* are at present recognized, *Francisella tularensis*, with its three biogroups *tularensis*, *novicida* and *palaearctica*, and *Francisella philomiragia*. *Francisella philomiragia* was first isolated from a dying Muskrat (*Ondatra zibethica*). This bacterium appears to be associated with human disease, especially in immunocompromised patients with underlying diseases.

Distribution

Francisella tularensis is widely distributed in nature and occurs throughout the northern hemisphere. The two main regions of the world where tularaemia is most reported are the USA and southern regions of the former Soviet Union. In March 1999, it was reported in ProMed that 19–25 people in Serbia became ill with tularaemia, which had not been reported previously in humans in that country. It was also reported that the number of people exposed to the infection had risen to 1431. Such numbers indicate that, when conditions are favourable, tularaemia can arise in geographical areas in which it was not previously known to occur.

Bacterium

Francisella tularensis is a non-motile, non-piliated and non-spore-forming pleomorphic coccobacillus, 0.2 μm by 0.2–0.7 μm in size. It is Gram-negative; staining with polychrome stains, e.g. Giemsa's stain, reveals a bipolar structure. The bacterium has a capsule, composed largely of lipids, that has been associated with the virulence of this bacterium. The mole% G + C of DNA is 33–36. The cellular fatty acid composition of *Francisella* is unique to this genus and is different from other Gram-negative bacteria. It is characterized by the presence of long-chain saturated and monounsaturated C_{18} to C_{26} fatty acids; relatively large amounts of even-chain saturated fatty acids, C_{10}, C_{14} and C_{16}; and two long-chain C_{16} and C_{18} hydroxy-acids. The fatty acid content of its cell wall is higher than that of other Gram-negative bacteria. The bacterium is relatively stable in nature, is viable for weeks in water, mud and soil or animal carcasses and remains viable for years in frozen meat.

Culture

Because it is highly infectious, a minimum biosafety level 2 is recommended for clinical laboratory work with suspected material. The bacterium is an obligate aerobe and grows in culture over a temperature range of 24–39°C. The bacterium is killed after exposure for 10 min at 56°C, but freezing does not inactivate it. The medium of choice is cystine–glucose blood agar, chocolate agar enriched with iso-VitaleX and modified charcoal–yeast agar. It is a slow-growing organism that requires 2–4 days for optimum colony formation.

Clinical symptoms

Clinical presentation takes various forms, depending on the site of entry of the bacterium into the host. Regardless of portal of entry, the onset and general features of tularaemia tend to be the same. The usual incubation period is 3–5 days. There is an abrupt onset, with fever, chills, headache, cough, myalgias and vomiting. The initial symptoms usually disappear in 1–4 days, followed by remission for 1–3 days, and then recurrence of the disease for 2–3 weeks.

The clinical picture of tularaemia is: ulceroglandular, most common form, characterized by the formation of an ulcer and lymphadenopathy; glandular, with lymphadenopathy; oculoglandular, with conjunctivitis and lymphadenopathy; oropharyngeal, with ulceration in the oropharynx; systemic/typhoidal tularaemia, with septicaemia, no ulcer and no lympha-denopathy; intestinal tularaemia, with intestinal pain, vomiting and diarrhoea; and pneumonic tularaemia, contracted by inhalation of infected aerosol or by dissemination from blood. Death may occur in 35% of untreated cases of septicaemic tularaemia and 5% in untreated cases of ulceroglandular tularaemia. Death occurs as a result of septicaemia or a lower nephron syndrome, manifested by uraemia, oliguria and acidosis. Septicaemic tularaemia accounts for 10–15% of tularaemia infec-tion. It occurs after inhalation exposure of, for example, contaminated dust or ingestion of contaminated food. It is difficult to diagnose because the signs and symptoms are non-specific. The overall clinical manifestation is fever, prostration, weight loss, pharyngitis and pneumonia. A non-productive cough may occur. Evidence of pneumonia may be seen on radiographs. About half the patients with septicaemic tularaemia have pulmonary infiltrates, which may be misdiagnosed as legionel-losis. No adenopathy is observed in septicaemic tularaemia.

Ulceroglandular tularaemia accounts for most tularaemia cases, ~80%. It is acquired through inoculation of skin and mucous membrane or through the bites of infected ixodid ticks or deer-flies (*Chrysops* species). Adenopathy is common in ulcero-glandular tularaemia. The bacterium invades the regional lymphatics and produces a necrotizing inflammation and enlargement of lymph glands. These lesions are called buboes.

Pathology

This bacterium is extremely invasive. It is one of the very few microorganisms that can penetrate intact skin. The infective dose in humans can be as low as 50 bacteria. Due to the capsule, the bacterium avoids destruc-tion by polymorphonuclear neutrophils upon entry. *Francisella tularensis* is a facultative intracellular organism that survives in the reticuloendothelial system. Macrophages and epithelioid cells afford the bacterium more protection from the host immune system. After infection with *F. tularensis*, through cuts or arthropod bites, a lesion appears at the site and progressively ulcerates. Lymph nodes next to the sites of inoculation become enlarged and progress to necrosis. The early acute inflammatory response to infection induces the migration of neutrophils and macro-phages into clusters of degenerating and necrotic inflammatory cells. Later, these clusters are surrounded by lymphocytes and epithelioid cells. The bacteria, although concentrated in areas of necrosis and inflammation, are difficult to detect in tissue sections. Once the bacterium enters the bloodstream, the patient becomes sys-temically ill. Thrombosis and necrosis of veins and arteries are frequent and necrotic areas may resemble infarcts. In the lung there may be extensive necrosis and cavita-tion. Lasting lesions of pulmonary tularae-mia include areas of caseation, calcification and fibrosis. In the kidney, acute interstitial nephritis has been described.

Diagnosis, laboratory

Because it is highly infectious, a minimum biosafety level 2 is recommended for clinical laboratory work with suspected material. The specimens of choice are lymph node aspirate, sputum, throat swab, bronchial washing and biopsies from edge of the lesion, not the central necrotic area. If it is necessary to hold specimens for more than a few hours, specimens must be kept moist with sterile broth or saline and frozen. Frozen specimen must be shipped to the reference laboratory. All specimens are to be placed in approved UN 10 double-mailing containers and then packed in UNC1177 cartons labelled and shipped according to the International Airline Transport Association (IATA) regulations or the Centers for Disease Control and Prevention (CDC) Federal Regulation 42 CFR part 72. Inoculation of selective media is best done with aspirates, using a syringe or small pipette, of the suppurative material from a necrotizing lesion or a bubo. A presumptive identification can be made upon observation on the cysteine–blood–dextrose agar of 1–2 mm, clear, drop-like colonies, which are visible within 48–72 h after inoculation, with slight greening of the agar immediately beneath the colony due to alpha haemolysis of the blood, particularly after prolonged incubation. Confirmatory differential characteristics include the formation of acid but no gas from glucose, maltose and mannose.

Francisella tularensis is weakly catalase-positive and oxidase-negative. Also, *F. tularensis* grown on a culture medium enriched with cysteine in a flask will release H_2S, as indicated by the blackening of a moistened lead acetate filter-paper exposed to the atmosphere in the flask. Isolates of the bacterium should be further identified serologically by slide or tube agglutination, using an affinity-purified polyclonal antibody, or by direct fluorescent antibody, using a monoclonal antibody specific to *F. tularensis*. A fourfold increase in titre to ≥80 is indicative of active infection on paired or multiple serum specimens collected at time intervals of at least 1 week. A single titre by slide/tube agglutination of ≥160 is presumptive evidence of infection at an unknown time period. Titres ≤80 are indicative of past infection or of cross-reactivity due to the presence of cross-reacting antibodies.

Transmission and epidemiology

Wild animals, especially Rabbits (*Oryctolagus cuniculus*) and hares (*Lepus* species), but also beavers (*Castor* species), Woodchucks (*Marmota monax*), Opossums (*Didelphis marsupialis*), Mule deer[1] (*Odocoileus hemionus*) and foxes (*Vulpes* species) are the reservoir hosts of *F. tularensis*. Humans become infected by handling rabbit carcasses, eating undercooked infected wild rabbit meat or being bitten by ixodid ticks or tabanids, especially by *Chrysops* species, such as *C. discalis* in North America. In ticks the infection is long-lasting and the bacterium multiplies in the gut and haemolymph and is transmitted by biting. Transovarial transmission occurs. With other vectors, such as tabanids and mosquitoes, transmission is mechanical, not cyclical.

Infection also occurs through contamination of the skin, mucous membrane or lining of the eyes, nose or mouth with contaminated fluids from infected animals. Other methods of transmission include drinking contaminated water, breathing in dust particles or handling contaminated pelts of infected animals.

Treatment

Tularaemia is fatal, especially in the typhoidal form, if there is delayed treatment or inappropriate treatment. There is no standardized antimicrobial susceptibility test for *F. tularensis*. The aminoglycoside antibiotic streptomycin, when begun promptly, cures the patient with low probability of relapse. Dramatic improvement is seen within 3 days when 7.5 mg kg^{-1} body weight is given intramuscularly every 12 h for 10 days. Erythromycin, tetracycline, gentamycin and chloramphenicol are also effective; however, patients may relapse. Doxycycline has been used successfully intravenously in patients with renal impairment.

Prevention and control
Vector control

The golden rule for preventing infection is to minimize arthropod bites by wearing protective clothing and by using protective gloves when carefully handling carcasses. Use of insect repellents will also reduce the likelihood of being bitten by potential vectors.

Vaccines

An investigative, live, attenuated vaccine is available and appears to protect against exposure to aerosolized *F. tularensis*. A whole-cell killed vaccine was found to be ineffective against exposure to aerosolized bacterium. The live vaccine is recommended for persons working with the agent in a laboratory. Laboratory infections have been known to occur, due, for example, to aerosolized *F. tularensis*, which is highly infectious. The live vaccine is also recommended for persons working with infected animals or carcasses.

Tularaemia in farm and domesticated animals

Tularaemia is a highly contagious disease, which may spread from rodents to domestic animals, inducing a severe septicaemia and a high mortality rate. Infection in farm and domesticated animals can occur, especially in sheep, piglets and cats. Tularaemia is rarely seen in dogs. Domestic fowl can act as reservoir hosts of infection. There is a sharp seasonal incidence, with most cases occurring in the spring months. Transmission occurs mainly by the bites of the wood tick, *Dermacentor andersoni*, but other ixodid ticks, such as *Amblyomma americanum*, *Dermacentor variabilis* and *Haemaphysalis leporispalustris*, are also vectors. Ticks become infected in the early part of their life cycle when they feed on rodents; there is both trans-stadial and transovarial transmission.

After infection a bacteraemia develops, with localization and granuloma formation in parenchymatous organs and lymph nodes. The characteristic gross lesions seen in rabbits and other wild animals are small necrotic granulomatous foci in the spleen, liver and lymph nodes.

Note

1   Mule deer and Black-tailed deer are usually considered to be the same species.

Selected bibliography

Forbes, B.A., Sahm, D.F. and Weissfeld, A.S. (1998) *Francisella*. In: Bailey, W.R. and Scott, E.J. (eds) *Diagnostic Microbiology*, 10th edn. Mosby, St Louis, Missouri, pp. 590–592.

Franz, D.R. and Zajtchuk, R. (2000) Biological terrorism: understanding the threat, preparation and medical response. *Disease of the Month* 46, 129–190.

Geyer, S.J., Burkey, A. and Chandler, F.W. (1997) *Tularaemia*. In: Connor, D.H., Chandler, F.W., Schwartz, D.A., Manz, H.J. and Lack, E.E (eds) *Pathology of Infectious Diseases*, Vol. 1. Appleton & Lange, Stamford, Connecticut, pp. 869–873.

Quinn, P.J., Carter, M.E., Markey, B. and Carter, G.R (eds) (1994) *Francisella tularensis*. In: *Clinical Veterinary Microbiology*. Mosby, London, pp. 259–260.

Wong, J.D. and Shapiro, D.S. (1999) *Francisella*. In: Murray, P.R., Baron, E.J., Pfaller, M.A., Tenover, F.C. and Yolken, R.H (eds) *Manual of Clinical Microbiology*, 7th edn. American Society for Microbiology, Washington, DC, pp. 647–651.

Typhoid *see* Flies.

Typhus *see* Endemic typhus, Epidemic typhus, Rocky Mountain spotted fever, Scrub typhus *and* Tick-borne typhuses.

Valtice fever *see* **Tahyna virus.**

Venezuelan equine encephalitis

Scott C. Weaver

Venezuelan equine encephalitis is the most important New World alphaviral disease, affecting both humans and equines. Because equines remain important in Latin America for agriculture and transportation, Venezuelan equine encephalitis outbreaks have had profound social and economic effects, in addition to direct effects on human health. Several recent outbreaks in northern South America and Mexico underscore the continued threat of Venezuelan equine encephalitis.

Distribution and history

Equine epizootics consistent with Venezuelan equine encephalitis were first recognized in Venezuela during 1936, and Venezuelan equine encephalitis (VEE) virus was first isolated and characterized in 1938. However, retrospective examination of epidemiological data suggests that equine outbreaks consistent with Venezuelan equine encephalitis had occurred at least since the 1920s. Venezuelan equine encephalitis activity continued periodically and sporadically for much of the 20th century. Epizootics and epidemics occurred primarily in northern South America, with northern Colombia and Venezuela being the site of many major outbreaks (Fig. 1). The Guajira Peninsula has been subject to a disproportionate amount of disease, probably owing to its large population of feral donkeys, which serve as excellent amplification hosts and are difficult to control or vaccinate. Other major outbreaks have occurred in the Colombian valleys of the Andes mountains, as well as on the Pacific coasts of Ecuador and Peru. The most geographically widespread Venezuelan equine encephalitis outbreak on record began on the Pacific coast of El Salvador and Guatemala in 1969 and spread southward to Costa Rica in 1972 and northward to Texas, USA, in 1971. This outbreak may very well have been an extension of one that began in coastal Peru and Ecuador earlier in 1969.

Equine avirulent, enzootic viruses in the VEE antigenic complex occur throughout much of the tropical and subtropical New World, extending from Florida and Colorado in the USA to northern Argentina (Fig. 2). The distribution of these viruses is mostly non-overlapping, with the exception of certain regions in the Amazon basin, where multiple subtypes or varieties circulate. Typical enzootic habitats include primary lowland forest and swamp habitats. The distribution of enzootic viruses can change over time, as evidenced by the apparent introduction of a lineage of subtype ID virus into the Amazon basin of Peru between 1970 and 1994. This lineage of enzootic viruses had previously been isolated only in Panama.

VEE virus

Venezuelan equine encephalitis virus, as are other alphaviruses in the family Togaviridae, is an enveloped RNA virus, c. 70 nm in diameter, with a plus or messenger-sense RNA genome of c. 11,400 nucleotides (Fig. 3). The genome encodes four non-structural proteins (nsP1–4) and three structural proteins (capsid, E1 and E2 glycoproteins). A cytoplasmic, subgenomic 26S messenger RNA (mRNA), identical to the 3′ one-third of the genome, encodes only the structural proteins. Like other alphaviruses, VEE virus is believed to enter the cytoplasm of vertebrate cells via receptor-mediated endocytosis. The high-affinity laminin receptor serves as a mosquito cell receptor *in vitro*, although the mechanism of entry into mosquito cells *in vivo* has not been identified. The highly specific

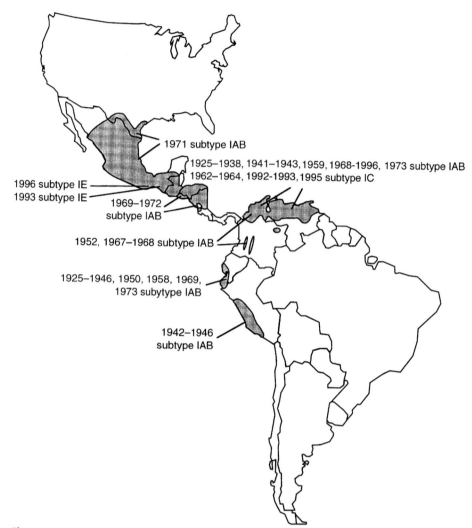

Fig. 1. Map of the Americas showing the locations, years and subtypes of major Venezuelan equine encephalitis epizootics and epidemics.

infectivity patterns of some VEE viruses for their mosquito vectors suggests the use of a less conserved protein receptor or the involvement of co-receptors during initial mid-gut infection.

Genomic VEE viral RNA is translated by cellular components to produce a non-structural polyprotein, and is the template for minus-strand RNA synthesis involving non-structural proteins. The 26S mRNA is also translated as a polyprotein; the capsid protein is cleaved in the cytoplasm and the remaining polyprotein is processed and cleaved in the secretory pathway to yield the E1 and E2 glycoproteins, which are inserted into the plasma membrane as a heterodimer. Following encapsidation of genomic RNA in the cytoplasm, enveloped virions mature when nucleocapsids bud through the plasma membrane. Venezuelan equine encephalitis virus replicates in and causes extensive cytopathic effects (CPE) in many different vertebrate cells *in vitro*. In contrast, infection of mosquito cells *in vitro* leads to persistent infection that is usually not accompanied by CPE. Alphavirus

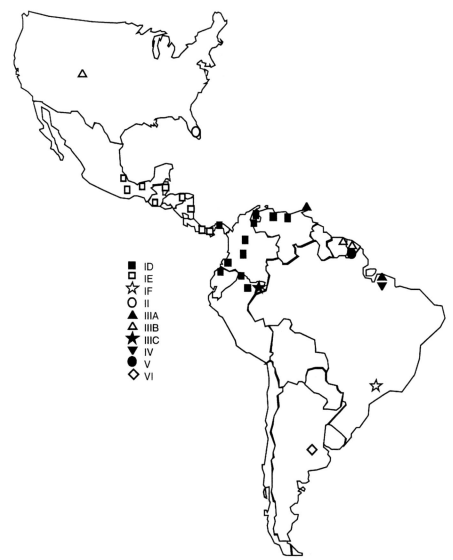

■	ID
□	IE
☆	IF
○	II
▲	IIIA
△	IIIB
★	IIIC
▼	IV
●	V
◇	VI

Fig. 2. Map of the Americas showing the distribution of the enzootic VEE complex viruses.

maturation in mosquito cell cultures occurs within cytoplasmic membrane-bound 'virus factories', which are extruded from the cell to release progeny virus. These 'virus factories' have not been observed in mosquitoes *in vivo*, where maturation occurs via plasma membrane budding.

Classification of VEE viruses

Venezuelan equine encephalitis virus is a member of the VEE antigenic complex, one of three major serogroups of New World alphaviruses (Table 1). The first systematic study of VEE-like viruses in the 1960s determined that all isolates from major outbreaks belong to specific serotypes, which were designated antigenic subtype I, varieties A, B and C. Recent serological tests and genetic analyses fail to distinguish varieties IA and IB, which are now grouped into variety IAB. The IAB and IC viruses are designated 'epidemic' or 'epizootic', because they have been isolated only during equine and human outbreaks; they are distinct from

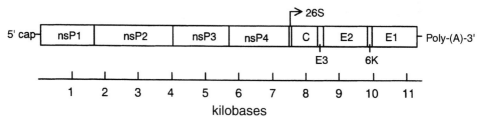

Fig. 3. Organization of the VEE virus genome.

enzootic strains (subtypes/varieties ID–F, II–VI), which circulate in sylvatic or swamp habitats and only occasionally cause overt disease in humans or domestic animals. Additional, serologically distinct, enzootic VEE viruses have been identified, which now comprise six subtypes and multiple varieties within subtypes I and III (Table 1). Transmission cycles have been described for five of the enzootic VEE subtypes/varieties (ID, IE, II, IIIA and IIIB (Bijou Bridge)); all except one are transmitted among rodents by *Culex* mosquitoes in the subgenus *Melanoconion*, the exception being Bijou Bridge, which is transmitted among birds in western North America by the cliff swallow bug, *Oeciacus vicarius* (family Cimicidae). Interestingly, all mosquito vectors are members of the *spissipes* section of the *Melanoconion* subgenus, suggesting the possibility of coevolution of VEE complex viruses with their vectors. However, phylogenetic studies (Fig. 4) of the viruses do not show concordant relationships with the known vectors, discounting this cospeciation hypothesis.

Clinical symptoms

In equines and humans, VEE viruses, in addition to causing inapparent infections, cause a spectrum of disease, ranging from fever to acute encephalitis. Most enzootic VEE strains in subtypes ID, IE, II, III and IV are avirulent for equines, producing little or no viraemia or illness. The lack of viraemia during equine infections results in their inability to exploit equines as amplification hosts and to cause extensive human outbreaks. However, at least some of the enzootic viruses can be pathogenic for humans, and have caused fatal disease when people become infected in enzootic

transmission foci. In contrast, epizootic IAB and IC viruses are virulent for both humans and equines. Equine mortality rates during epizootics have been estimated at 19–83%, while human fatalities occur infrequently, with neurological disease appearing in only 4–14% of cases. Venezuelan equine encephalitis occurs in all human age groups, with no preference between the sexes. However, children are more likely to develop neurological disease and fatal encephalitis than are adults.

The incubation period in humans is usually 2–3 days, although some cases have had an onset as few as 12 h after laboratory exposure. Human infection with either enzootic or epizootic VEE viruses is usually accompanied by an abrupt onset, with moderate fever, chills, severe headache and myalgia. Prostration and vomiting are also common, along with diarrhoea, inflammation of the throat and lymphadenitis. Neurological signs occur most often in children and the elderly, and typically include convulsions, dizziness, disorientation, drowsiness and mental depression. Motor weakness and paralysis, meningismus and cranial nerve palsy occur in 5–10% of hospitalized cases, with stupor and coma occurring at lower rates.

Laboratory findings of Venezuelan equine encephalitis include leucopenia, with early lymphopenia and a later decline in neutrophil counts. Pleocytosis in the cerebral spinal fluid is predominantly lymphocytic, and is sometimes accompanied by elevated glucose. Mortality rates during epizootic outbreaks are generally about 0.2–1.7%, with a case fatality rate of 10–25% among encephalitis cases.

Teratogenic effects have also been attributed to maternal infection with VEE

Table 1.   VEE antigenic complex viruses.

Subtype	Variety	Transmission pattern	Equine virulence	Location	Vertebrate amplification/reservoir host	Vector
I	AB	Epizootic	Yes	C., S., N. America	Equines	Mammalophagic mosquitoes
	C	Epizootic	Yes	S. America	Equines	Mammalophagic mosquitoes
	D	Enzootic	No	C., S., America	*Sigmodon, Proechimys* species	*Culex (Melanoconion) ocossa, Culex (Melanoconion) panocossa*
	E	Enzootic	No	C. America, Mexico	*Sigmodon, Proechimys* species	*Culex (Melanoconion) taeniopus*
	F	Enzootic	Unknown	Brazil	Unknown	Unknown
II		Enzootic	No	Southern Florida	*Sigmodon, Peromyscus* species	*Culex (Melanoconion) cedecei*
III	A	Enzootic	No	S. America	*Oryzomys, Heteromys, Proechimys, Zyodontomys* species	*Culex (Melanoconion) portesi*
	B	Enzootic	Unknown	S., N. America	Birds	Swallow bug (*Oeciacus vicarius*)
	C	Enzootic	Unknown	Peru	*Proechimys* species	Unknown
IV		Enzootic	Unknown	Brazil	Unknown	Unknown
V		Enzootic	Unknown	French Guiana	Unknown	Unknown
VI		Enzootic	Unknown	Argentina	Unknown	Unknown

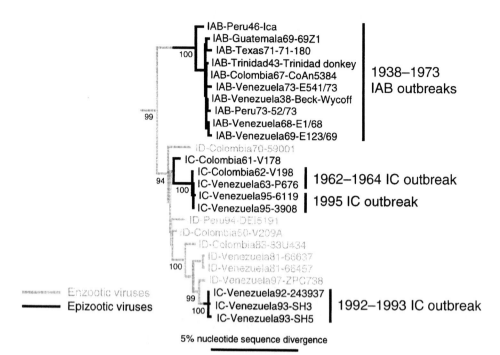

Fig. 4. Phylogenetic tree, generated using maximum parsimony and E2 envelope glycoprotein gene nucleotide sequences, showing the evolution of the epizootic subtypes IAB and IC VEE viruses from enzootic, subtype ID progenitors. Virus strains are listed by subtype, country of isolation and strain name. Grey branches represent the enzootic phenotype and black branches represent epizootic, based on minimizing phenotypic change in the tree. Numbers indicate bootstrap value for monophyletic groups to the right, and the scale shows genetic distance.

virus, and the virus has been recovered from stillborn foetuses during outbreaks. Among survivors of encephalitis, neurological sequelae often include recurrent seizures, motor impairment, forgetfulness, nervousness, asthenia and headache. Behavioural disorders are seen in some children.

Diagnosis

Clinical diagnosis of Venezuelan equine encephalitis is unreliable for two reasons: (i) human signs and symptoms of Venezuelan equine encephalitis are often indistinguishable from those of other viral diseases common in the tropics and subtropics, such as dengue (see entry). In fact, some recent Venezuelan equine encephalitis outbreaks were initially characterized as dengue, due to its prevalence in the affected regions; and (ii) equine disease caused by VEE virus can also be confused with encephalitis caused

by other viruses, such as eastern equine encephalitis (see entry), which have an overlapping distribution in the New World, or even with toxicological diseases. The absence of a rash is somewhat useful in ruling out dengue and Mayaro fevers (see entries). Definitive diagnosis of human infection generally relies on virus isolation from the serum or by pharygeal swabs, most easily accomplished during the first 3 days of illness. Detection of VEE virus-specific immunoglobulin M (IgM) antibodies or demonstration of seroconversion is also diagnostic. Detection of viral RNA has also been described, using reverse transcription–polymerase chain reaction (RT-PCR)-based approaches. Virus isolation can be accomplished using a variety of cell cultures or by inoculation of newborn mice. Virus isolation from equines is more problematic, because mortality rates sometimes exceed

50% and viraemia has often waned by the time signs of encephalitis first appear. At this time and soon after death, VEE virus can sometimes be isolated from the equine brain and occasionally from other tissues, such as spleen and blood. A highly specific and sensitive IgM capture enzyme-linked immunosorbent-assay (ELISA) is available for detecting early antibodies in human or equine serum and has proved useful in recent outbreaks. Seroconversion is generally demonstrated by detecting a fourfold or greater rise in IgG antibody titres between acute and convalescent serum samples. Plaque reduction neutralization is commonly used for IgG detection, because it is highly specific, although ELISA may also be used provided that antigens to related alphaviruses, such as eastern equine encephalitis (EEE) virus, are included in the assay. Identification of VEE virus antigenic subtypes can be accomplished, using an indirect immunofluorescence assay with a battery of specific and cross-reactive monoclonal antibodies. Subtyping of isolates is critical in determining the potential for a widespread epidemic, as the IAB and IC subtypes are the only ones known to be capable of amplification in equids.

Transmission

Enzootic transmission

Transmission cycles have been characterized for five of the enzootic VEE complex serotypes. These viruses generally circulate almost continuously in discrete, wet tropical forest or shaded swamp habitats. Transmission can be remarkably focal, varying dramatically within distances of only metres. Rodents in the genera *Sigmodon*, *Oryzomys*, *Zygodontomys*, *Heteromys*, *Peromyscus* and *Proechimys* are believed to be the principal vertebrate amplifying hosts of enzootic VEE viruses, because they are frequently infected in nature, have high rates of antibody and develop high-titre viraemia after experimental infection. Other mammals, such as Opossums (*Didelphis marsupialis*) and other marsupials, are also frequently involved, and bats and shore birds may be involved in dispersal of enzootic viruses.

Natural hosts usually show little adverse effect from enzootic VEE virus infection. Human infections occur sporadically when people enter enzootic transmission foci, but outbreaks involving hundreds of people have also been described. Enzootic mosquito vectors have been identified for four enzootic VEE serotypes: (i) *Culex* (*Melanoconion*) *portesi* transmits Mucambo virus (VEE subtype IIIA) in Trinidad; (ii) *Culex* (*Melanoconion*) *cedecei* transmits Everglades virus (VEE subtype II) in southern Florida; (iii) *Culex* (*Melanoconion*) *ocossa* and *Culex* (*Melanoconion*) *panocossa* transmit variety ID VEE viruses in Panama (formerly the name *Culex aikenii* was given as the vector, but this is a *nomen nudum*); and (iv) *Culex* (*Melanoconion*) *taeniopus* is the primary enzootic vector of variety IE viruses in Guatemala. Over 70% of enzootic VEE virus field isolations have come from the subgenus *Melanoconion*, suggesting that these mosquitoes are the principal vectors of most or all enzootic strains.

Epizootic/epidemic transmission

Epizootic/epidemic transmission relies on equines as the principal amplification hosts. Horses, donkeys and mules produce high-titre viraemias following infection, allowing mosquitoes that engorge to become infected and transmit after an extrinsic incubation of about 1 week or possibly less. A wide variety of mammalophagic mosquitoes in the genera *Aedes*, *Ochlerotatus*,[1] *Mansonia*, *Psorophora* and *Deinocerites* are believed to transmit epidemic/epizootic viruses during epizootics. Enzootic vectors (see above) have not been implicated in epizootic/epidemic transmission. Only *Psorophora confinnis* and *Ochlerotatus taeniorhynchus* are confirmed vectors of epizootic viruses according to established criteria, including experimental susceptibility to oral infection and appropriate host contacts. Because infected equines develop high-titre viraemias of up to 10^8 infectious units ml^{-1} serum and are extremely attractive to many mosquito species, many different species of mosquitoes, some only marginally susceptible, can probably become infected by biting equines.

Mosquito vectorial capacity probably depends more on mosquito abundance, longevity and host preferences than on intrinsic differences in susceptibility.

Mechanical transmission (infection via contaminated vector mouthparts, without viral replication) by black-flies (Simuliidae) has been implicated in at least one outbreak, and the chicken mite, *Dermanyssus gallinae*, is also capable of mechanical transmission. Experimental studies have also shown that larvae of *Amblyomma cajennense* ticks can be infected orally and transmit trans-stadially to nymphs, which can transmit horizontally to a vertebrate. The significance of these findings with regard to natural VEE virus transmission is unknown. The swallow bug, *O. vicarius*, is a vector of Bijou Bridge subtype among birds (see p. 541).

During extrinsic incubation, VEE virus replicates in the mid-gut of mosquitoes, disseminates via the haemolymph and replicates in the salivary glands. Transmission occurs during salivation accompanying a subsequent blood meal from a naïve host. Epidemic/epizootic Venezuelan equine encephalitis usually occurs following heavy rainfall and the production of large numbers of floodwater or salt-marsh mosquitoes, which serve as vectors. A large supply of susceptible equines is also a prerequisite for major outbreaks, and people who live in agricultural areas appear to be tangentially infected. Infected people develop viraemia titres similar to those of equines and can potentially serve as amplification hosts in the absence of equines. However, epidemiological data indicate that humans play a lesser role in amplification, probably due to their more limited attraction and exposure to mosquito vectors. *Aedes aegypti* can transmit VEE virus from naturally infected people to experimental animals, suggesting the possibility of urban transmission.

Direct human-to-human transmission without vector involvement has long been suspected during Venezuelan equine encephalitis epidemics, because the virus can be isolated from pharyngeal swabs of many infected people. However, household studies and rates of infection in health-care workers have failed to provide evidence for this mode of transmission.

Venezuelan equine encephalitis outbreaks spread rapidly, often in an irregular wave-like manner over large distances. This might be explained by the movement of infected equines or humans from epizootic locations into, as yet, disease-free regions or by the great dispersal potential of some epizootic vector mosquitoes. Flying 'transport hosts', such as birds or bats, are another possibility.

Because Venezuelan equine encephalitis epizootics have historically been interrupted by many years without any evidence of the circulation of the IAB and IC viruses, their source remained an enigma for much of the 20th century. Recent genetic studies indicate that the epizootic IAB and IC serotypes have evolved recently from enzootic subtype ID viruses, which circulate in northern South America. At least three different genotypes of these epizootic viruses have emerged from one particular enzootic ID lineage, which is known to circulate in western Venezuela, central and eastern Colombia and northern Peru (Fig. 3). The IAB viruses probably arose early in the 20th century and caused all known outbreaks until 1962. Several outbreaks during the 1960s to 1973 were probably caused by the use of inadequately inactivated equine vaccine preparations made from early, virulent IAB isolates in several countries. These vaccines were eventually replaced by the live, attenuated TC-83 vaccine, which is still used for equine vaccination. The other epizootic subtype, IC, emerged in 1962 and caused a major outbreak in northern Colombia and Venezuela. This same genotype of IC virus re-emerged in 1995 to cause a major epizootic and epidemic in the same locations of Colombia and Venezuela. However, a small 1992–1993 epizootic and epidemic in western Venezuela was caused by a different genotype of IC viruses, which apparently emerged very recently via mutation of sympatric, enzootic ID viruses. Some of these ID strains from the Catatumbo region of western Venezuela differ from the 1992–1993 IC epizootic/epidemic isolates by only 12 amino acids in the entire deduced sequence of the viral proteins. Because these enzootic strains are avirulent for equines, as are other enzootic strains, and produce little or no viraemia, the 1992 emergence has provided a useful model system for determining the mutations that can generate epizootic strains from enzootic progenitors. Preliminary results indicate that mutations in the E2 envelope protein are at least partly responsible for the equine viraemia phenotype and epizootic emergence.

Treatment

Like that of most arboviral infections, treatment of Venezuelan equine encephalitis is largely supportive and palliative in nature, typically relying on analgesics and bedrest. Anticonvulsive therapy is important in reducing morbidity and mortality. Secondary pneumonia should be treated aggressively, and antibacterial treatment should be considered because lymphoid depletion may predispose patients to gastrointestinal infections. Experimental work with mice has shown that the immunomodulators, ridotin and reaferon, can decrease mortality when administered soon after infection. Melatonin also reduces the death rate and evolution of the disease in mice. Prophylactic administration of ribamydil (an analogue of ribavirin) has also been shown to reduce disease manifestation in baboons.

Control

Control of Venezuelan equine encephalitis relies largely on vaccination of equines and control of mosquito vector populations.

Vaccines

Early VEE virus isolates were used to produce formalin-inactivated vaccines in several South American countries, as well as the USA. However, because virulent IAB viruses were used for these vaccines, incomplete inactivation may have initiated some outbreaks; sequencing studies support this hypothesis. Beginning in the 1960s, a live, attenuated vaccine, TC-83, was used to vaccinate equines, and also people at risk from laboratory exposure. The TC-83 vaccine has proved safe and effective for equines, although its efficacy in humans is limited; the vaccine is reactogenic in 23% of vaccinees and 18% do not seroconvert. A formalin-inactivated version, C-84, induces neutralizing antibodies in 76% of persons who do not respond to TC-83, but does not protect well against aerosol challenge. Another concern related to vaccination is that protection against heterologous VEE subtypes may be lower than against IAB strains. A newer live, attenuated vaccine with attenuating mutations, generated by the genetic engineering of an infectious complementary DNA (cDNA) clone, is now under testing and appears to be superior to TC-83. Because it induces mucosal immunity, VEE virus is also being used as a vaccine vector to express other viral proteins.

Continuous vaccination of equines in neotropical regions subject to frequent Venezuelan equine encephalitis outbreaks could probably eliminate the occurrence of outbreaks. However, vaccination is often reduced or discontinued when epizootic activity has not occurred for several years, resulting in the re-establishment of susceptible equine amplification populations. This temporal pattern repeated itself many times during the 20th century, resulting in periodic outbreaks.

During epizootics, control is difficult and often ineffective. Vaccination efforts usually begin several weeks after equine and/or human cases are documented, when the outbreak may already be widespread. The ability of epizootics to bypass some geographical regions and sequentially affect locations over 100 km apart makes effective vaccination barriers difficult to establish. Owners of equines in affected regions often attempt to transport their animals to unaffected regions, undoubtedly contributing to dissemination when some transported animals are at an early stage of infection preceding signs of disease.

Vector control

Control of mosquito vector populations is difficult because of the large geographical regions affected and the large mosquito populations usually present. However, aerial ultra-low-volume (ULV) adulticiding in the early mornings with insecticides such as malathion may help interrupt epidemics. Such spraying during the 1971 Texas outbreak may have reduced the spread of the virus.

As with many arthropod-borne diseases, personal protection against mosquito bites is often the most effective means of disease prevention. This is especially important for individuals who reside or work near equine herds during epizootics, or those who contact tropical forest or swamp habitats where enzootic VEE viruses circulate continuously. *N*,*N*-diethyl-*m*-toluamide (DEET) (≤35% formulations recommended, ≤10% for children) is the most effective mosquito repellent generally approved for use on the skin. Pyrethroid insecticides, such as permethrin, or insect repellents can be applied to clothing and camping gear to enhance protection.

Note
[1] *Ochlerotatus* was formerly in the subgenus *Aedes*.

Selected bibliography
Johnson, K.M. and Martin, D.H. (1974). Venezuelan equine encephalitis. *Advances in Veterinary Science and Comparative Medicine* 18, 79–116.

Johnston, R.E. and Peters, C.J. (1996) Alphaviruses. In: Fields, B.N., Knipe, D.M. and Howley, P.M. (eds) *Virology*, Vol. 1, 3rd edn. Lippincott-Raven, New York, pp. 843–898.

Oberste, M.S., Fraire, M., Navarro, R., Zepeda, C., Zarate, M.L., Ludwig, G.V., Kondig, J.F., Weaver, S.C., Smith, J.F. and Rico-Hesse, R. (1998) Association of Venezuelan equine encephalitis virus subtype IE with two equine epizootics in Mexico. *American Journal of Tropical Medicine and Hygiene* 59, 100–107.

Rivas, F., Diaz, L.A., Cardenas, V.M., Daza, E., Bruzon, L., Alcala, A., De la Hoz, O., Caceres, F.M., Aristizabal, G., Martinez, J.W., Revelo, D., De la Hoz, F., Boshell, J., Camacho, T., Calderon, L., Olano, V.A., Villarreal, L.I., Roselli, D., Alvarez, G., Ludwig, G. and Tsai, T. (1997) Epidemic Venezuelan equine encephalitis in La Guajira, Colombia, 1995. *Journal of Infectious Diseases* 175, 828–832.

Tsai, T.F. and Monath, T.P. (1997) Alphaviruses. In: Richman, D.D., Whitley, R.J. and Hayden, F.G. (eds) *Clinical Virology*. Churchill Livingstone, New York, pp. 1217–1255.

Walton, T.E. and Grayson, M.A. (1988). Venezuelan equine encephalomyelitis. In: Monath, T.P. (ed.) *The Arboviruses: Epidemiology and Ecology*, Vol. IV. CRC Press, Boca Raton, Florida, pp. 203–231.

Wang, E., Barrera, R., Boshell, J., Ferro, C., Freier, J.E., Navarro, J.C., Salas, R., Vasquez, C. and Weaver, S.C. (1999). Genetic and phenotypic changes accompanying the emergence of epizootic subtype IC Venezuelan equine encephalitis viruses from an enzootic subtype ID progenitor. *Journal of Virology* 73, 4266–4271.

Watts, D.M., Callahan, J., Rossi, C., Oberste, M.S., Roehrig, J.T., Wooster, M.T., Smith, J.F., Cropp, C.B., Gentrau, E.M., Karabatsos, N., Gubler, D. and Hayes, C.G. (1998) Venezuelan equine encephalitis febrile cases among humans in the Peruvian Amazon River region. *American Journal of Tropical Medicine and Hygiene* 58, 35–40.

Weaver, S.C. (1998) Recurrent emergence of Venezuelan equine encephalomyelitis. In: Scheld, W.M. and Hughes, J. (eds) *Emerging Infections I*. ASM Press, Washington, DC, pp. 27–42.

Weaver, S.C., Salas, R., Rico-Hesse, R., Ludwig, G.V., Oberste, M.S., Boshell, J. and Tesh, R.B. (1996) Re-emergence of epidemic Venezuelan equine encephalomyelitis in South America. *The Lancet* 348, 436–440.

Vesicular stomatitis

James A. Comer

Vesicular stomatitis is a viral disease caused by vesicular stomatitis (VS) virus that primarily affects domestic livestock, although humans and many species of wildlife may also be infected. Vesicular stomatitis takes its name from the vesicles (blisters) that are formed at any of various locations during the acute phase of the disease. Vesicular stomatitis is a zoonosis; veterinarians, dairymen, others who handle animals with clinical disease and people who are exposed to arthropod vectors are all at risk for infection. Laboratory infections, primarily due to inhalation of aerosols, are well documented.

The first recognized outbreak of vesicular stomatitis occurred in the USA in 1916 among cavalry horses in the Denver, Colorado, stockyards. The Indiana (VSI) and the New Jersey (VSNJ) serotypes are the most widely distributed and important causes of disease. They were first isolated in 1925 and 1926, respectively.

Distribution

Vesicular stomatitis is known only in the western hemisphere. Vesicular stomatitis in animals occurs in both enzootic and epizootic forms. The VSNJ and VSI viruses are enzootic in eastern Mexico, Venezuela, Colombia, Panama and Costa Rica, mostly in lowland tropical areas. In the USA, a band of enzootic VSNJ virus formerly affected animals in the coastal plains of South Carolina, Georgia and Florida in the 1950s, but only one well-documented focus of vesicular stomatitis remains in this region; VSNJ virus is enzootic on Ossabaw Island, Georgia.

In more temperate areas, vesicular stomatitis occurs as epizootics. Large-scale epizootics of vesicular stomatitis have been reported from Argentina to Canada and have occurred numerous times in the USA. As a general rule, outbreaks tend to occur with decreasing frequency and increasing magnitude as latitude increases in both North and South America. These outbreaks have been spectacular in appearance. In the USA, major epizootics of VSI virus were recorded in 1942, 1956, 1964 and 1965; VSNJ virus epizootics were observed in 1944, 1949, 1957, 1959, 1963, 1982–1983, 1985 and 1995. Most outbreaks have occurred in western states; both serotypes were identified there in 1997. Subclinical infections with these viruses also occur during epizootics. An enzootic cycle in the western USA has been suggested, based on the presence of antibodies in wildlife during periods when no outbreaks were occurring, but such a cycle has never been demonstrated.

Two outbreaks of vesicular stomatitis may have occurred in the Old World, but

their aetiology was never confirmed and vesicular stomatitis did not persist in either locale. One of these was apparently introduced into France by transport of infected army horses during the First World War (1914–1918). An earlier report of a disease resembling vesicular stomatitis in South Africa in the late 1800s was not supported by a history of recent importation of livestock from enzootic or epizootic areas, and moreover the aetiology was never determined.

Aetiological agents

Vesicular stomatitis is caused by any of four RNA viruses in the family Rhabdoviridae, genus *Vesiculovirus*. The viruses are sensitive to ether and other organic solvents and are not stable in the environment outside living hosts. They are inactivated at 58°C for 30 min but survive for years at ultralow temperatures (−70°C).

In addition to VSI and VSNJ viruses, two additional serotypes, VS Alagoas and Cocal, occur only in South America. Antigenically, VSI, VS Alagoas and Cocal viruses are closely related; the original Indiana isolate is sometimes referred to as Indiana subtype 1, and Cocal is sometimes referred to as Indiana subtype 2 and Alagoas as Indiana subtype 3. They are distinct viruses, however, and, although their natural cycles are incompletely known, they are likely to be substantively different and involve different vector species. Cocal virus has been associated with vesicular disease in horses in Argentina, whereas VS Alagoas virus has been associated with vesicular disease in horses, mules and plantation workers in Brazil. Seven other members of the genus *Vesiculovirus* have not yet been associated with vesicular disease.

Clinical symptoms

As a zoonosis, vesicular stomatitis has an undefined health impact. Vesicular stomatitis in humans results from contamination of mucous membranes or abrasions in the skin, from inhalation of aerosols or from the bite of an infected vector. Disease in humans presents as an acute, self-limiting, influenza-like illness, characterized by fever, headache, myalgia and malaise. Vesiculation can occur but normally does not. Natural human infections are common in rural areas throughout much of tropical America. Serosurveys indicate that prevalence of infection increases with age, and as many as 90% of the inhabitants in certain areas have neutralizing antibodies to VS viruses. Because symptoms are non-specific and the duration of the illness is short and because most infections tend to occur in tropical areas with decreased access to health care, most human cases are mild and go unrecognized.

Vesicular stomatitis is of great economic importance in veterinary regulatory medicine, because it is clinically indistinguishable from foot-and-mouth disease in cattle, sheep, goats, other ruminants and pigs. Vesicular stomatitis complicates eradication programmes in areas where foot-and-mouth disease occurs. Horses are susceptible to vesicular stomatitis but are resistant to foot-and-mouth disease. In addition, vesicular stomatitis lesions in pigs are clinically indistinguishable from lesions of vesicular exanthema and pig vesicular disease.

Vesicular stomatitis is a disease of high morbidity but low mortality. Following infection, vesicles are formed in the oral cavity, on the muzzle and snout, on the udder, around the coronary band and in interdigital areas. Lesions in the oral cavity result in decreased feed consumption and loss of weight. Milk production is decreased dramatically, which may result in early weaning and calves of low weight. Fever is of short duration and thus usually not detected in horses and cattle. Viraemia is low-level and ephemeral. As vesicles rupture, excessive salivation (drooling) is a common sign, and cattle make a characteristic smacking sound.

Economic losses associated with vesicular stomatitis in dairy cattle can occur because of bacterial mastitis secondary to infected teat lesions. Lameness can develop in horses and swine. Complete recovery normally occurs in about 2 weeks in uncomplicated cases. Lesions of the oral cavity can take as long as a month to heal; lesions on the hooves and teats take longer to heal if they become secondarily infected. Immunity to the infecting serotype is incompletely protective, and reinfection with the same serotype can occur. Infection with one serotype confers no protection against infection with other serotypes.

Diagnosis

As detected by serosurveys, enzootic areas are characterized by predominantly subclinical infection in domestic livestock, wildlife and humans. Characteristic but non-pathognomonic lesions occur in cattle and pigs, for which a diagnosis of foot-and-mouth disease must be excluded.

Virus is readily isolated from throat swabs, vesicle fluid, or the epithelium of vesicles by inoculation of VERO, BHK-21, chick fibroblast or pig kidney cell cultures. Vesicular fluid especially contains large concentrations of virus. Virus can also be isolated in suckling or weanling mice and in embryonated chicken eggs.

The complement fixation test, confirmed by virus isolation in tissue culture, is the current method of diagnosis. The serum dilution plaque-reduction neutralization test and the indirect immunofluorescence antibody test, with paired acute- and convalescent-phase serum samples demonstrating a fourfold increase in titre, are also used for serological diagnosis.

An immunoglobulin M (IgM) capture enzyme-linked immunosorbent assay (ELISA) has been developed to detect recent infections with these viruses. Polymerase chain reaction (PCR) assays of clinical material have been developed and offer sensitive and rapid diagnosis. These assays will probably be used increasingly in the future.

Transmission

Both VSI and VSNJ viruses have been isolated from a wide variety of biting and non-biting insects, including house-flies (*Musca* species), face-flies (*Musca autumnalis*), eye-gnats or eye-flies (*Hippelates* species), mosquitoes (e.g. *Aedes*, *Culex*, *Mansonia* species), ceratopogonid midges (*Culicoides* species), simuliid black-flies (*Simulium* species) and phlebotomine sand-flies (*Lutzomyia* species). In only a few instances has viral load been quantified, and few transmission studies have been done. Despite intensive studies, vertebrate amplifying hosts (those that have sufficient viraemia to infect subsequently feeding vectors) have never been identified. How vectors become infected in nature in sufficient quantities to initiate and maintain epizootics is not yet known.

In the USA, major outbreaks have the following features: (i) they tend to occur at sporadic intervals; (ii) they begin in late spring or early summer; (iii) clinical cases occur along natural drainages, but can spread rapidly to distant areas and yet exclude large populations of susceptible animals; and (iv) outbreaks cease with the onset of frosts. These characteristics are suggestive of arthropod transmission.

The origin of epizootics is not understood. It is not known whether silent enzootic foci exist (foci that occasionally cause outbreaks) or whether these viruses are periodically reintroduced into areas from which they have been absent for long periods. Serological evidence of infection of these viruses in wildlife in the USA and Panama suggests that there are separate, sylvatic maintenance cycles for each virus. Wind-borne carriage of infected biting flies or movement of infected cattle northward from Mexico has been postulated as a means whereby the viruses gain entry into areas in the USA. Molecular studies reveal that the strains of virus circulating in Mexico are similar to the strains isolated in western states, supporting the view that viruses causing these outbreaks originate in Mexico.

Field and laboratory investigations have shown that phlebotomine sand-flies of the genus *Lutzomyia* may serve as reservoir hosts, as well as vectors, for VSI virus in Panama, VSNJ virus on Ossabaw Island, Georgia, and VS Alagoas virus in Colombia. Sand-flies have been shown to transmit these viruses transovarially in the laboratory. Isolates of VSNJ virus of high titre have been made from wild-caught male sand-flies, which has been interpreted as evidence of transovarial transmission, because males do not feed on vertebrate blood. Together, these observations suggest

that sand-flies may be reservoir hosts of the viruses and may serve as vectors.

A high titre of VSNJ virus has been isolated from pools of *Simulium* species (black-flies) collected in Colorado in 1982, suggesting that black-flies may also be involved as biological vectors. Recent experimental studies with black-flies indicated that uninfected black-flies could become infected by co-feeding beside an infected black-fly on a non-viraemic mouse. Infection by co-feeding is more likely to be involved with epizootic spread of these viruses, rather than with their enzootic maintenance.

Other forms of transmission of VS viruses are likely to be important under certain conditions. A large number of isolations of VSNJ virus from muscoid flies (*Musca autumnalis*, *Musca domestica*) in Colorado in 1982 suggests that mechanical transmission by non-biting flies may occur. Virus-laden flies may be transported from infected to uninfected premises in the interiors of vehicles. Contact transmission from infected to uninfected vertebrates has been demonstrated experimentally, but the importance of this type of spread under natural conditions has not been determined. Vesicular stomatitis viruses can be spread by fomites, especially among dairy cattle, where outbreaks have been associated with the transfer of virus through the use of contaminated milking machines or milkers' hands.

The epizootiology of VS viruses has been difficult to elucidate, because of the inability to identify viraemic vertebrate hosts and because transovarial transmission alone does not seem to be sufficient to maintain infection in vector populations. The recognition that infection of arthropods may occur by co-feeding is recent. This mechanism of infection obviates the need for a viraemic vertebrate host; however, this possibility has not been evaluated fully in the laboratory and not at all in the field. There has been speculation that VS viruses are plant viruses, but no convincing evidence has been presented to support this hypothesis. Another hypothesis suggests that VS viruses are stabilized in their insect vectors (100% efficiency in transovarial transmission) and thus the insects represent the only reservoir. If this were the case, vertebrates would merely represent dead-end hosts for the viruses; most epidemiological studies support this view. Clearly, much additional fieldwork will be required to effectively understand how the viruses are maintained in enzootic conditions, how viruses from enzootic areas spread to initiate epizootics and how epizootics are maintained.

Treatment

No specific treatment is available for vesicular stomatitis. Infections are usually self-limiting and generally mild, and most affected animals recover fully within 2 weeks. Lost weight is regained following recovery. Soft feeds make it easier for affected animals to eat. Mastitis can be treated with antibiotics.

Control

Because enzootic and epizootic maintenance cycles are not well understood, there is no practical, effective control for vesicular stomatitis. Experimental inactivated and attenuated vaccines have been tried with variable success, but are not commercially available. In enzootic areas, protection of humans and livestock from arthropod vectors is usually not possible. In epizootic areas, interest in the disease wanes because the interepizootic intervals are often long and outbreaks are unpredictable. Because of contact transmission between infected and uninfected animals, restrictions in animal movements is helpful in limiting spread, although it leads to economic hardship. Workers who have to handle infected animals should wear protective gloves and clothing. Disinfection of fomites and decontamination of vehicles help minimize spread. A 1% solution of formalin is an effective disinfectant. Avoiding the production of aerosols is important in preventing laboratory infections.

Selected bibliography

Comer, J.A., Kavanaugh, D.M., Stallknecht, D.E. and Corn, J.L. (1994) Population dynamics of *Lutzomyia shannoni* (Diptera: Psychodidae) in relation to the epizootiology of vesicular stomatitis on Ossabaw Island, Georgia. *Journal of Medical Entomology* 29, 178–182.

Cupp, E.W., Mare, J., Cupp, M.S. and Ramberg, F.B. (1992) Biological transmission of vesicular stomatitis virus (New Jersey) by *Simulium vittatum* (Diptera: Simuliidae). *Journal of Medical Entomology* 29, 137–140.

Hanson, R.P. (1952) The natural history of vesicular stomatitis. *Bacteriological Review* 16, 179–204.

Johnson, K.M., Vogel, J.E. and Peralta, P.H. (1966) Clinical and serological response to laboratory-acquired human infection by Indiana type vesicular stomatitis virus. *American Journal of Tropical Medicine and Hygiene* 15, 244–246.

Mead, D.G., Ramberg, F.B., Besselsen, D.G. and Mare, J.C. (2000) Transmission of vesicular stomatitis virus from infected to noninfected black flies co-feeding on nonviremic deer mice. *Science* 287, 485–487.

Rodriguez, L.L., Bunch, T.A., Fraire, M. and Llewellyn, Z.N. (2000) Re-emergence of vesicular stomatitis in the western United States is associated with distinct viral genetic lineages. *Virology* 271, 171–181.

Stallknecht, D.E., Fletcher, W.O., Erickson, G.A. and Nettles, V.F. (1985) Enzootic vesicular stomatitis New Jersey type in an insular feral swine population. *American Journal of Epidemiology* 122, 876–883.

Tesh, R.B., Peralta, P.H. and Johnson, K.M. (1969) Studies of vesicular stomatitis. 1. Prevalence of infection among animals and humans living in an area of endemic V.S.V. activity. *American Journal of Epidemiology* 90, 255–261.

Tesh, R.B., Chaniotis, B.N. and Johnson, K.M. (1971) Vesicular stomatitis virus (Indiana serotype): multiplication in and transmission by experimentally infected phlebotomine sand flies (*Lutzomyia trapidoi*). *American Journal of Epidemiology* 93, 491–495.

Tesh, R.B., Chaniotis, B.N. and Johnson, K.M. (1972) Vesicular stomatitis virus, Indiana serotype: transovarial transmission by phlebotomine sand flies. *Science* 175, 1477–1479.

Tesh, R.B., Boshell, J., Modi, G.B., Morales, A., Young, D.G., Corredor, A., Carrasquilla, C.F., Rodriguez, C., Walters, L.L. and Gaitan, M.O. (1987) Natural infection of humans, animals, and phlebotomine sand flies with the Alagoas serotype of vesicular stomatitis virus in Colombia. *American Journal of Tropical Medicine and Hygiene* 36, 653–661.

Vibrios

C.A. Hart

The genus *Vibrio* is one member of the family *Vibrionaceae*, which also includes the genera *Photobacterium*, *Aeromonas* and *Plesiomonas*. *Vibrio cholerae* is the aetiological agent of cholera. It is a Gram-negative, curved or straight rod (0.5 μm × 3 μm) that is motile by means of a polar flagellum. It is part of the autochthonous flora of brackish water and is able to persist and grow in a variety of aquatic environments in association with aquatic plants, zooplankton and blue-green algae. There have been eight pandemics of cholera. The first seven have been due to *V. cholerae* O1 serotype (biotypes classical and El Tor). The most recent pandemic is due to the newly emerged *V. cholerae* O139 serotype. It causes acute, frequently fatal, secretory diarrhoea mediated by three enterotoxins. Infection is predominantly spread by faeco-oral transmission person to person or via food and water. However, house-flies and other Muscidae can be mechanical vectors (see Flies).

Selected bibliography

Drasar, B. (1997) Vibrios. In: Emmerson, M.A., Hawkey, P.M. and Gillespie, S.H. (eds) *Principles and Practice of Clinical Bacteriology*. John Wiley & Sons, Chichester, UK, 449–466.
Shears, P. (1994) Cholera. *Annals of Tropical Medicine and Parasitology* 88, 109–122.

Viruses

C.A. Hart

Viruses are obligate intracellular pathogens, ranging in size from 20 to 350 nm. They are classified by the composition and organization of their genomes, the symmetry of their nucleocapsid, the presence of a lipid envelope and size; they are further subdivided by biological properties and antigenic make-up. Viruses have genomes of either RNA or DNA. The genomes can be single- or double-stranded and looped or linear, and the linear genome can be one long chain or present as a number of segments. For viruses with single-stranded RNA genomes, their sense can be positive (i.e. directly translated to produce protein) or negative (must be transcribed to messenger RNA (mRNA) before serving as a template for protein production). Viral nucleocapsid can be helical (one plane of symmetry) or cuboidal (usually an icosahedron, 20 facets with three planes of symmetry). Some viruses have a lipid envelope (derived from the host cell membrane for flaviviruses, togaviruses and bunyaviruses, but from the nuclear membrane for herpesviruses), while others are unenveloped (e.g. reoviruses, enteroviruses, parvoviruses and papillomaviruses).

These characteristics serve to place viruses into families, subfamilies and genera. Individual viruses within a family are usually defined by biological characteristics, antigenic structure or genome sequence. Arthropod-borne viruses, or arboviruses (see entry), do not comprise a taxon but are a collection of viruses belonging to many families, all of which are maintained by biological transmission between haematophagous arthropods and vertebrates, including humans and livestock.

Selected bibiography

Fields, B.N., Knipe, D.M. and Howley, P.M. (eds) (1996) *Fields Virology*, Vol. 1, pp. 1–1504, Vol. 2, pp. 1505–2950, 3rd edn. Lippincott, Philadelphia.
Murphy, F.A., Fauquet, C.M., Bishop, D.H.L., Ghabrial, S.A., Jarvis, A.W., Martelli, G.P., Mayo, M.A. and Summers, M.D. (eds) (1995) Sixth report of the International Committee

on Taxonomy of Viruses. *Archives of Virology* Suppl. 10, 1–586.

Murphy, F.A., Gibbs, E.P.J., Horzinek, M.C. and Studdert, M.J. (1999) *Veterinary Virology*, 3rd edn. Academic Press, San Diego, California, 629 pp.

Porterfield, J.S. (ed.) (1989) *Andrewes' Viruses of Vertebrates*. Baillière-Tindall, London, 457 pp.

Richman, D.D., Whitley, R.J. and Hayden, F.G. (eds) (1997) *Clinical Virology*. Churchill Livingstone, Edinburgh, 1355 pp.

Webster, R.G. and Granoff, A. (eds) (1998) *Encyclopedia of Virology*. Academic Press, London, 1997 pp.

White, D.O. and Fenner, F.J. (1994) *Medical Virology*, 4th edn. Academic Press, London, 603 pp.

Weak back *see* **Setariosis.**

Wesselsbron virus

Jack Woodall

Wesselsbron (WSL) virus causes an infection of humans and other mammals.

Wesselsbron virus disease, human
Distribution

Sub-Saharan Africa, Madagascar and Thailand. The virus has been isolated in the Republic of South Africa, Zimbabwe, Senegal, Nigeria, Kenya, Guinea, Cameroon, the Central African Republic, Botswana and Madagascar. Antibody evidence suggests it may also be present in Angola, Mozambique, Namibia and possibly Ethiopia. It is prevalent in lowland, humid areas where there are many mosquitoes. The virus has also been isolated from mosquitoes in Thailand, and a subtype, Sepik virus (see entry), has been isolated in Australia and Papua New Guinea.

Virus

Isolated from the liver of an 8-day-old Merino lamb in the Republic of South Africa in March 1955, during an outbreak of abortion in ewes and mortality in lambs. It is an enveloped RNA virus, diameter 45 nm, in the genus *Flavivirus*, family Flaviviridae, and related to yellow fever (see entry) but distinct from it and from more than 60 other known flaviviruses.

Clinical symptoms

The high prevalence of neutralizing antibodies in endemic areas suggests that the infection is usually mild or subclinical. After an incubation period of 2–4 days, there is biphasic fever for 2–3 days, headache, eye pain, body pains, anorexia, insomnia, hepatomegaly, splenomegaly, disturbances in speech, hearing and vision and a rise in serum transaminases. Occasionally, there is cutaneous hyperaesthesia and a mild rash. Myalgia may persist. Infections in laboratory and field workers have occurred; masks and other precautions against aerosol infection should be taken when performing animal autopsies or laboratory tests.

Diagnosis

By virus isolation in newborn mice or a variety of tissue cultures (PS, VERO, LLC-MK2, MA-104, PS-C1, BHK-21), from acute blood, serum or throat washings. The virus cross-reacts widely in the haemagglutination inhibition (HI) test with other flaviviruses common in Africa; therefore serosurveys using only HI are not definitive. Nevertheless, one recent (1997) report comparing tests claimed that in sheep sera the specificity of the HI test was 100% versus only 95.7% for the indirect enzyme-linked immunosorbent assay (ELISA), compared with sensitivities of 87.5% and 97.9%, respectively.

Transmission

The virus has been isolated from many species of mosquitoes. These include *Aedes mcintoshi/luridus* and *Ochlerotatus*[1] *juppi/caballus* in South Africa, *Aedes circumluteolus* in Madagascar, *Aedes lineatopennis* in Zimbabwe, *Aedes dentatus* in Kenya, *Aedes dalzieli* in Senegal, *Aedes tarsalis* and five other species in Cameroon, and *Aedes abnormalis* and two other species in the Central African Republic. Laboratory transmission has been obtained with *O. juppi/caballus*, *A. circumluteolus* and *Culex zombaensis*. In Thailand the virus was isolated from *Aedes mediolineatus* and *Aedes lineatopennis*, and in Papua New Guinea the Sepik strain was isolated from *Mansonia septempunctata*, *Ficalbia flavens* and other *Ficalbia* and also *Armigeres* species. The virus has been isolated from an African rodent and produces viraemia in birds (see below under Wesselsbron disease in wildlife), so those may be the natural hosts.

Treatment

Symptomatic. There are no reports of the effects of antivirals on this disease.

Control

There is no vaccine for human use. Given the wide variety of mosquito vectors and virus circulation in livestock, no control measures seem practicable.

Wesselsbron virus disease, animal

A mosquito-borne disease causing abortions and death in livestock, with possibly a rodent and/or avian reservoir host.

For information on distribution, viral morphology, diagnosis and transmission, see under human infections of Wesselsbron.

Bovine Wesselsbron disease

Of 15 pregnant cows inoculated during gestation with the wild-type WSL virus there was a brief rise in temperature reaction in some, but no other clinical symptoms were recorded. Abortion occurred in three animals. A viraemia was not always present in these cows and, when detected, was of low magnitude and short duration. One cow, in which the fetus was inoculated at 115 days of gestation, aborted at 231 days. The fetus showed marked porencephaly and cerebellar hypoplasia.

Caprine Wesselsbron disease

In red Sokoto goats experimentally infected with the Nigerian strain of WSL virus, viraemia commenced 24–72 h after infection and lasted for 3–4 days. A mainly biphasic febrile reaction accompanied viraemia, and the mortality rate was 50%. The virus was isolated from liver, spleen, lungs, brain, kidney, adrenal glands, lymph node and heart tissues. Complement-fixing (CF) antigens were detected in the tissues of dead goats, the titre of which correlated positively with the infectivity titre. All infected animals developed CF and HI antibodies to WSL virus. However, neutralizing antibody was detected only in goats that survived the infection.

In experimentally infected West African dwarf goats, viraemia was detected 2 days after infection and lasted for 1 day. All the animals died; the virus was isolated from almost every tissue in mice. In addition, the infected goats developed CF and HI antibodies to WSL virus.

Ovine Wesselsbron disease

In early March 1996, WSL virus caused mortality among lambs on a farm near Bultfontein in the northern Free State Province, South Africa. Among a sample of 44 sheep bled on 4–5 September, 59% were antibody-positive by the HI test against WSL virus. In South Africa, autopsy of 13 lambs revealed mild to severe icterus and a slight to moderate hepatomegaly, with discoloration of the liver. Except for petechial and ecchymotic haemorrhages in the mucosa of the abomasum and generalized lymphadenopathy, no obvious macroscopic lesions were seen. There was mild to extensive necrosis of the liver parenchyma, with degenerated and necrotic hepatocytes diffusely scattered throughout. Mitotic figures and hepatocytes with large nuclei indicated that active regeneration of parenchymal cells had occurred in some of the livers. Kupffer cell proliferation, sinusoidal leucostasis, bile-duct proliferation and infiltration of mononuclear cells in the portal triads were frequently encountered. Moderate to severe cholestasis was a feature in 66% of the livers examined, while intranuclear inclusions and intracytoplasmic acidophilic or Councilman-like bodies were frequently observed.

In laboratory experiments, WSL viraemia in lambs commenced approximately 27 h after infection and lasted on the average for 50 h. A febrile reaction, which was mostly biphasic, commenced several hours after the viraemia and continued for another 50 h. The viraemia in adult animals began about 50 h after infection and lasted for 30 h. The fever usually commenced several hours after the viraemia and, in three cases out of four, it outlasted the viraemia by at least 30 h. The virus was isolated in mice from every tissue examined, but pathological lesions are restricted to the liver and lymphatic tissues.

During the 1974–1975 lambing season numerous reports were received from various parts of South Africa and South West Africa (now Namibia) of severe abdominal distension in ewes after vaccination with attenuated Wesselsbron disease vaccine. The ewes were vaccinated at different stages of gestation, in spite of recommendations to the contrary, the syndrome being especially obvious in ewes immunized during the first trimester of pregnancy. In some of the flocks, *Hydrops amnii* was recorded in as many as 15% of the ewes. Many of the ewes so affected showed a prolonged gestation of up to 6–7 months and, towards the end of gestation, were unable to rise or walk. They eventually died of ketosis, hypostatic pneumonia and complications due to dystocia. The fetuses examined were malformed and larger than normal. They usually showed arthrogryposis, brachygnathy inferior, hydranencephaly, hypoplasia or segmental aplasia of the spinal cord and neurogenic muscular atrophy. No definite conclusions as to the aetiology of the syndrome could be drawn from serological tests performed on the ewes, lambs or fetuses. Preliminary experimental work confirmed previous observations that the attenuated Wesselsbron disease vaccine virus is responsible for this syndrome and that the wild-type virus is also implicated.

Wesselsbron disease in other domestic animals

Isolations have been reported from a camel in Nigeria and from a fatal case in a dog in South Africa. Experimental inoculation of pigs produces fever without any other symptoms. In the late 1980s, 62 horse sera collected from two stables at Lagos, Nigeria, were tested for CF antibody to eight arbovirus antigens, including the flaviviruses yellow fever, Wesselsbron, West Nile and Uganda S. Ten per cent of the sera contained CF antibody to one or more of those antigens; reactions with the flavivirus antigens were the commonest, and the highest antibody titres were for WSL and yellow fever viruses. Since yellow fever virus was not circulating in Lagos at that time,

it is likely that the antibodies indicated infection with WSL virus.

Wesselsbron disease in wildlife

The virus was isolated from Ostriches (*Struthio camelus*) and the Cape short-eared or Namaqua gerbil (*Desmodillus auricularis*) in South Africa, and this rodent species has produced a viraemia lasting 1 week in the laboratory, indicating that it could infect mosquitoes. In a survey of South African wild animals, antibodies against WSL virus were present in 16 species, including zebras (*Equus* species), but no disease was associated with these. Antibodies have been found in lemurs (Lemuridae) in Madagascar and in several species of wild birds; experimentally infected birds have shown viraemia.

Treatment of animal Wesselsbron disease

There is no specific treatment.

Control of animal Wesselsbron disease

There are no specific control measures other than vaccination. The attenuated, live virus vaccine should be given 3 weeks before breeding to avoid the problems listed under Ovine Wesselsbron disease above. Lambs can acquire maternal antibody through the colostrum, but should be vaccinated after 6 months of age.

Note

[1] *Ochlerotatus* was formerly a subgenus of *Aedes*.

Selected bibliography

Baba, S.S., Fagbami, A.H., Ojeh, C.K., Olaleye, O.D. and Omilabu, S.A. (1995) Wesselsbron virus antibody in domestic animals in Nigeria: retrospective and prospective studies. *New Microbiology* 18, 151–162.

Barnard, B.J. (1997) Antibodies against some viruses of domestic animals in southern African wild animals. *Onderstepoort Journal of Veterinary Research* 64, 95–110.

Blackburn, N.K. and Swanepoel, R. (1980) An investigation of flavivirus infections of cattle in Zimbabwe Rhodesia with particular reference to Wesselsbron virus. *Journal of Hygiene* 85, 1–33.

Brès, P. (1965) Infection humaine à virus Wesselsbron par contamination au laboratoire. *Bulletin de la Société de Pathologie exotique* 58, 994–999.

Coetzer, J.A.W. and Barnard, B.J. (1977) *Hydrops amnii* in sheep associated with hydranencephaly and arthrogryposis with Wesselsbron disease and Rift Valley fever viruses as aetiological agents. *Onderstepoort Journal of Veterinary Research* 44, 119–126.

Coetzer, J.A.W. and Theodoridis, A. (1982) Clinical and pathological studies in adult sheep and goats experimentally infected with Wesselsbron disease virus. *Onderstepoort Journal of Veterinary Research* 49, 19–22.

Coetzer, J.A.W., Theodoridis, A., Herr, S. and Kritzinger, L. (1979) Wesselsbron disease: a cause of congenital porencephaly and cerebellar hypoplasia in calves. *Onderstepoort Journal of Veterinary Research* 46, 165–169.

Jupp, P.G. and Kemp, A. (1998) Studies on an outbreak of Wesselsbron virus in the Free State Province, South Africa. *Journal of the American Mosquito Control Association* 14, 40–45.

Justines, G.A. and Shope, R.E. (1969) Wesselsbron virus infection in a laboratory worker, with virus recovery from a throat washing. *Health Laboratory Science* 6, 46–49.

Morvan, J., Fontenille, D., Digoutte, J.P. and Coulanges, P. (1990) Le virus Wesselsbron, un novel arbovirus pour Madagascar. *Archives d'Institut Pasteur Madagascar* 57, 183–192.

Mushi, E.Z., Binta, M.G. and Raborokgwe, M. (1998) Wesselsbron disease virus associated with abortions in goats in Botswana. *Journal of Veterinary Diagnostic Investigation* 10, 191.

Theiler, M. and Downs, W.G. (1973) *The Arthropod-borne Viruses of Vertebrates.* Yale University Press, New Haven, Connecticut, 578 pp.

Western equine encephalitis

William K. Reisen

Neurological complications resulting from an infection of humans, equines and other vertebrates with western equine encephalitis (WEE) virus, an arbovirus in the family Togaviridae.

Distribution

Western equine encephalitis virus was isolated originally in 1930 from Merced County, California, from the brain of an encephalitic horse collected during a large equine epizootic in the Central Valley of California. Human involvement was documented for the first time in 1938, when WEE virus was isolated from the brain of a fatal human case in Bakersfield, California. Western equine encephalitis virus was subsequently discovered to be one of the contributing aetiological agents responsible for the large number of polioencephalitis cases diagnosed during summer in western North America.

Historically, WEE virus was thought to be distributed throughout the western hemisphere, from the Arctic Circle to Argentina and from the Pacific to the Atlantic coasts. However, this virus now is recognized as a complex of at least six closely related viruses, with WEE virus found in North America west of the Mississippi River and in Central and South America, wherever detailed investigations have been conducted. Western equine encephalitis virus isolates previously reported from mosquitoes and birds in eastern North America have now been shown to be the closely related Highlands J virus, whereas some infections in western birds (especially swallows; Hirundinidae) may have been due to infection with Fort Morgan virus. Other viruses in this complex include Sindbis (see entry), which is distributed widely throughout Europe, Africa and Asia, and Aura from South America.

Virus

Western equine encephalitis virus is classified in the genus *Alphavirus* of the family Togaviridae. Recent sequence studies indicate that WEE virus may be a genetic construct of eastern equine encephalitis (EEE) (see entry) and Sindbis viruses. The genome consists of a single-stranded, plus-sense RNA containing over 11,000 nucleotides, which serve as a messenger RNA for the translation of three or four non-structural polypeptides. A subgenomic message identical in sequence to the 3' one-third of the viral genome codes for the three structural proteins, C, E1 and E2. Virus particles are typically spherical (60–65 nm in diameter) and contain a 35–39 nm capsid, surrounded by a lipo-protein envelope with 6–10 nm surface projections.

Clinical symptoms

Humans

The onset of illness is rapid and follows a 7–10-day incubation period. Clinical presentation is vague, ranging from inapparent to flu-like to meningitis, encephalitis and, occasionally, death. Because cases occur infrequently in time and space and present with varying symptoms, this disease is probably underdiagnosed and under-reported. Despite the dramatic increase in the human population in the western USA in the past few decades, the number of clinical western equine encephalitis cases reported to the US Centers for Disease Control have decreased progressively and few are currently reported annually (Fig. 1). Cases typically appear in summer and disappear in the autumn, in conjunction with the onset of diapause in the primary

mosquito vector, *Culex tarsalis*. The ratio of apparent to inapparent infection varies widely, depending upon strain virulence and endemicity, but is in the order of 1 : 100 to 1 : 500. The severity of illness appears to decrease with age, with >50% of the reported cases in patients <10 years of age. About 30% of infants <1 year of age develop debilitating neurological sequelae and require institutional care due to seizure disorders, spastic paresis and mental retardation. In older patients, recovery is the rule, with case fatality rates ranging from 3 to 4%. The economic burden of encephalitis case management is great and has been estimated to be >US$3 million per case for eastern equine encephalitis.

Equines

Onset of illness in horses and mules occurs 1–3 weeks post-infection. Symptoms parallel other neurological equine disease and include fever, restlessness, irritability and ataxia. Other symptoms include head drooping and pressing, blindness, excessive salivation, involuntary movements and paralysis. During the terminal stages, animals frequently lie on their side, are unable to stand and exhibit 'paddling' movements. Case fatality rates have historically ranged from 10 to 50%; however, comparably severe disease has been difficult to reproduce experimentally in horses, ponies and burros (i.e. donkeys). Early epizootics in

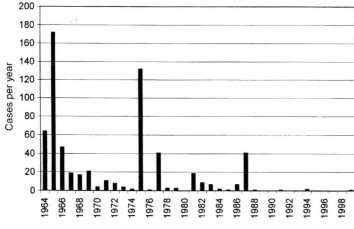

G.L. Cambell, CDC, unpublished data

Fig. 1. Number of human cases of western equine encephalitis in the USA detected by passive case detection.

the Central Valley of California reportedly decimated the equine population, having a severe impact on agricultural production and the economics of rural communities.

Other vertebrates

Other domestic animals show little illness. Experimentally infected pigs developed a mild viraemia, but did not show clinical symptoms. Inoculated cattle failed to show symptoms and did not produce a viraemia, but developed detectable antibody. Poultry frequently are infected and show antibody, but illness seems minimal, especially in mature birds. Adult Leghorn chickens (>22 weeks of age) do not develop a detectable viraemia following experimental infection. However, neurological illness has been reported in turkeys and mortality in Ring-necked pheasants (*Phasianus colchicus*), Chukar partridges (*Alectoris chukar*) and Emus (*Dromaius novaehollandiae*). White-crowned sparrows (*Zonotrichia leuco-phrys*), Golden-crowned sparrows (*Zono-trichia atricapilla*) and, to a lesser extent, Tricolored blackbirds (*Agelaius tricolor*) and Red-winged blackbirds (*Agelaius pho-eniceus*) frequently succumb to experimental infection. Mortality has been reported in sentinel Pigeons (*Columba livia*), but could not be repeated experimentally.

Diagnosis

Clinical symptoms are vague and diagnosis must be based on sound virology or serology. Virus isolation from human or equine clinical material is rare, because samples typically are taken late in the course of infection. Western equine encephalitis virus can be isolated readily from infected mosquitoes and vertebrates during the acute phase of infection, which in wild birds occurs 1–2 days post-infection. Western equine encephalitis virus is lethal for suckling or weanling mice inoculated intra-cranially and newly hatched chickens, both of which are useful in isolation attempts. Western equine encephalitis virus also grows readily on monkey, hamster or por-cine kidney cell cultures and produces large plaques and other cytopathic effects within 3–4 days after inoculation. Virus also grows

well in insect cell lines, such as C6/36 from *Aedes albopictus*. Reverse transcription–polymerase chain reaction (RT-PCR) and genetic sequencing provide a useful alterna-tive or adjunct to isolation in diagnosis, especially for clinical or autopsy samples.

Clinical diagnosis is most frequently confirmed by serology and is either pre-sumptive, based on the demonstration of elevated immunoglobulin M (IgM) antibody titre in cerebrospinal or serum samples, or confirmed, based on a > fourfold rise in IgG titre between acute and convalescent (4–6 weeks post-infection) serum samples. Serological diagnosis in horses is usually confounded, because equines in endemic areas are vaccinated annually against WEE and EEE viruses. Serology using enzyme immunoassays (EIA) or complement fixa-tion (CF) tests may also be confounded when more than one alphavirus is circulating con-currently in an area. An immunofluorescent antibody test using monoclonal antibodies or end-point cross-neutralization assays are useful for confirmation of positive screening assay results.

Transmission

In western North America, WEE virus is maintained and amplified during summer in an enzootic cycle involving wild bird reservoir hosts and the primary mosquito vector, *C. tarsalis* (Fig. 2). During spring and early summer *C. tarsalis* females feed most frequently on perching birds, especially House finches (*Carpodacus mexicanus*) and House sparrows (*Passer domesticus*). However, as summer progresses, *C. tarsalis* expands its host range to include progres-sively more bird species, including chick-ens, as well as mammals, including rodents, rabbits, horses and humans. Avian host competence varies markedly, with species such as chickens and quail (*Callipepla* species) producing low-titre viraemias as adults, columbiforms producing a moderate but varied response and passeriforms pro-ducing elevated viraemias, which some-times result in fatal infections. Most imma-ture birds produce an elevated viraemia and may be important in virus amplification. Mammals, such as rodents, equines and

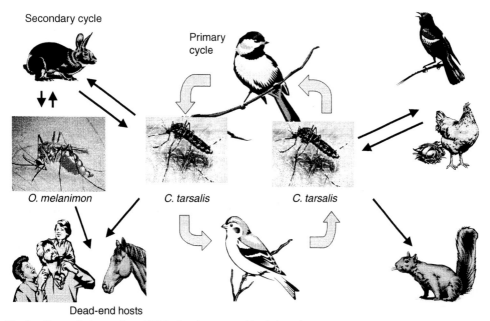

Fig. 2. Transmission cycles of WEE virus in western North America.

humans, appear to be dead-end hosts for WEE virus, because they produce low-titre viraemias, whereas lagomorphs, especially *Lepus californicus* (Black-tailed jackrabbits), produce moderate viraemias of sufficient titre to infect competent *Ochlerotatus*[1] mosquitoes of the *O. dorsalis* complex. In the Central Valley of California, a secondary rabbit–*Ochlerotatus melanimon* cycle has been documented and the isolation rate in *Ochlerotatus* populations has exceeded that in *C. tarsalis* in some years in the Sacramento Valley. *Ochlerotatus* mosquitoes may be very important in transmitting WEE virus to equines and humans, because they feed predominantly on mammals during the day, as well as during the crepuscular periods. Western equine encephalitis virus has been isolated from a total of 27 North American mosquito species, but most of these infections are considered to be incidental to the transmission cycles described above.

Vector competence of *C. tarsalis* has been related genetically to a mesenteronal infection barrier. Population susceptibility to infection varies spatially and temporally. Females are most susceptible to infection when reared under cool conditions

during spring, after which their susceptibility decreases by as much as 1000 times during the course of summer. Interestingly, populations are least susceptible during midsummer, when WEE virus is most active, emphasizing the importance of temperature-driven viral replication rates in the vector in the dynamics of virus amplification.

Transmission cycles of WEE virus in South America are less well understood. In the tropical Amazon rain forest and subtropical northern Argentina, *Culex* (*Melanoconion*) species transmit a subtype of WEE virus not involved in outbreaks among equines, whereas in the temperate regions of Argentina *Ochlerotatus albifasciatus* may be important in transmitting a virulent strain to hares and horses.

Mechanisms to explain WEE virus persistence in temperate ecosystems have remained cryptic, despite over 50 years of intensive investigation. Sequencing studies have recently compared the genomic composition of a large number of strains in time and space. In California, strains isolated from *Culex tarsalis* collected in the Central Valley remained identical from 1938 through 1961, implying local persistence, but then changed during 1968–1971 and 1993–1998, implying regional extinction and subsequent replacement by newly established strains. Recent research on persistence mechanisms has focused on transgenerational transmission among *Ochlerotatus* mosquitoes, alternative verte-brate–*Ochlerotatus* transmission cycles and chronic infections in wild birds. To date, data supporting all three persistence mechanisms are limited. Vertical transmission was reported in coastal California by the isolation of WEE virus from *O. dorsalis* collected as larvae, but this finding could not be confirmed by subsequent field studies at the same locality or by vertical transmission attempts using the same sympatric virus–mosquito combination. Rabbit–*Ochlerotatus* and reptile–mosquito cycles have been reported or inferred in the absence of *Culex*–bird transmission, implying maintenance by other cycles. However, these reports have not been well substantiated by subsequent research, and the primary vector feeds primarily upon avian hosts during the spring amplification period. Chronic infections have been detected at a low rate in experimentally infected passeriform birds; however, attempts to infect mosquitoes by xenodiagnostic feeds on these birds were not successful and natural relapses have yet to be detected by infectious assays or RT-PCR. Chronic infections in birds appear to be the most likely mechanism for long-range WEE virus dispersal and the introduction of new virus strains after regional extinctions; however, this must occur infrequently in migratory species, because southern hemisphere WEE virus isolates appear to be genetically distinct from northern hemisphere strains and antibodies are rarely detected in migrant species during serosurveys. If genetic exchange occurred frequently, genetic similarity would be expected.

Treatment

Therapeutic agents are not currently available for any of the encephalitides, including western equine encephalitis.

Control

Prevention and control are limited to mosquito abatement, implemented using sound integrated pest management practices. In western North America, surveillance programmes have been established, which integrate information on weather, vector abundance, virus enzootic amplification and human and equine cases. In California, the water content of snow-pack in the Sierra Nevada is highly predictive of vernal runoff, as well as the availability of water for agriculture, which creates surface-water habitats for mosquito production. Increased spring vector population size is directly related to area receptivity for WEE virus amplification and the risk of horse and human infections.

In recent years, extensive water management, improved irrigation methodology, expanded mosquito control and widespread vaccination of equines have combined to limit human infection. For example, in the late 1940s serological surveys showed that 30% of rural residents >20 years of age in the southern Central Valley of California had naturally acquired neutralizing immunity to WEE virus, whereas by the mid-1990s populations sampled in the Coachella and Sacramento Valleys were <1% antibody-positive. These data indicated that the decrease in the number of reported human cases has probably paralleled a decline in the human infection rate. This decline has been related to changes in human behaviour, associated with increased ownership of television and air-conditioning, which has essentially moved the human population from outdoors, where they were historically exposed to mosquitoes during the evening, to the screened house, where they are now protected from mosquitoes and therefore from virus infection.

Note

[1]   *Ochlerotatus* was formerly a subgenus of *Aedes*.

Selected bibliography

Kramer, L.D. and Fallah, H.M. (1999) Genetic variation among isolates of western equine encephalomyelitis virus from California.

American Journal of Tropical Medicine and Hygiene 60, 708–713.

Reeves, W.C. (1990) Epidemiology and Control of Mosquito-borne Arboviruses in California, 1943–1987. California Mosquito and Vector Control Association, Sacramento, 508 pp.

Reeves, W.C. and Hammon, W.M. (1962) Epidemiology of the Arthropod-borne Viral Encephalitides in Kern County, California, 1943–1952. Publications in Public Health 4, University of California, Berkeley 257 pp.

Reisen, W.K. and Monath, T.P. (1989) Western equine encephalomyelitis. In: Monath, T.P. (ed.) The Arboviruses: Epidemiology and Ecology, Vol. V. Boca Raton, Florida, pp. 89–138.

Weaver, S.C., Kang, W., Shirako, Y., Rumanapf, T., Strauss, E.G. and Strauss, J.H. (1997) Recombinational history and molecular evolution of western equine encephalomyelitis complex alphaviruses. Journal of Virology 71, 613–623.

West Nile virus

Vincent Deubel and Hervé Zeller

West Nile (WN) virus is a member of the Japanese encephalitis (JE) serogroup (see entry) in the genus *Flavivirus*, family Flaviviridae.

Distribution

West Nile virus has a wide distribution, which includes Africa and Madagascar, south-western Europe to Russia, Asia and the Middle East (Fig. 1). In 1999 WN virus was identified for the first time in the Americas, in the USA. Table 1 shows the distribution of WN virus in emerging areas in 1999–2000. West Nile virus can infect a wide variety of species of mosquitoes and ticks, as well as vertebrates, as determined by virus isolation and detection of antibodies, and by experimental infection. The virus is endemic in Africa and Asia, where it is transmitted in natural cycles between bird-feeding mosquitoes and wild animals, mainly birds (Fig. 2). Human disease associated with WN virus was first recognized in the West Nile district of Uganda in 1937, with a virus isolate from a febrile woman. The virus was subsequently isolated from febrile children and from birds during the first recognized West Nile virus epidemic, in Egypt in 1950. Large epidemics involving hundreds of cases and several human deaths were recorded in Israel in the 1950s, South Africa in 1974, Algeria in 1994, Romania in 1996, Tunisia in 1997, the USA in 1999 and southern Russia in 1999 (Table 1). Sporadic human cases, with apparently lower case/fatality rates, occurred in many countries of Europe, Africa and Asia. West Nile encephalitis in equines is a rare occurrence and has been reported only in Egypt in the early 1950s, France in the early 1960s and 2000, Morocco in 1996, Italy in 1998 and the USA in 1999 and 2000. In the USA WN virus has been recorded from New York, New Jersey, Connecticut, Pennsylvania, Maryland, New Hampshire and Massachussetts. Several human cases of West Nile encephalitis were recorded concomitantly in horses in Egypt, France and the USA, but not in Italy. West Nile virus was isolated in a sick pigeon (*Columba livia*) in Egypt in 1950 and has recently been isolated in Israel from a sick stork (Ciconiidae) and from dead geese (Anatidae), in 1998, and from dead crows (Corvidae), from other endemic bird species and from several exotic birds in New York City, in 1999 and 2000. High levels of mortality were also observed in crows during the outbreak in Astrakhan in southern Russia in 1999.

Virus

Virion structure and replication

The virus is a small (50–60 nm in diameter) enveloped virus, which contains a single plus-strand 11-kilobase RNA genome. The genomic RNA has a type 1 cap at the 5′ end, and the 3′ terminus lacks a poly-(A) tract. The 5′ and 3′ extremities, of about 96 and 630 nucleotides in length, respectively, are not translated and contain *cis*-acting signals and stem–loop structures, which are involved in the

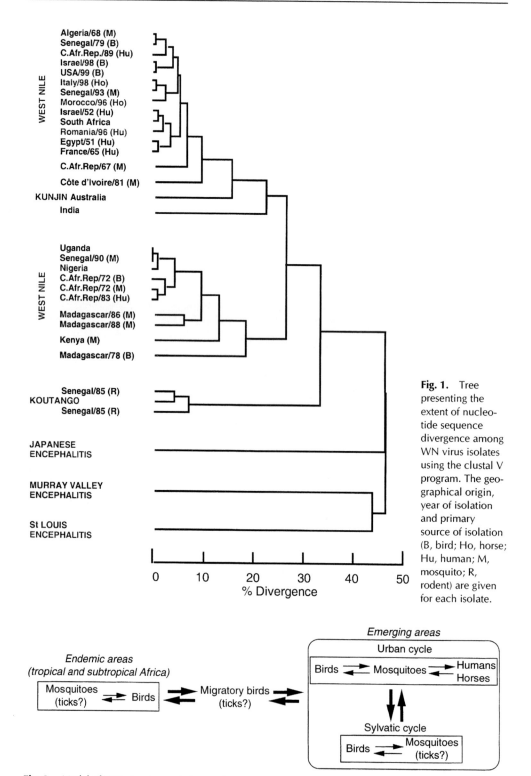

Fig. 1. Tree presenting the extent of nucleotide sequence divergence among WN virus isolates using the clustal V program. The geographical origin, year of isolation and primary source of isolation (B, bird; Ho, horse; Hu, human; M, mosquito; R, rodent) are given for each isolate.

Fig. 2. Model of WN virus transmission cycle.

initiation of translation and transcription. The genome encodes a single polyprotein of about 3400 amino acid residues in the gene order 5'-C-prM-E-NS2A-NS2B-NS3-NS4A-NS4B-NS5-3', which is co- and post-translationally processed by cellular and virus-encoded proteases, in strong association with the endoplasmic reticulum membranes. Upon infection, the plus-strand genomic RNA is transcribed into a complementary minus-strand RNA, which in turn serves as the template for the transcription of plus-strand genomic RNA.

Table 1. West Nile virus in emerging areas (1960–2000)

Country	Year	Species infected				
		Animals*	Horses	Birds	Arthropods†	Human
Albania	1958	D				+
Algeria	1994					+
Austria	1964–1977	D, W		+		+
Belanus	1972–1973			+		
	1977					+
Bulgaria	1960–1970	D		+		+
	1978				M	
Czech Republic	1978	D, W				
	1980–1990	W		+		
	1997				M‡	+‡
Egypt	1951			+‡	M	+‡
	1959		+‡			
	1963		+			
France	1962–1965		+‡	+‡	M‡	+‡
	2000		+‡			
Greece	1970–1978	D		+		+
Hungary	1970	R‡, C				+
India	1955					+‡
Israel	1950–1954					+‡
	1997–2000	P‡	+‡	+‡		+‡
Italy	1965–1969	D, R, P		+		+
	1981	R				
	1998		+‡			
Moldavia	1970				T, M‡	+
Morocco	1997		+‡			+
Poland	1996			+		
Portugal	1967–1970	C	+	+	M‡	+
Romania	1966–1970				M‡	
	1980					+
	1996–1998	W, D		+		+‡
Russia	1963–1968			+‡	T‡, M‡	+‡
	1999			+‡		+‡
Slovakia	1970–1973	W, D		+‡	M‡	+
South Africa	1974				M‡	+‡
Tunisia	1997			+		+
Ukraine	1970			+‡	M‡	+‡
	1985					+
USA	1999–2000	W‡	+	+‡	M‡	+‡

*C, cattle; D, domestic animal; P, poultry; R, rodent; W, wild animal.
†M, mosquito; T, tick.
‡Virus isolation.

The mature virion contains three structural proteins. The core protein C is associated with the genomic RNA to form the nucleocapsid. The membrane protein M and the envelope protein E, which may or may not be glycosylated, are both associated with the lipid envelope by means of hydrophobic membrane anchors. The E protein is layered on the surface of the virus particle as a head-to-tail dimer. It contains important antigenic determinants involved in haemagglutination inhibition and neutralization activities and elicits immunological responses in the infected host. Structural sequences in the E protein are involved in cell receptor recognition and intraendosomal fusion at acidic pH.

Some functions have been recognized in the non-structural proteins. The intracellular homodimeric form of the glycoprotein NS1 is maintained in an early cell compartment of secretion, where it is presumably recruited for viral replication. A secreted form of NS1 is associated in hexamers during its transport within mammalian cells. The role of the secreted form of NS1 remains unknown. The NS3 protein is the viral protease and contains protease and NTPase (nucleotide triphosphatase) activities. Protein NS5 is the RNA-dependent RNA polymerase and may have methyl-transferase activities for the capping of the 5′ extremity.

Genetic variability

Genetic analysis of strains of WN virus from different parts of Africa, Europe, Asia, the Middle East, Australia and the USA showed close relationships between WN viruses from Africa, northern and western hemispheres and the Australian virus Kunjin (see entry). A genetically distinct cluster of viruses, showing more than 30% nucleotide divergence, is also circulating in a mosquito–bird wild cycle in Africa, including Madagascar, but has never been isolated outside Africa (Fig. 1).

West Nile/Kunjin viruses are classified by antigenic variation of the envelope E protein, using standard serological tests and monoclonal antibodies. Amino acid differences among WN virus strains are as great as 25%. The most notable differences are observed on the N_{153}-glycosylation site, which may not be occupied after substitution or deletion of amino acids in the 154–157 positions.

Clinical symptoms

Infection with WN virus is asymptomatic in most human infections. When symptomatic, West Nile fever is characterized by sudden onset and mild to high fever in humans for 3–5 days. Frontal headache, malaise, myalgia, arthralgia, abdominal pain, gastrointestinal disturbance, nausea, sore throat, conjunctivitis, lymphadenopathy and a maculopapular rash have been observed to occur. Meningoencephalitis may occur in less than 10% of the cases; it is associated with neck stiffness, confusion, convulsions, impaired consciousness and coma. In some cases, anterior myelitis, hepatosplenomegaly, hepatitis, pancreatitis and myocarditis might also occur. Neurological disorders usually occur in young children and elderly patients. Recovery is complete without permanent sequelae, although a long-term weakness may occur.

Horses with encephalitis show ataxia, weakness, tremor, paraparesis, tetraplegia and muscle rigidity. Specific neurological symptoms in birds consist of ataxia, tremors, abnormal head posture, circling or convulsions. Non-specific signs include weakness or sternal recumbency.

Pathology

General observations in autopsy materials from humans and animals show focal necrotic areas, with predominantly polymorphonuclear leucocytes and mononuclear macrophages, in the central nervous system. Grey and white matters are usually involved in the brain and in the spinal cord. Haemorrhagic manifestations may be seen in the lumbar and thoracic regions of horses and in the gastrointestinal tract of dead birds. Laboratory tests show a slight elevation of the sedimentation rate and a mild leucocytosis. The cerebrospinal fluid is clear, with moderate pleocystosis and elevated protein. Experimental infection of laboratory mice shows susceptibility of adults inoculated by the intracerebral route (neurovirulence). West Nile virus strains show variations in virulence when inoculated into adult mice by peripheral routes (neuroinvasiveness). Death occurs between 2 and 5 days in baby mice and 6 and 9 days in adult mice. Fatal disease is observed in hamsters inoculated intracerebrally and intraperitoneally. West Nile virus replicates in rabbits, adult albino rats and guinea-pigs, but does not induce disease. Monkeys develop various symptoms according to the route of inoculation and species of monkey. West Nile virus persistence in the brain of monkeys has been observed, resulting in subacute central nervous system (CNS) disease at a later date. West Nile virus produces lethal infection in chicken embryos. Several species of birds are susceptible to WN virus encephalitis and show fatal disease or long-term virus persistence. Horses experimentally infected experience fever and/or diffuse encephalomyelitis.

Pathogenesis

Experimental rodent models of West Nile encephalitis have provided data that are important in understanding the infectious process. Injected virus is carried by dendritic cells to the regional lymph node, where initial replication occurs; other extraneural tissues can also become infected. Released virus enters the vascular compartment via lymphatic channels. Sites of virus replication outside lymph nodes may depend on the virus and on the viraemia. The mode of entry of virus into the neuroparenchyma remains unknown. Infection of the olfactory endothelium may be important in neuroinvasion. Alternatively, if the virus does not replicate in vascular endothelium, it may be passively transported across the capillary endothelium within pinocytotic vesicles. Damage to the blood–brain barrier may increase its permeability, thus allowing virus access to the CNS. In susceptible rodents, a large proportion of neurons are infected (Fig. 3), while, in resistant murine models, less than 1% of cells are involved. West Nile encephalitis consists mainly of necrosis of neurons and inflammatory changes. Lymphocytes and mononuclear cells appear as perivascular cuffs in the space between the endothelium and basement membrane, with diffuse infiltrates into the neuronal parenchyma.

The humoral immune response to WN virus infection is detectable 4–6 days following infection. Detection of neutralizing and haemagglutination–inhibiting antibodies is associated with termination of viraemia. Immunoglobulin M (IgM) antibodies appear 1 day earlier than IgG antibodies. Treatment of mice with cyclophosphamide 24 h after infection converted inapparent infection into lethal encephalitis, supporting the concept that humoral responses represent an important part of the host defence system in WN virus infection. However, subneutralizing levels of antibody or antibody from both close and distantly related flaviviruses may enhance WN virus infection in the monocyte–macrophage

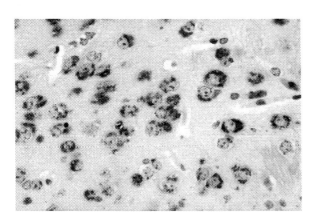

Fig. 3. Experimental encephalitis in susceptible adult mice inoculated intraperitoneally with a neuroinvasive strain of WN virus. Immunolabelling reveals WN virus antigens in the cytoplasm of neurons.

lineage by the so-called antibody-dependent enhancement.

Cytotoxic T-cell response is elicited by WN virus infection 4 days post-infection, peaking on days 5 and 6. Flavivirus infection up-regulates major histocompatibility complex (MHC) I and II surface expression of various cell types, and MHC II primarily recognizes epitopes in the NS3 protein. However, suppression of cytotoxic cells by anti-lymphocytes does not potentiate viral infection. Indeed, WN virus encephalitis in mice is associated with an inflammatory response consisting primarily of T cells, which may play a role in the pathogenesis.

Diagnosis

Several assay systems can be used to isolate WN virus from the blood of febrile patients and sick animals or from the CNS taken at autopsy. Suckling mice inoculated intracerebrally or intraperitoneally are highly susceptible to WN virus. Several mammalian (Vervet monkey kidney (VERO), baby hamster kidney (BHK-21) or pig kidney (PS)) and mosquito (*Aedes albopictus* C6/36 or *Aedes pseudoscutellaris* AP61) cell lines show cytopathic effects 4–6 days after infection with WN virus. Due to the considerable cross-reactivity among viruses of the JE complex, to which this virus belongs, WN virus identification should be performed by indirect fluorescent antibody (IFA) or other assays, using WN virus-specific monoclonal antibodies. West Nile viruses have been identified directly in biological specimens, using either WN virus-specific oligonucleotides or flavivirus-specific primers to prime reverse transcription–polymerase chain reaction (RT-PCR), followed by direct sequencing of the amplified products.

Neutralization, complement fixation, haemagglutination inhibition and indirect enzyme-linked immunosorbent assays have been successfully employed to diagnose WN virus infections. Although antibodies cross-react with other flaviviruses and can be detected by these methods, the titres are substantially lower than are titres to antibody to WN virus in primary flavivirus-infected patients. High levels of heterologous antibody titres may be noticed in

secondary-infected as well as yellow fever- or JE-vaccinated individuals (see entries on yellow fever and Japanese encephalitis). Immunoglobulin M detection by capture enzyme-linked immunosorbent assays of serum and cerebrospinal fluid of WN virus-infected patients have been detected 4 days after the onset of the disease and showed specificity to WN virus.

Transmission

The virus has been isolated from 43 mosquito species, predominantly from the genus *Culex*. In addition, species of *Anopheles*, *Aedeomyia*, *Aedes*, *Coquillettidia*, *Mansonia* and *Mimomyia* have been found infected. Bird-feeding ticks (e.g. *Argas hermanni* and *Hyalomma asiaticum*) may serve as substitute vectors for virus maintenance and a bird–tick cycle in some areas. West Nile virus replicates to high levels in wild birds and has been hypothesized to persist for months, but the infection is usually inapparent and rarely lethal. Thus, migratory birds may be instrumental in introducing the virus into temperate regions crossed by their migratory routes. Only rarely has WN virus been isolated from mammals, but horses and camels (*Camelus* species) show moderate viraemia and may support WN virus circulation locally. West Nile virus has been isolated from bats (Chiroptera) in India. In Israel antibodies against WN virus have been detected in some rodents, in cattle and in dogs, but the role of these animals in the virus cycle remains unknown.

Humans acquire WN virus from infected mosquitoes, including *Culex univittatus*, *Culex antennatus*, *Culex pipiens*, *Culex modestus* and the *Culex vishnui* group, which feed on both birds and humans. The principal cycle is rural, but the urban cycle predominated during the 1996–1997 outbreak in Bucharest and in the 1999–2000 outbreak in New York. The reason so many countries have experienced outbreaks with severe meningoencephalitis in humans, horses and birds in the past few years is unknown. Environmental and climatic factors have not been investigated and further monitoring of ecological factors related to mosquito and bird populations should be carried out. The unusual pathogenicity for animals and humans observed during recent outbreaks may also be attributed to the introduction of new virus strains with increased virulence or to infection of evolutionarily näive local vertebrates.

West Nile virus may be transmitted by aerosol, as demonstrated experimentally with adult mice and through laboratory infections in humans. This viral agent requires efficient safety conditions, including a level 3 laboratory, for its manipulation.

Treatment and prophylaxis
Treatment is supportive and consists of good general management and nursing care, especially during the comatose period. Anticonvulsants may be required. No vaccine against WN virus is available.

Surveillance and control
When a West Nile virus epidemic is recognized, a mosquito surveillance and control programme should be part of the emergency response. Control efforts are focused on larval source reduction, when applicable, and, more importantly, especially in epidemic situations, insecticidal space-spraying, such as aerial ultra-low-volume applications of malathion or pyrethroids, such as permethrin, to kill adult mosquitoes. These efforts must be accompanied by an intensive public outreach programme to educate the public about the disease and how to protect themselves against infection with WN virus.

A surveillance system can employ virus isolation from, or virus detection in humans, horses and birds using RT-PCR assays. Sentinel flocks of pigeons and chickens placed on the route of migratory birds and bled at frequent intervals have been used to detect seroconversions (evidence of virus infection). Such sentinels may provide a sensitive indicator of WN virus activity and help to predict impending human epidemics.

Individual protection against mosquito bites by using insect repellents on exposed skin and wearing protective clothes treated with repellents or insecticides, such as permethrin, may reduce exposure to mosquito bites. However, the value of such protection may be limited.

Selected bibliography
Berthet, F.X., Zeller, H., Drouet, M.T., Rauzier, J., Digoutte, J.P. and Deubel, V. (1997) Extensive nucleotide changes and deletions within the envelope glycoprotein gene of Euro-African West Nile viruses. *Journal of General Virolology* 78, 2293–2297.

Cantille, C., Di Guardo, G., Eleni, C. and Arispici, M. (2000) Clinical and neuropathological features of West Nile virus equine encephalomyelitis in Italy. *Equine Veterinary Journal* 32, 31–35.

Hayes, C.G. (1988) West Nile fever. In: Monath, T.P. (ed.) *The Arboviruses: Epidemiology and Ecology*, Vol. V. CRC Press, Boca Raton, Florida, pp. 58–89.

Hubalek, Z. and Halouzka, J. (1996) Arthropod-borne viruses of vertebrates in Europe. *Acta Scientiarum Naturalium Brno* 30(4–5), 1–95.

Lanciotti, R.S., Roehrig, J.T., Deubel, V., Smith, J., Parker, M., Steele, K., Crise, B., Volpe, K.E., Crabtree, M.B., Scherret, J.H., Hall, R.A., Mackenzie, J.S., Cropp, C.B., Panigrahy, B., Ostlund, E.B.S., Malkinson, M., Banet, C., Weissman, J., Komar, N., Savage, H.M., Stone, W., McNamara, T. and Gubler, D.J. (1999) Origin of the West Nile virus responsible for an outbreak of encephalitis in the northeastern United States. *Science* 286, 2333–2337.

Monath, T.P. and Heinz, F.X. (1996) Flaviviruses. In: Fields, B.N., Knipe, D.M. and Howley, P. (eds) *Fields Virology*, Vol. 1, 3rd edn. Lippincott-Raven Press, Philadelphia, pp. 961–1034.

Rice, C.M. (1996) Flaviviridae: the viruses and their replication. In: Fields, B.N., Knipe, D.M. and Howley, P. (eds) *Fields Virology*, 3rd edn. Lippincott-Raven Press, Philadelphia, pp. 931–959.

Steele, K.E., Linn, M.J., Schoepp, R.J., Komar, N., Geisbert, T.W., Manduca, R.M., Calle, P.P., Raphael, B.L., Clippinger, T.L., Larsen, T., Smith, J., Lanciotti, R.S., Panella, N.A., Tsai, T.F., Popovici, F., Cernescu, C., Campbell, G.L. and Nedelcu, N.I. (1998) West Nile encephalitis epidemic in southeastern Romania. *The Lancet* 352, 767–771.

Steele, K.E., Linn, M.J., Schoepp, R.J., Komar, N., Geisbert, T.W., Manduca, R.M., Calle, P.P., Raphael, B.L., Clippinger, T.L., Larsen, T.,

Smith, J., Lanciotti, R.S., Panella, N.A., McNamara, T.S. (2000) Pathology of fatal West Nile virus infections in native and exotic birds during the 1999 outbreak in New York City, New York. *Veterinary Pathology* 37, 208–224.

Wuchereria bancrofti *see* **Bancroftian filariasis.**

Yellow fever

Thomas P. Monath

Infection of humans and non-human primates with yellow fever (YF) virus, the prototype of the genus *Flavivirus*, family Flaviviridae.

Yellow fever is the original 'viral haemorrhagic fever', a systemic illness characterized by hepatic, renal and myocardial injury, haemorrhage and high lethality. The virus causing the disease is transmitted by mosquitoes. Yellow fever is endemic and epidemic in tropical regions of Africa and South America, where approximately 200,000 cases occur annually, of which only about 1% are officially reported. Between 1986 and 1995, 23,543 cases and 6421 deaths were reported. Africa accounted for 21,541 cases (91%), with an annual incidence of 200–5000 reported cases. Between 1996 and

1999, four unvaccinated persons from the USA and Europe developed fatal infections after travel to South America or Africa.

Distribution

Transmission of YF virus occurs throughout tropical regions of Africa, with the highest intensity in West Africa (Fig. 1). In South America, transmission is limited to the tropical rain forest and grasslands in the Amazon and Orinoco river basins. Areas infested with the urban vector, *Aedes aegypti*, are receptive to introduction and spread of the virus by viraemic travellers. Yellow fever virus does not occur in Asia, although this region is receptive to introduction. The precise geography of virus activity is important for application of YF

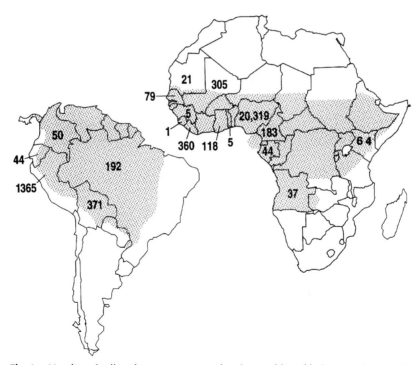

Fig. 1. Number of yellow fever cases reported to the World Health Organization (WHO), by country, 1986–1995. Regions endemic for yellow fever are shaded. (Figure reproduced from Monath (1999), with permission.)

vaccine in residents and travellers; yellow fever is a quarantinable disease subject to International Health Regulations. Current YF viral activity is published in the World Health Organization (WHO) *Weekly Epidemiological Record* and by the Centers for Disease Control and Prevention. Current information can also be found in the Centers for Disease Control and Prevention home page (http://www.cdc.gov/travel/travel.html).

Virus

Yellow fever virus is a small (40–60 nm) positive-sense, enveloped, single-stranded RNA virus. The viral envelope is comprised of a lipid bilayer derived from the host cell, with dimers of the flavivirus envelope (E) protein on the surface. The virus is inactivated by organic solvents and detergents. The E protein plays a central role in cell tropism, virulence and immunity. The E protein mediates attachment to cell receptors and internalization by membrane fusion, and antibodies interfere with these functions, neutralizing the virus. Yellow fever virus replicates intracellularly, with assembly of virus particles in close association with endoplasmic reticulum. Cellular functions are maintained until late in the virus replication phase. The virus principally targets monocytes/macrophages, hepatocytes and neurons. Differences in genome sequence distinguish geographical strains of YF virus. Five virus genotypes have been recognized, three in Africa and two in South America.

Yellow fever is a zoonotic disease. The natural transmission cycle involves tree hole-breeding aedine mosquitoes and a wide array of monkeys, apes and marmosets. Some Neotropical monkeys, e.g. howler monkeys (*Alouatta* species), develop fatal infections similar to the human disease.

Clinical symptoms

The clinical spectrum includes subclinical infection, abortive infection, with non-specific influenza-like illness, and lethal systemic disease, with fever, jaundice, renal failure and haemorrhage. As for many other infections, the variability in disease expression is due to intrinsic and acquired host resistance factors, and probably to differences in the virulence of virus strains. The illness : infection ratio is 3.8–7.4 : 1. After an incubation period of 3–6 days, the onset is abrupt, with chills and headache.

The disease is characterized by three stages. The first 'period of infection', lasting 3–4 days, is characterized by fever, malaise, prostration, headache, photophobia, lumbosacral pain, generalized myalgia, nausea, vomiting, restlessness, irritability and dizziness. On physical examination the patient appears toxic, with congestion of the conjunctivae, gums and face, epigastric tenderness, and tenderness and enlargement of the liver. The tongue is characteristically bright red at the tip and sides, with a white coating in the centre. The pulse rate is slow relative to fever (Faget's sign). The average fever is 38.9–39.4°C and lasts 3.3 days, but temperature may rise as high as 40.6°C, a bad prognostic sign. Laboratory abnormalities include leucopenia ($1.5–2.5 \times 10^9$ l^{-1}) with a relative neutropenia. Elevation of serum transaminases may precede the appearance of jaundice, the levels often predicting the severity of hepatic dysfunction later in the illness. Virus is present in the blood and the patient is infectious for mosquito vectors. Peak viraemia occurs on days 2–3 of illness, with titres of up to 5.6 log_{10} mouse intracerebral (i.c.) lethal dose (LD_{50}) ml^{-1} (approximately equivalent to 7 log_{10} plaque-forming units ml^{-1}).

The second phase or 'period of remission' is characterized by resolution of fever and symptoms lasting up to 48 h. In abortive infections, the patient simply recovers at this stage. Approximately 15% of infected persons progress to the third stage of the disease, the 'period of intoxication' on the third to sixth days after onset. Fever reappears, accompanied by nausea, vomiting, epigastric pain, jaundice, oliguria, albuminuria and a haemorrhagic diathesis. Virus disappears from blood and antibodies appear. The clinical course reflects the dysfunction and failure of multiple organ systems, including the liver, kidneys and cardiovascular system. The clinical picture is characterized by fulminating hepatitis, acute renal failure and a haemorrhagic diathesis (typically manifested as coffee-grounds haematemesis), hypotension, shock and metabolic acidosis. Central nervous system signs include delirium, agitation, convulsions, stupor and coma, reflecting metabolic encephalopathy rather than viral encephalitis. The critical phase of the illness occurs between the fifth and tenth day, at which point the patient either dies or rapidly recovers. The case–fatality rate in patients with jaundice approximates 20%. Recovery is usually complete, but convalescence may be prolonged for several weeks, with increased fatiguability. Some patients who survive the acute phase may require dialysis for a brief period. Complications of yellow fever include superimposed bacterial pneumonia, parotitis and sepsis. Late deaths during convalescence have been ascribed to myocarditis, arrhythmia or heart failure, but documentation is poor.

Diagnosis

Mild yellow fever infections may resemble many other arboviral infections and influenza characterized by fever, headache, malaise and myalgia. The differential diagnosis of the individual case with severe yellow fever includes leptospirosis (Weil's disease), louse-borne relapsing fever (*Borrelia recurrentis*) (see entry), viral hepatitis (especially hepatitis E in pregnancy and delta hepatitis), Q fever, West Nile virus hepatitis, Rift Valley fever (see entries), typhoid and severe malaria (see Malaria, human). Malaria (blackwater fever) may be distinguished by the absence of proteinuria. Dengue haemorrhagic fever (see dengue), Lassa, Marburg and Ebola virus diseases, Bolivian haemorrhagic fever and Crimean–Congo haemorrhagic fever (see entry) are not usually associated with jaundice.

Specific laboratory diagnosis is by detection of virus or viral antigen in blood or by serology. Virus is readily isolated from blood during the first 4 days after onset, but isolations as late as 12 days or longer are possible. The virus may also be recovered from post-mortem liver, heart or kidney tissue. Virus isolation methods include intracerebral inoculation of suckling mice,

intrathoracic inoculation of *Toxorhynchites* mosquitoes or inoculation of mosquito cell cultures, of which *Aedes pseudoscutellaris* (AP61) cells are the most sensitive cell line. Virus is identified by immunofluorescence or other serological methods. The polymerase chain reaction (PCR) is likely to replace more cumbersome methods in the future, and is applicable to the rapid detection/identification of virus in blood or in cell cultures inoculated with clinical samples.

Post-mortem examination of liver reveals a unique and diagnostic pattern characterized by midzonal necrosis (sparing of the portal areas and cells surrounding the central vein), eosinophilic degeneration of hepatocytes (Councilman bodies), microvesicular fatty change, and absence of inflammation. Liver biopsy during the illness should never be performed, as fatal haemorrhage may occur. Immunohistochemical staining for YF antigen in liver, heart or kidney or detection by PCR provides a definitive diagnosis.

Serological diagnosis is accomplished by classical methods (haemagglutination inhibition, complement fixation or neutralization tests) or, most efficiently, by immunoglobulin M (IgM)-capture enzyme-linked immunosorbent assay (ELISA). Immunoglobulin M antibody in a single sample provides a presumptive diagnosis, and a rise in titre between paired acute and convalescent samples or a fall between early and late convalescent samples is confirmatory. Cross-reactions complicate the serological diagnosis of YF virus in patients who have sustained prior infections with other flaviviruses.

Transmission

The basic enzootic transmission cycle involves non-human primates and diurnal tree hole-breeding mosquitoes (*Haemagogus janthinomys*, other *Haemagogus* species and *Sabethes chloropterus* in South America; *Aedes africanus* in Africa) (Figs 2 and 3). Infection of mosquitoes begins after ingestion of blood containing a threshold concentration of virus (~3.5 $\log_{10}$ ml^{-1}), resulting in infection of the mid-gut epithelium. The virus is released from the mid-gut into the haemolymph and spreads to other tissues, notably the reproductive tract and salivary glands. Seven to 10 days are required between ingestion of virus and virus secretion in saliva (the so-called 'extrinsic incubation period'), at which point the female mosquito is capable of transmitting virus to a susceptible host. Vertical (transovarial) transmission of virus occurs from the female mosquito to her progeny and from congenitally infected males to females during copulation (i.e. venereal transmission). The presence and stability of virus in the egg stage provide a

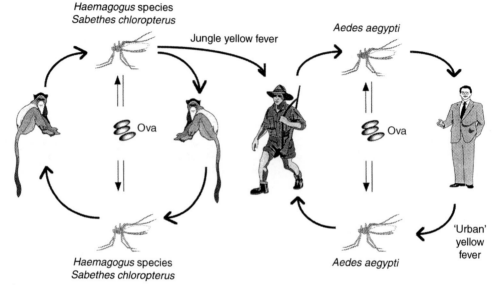

Fig. 2.   Transmission cycles of yellow fever virus in South America.

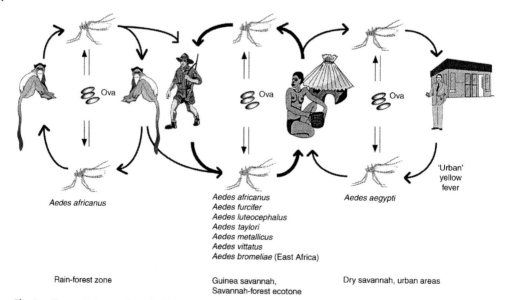

Fig. 3.   Transmission cycles of yellow fever virus in Africa.

mechanism for survival across the long dry season, when adult mosquito activity and horizontal virus transmission subside. Ticks (*Amblyomma variegatum*) may play a secondary role in virus transmission between monkeys in Africa.

In South America and in the rain-forest zone of Africa, humans develop 'jungle yellow fever' when exposed to infected mosquitoes in forested areas. Occupations associated with exposure include hunting, clearing forest for agricultural purposes and logging. Consequently, the disease incidence is highest in adult males. The ecology of YF virus differs in the ecotone bordering the rain-forest block in Africa and in the Guinea savannah zones, where a wide variety of tree hole-breeding mosquito vectors are involved in transmission between monkeys, from monkeys to humans and sometimes between humans. In West Africa, the principal vectors are *Aedes furcifer* and *Aedes luteocephalus*, as well as *Aedes africanus*, and less important are *Aedes taylori* and *Aedes metallicus*. In East Africa, the vectors are *A. africanus* and anthropophagic populations of what was formerly regarded as *Aedes simpsoni* but is now known as *Aedes bromeliae,* a species that breeds in leaf axils of bananas, plantains and other plants, such as coco-yams (*Colocasia*) and pineapples. As might be expected adults of *A. bromeliae* are active in plantation areas in proximity to human dwellings and even occasionally indoors. During the wet and early dry seasons, vector density reaches a high level. In certain areas, such as Sudan, *Aedes vittatus*, a rock pool-breeding mosquito, has been incriminated in transmission. The disease incidence is highest in children <15 years, and there is no significant gender difference in incidence. The savannah–forest ecotone and Guinea savannah are dubbed the 'zone of emergence' of yellow fever, and are the regions principally affected by epidemics.

In both South America and Africa, a distinct transmission cycle, the urban cycle, involves *A. aegypti*, breeding principally in artificial containers used to store water (Fig. 4). *Aedes aegypti* transmits YF virus between humans. The vector occurs in dry areas and heavily settled areas, but may also be widely dispersed in settlements in rural areas. Urban outbreaks have followed virus introductions by viraemic persons from areas of jungle/forest YF virus activity. In the Americas, urban yellow fever was common through the 1930s. The risk of future re-emergence of the urban disease has increased due to reinfestation of much of South America by *A. aegypti* in the last 30 years. For example, a small urban outbreak occurred in Santa Cruz, Bolivia, in 1997–1998. In contrast, Africa suffers many *A. aegypti*-borne epidemics. *Aedes aegypti*-borne epidemics in the past 40 years include those in Senegal in 1965; Angola in 1971; Ghana in 1969, 1977–1980 and 1983; Côte d'Ivoire in 1982; and multiple outbreaks in Nigeria between 1987 and 1994.

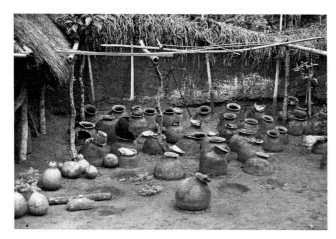

Fig. 4. Village water-storage pots in eastern Nigeria, typical peridomestic larval habitat of *Aedes aegypti* (courtesy of M.W. Service).

The introduction and spread of *Aedes albopictus* from its native Asia to the Americas and West Africa initially raised concerns that it could become involved in YF (and dengue) virus transmission. *Aedes albopictus* has become a prevalent pest species in many areas. Although the host and habitat preferences and the biting habits of this mosquito suggest that field studies of its role in virus transmission should be undertaken, experimental studies indicate that it is not an efficient vector of YF virus.

There is justified concern over the future re-emergence of *A. aegypti*-borne epidemics in heavily populated coastal regions of South America and the spread of YF virus to other *A. aegypti*-infested areas (e.g. the Caribbean, North America, the Middle East, coastal East Africa, the Indian subcontinent, Asia and Australia). Factors increasing this risk include: the recent upsurge of YF virus activity; the reinfestation by *A. aegypti* of South American countries from which the vector had been eliminated or its population greatly reduced; expanding human populations in urban centres; the opening up of remote rural areas to commerce within countries in the endemic zone; the marked increase in air travel; poor enforcement of vaccination certification for travellers; and global warming.

Treatment

There is no specific treatment. Intensive care of patients has not been optimized, because the disease occurs in remote areas. Supportive care includes: maintenance of nutrition and prevention of hypoglycaemia; nasogastric suction to prevent gastric distension and aspiration; treatment of hypotension by fluid replacement and, if necessary, vasoactive drugs; administration of oxygen; correction of metabolic acidosis; treatment of bleeding with fresh-frozen plasma; dialysis, if indicated by renal failure; and treatment of secondary infections with antibiotics.

Administration of antibody to YF virus or interferon is ineffective after appearance of symptoms. Although no antiviral drugs have been clinically tested, molecular targets have been defined and *in vitro* activity

demonstrated for a number of compounds. It is likely that antiviral therapy would be effective only during the early phase of infection. Future therapeutic interventions in yellow fever will probably involve drugs that inhibit cytokine mediators of shock.

Control
Vectors

Epidemics of *A. aegypti*-borne YF virus may be prevented by control or elimination of breeding sites. It is generally accepted that reduction of *A. aegypti* to a Breteau index (no. containers with larvae per 100 households) below 5.0 will prevent yellow fever epidemics. Control of *A. aegypti* is increasingly difficult, due to poor sanitation in expanding human urban environments and generally poor community participation in reducing larval breeding in water-storage pots. Furthermore, such environmental control measures are not usually sustainable, although there are a few reported successes. In the event of an urban epidemic, adulticiding with organophosphate (e.g. malathion, bendiocarb, pirimiphos-methyl) or pyrethroid (e.g. permerthrin, deltamethrin, lambdacyhalothrin) insecticides delivered by thermal fogging or ultra-low-volume applications, especially from aircraft, may be effective. Adulticiding has also been investigated for the control of sylvatic yellow fever, but the large areas affected and dense vegetation represent significant obstacles.

Vaccines

Since yellow fever is a zoonosis with a natural reservoir host that cannot be eliminated, the most efficient control method is preventive immunization of the human population. Current recommendations are for routine immunization of all inhabitants at age 9 months of countries, or in areas within countries endemic for yellow fever. The live, attenuated 17D vaccine produced in embryonated chicken eggs is an extremely effective and safe product, which has been in use for over 60 years. Yellow fever virus vaccine is given by the subcutaneous route in a volume of 0.5 ml. The minimum dose requirement is 1000 mouse i.c. LD_{50} ml^{-1}, or the equivalent in plaque-forming units.

The vaccine is distributed as a lyophilized product, which requires a cold chain and must be stored at point of use at 2–8°C. After reconstitution with a diluent, it must be discarded within 1 h (longer times may be allowed under field conditions). The vaccine is highly immunogenic. In controlled trials, 99% of subjects develop immunity, and under field conditions seroconversion rates exceed 90%. Following inoculation, neutralizing antibodies appear rapidly and the majority of subjects are immune by days 8–9. The International Health Regulations (IHR) stipulate that the vaccination certificate for yellow fever is valid 10 days after administration of 17D vaccine. Immunity is extremely durable, and probably persists for life. However, the IHR specify that the yellow fever immunization certificate for international travel is valid for 10 years, whereupon revaccination is required. Revaccination is associated with a boost in antibody titres. Malnutrition, pregnancy and human immunodeficiency virus (HIV) infection reduce the effectiveness of immunization.

Yellow fever 17D is widely acknowledged as one of the safest vaccines in use. Over 300 million persons have been immunized, with an excellent record of tolerability and safety. Local reactions, headache and feverishness occur in up to 20% of subjects, but are typically mild and do not interfere with normal activities. Contraindications include young age (<9 months), known egg allergy, immunosuppression and (on theoretical grounds) pregnancy. Rare serious adverse events include post-vaccinal encephalitis, generalized allergic reactions and multisystemic illness resembling yellow fever. Post-vaccinal encephalitis has occurred almost exclusively in very young infants, leading to the recommendation that vaccination should not be given to infants <9 months of age. The risk of encephalitis in persons over 9 months of age is extremely low, probably 1 in 8 million. Since the vaccine is made in eggs, allergy to eggs is a contraindication. Generalized hypersensitivity reactions are uncommon and have been reported at an incidence of 1 in 131,000. Fatal, multisystem disease temporally associated with vaccination and resembling wild-type YF virus has been extremely rare, with only six such cases reported. In a recent analysis, severe adverse reactions were found to be more frequent in elderly subjects (>65 years) than in young persons.

Selected bibliography

Barrett, A.D.T. (1997) Yellow fever vaccine. *Biologicals* 25, 17–30.

Digoutte, J.-P., Cornet, M., Deubel, V. and Downs, W.G. (1995) Yellow fever. In: Porterfield, J.S. (ed.) *Exotic Virus Infections.* Chapman & Hall, London, pp. 67–102.

Gessner, B., Fletcher, M., Parent du Chatelet, I., Schlumberger, M., Da Silva, A. and Stœckel, P. (eds) (1999) *International Seminar on Yellow Fever in Africa (Dakar, 25–27 June 1998).* Collection Fondation Marcel Mérieux, Marnes la Coquette, France, 230 pp.

Monath, T.P. (1988) Yellow fever. In: Monath, T.P. (ed.) *The Arboviruses: Epidemiology and Ecology,* Vol. V. CRC Press, Boca Raton, Florida, pp. 139–231.

Monath, T.P. (1995) Yellow fever and dengue – the interactions of virus, vector and host in the re-emergence of epidemic disease. *Seminars in Virology* 5, 1–13.

Monath, T.P. (1997) Epidemiology of yellow fever: current status and speculations on future trends. In: Saluzzo, J.-F. and Dodet, B. (eds) *Factors in the Emergence of Arbovirus Diseases.* Elsevier, Paris, pp. 143–156.

Monath, T.P. (1999) Yellow fever vaccine. In: Plotkin, S. and Orenstein, W. (eds) *Vaccines.* W.B. Saunders, Philadelphia, pp. 815–879.

Robertson, S.E., Hull, B.P., Tomori, O., Bele, O. and LeDuc, J.W. (1996) Yellow fever. A decade of reemergence. *Journal of the American Medical Association* 276, 1157–1164.

Strode, G.K. (ed.) (1951) *Yellow Fever.* McGraw Hill, New York, 710 pp.

Tomori, O. (1999) Impact of yellow fever on the developing world. *Advances in Virus Research* 53, 5–34.

World Health Organization (1986) *Prevention and Control of Yellow Fever in Africa.* WHO, Geneva, 94 pp.

Yersinia pestis see **Plague.**

Zika virus

Oyewale Tomori

Distribution

Zika (ZIKA) virus was first isolated in 1947 from the blood of a sentinel Rhesus monkey (*Macaca mulatta*) in Zika forest, near Entebbe in Uganda. Subsequently, the virus was recovered from humans and mosquitoes in Uganda, Senegal, Nigeria, Côte d'Ivoire, the Central African Republic and Malaysia.

Serological surveys have confirmed the geographical distribution of Zika virus infection in Uganda, Tanzania, Ethiopia, Mozambique, Nigeria, Senegal, Ghana, Côte d'Ivoire, Liberia, Cameroon, Democratic Republic of Congo (Zaire), Egypt, India, Malaysia, Borneo, Philippines, Vietnam and Thailand. This suggests the likelihood that the ecology of Zika virus is considerably more complex than originally thought, and is not as yet fully understood.

Virus

Zika virus, a single-stranded RNA virus, is an unassigned member of the *Flavivirus* genus of the Flaviviridae family. It is most closely related to Spondweni (see entry), Uganda S and yellow fever (see entry) viruses. It is an enveloped spherical virus, measuring 18–45 nm in diameter. Zika virus is stable for up to 6 months at 4°C in glycerol, but is easily inactivated by chloroform, ether and sodium deoxycholate. The virus is also inactivated by p-chloromercuribenzoate. The brains of virus-infected suckling mice contain haemagglutinin activity with goose and chick erythrocytes. The haemagglutinin activity is inactivated by trypsin, chymotrypsin and papain.

Clinical symptoms, pathogenesis and pathogenicity

The response of laboratory and experimental animals to infection with Zika virus depends on the strain, passage level and route of inoculation. Intracerebral inoculation of suckling mice with mouse-brain passage level 4 of Lunyo V strain of Zika virus results in paralysis and death, with the development of a high virus titre ($>10^{8.0}$ 0.1 ml^{-1}) in the brain. Mice up to 5 weeks old are paralysed and die from intracerebral inoculation with high passage level 10 of Zika virus, but with an extended average survival time of 11–12 days and a lower virus titre ($10^{5.9}$ 0.1 ml^{-1}) in the brain.

The E/1 strain of Zika virus at high (>50) mouse-brain passages is pathogenic for suckling and adult mice inoculated by the intracerebral or intraperitoneal route. Cellular degeneration and the presence of Cowdry type A inclusion bodies in the central nervous system (CNS) are characteristic histopathological lesions in mice dying from Zika virus infection. Other lesions include myocarditis and skeletal myositis. Rhesus (*M. mulatta*) and wild monkeys develop viraemia and antibodies when inoculated by either the intracerebral or subcutaneous route with Zika virus. Guinea-pigs died from intracerebral inoculation with the third passage level of Zika virus, but no virus was recovered from the animals that succumbed to infection. Rabbits and guinea-pigs inoculated by peripheral routes develop antibody, but do not die. Experimentally infected donkeys developed viraemia and antibodies, but no clinical disease. There is virus multiplication in 6–12-day-old chick embryos inoculated with Zika virus. Cotton rats (*Sigmodon hispidus*) are resistant to experimental infections with Zika virus. Zika virus replicates and causes cytopathic effects in human (HeLa) and primary duck embryo cell cultures. Plaques develop in rhesus kidney and primary duck and chick embryo cells inoculated with Zika virus.

Adult *Aedes aegypti* mosquitoes, exposed to Zika virus by feeding, successfully transmitted the virus to mice and monkeys. Zika virus was serially passaged in *A. aegypti*, *Anopheles quadrimaculatus* and *Culex quinquefasciatus* inoculated by the intrahaemocoelic route. Five human illnesses with Zika virus have been reported. These include three natural infections in Nigeria, a laboratory-acquired infection in Senegal and an infection in a male collecting mosquitoes for laboratory studies. The symptoms of Zika virus infection are fever, malaise, headache, stomach-ache, dizziness, anorexia and maculopapular rash. Considering the high prevalence of antibody Zika virus in Africa, South-East Asia and India, it would appear that most Zika virus infections in humans are febrile benign illnesses of short duration.

Diagnosis

Diagnosis is by virus isolation from blood or by serology. However, cross-reactions may confuse interpretation of serological results, especially in persons with previous exposures to other flaviviruses.

Transmission

In addition to the isolation of Zika virus from naturally infected humans in Nigeria and Senegal, the virus has been isolated from sentinel monkeys in Uganda and from mosquitoes of various species, such as from *Aedes africanus* in Uganda and the Central African Republic, *Aedes luteocephalus* in Nigeria and *A. aegypti* in Malaysia, as well as from other *Aedes* species in Côte d'Ivoire and Senegal. Explosive epizootics (without recognized disease) have been reported in monkey populations in East and West

Africa. In addition, an isolate of Zika virus was recovered from a gerbil (*Taterillus* species) in Senegal.

Control

There is currently no specific control measure available.

Selected bibliography

Dick, G.W.A., Kitchen, S.F. and Haddow, A.J. (1952) Zika virus. I. Isolation and serological specificity. *Transactions of Royal Society of Tropical Medicine and Hygiene* 46, 509–520.

Karabatsos, N. (ed.) (1985) *International Catalogue of Arboviruses Including Certain Other Viruses of Vertebrates*, 3rd edn. American Society of Tropical Medicine and Hygiene, San Antonio, Texas, 1147 pp.

Marchette, N.J., Garcia, R. and Rudnick, A. (1969) Isolation of Zika virus from *Aedes aegypti* mosquitoes in Malaysia. *American Journal of Tropical Medicine and Hygiene* 18, 411–415.

Monath, T.P. and Heinz, F.X. (1996) Flaviviruses. In: Fields, B.N., Knipe, D.M., Howle, P.M., Chanock, R.M., Melnick, J.L., Monath, T.P., Roizman, B. and Straus, S.E. (eds) *Fields Virology*, Vol. 1, 3rd edn. Lippincott-Raven, Philadelphia, pp. 961–1034.

Moore, D.L., Causey, O.R., Causey, D.E., Reddy, S., Cooke, A.R., Akinkugbe, F.M., David-West, T.S. and Kemp, G.E. (1975) Arthropod-borne viral infection of man in Nigeria (1964–1970). *Annals of Tropical Medicine and Parasitology* 69, 49–64.

Simpson, D.I.H. (1964) Zika virus infection in man. *Transactions of the Royal Society for Tropical Medicine and Hygiene* 58, 335–338.

Zimbabwe theileriosis *see* **Theilerioses.**

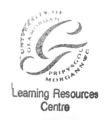